BIOMECHANICS IN APPLICATIONS

Edited by **Václav Klika**

Biomechanics in Applications
Edited by Václav Klika

Published by InTech
Janeza Trdine 9, 51000 Rijeka, Croatia

Publishing Process Manager Iva Simcic

Technical Editor Teodora Smiljanic

Cover Designer InTech Design Team

Additional hard copies can be obtained from orders@intechopen.com

Biomechanics in Applications, Edited by Václav Klika
p. cm.
978-953-307-969-1

For EU product safety concerns:
IN TECH d.o.o., Prolaz Marije Krucifikse Kozulić 3, 51000 Rijeka, Croatia,
info@intechopen.com or visit our website at intechopen.com.

Meet the editor

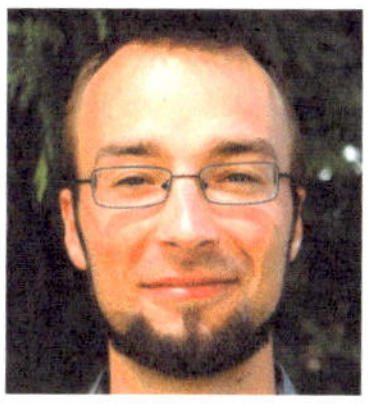

Dr. Václav Klika, received his MS (2006) and PhD (2009) from the Czech Technical University in Prague, FNSPE, Mathematical Engineering. Since 2004, he has gained valuable experience as a researcher at Institute of Thermomechanics, Academy of Sciences of Czech Republic. He is currently an assistant professor at Department of Mathematics, FNSPE, Czech Technical University in Prague. His research interests include non-equilibrium thermodynamics, mathematical biology, biomechanics, and analytical solutions in fluid dynamics. Dr. Václav Klika has published more than 15 journal and conference papers, is a reviewer in Journal of Physical Chemistry and has active collaborations with groups in University of Zaragoza, Spain and University of Oxford, UK.

Contents

Preface

During last couple of years there has been an increasing recognition that problems arising in biology or related to medicine really need a multidisciplinary approach. One simply cannot treat evolving and adapting living tissues as rigid rods or as a material with some inner structure. Although they do bring some insight into the treated problem it remains a rather limited source of understanding.

For this reason some special branches of both applied theoretical physics and mathematics have recently emerged such as biomechanics, mechanobiology, mathematical biology, biothermodynamics. The ultimate goal of all these approaches and models is to help in clinical applications, to improve medicine. This is actually a very long process to follow with many intermediate steps involving many approaches and specialists as for example experts in theoretical biomechanics and mathematical modelling, biologists, and finally clinicians. It was intended to preserve generality in the modelling and viewpoints of problems related to biomechanics. The same holds for its applications.

The book Biomechanics in Applications, is focusing on experimental praxis and clinical findings. Namely, the first section is devoted to Injury and clinical biomechanics starting with an overview of the biomechanics of musculoskeletal injury including biological background, mechanical properties of bone, motor vehicle collision and anterior cruciate ligament tear. Further there are chapters about distraction osteogenesis in mandible and a mechanism allowing direct assessment and monitoring of distraction forces, consequences of drilling in bone and how bone tissue is insulted by heat arising from friction and breakage of molecular bonds, effects of growth factors on performance of grafted tendons in anterior cruciate ligament reconstruction, and current available treatment techniques for long bone fractures with differences among them from biomechanical point of view. The next section is on Spine biomechanics. It is dealing with different applications of clinical studies and biomechanical models for upper limb after spinal cord injury, further with an animal model bringing new insights into changes occurring as a consequence of spinal cord injury and affecting the physiology of the whole motor system, biomechanical analysis of craniovertebral junction including stability, fractures and fixation, and finally a pure moment based tester for assessing mechanical properties of spine column. Section Musculoskeletal Biomechanics has one contributor, whose chapter is devoted to dynamical stability of lumbo-pelvi-femoral complex which involves analysis of relationship among appropriate anatomical structures in this region. The fourth section is on Human and Animal Biomechanics in general with contributions from area of foot biomechanics (and the importance of used pressure measurement techniques), a very complex problem of chewing rhythms in mammals which cannot be tackled as a whole due to its complexity but still some advancements in understanding have been made, extraordinary adaptations of bats as a mammalian species with focus on biomechanical aspects of this adaptation, and also from proprioception and its role in musculoskeletal functioning. The last section, Sport Biomechanics, is another typical example of application of biomechanics. It is being documented by three chapters. One is devoted to kinesiological non-invasive measurement techniques (electromyography) for qualitative assessment and analysis of dynamic human movement and the other two are dealing with applications in swimming: flow visualisation and motion analysis with aim to investigate the propulsive forces involved in swimming strokes, and an overview of competitive swimming strokes and the role of biomechanics in optimizing them.

I would like to take this opportunity to acknowledge the Czech Technical University in Prague (CTU) as well as Institute of Thermomechanics, Academy of Sciences of the Czech Republic (IT AS CR) for their support. My thanks also go to prof. František Maršík from the Department of Thermodynamics at IT AS CR and to my family.

Václav Klika
Dept. of Mathematics, FNSPE Czech Technical University in Prague
Czech Republic

Part 1

Injury and Clinical Biomechanics

1

Biomechanics of Musculoskeletal Injury

IL Gitajn[1] and EK Rodriguez[2]
[1]*Harvard Combined Orthopaedic Surgery Residency Program, Massachusetts General Hospital*
[2]*Beth Israel Deaconess Medical Center, Department of Orthopaedic Surgery, Harvard Medical School*
United States

1. Introduction

Fracture as a result of traumatic injury is a major contributor to long-term disability and loss of work and is therefore an important health concern, as well as contributor to overall societal economic burden. Finklestein et al reported that the annual medical cost of traumatic injury in 2000 in the US was $80.2 billion and that the cost of productivity losses was $326 billion (Finklestein et al, 2006). A total of 1.5 million fractures occur each year, including 280,000 hip fractures and 500,000 vertebral fractures (Bouxsin et al, 2006). Because the human musculoskeletal system is a living organ with predominantly a mechanical role, physiology and engineering principles are critical for its study and understanding. Fracture and musculoskeletal injury occur when local stresses or strains exceed the ultimate strength of bones, tendons, ligaments and muscles. These tissues regenerate, heal, or fail to heal according to both mechanical and biological stimuli. This chapter will provide an overview of the biomechanics of musculoskeletal injury.

2. Acute injury and inflammation

Injury occurs when local stress or strain exceed the ultimate strength of bones and soft tissue. Since all tissues are to some degree viscoelastic, the rate at which energy is dissipated also contributes to the degree of tissue injury since tissue stiffness, which often defines failure modes, is dependent on rate of deformation. Unlike most materials, living tissues also respond to a traumatic event, not only with mechanical failure, but with an acute inflammatory response. This inflammatory response results in the sudden and extended release of inflammatory mediators, cytokines, and other factors that act, not only locally to define the injury and to initiate what ultimately will be the healing response, but also may have significant systemic effects, potentially resulting in severe pulmonary injury or end stage organ failure. Inflammatory cascades are initiated, not only in traumatized tissues, but also by pathogens, or other foreign irritants. In the setting of trauma, these inflammatory mediators are intimately associated with the healing process. They attract precursors for cell growth, and they modulate repair mechanisms. Inflammation also stimulates and increases the sensitivity of pain receptors, which serve a protective purpose, causing trauma patients to limit motion around the damaged tissue.

Inflammation is an acute immune response, designed to rid the organism of both the initial cause of cell injury and the consequences of such injury. In trauma, inflammation is triggered by pathogens, tissue necrosis, and foreign bodies. The inflammatory cascade is amplified by early recruitment of inflammatory cells, which in turn release further mediators. In the setting of trauma, the amount of inflammation is usually determined by the amount of energy transferred to the soft tissue and bone, the degree of contamination, and type of bacteria, if any, present, as well as patient factors, such as preexisting immunodeficiency, diabetes, or steroid use. The magnitude of the inflammatory response depends on the severity of the injury and the degree of vascularization of the tissue that is injured (Smith et al, 2008). Inflammation is likely initiated by cellular damage and subsequent leakage of intracellular contents, as well as by capillary damage, leading to blood flow into the site of injury and initiation of the injury hematoma.

Inflammation is primarily represented by four major events: vasodilatation, increased micro vascular permeability, cellular activation and adhesion of immune cells, and coagulation (Kumar et al, 2009). Vasodilatation and increased permeability of microvasculature permit extravasations of protein-rich fluid into tissues. This fluid consists of macrophages and monocytes, which release and stimulate cytokines and growth factors. Loss of fluid and increased vessel diameter lead to slower blood flow and vascular congestion (Kumar et al, 2009; Schroeder et al, 2009). Once leukocytes have been recruited to the site of injury, they are activated by intracellular components in the extracellular space, by proteins expressed on the surface of dead cells, or by cytokines.

2.1 Inflammatory mediators

There are several important mediators in inflammation, and a complete discussion is beyond the scope of this chapter. They can be categorized into cell-derived mediators, which may be sequestered into granules (histamine) or synthesized de novo (prostaglandins, cytokines), and plasma-derived mediators, which circulate as inactive precursors. Active mediators are produced in response to substances released from necrotic cells or microbes, and one mediator can stimulate the release of others. Platelets are an important source of cytokines and growth factors, and they are stimulated to release these cellular products during clotting, which occurs when platelets come in contact with collagen immediately after trauma is sustained (Diegelmann & Evans, 2004). There is increasing interest in the orthopedic community on the use of platelet enriched products as a therapeutic option for a variety of musculoskeletal conditions, ranging from tendon injury to bony nonunions (Hamilton et al, 2011; Mei-Dan et al, 2010; Sanchez et al, 2009). Histamine is present in mast cell granules and can be released in response to trauma, producing dilatation of arterioles and increased permeability of venules. Prostaglandins are a group cell derived mediators that can cause vasodilation, fever, and pain. The mechanism of NSAIDs' (non steroidal anti-inflammatory) anti-inflammatory action is by inhibiting cyclooxygenase, which is an enzyme that is critical in prostaglandin formation. Leukotrienes increase vascular permeability and cause chemotaxis and leukocyte adhesion.

Cytokines exert their effects by binding to specific cellular receptors and are thus able to regulate gene transcription and modify intracellular signally pathways, both locally and systemically. They have small molecular weight and are active in extremely low concentrations. They have overlapping functions, multiple targets, and pleiotrophic actions. TNFa and IL-1 are two important early pro-inflammatory cytokines. They affect a wide variety of cells to induce fever, production of cytokines, endothelial gene regulation, chemotaxis, leukocyte adherence, and activation of fibroblasts. They are responsible for the systemic effects of inflammation, such as loss of appetite and tachycardia (Reikeras, 2010). IL-6 is another cytokine that appears to be critical in the inflammatory cascade in the setting of trauma. IL-6 levels are elevated 60 minutes after trauma (or surgery) and decline over days 2 to 5 after trauma. Importantly, the magnitude of IL-6 elevation after mechanical trauma can be used as a reliable marker for the magnitude of systemic inflammation and correlates with the risk of post-injury complications (Reikeras, 2010; Biffl et al, 1996; Pape et al, 2007). IL-6 appears to be responsible for regulating the acute phase response (Reikeras, 2010).

2.2 Systemic response

The inflammatory cytokines act locally, as well as systemically, and can lead to signs and symptoms similar to sepsis, including hypotension, fever, fatigue, anorexia, headache, activation of coagulation, and other systemic changes known together as the Systemic Inflammatory Response Syndrome (SIRS). This syndrome is most commonly seen in the setting of a serious bacterial infection and is initiated by circulating bacteria triggering an intense systemic inflammatory response. SIRS however does not require a setting of infection and can occur only as the result of injury and an inflammatory cascade. There is recent evidence that the systemic release of mitochondrial DNA and mitochondrial molecular patterns, which can occur with cellular breakdown in trauma, play a role in activating systemic inflammation in SIRS that is not a result of bacterial infection. Mitochondrial DNA and molecular patterns are similar to that of bacteria because they were likely derived from similar ancestors prior to the incorporation of mitochondria into human cells. Because of this similarity mitochondrial DNA and molecular patterns may trigger this intense inflammatory response by binding to the same immune receptors that recognize circulating bacteria (Zhang et al, 2010).

SIRS can be of severe consequence to the already debilitated trauma patient, resulting in pulmonary function collapse and organ failure. Careful consideration of timing is critical in the care of the trauma patients since further surgical intervention can worsen the inflammatory response. In severe polytrauma patients, it is often preferable to perform limited fracture stabilization, rather than definitive orthopaedic repair immediately, since surgery can function as a second traumatic event with a second wave of inflammatory cytokine release, which can augment the initial systemic inflammatory response to the trauma with increased potential to cause systemic disease including SIRS and ARDS (Second hit theory) (Reikeras, 2010; Pape et al, 2003; Sears et al, 2009). Hauser et al reports that SIRS is universal after traumatic injury and that the clinical presentation differs only in intensity (Hauser et al, 2010). One study showed that combined fracture and soft tissue injury caused higher levels of systemic inflammatory mediators (IL-6 and IL-10) than either fracture of soft tissue injury alone. The literature on SIRS and orthopedic trauma is extensive (Hardwood et al, 2005; Seibel et al, 1985; Scalea 2000; Olson, 2004; Schroeder et al, 2009; Sears et al, 2009; Weninger et al, 2007) with the femoral fracture being the primary model since it is a long bone fracture and is often most related with systemic and pulmonary collapse secondary to injury and surgery. Concern about the timing of definitive intramedullary fixation, which includes intramedullary reaming and further release of marrow contents and inflammatory mediators, is an ongoing debate in the orthopedic trauma community. It has been clear for several decades that early surgical

stabilization of long-bone fractures reduces pulmonary complications when compared to limb placed in a splint or skeletal traction. However, patients who are hemodynamically unstable, hypothermic, who have coagulation abnormalities or poor oxygenation due to traumatic lung injury have increased rates of acute lung injury after intermedullary reaming. If these conditions cannot be reversed with adequate resuscitation, these patients benefit from a protocol of damage control orthopaedics consisting of initial external fixation for transient stabilization followed by delayed definitive fracture fixation stabilization followed by delayed definitive fracture fixation (Bone & Giannoudis, 2011; Giannoudis et al, 2009; O'Toole et al, 2005, Hardwood et al, 2005; Sears et al, 2009; Pape et al, 2009; Pape et al, 2007; Pape et al, 2003).
Although inflammation is potentially harmful, with the ability to induce both local and systemic responses, it is also necessary to initiate the healing process. The inflammatory cells and proteins release growth factors and chemokines that recruit stem cells and other precursors and immune cells to the site of injury. These are then activated and stimulate others into becoming mitogenically active and proliferative. Even the hematoma and fibrin clot that occurs at the time of injury is important, likely providing a provisional structure for regenerative cells (Diegelmann & Evans, 2004). Studies demonstrate that when inflammation is limited, either in knockout mice or by pharmacological intervention, healing does not occur normally or is disrupted in time and sequence (Pape et al, 2007).

3. Bone material and structural properties

3.1 Introduction

Because the human musculoskeletal system is a living organ with predominantly a mechanical role, both physiology and engineering principles are critical for its study and understanding. The critical feature of any structural design is to consider what loads the structure must sustain and to adjust the overall geometry and the materials used to achieve the desired function. This is true in the musculoskeletal system as well.
The main function of the musculoskeletal system is to support and protect soft tissues and to assist with movement. Bones, muscle, tendons, ligaments and joints function to generate and to transfer forces so that our limbs can be manipulated in three-dimensional space. The musculoskeletal system also has a metabolic role in calcium handling, as well as hematopoiesis. To optimize function, bones must be rigid enough that they don't fail when loaded or demonstrate unnatural elastic behavior. They must also be elastic enough to absorb energy when loaded, but not so elastic that they are subject to plastic deformation (Seeman, 2003, 2006). The primary function of the musculoskeletal system is to manage applied load. The ability of a bone to resist fracture depends on the intrinsic properties of the material and the spatial distribution of bone mass (geometry and micro architecture) (Bouxsein & Karaski, 2006).

3.2 Material properties

Material properties characterize the behavior of materials comprising the tissue and to a first approximation, are independent of the size of the tissue. They are usually expressed in terms of the stress-strain relationship of the material. Stress is the amount of force applied per unit area, and strain represents the degree of deformation in response to a specific stress. Elastic deformation is the component of the stress-strain relationship in which the material deforms as load is applied yet returns to its original shape when the load is removed. The slope of this curve is the elastic modulus or Young's modulus and it is a measure of stiffness. The stiffer the material is, the steeper the slope (the less it deforms under stress). Bone is an anisotropic material with a nonlinear stress-strain relationship that can be approximated as linear in its elastic region. When bone is loaded in the elastic range it absorbs the energy by shortening and widening in compression, lengthening and narrowing in tension, and then returning to its original length when unloaded (Chavassioux et al, 2007). Plastic deformation describes the condition in which some permanent deformation remains after the load is removed. With regards to bone, deformation in the plastic zone includes micro-cracks and disruption of collagen fibrils and its trabecular architecture. The anelastic modulus describes the slope of the stress-strain curve in the plastic range. Once the load exceeds the plastic deformation zone, the energy is dissipated in fracture or tissue failure. The yield point is the point at which elastic behavior changes to plastic, and it essentially describes the safe functional load. Subtle changes in density, which can occur with aging, disease, use and disuse, greatly change strength and elastic modulus (Browner et al, 2009; Bucholz et al, 2005).

Material properties of bone are generally separated into the material properties of the outer cortex and material properties of trabecular bone, which is found inside the cortex. These structures serve slightly different purposes and this is reflected by their material properties as well as the architecture. Bone is an anisotropic material; the stress-strain behavior differs with different directions of loading. Cortical bone is stronger and stiffer when loaded in the longitudinal direction than in the transverse direction. This is related to the orientation of bone microstructure (Browner et al, 2009). The orientation of orbicular architecture corresponds with the orientation of the principle stress sustained by the tissue (Huiskes, 2000). In less anisotropic bone, trabecular bone consists of cylindrical struts extending about 1mm before making connection with other struts, usually at right angles. In more highly anisotropic bone, trabeculi are more sheet-like than cylindrical, and they are longer and preferentially aligned in one direction (Currey, 2002). On a molecular scale, regions of bone loaded in tension tend to have their collagen fibers oriented longitudinally, while those loaded in compression tend to be oriented obliquely to transversely and collagen fibrils have been found to be oriented in the direction of the trabeculae (Rupple, et al, 2008; Chavassioux et al, 2007). Because of the anisotropic nature of bone, there is not a single value for elastic modulus and hardness of cortical or trabecular bone. This anisotropic nature will play an important role in bone resistance to failure or fracture.

Bone mineral content contributes to stiffness of bone at the expense of flexibility, and it also has an effect on bone toughness. As mineral content increases up to 65%, toughness increases, and as mineral content exceeds about 65%, toughness begins to decline (Seeman 2003; Xiaodu & Puram, 2003). Toughness is determined by the material composition and the ability of the microstructure to dissipate deformation energy without propagation of a crack. Energy can be dissipated by viscoelastic flow and by the formation of non-connected micro-cracks (Petterlik et al, 2006). Collagen cross-links are known to limit crack propagation, thus increasing bone toughness. Collagen structure is another important contributor to bone material properties. The triple helix of collagen and its cross-links confer strength in tension and are closely related to post-yield properties of bone, particularly bone toughness and ductility (Seeman & Delmas, 2006; Ruppel et al, 2008; Xiaodu & Puram, 2003). Water content also plays a role in relative stiffness and toughness of bone. The collagen network is very sensitive to the condition of hydration (Seeman & Delmas, 2006). Dehydrated bone exhibits increased stiffness and decreased toughness (Xiaodu & Puram, 2003). The literature on documenting the mechanical properties of bone in various forms of loading is extensive (Turner et al, 1998; Choi, 1990; Morgan et al, 2003; Rho et al, 1997; Nyman et al, 2006; Bonfield, 1987)

Bone also exhibits viscoelastic behavior; bone strength depends on rate of loading and it exhibits creep and stress-relaxation. At higher strain rates, both ultimate strength and elastic modulus increase (Browner et al, 2009; Courtney et al, 1994; Bucholz et al, 2005; Currey, 2002). Under constant loads, bone will continue to deform or creep. If the strain is held constant, the stress decreases with time (relaxation). If cyclic loading is applied hysteresis (a phase lag in which the shape of the unloading curve is different from the shape of the loading curve), occurs leading to a dissipation of mechanical energy. More simply, some solid materials can flow slightly , but not indefinitely, and the rate of flow is proportional to the load being imposed but also inversely proportional to some function of time that the load has been imposed (Currey, 2002).

Bone also exhibits fatigue, in which loads below the yield point applied in succession progressively create a crack that grows until the material fails at a stress that is below the yield point. The fatigue resistance of a material depends more on limiting micro-crack growth than micro-crack initiation, and in bone, fatigue resistance also depends how quickly the material is able to restore micro-cracks, or heal. Micro-crack propagation is limited by bone heterogeneity and microstructural features, like cement lines around each osteon and the interface between loose and dense lamellae (Chapuriat & Delmas, 2009; Chavassioux et al, 2007). However, unlike inert materials, bone is able to sense accumulation of micro damage and to repair it. The phenomenon of fatigue is responsible for stress fractures, which are commonly seen in athletes, like runners, who do not provide frequently loaded bones with the opportunity to repair micro-damage (Hughes & Petit, 2010).

3.3 Structural properties

Structural properties of the musculoskeletal system, which characterize the tissue in its intact form, also play a critical role in managing applied loads and particularly in transferring stress through the skeletal system. This takes into account the material properties of each type of tissue in the structure, as well as the geometry and architecture of the system. Overall strength of the system depends on the size and shape of the bone (cortical thickness, cross sectional area and moment of inertia), the micro-architecture of the bone (cortical porosity, trabecular morphology), and the amount of accumulated damage.

Moment of inertia is a measure of how the material is distributed in the cross-section of the object relative to the load applied to it, and moment of inertia can be used to predict the resistance of the structure to bending and deflection (Bucholz et al, 2005; Bouxsein & Karasik, 2006).

$$\begin{aligned}&\text{Moment of inertia } = P\left(R^4 - r^4\right)/\,4\\&R = \text{cortical outer diameter; } r = \text{cortical inner diameter}\end{aligned} \qquad (1)$$

Since moment of inertia is proportional to the diameter of the structure to the 4th power (Browner et al, 2009) small increases in external diameter of a long bone can markedly improve its resistance to bending and torsional loading (Bouxsein & Karasik, 2006). Resistance to compressive loading depends on the cross sectional area of bone; resistance to bending and torsional loads involves distributing bone material far from the neutral axis of bending or torsion (generally this axis is near the center of bone) (Bouxsein & Karasik, 2006). This is highly relevant for understating changes in bone properties with aging. Osteoporosis as a result of aging, not only results in decreased mineral bone content, but aging causes a architectural remodeling which affects the moment of inertia of bone. Geriatric patients have long bones characterized by an increase in external diameter and a larger increase in internal diameter, resulting in a thinner cortex (figure 1). The increased inner diameter (and thinner cortex) results in significant decreases in bone bending resistance since moment of inertia is directly related to (R^4 - r^4). This is countered, to some degree by the increase in outer cortical diameter.

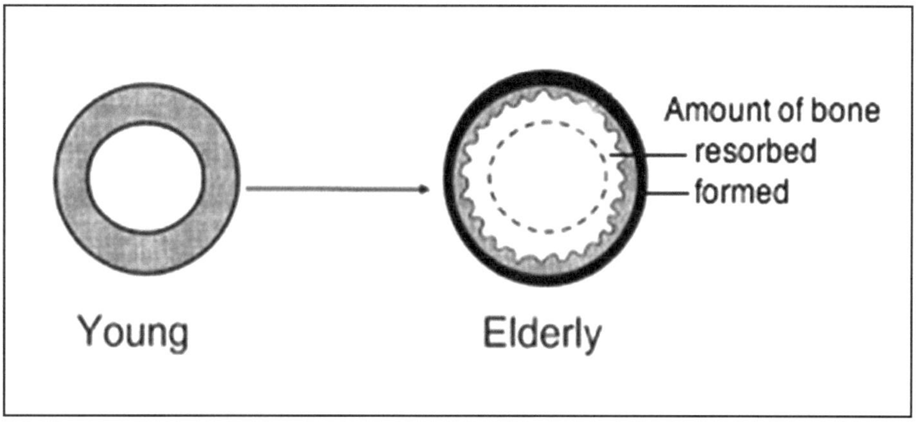

Fig. 1. Change in bone cortical diameter with age. Figure adapted from Seeman, 2003, with permission of Elsevier Limited.

Geometry is difficult to discuss in general over the entire skeleton because it is not uniform; skeletal structure and geometry is specific to the needs of each anatomical region. For example, long bones are needed for loading and movement, and rigidity in these bones is therefore favored over flexibility (Seeman & Delmas, 2006; Chavassioux et al, 2007). By shifting the cortical shell outward from the neutral axis, the long bones have increased bending strength. External and internal contours differ at each point along and around the shaft, reflecting local modeling and remodeling in response to regional loading needs (Chavassioux et al, 2007). The reverse is true in the vertebrae, where ability to deform in response to loading is favored over stiffness. Vertebral bodies with large volume of trabecular bone function more like springs than levers. Interconnecting trabecular plates achieve lightness and favor structural flexibility over stiffness (Seeman & Delmas, 2006; Chavassioux et al, 2007). Additionally the diameter and thickness of bones is different, depending on the types of stresses that are sustained by that bone. For example, the femoral neck adjacent to the shaft is elliptical, with the longer diameter in the superior-inferior direction with greater cortical thickness inferiorly. These geometrical features minimize bending. Near the femoral head, stresses are mainly compressive and the geometry reflects this. The femoral neck is more circular and largely trabecular, with a cortex of similar thickness around its perimeter (Seeman & Delmas, 2006). Later sections will elaborate on biomechanical changes that occur with age and how this affects propensity for musculoskeletal injury.

3.4 Remodeling

In 1982 Julius Wolff published a paper on bone remodeling, defining a phenomenon that would become known as Wolff's law--that bone changes external geometry and internal architecture in response to stresses acting on it (Wolff, 1986). Wolff's law has been quoted in numerous ways through the years and referenced for support whenever the argument of stress modulated bone remodeling was being made. However, Wolf's law is not a law in the quantitative sense but rather an insightful observation. There is no known growth law for bone or any other musculoskeletal tissue that is universally applicable or demonstrated. It is also unclear if bone remodeling is a stress- or strain-governed phenomenon.

During the remodeling process, osteoclasts (bone resorption cells) remove old bone tissue by resorption, and osteoblasts (bone forming cells) create new bone tissue. It is understood that bone is remodeled to meet its mechanical demands. There is evidence that micro damage initiates bone remodeling and that fracture repair is a form of load-induced bone remodeling in which damage serves as trigger (Chapuriat & Delmas, 2009; Burr et al, 1985; Mori & Burr, 1993). Stress fractures are often localized radiographically when patients complain of limb pain, and a radiograph demonstrates a reactive response or fracture callus that illustrates the remodeling process initiated by the injury. The principles of remodeling and bone fracture healing with callus often reflect the need to redistribute stress at the site of healing. A large callus that increases the cross sectional areal of the bone at the site of a transverse shaft fracture serves a means of increasing the moment of inertia and decreasing the bending stress sustained at the fracture site.

Evidence for exercise-induced osseous remodeling in adults is less clear. Data from intervention randomized control trials is limited. Follow-up times have been short, the quality of the conduction of intervention and reporting of outcomes has been poor, and there has been a lack of reporting on the specific exercise characteristics that are effective (Korpelainen et al, 2006; Bonaiuti, 2004). However, adaptation to loading in children and adolescents is well documented, and these changes in bone density and geometry persist into adulthood. Exercise, particularly weight-bearing impact exercises, in prepubertal boys increases estimates of bone strength at loaded sites, likely due to thicker cortices (Nikander et al, 2010; Nara-Ashizawa et al, 2002). Young tennis players have increased cortical thickness and increased cortical drift in the perosteal direction in their playing arm compared with their non-dominant arm. However, in middle-aged subjects, tennis did not stimulate cortical drift in the periosteal direction. In middle-aged subjects cross-sectional areas of the radius were actually smaller, suggesting that unilateral use of the arm after the third decade of life suppresses age-related changes in bone geometry since normally there is increased endocortical area and slower expansion of periosteal area resulting in decreased cortical thickness (Nara-Ashizawa et al, 2002). There is some evidence that exercise can increase bone mineral density (BMD) in post-menopausal women, particularly after one year or longer. The type of exercise and the amount of improvement is somewhat contested. A few studies, however, suggest that resistance training and low- to moderate-impact exercises are most effective. However the gains in BMD are generally small (1-2%) (Nikander et al, 2010; Korpelainen et al, 2006; Bonaiuti, 2004). Exercise has been shown to result in up to a 50% reduction in fracture incidence, but a large component of this reduction is likely due to improved muscle function and balance, combined with the small 1-2% increase in BMD (Nikander et al, 2010).

The cellular mechanism for remodeling control is a focus of research interest, but the details are still largely unknown. Osteocytes appear to be the primary mechanosensors that begin the remodeling cascade. There is evidence that pressure gradients within the bone matrix lead to interstitial fluid flow in the lacunar-canalicular system, which activates mechanosensory osteocytes that reside in lacunae. The osteocytes then transmit load-provoked signals via canaliculi and gap junctions (Chen et al, 2010; Ulstrup, 2008). There is evidence that osteocyte death is associated with remodeling as well (Seeman & Delmas, 2006). Death of cells likely creates biochemical and chemotactic signals, which indicate presence of damage and its location. Regions of micro damage contain apoptotic osteocytes whereas quiescent zones do not (Seeman & Delmas, 2006; Hughes & Petit, 2010).

3.5 Mechanics of bone regeneration

Under most circumstances bone is able to regenerate its baseline mechanical properties after sustaining a fracture. However, the mechanical environment is critical in establishing tissue formation patterns during fracture repair. There are two forms of bone healing: direct or primary healing and indirect or secondary healing, which occur depending on the mechanical environment. Direct healing occurs when the fracture is subjected to surgical fixation with absolute stability, fixation with absolute stability, with no interfragmentary motion or strain with no interfragmentary motion or strain. This direct healing is achieved by interfragmentary compression, most often achieved technically during surgery with lag screws and/or compression plates. In this setting, bone heals via intramembranous ossification without development of a fracture callus. This is most often applied to peri-articular fractures where perfect anatomic reduction is necessary for an optimal functional outcome. Indirect healing occurs when the fracture is subjected to relative stability, or when there is some degree of interfragmentary motion or strain. Bone heals with development of a fracture callus, which changes the mechanical properties and the geometry of the fracture site. This often produces optimal biological conditions for healing.

Interfragmentary strain theory, pioneered by Perren in 1979 is the basis for our understanding of how the mechanical environment impacts tissue differentiation in a fracture gap (Figure 2). He theorized that the magnitude of interfragmentary strain determines subsequent tissue differentiation of fracture gap tissue. Each tissue has different strain tolerances, and applied interfragmentary strain must be smaller than the strain tolerance of a tissue for it to form. According to Perren, strains below 2% permit direct bone formation (direct fracture healing), strains below 10% allow cartilage differentiation and subsequent endocondral ossification (indirect fracture healing), and strains between 10% and 100% lead to granulation tissue formation and non-union. Perren believed that differentiation of initial fracture gap tissue would stiffen the fracture gap leading to lower interfragmentary strain, allowing differentiation to the next stiffest tissue. (Perren, 1979; Perren, 2002; Isaksson et al, 2006).

Carter and Blenman supplemented Perren's theory with the idea that, in addition to strain magnitude, both the type of mechanical stimulus (cyclic, compressive, tensile or shear) and the degree of vascular supply would affect tissue differentiation. Prendergast et al later developed a different mechanoregulation concept that proposed two biophysical stimuli, shear strain in the solid phase and fluid velocity in the interstitial fluid phase. According to this concept, bone formed only when both stimuli were low enough. However, none of these models are flawless, and clinical results suggest that these theories are correct in the extremes, where they are similar: low strain leads to bone formation, and high strain leads to fibrous non-union. (Carter et al, 1998; Carter et al, 1988; Prendergast et al, 1997; Isaksson et al, 2006).

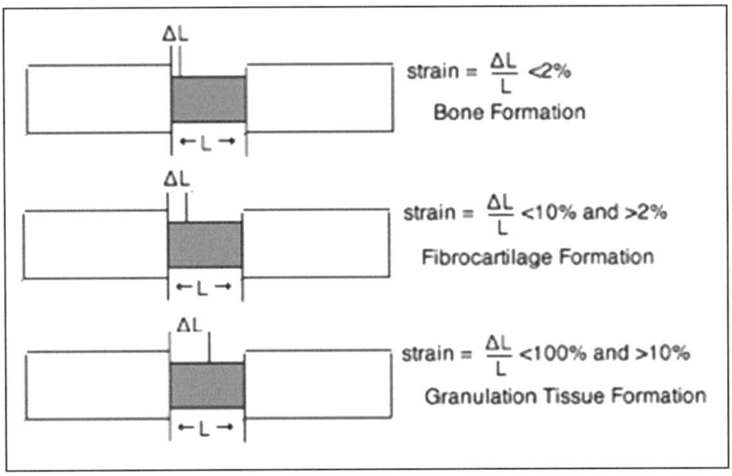

Fig. 2. Interfragmentary strain theory. The formation of tissue type based on strain at the fracture gap

4. Geriatric biomechanics

4.1 Osteoporosis

Osteoporosis is defined as a "systemic skeletal disease characterized by low bone mass and micro-architectural deterioration of bone tissue, leading to enhanced bone fragility and a consequent increase in fracture risk "(Alexeeva et al, 1994). In the US over 1.5 million fractures occur each year, including 280,000 hip fractures, and these numbers are expected to double or triple in the coming decades due to the aging population (Bouxsein & Karasik, 2006). There are several components of whole bone strength that change over time, including the intrinsic properties of the materials that form bone, the amount of bone (ie mass), and the spatial distribution of bone mass (ie geometry and microarchitecture) (Bouxsein & Karasik, 2006). The biggest challenge is determining the effects of these changes and identifying which change is most important in the development of osteoprosis.

4.2 Bone mechanical properties

Whole bone strength declines dramatically with age. Changes that occur in cortical, as well as trabecular bone collectively lead to decreased bone strength and increased risk of fracture. Between 30 and 80 years of age, elastic modulus of cortical bone decreases by 8%, bone strength decreases by 11%, and toughness declines by 34% (Bouxsein & Jepsen, 2003). All of these changes result in mechanical failure or fracture as a result of lower energy traumatic events. The specific changes that contribute to these events are a topic of investigation. It is clear that there is a reduction in overall bone mass with age. It is thought that thinning of cortical bone and increased porosity are major contributors to loss in stiffness, strength, toughness, and resistance to propagation of cracks (Silva, 2007; Seeman 2006). Studies have shown that there is a four-fold increase in cortical bone porosity from 20 to 80 years of age (Brockstedt et al, 1993). The elastic modulus of cortical bone in a longitudinal direction decreases significantly with increased porosity (Schaffler & Burr, 1988; Currey, 1988; Dong & Guo, 2004). Other factors that may contribute to decreased toughness include loss of bone mass, increased mineralization or development of hypermineralized regions, accumulation of micro damage, decreased integrity of collagen, and changes in collagen crosslinks (Xiaodu & Puram, 2003).

The changes in mechanical properties of trabecular bone are even more pronounced. Between 30 and 80 years of age, elastic modulus of trabecular bone decreases by 64%, strength decreases by 68%, and toughness decreases by 70% (Bouxsein & Jepsen, 2003). These changes are likely due to loss of trabecaular plates and connectivity, as well as micro damage. Studies have shown that loss of connectivity in trabecular plates produces a greater deficit in bone strength than thinned plates that continue to be well connected (Seeman & Delmas, 2006; Silva, 2007; Chavassioux et al, 2007).

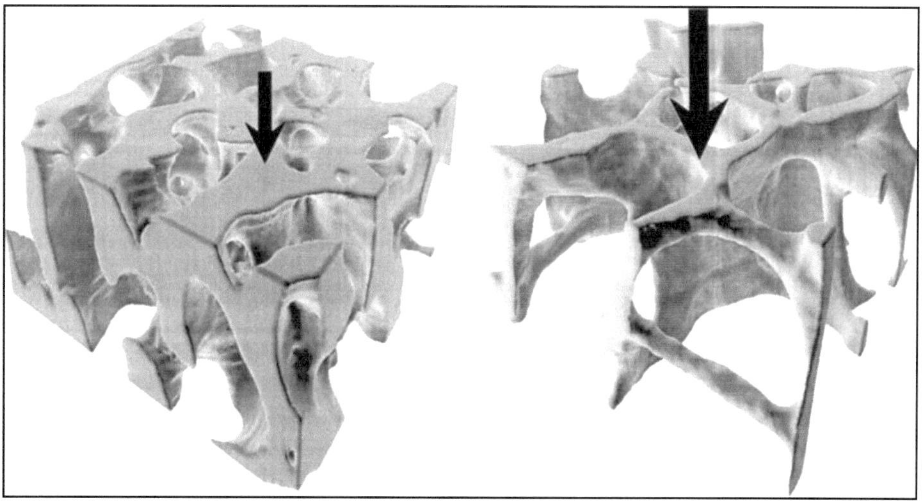

Fig. 3. Loss of trabecular bone mass and decreased trabecular connectivity ocurs with increasing age. Figure from Seeman, 2003, with permission from Elsevier Limited.

4.3 Bone geometry

The overall size and shape of bones play important roles in their mechanical behavior. Microarchitectural changes in trabecular bone, such as decreased number of trabecular plates and decreased connectivity between plates, appear to play a large role in decreased strength of trabecular bone. Decreases in bone mass and changes in distribution of bone mass also appear to play a large role in overall bone strength (McCreadie & Goldstein, 2000; Kreider & Goldstein, 2009). It is well established that endosteal expansion (increase in inner cortical radius due to loss of cortical bone) and perioesteal expansion (increase in external cortical radius due to deposition of new bone on the external surface of bone cortex) both occur, but that endosteal expansion exceeds periosteal expansion (Figure 1). This excess leads to age-related deceases in cortical thickness but increases in bone outer diameter. Decreased cortical thickness contributes to the decreases in strength, elastic modulus, and toughness of bone. However, the greater diameter increases moment of inertia and increases structural resistance to bending and torsional loads, which may offset decreases in cortical thickness and bone mineral density that occur with age. This effect explains how bone mineral density can decrease while bending resistance may not (McCreadie & Goldstein, 2000; Beck et al, 2000; Bouxsein et al, 2006; Silva, 2007; Seeman & Delmas, 2006; Mayhew et al, 2005).

Bone is known to be highly anisotropic at baseline and is strongest in the direction of habitual loading. There is emerging evidence to suggest that in hip-fracture patients, bone is more anisotropic and more highly oriented in the direction of habitual loading than control subjects, occurring at the expense of strength in other directions. One study examined specimens from hip fracture patients and un-fractured controls, and controlled for bone volume. The study found that hip fracture specimens of the same bone volume were more highly organized in the direction of habitual loading. This increased anisotropy leads to a reduced ability to withstand off-axis impact, during a fall in a direction different from the direction of habitual loading, such as a sideways fall. In these patients, bone reorganization may be overcompensating for the low mass status by increasing the degree of anisotropy so that strength of the bone is only maximized in the frequently loaded direction (Kreider & Goldstein, 2009; Ciarelli et al, 2000; McCreadie & Goldstein, 2000).

The rate of bone remodeling may also play a role in development of osteoporosis. During growth the balance between bone that is removed and bone that is formed is positive (more bone is added than removed). Once skeletal maturity is reached, this reverses and the balance becomes negative (more bone is removed than is added in the remodeling process). In general, the rate of remodeling, and therefore the rate of bone loss, is extremely slow later in life. However, there is evidence to suggest that estrogen deficiency increases the rate of remodeling and there may be other factors that modulate remodeling rate. It is possible that bone loss is driven more by increased rate of remodeling than by magnitude of bone loss during each remodeling event (Seeman & Delmas, 2006; Xiaodu & Puram, 2003). Another possible mechanism through which bone remodeling contributes to osteoporosis is through increasing dysfunction of mechanoreceptors, which drive the remodeling process. This could contribute to bone loss and could interfere with remodeling in response to micro damage or in response to changes in loading (Kreider & Goldstein, 2009).

4.4 Bone mineral density

Bone mineral density (BMD) is the attribute currently used in clinical practice to diagnose osteoporosis and to monitor efficacy of interventions. Dual-emission X-ray absorptiometry (DXA) is used to measure BMD clinically. BMD is bone mineral content (BMC) (measured as the attenuation of the X-ray by the bones being scanned) divided by area of the site being scanned. Osteoporosis is diagnosed by determining how many standard deviations the BMD of the patient is below the mean BMD of a healthy thirty year-old. Any BMD that is greater than two and a half standard deviations below the mean thirty year-old BMD is considered osteoporotic.

BMD explains a significant portion of the risk of osteoporotic fracture and correlates with bone strength. BMD is a strong predictor of fracture risk; risk of fracture increases 50-150% with each standard deviation decrease in bone mass as measured by DXA (McCreadie & Goldstein, 2000; Kreider & Goldstein, 2009; Bouxsein et al, 1999). However, it is clear that there are other factors that contribute to fracture risk. Studies have demonstrated that there is a significant overlap in BMD between osteoporotic individuals and healthy individuals who have not experienced osteoporotic fracture. The risk of fracture of the hip or forearm in a 75 year-old is 4-7 times that of a 45 year-old with an identical BMD. Risk for hip fracture actually doubles for each decade of age increase even after adjusting for bone density (Beck et al, 2000; Ruppel et al, 2008; Degoede et al, 2003). Additionally, current therapies are able to, at best, increase bone density by 10%, but the risk of fracture decreases by a much larger extent (McCreadie & Goldstein, 2000). The specific non-BMD factors that explain this discrepancy are not known.

BMD is used clinically because it represents a non-invasive, relatively inexpensive way, to predict fracture risk. It indirectly reflects bone geometry, mass, size, and mineralization. However, DXA does not provide information on cortical vs. cancellous density, 3D geometry, trabecular architecture, microstructure or strength parameters. It functions as a surrogate for these attributes, which are difficult to measure non-invasively (Kreider & Goldstein, 2009; Bouxsein et al, 1999).

4.5 Bisphosphonates

Bisphosphonates are a class of drugs that are commonly used to manage osteoporosis. They function by inhibiting bone resorption by osteoclasts, which occurs during remodeling. They mimic the structure of pyrophosphate and are incorporated into bone. They are then ingested by osteoclasts and ultimately result in osteoclast cell death. During bisphosphonate treatment bone remodeling rate is slower and there are a fewer number of osteoclast-induced excavation sites each with decreased depth, leading to slower bone loss. Fractures are less frequent but not eliminated in patients taking bisphosphonates (Seeman & Delmas, 2006). Maximum fracture risk reduction occurs in the first year of treatment. Observed fracture risk appears to be at least twice as large as would be expected from changes in BMD alone (Ruppel et al, 2008).

In recent years there has been some controversy with regard to safety of prolonged bisphosphonate administration. Several case series initially described cases of "atypical" subtrochanteric and diaphyseal femur fractures and suggested that the risk may be increased in long-term users of bisphosphonates (Black et al, 2010; Glusti et al, 2010; Capeci & Tejwani, 2009). Unique clinical features of these fractures in the literature include prodromal pain for weeks to months prior to fracture, complete absence of precipitating trauma, and bilateral fracture (either simultaneous or sequential) in some. Distinctive radiographic features include presence of a stress reaction on the affected and/or unaffected side, transverse or short oblique pattern (in contrast to the more common spiral fracture), thick femoral cortices, and unicortical breaking (Black et al, 2010; Glusti et al, 2010; Nieves & Crosman, 2010; Singer, 2011). The theory behind this concern is that long-term bisphosphonate use with prolonged suppression of bone turnover may lead to accumulation of micro damage due to impaired remodeling. It has also been suggested that long-term bisphosphonate use could create a more homogenous tissue with BMD more similar throughout, and this may offer less resistance to propagation of cracking (Glusti et al, 2010; Seeman & Delmas, 2006; Rupel et al, 2008). Fracture patterns and cortical thickening are reminiscent of osteopetrosis and fractures that occur in ostepetrosis in the subtrochanteric area (Armstrong et al, 1999; Golden & Rodriguez, 2010; Tolar et al, 2004; Singer, 2011). Osteopetrosis is a congenital malfunction of the osteoclast resulting in severe brittle and dense bone. There are several retrospective cohort studies that indicate that there is a correlation between atypical subtrochanteric and diaphyseal femur fractures and use of several bisphosphonates (Vestergaard et al, 2011; Lenart et al, 2009). However, it is difficult to determine whether this correlation is confounded by the fact that those taking bisphosphonates, particularly long-term, have significant osteoporosis that may account for these atypical fractures. Data from three large placebo controlled, randomized control trials have indicated that there is no association between bisphosphonate use and atypical subtrochanteric or diaphyseal femur fracture. Based on these three studies, it is likely that these subtrochanteric and femoral shaft fractures may be related to the underlying osteoporosis, which was the reason for long-term bisphosphonate use (Black et al, 2010; Nieves & Crosman, 2010; Rizzoli et al, 2010) or to an additional metabolic predisposition yet to be dignosed. However, confidence intervals in these studies were high due to the small number of events, and, although, one study followed patients for ten years, it is possible that this is not long enough to observe an effect. Additionally, it has been suggested that these fractures are associated with bisphosphonate use in a subset of patients, like those taking steroids or proton pump inhibitors. Future studies will investigate these possibilities and bisphosphonates remain a valuable tool in the standard of care of the osteoporotic patient.

5. Fracture mechanisms

Injury patterns sustained in trauma can often be inferred from bone radiographs after trauma with certain confidence and consistency (Linnau et al, 2007; Clare, 2008; Mubarak et al, 2009; Arimoto & Forrester, 1980; Browner et al, 2009). Knowledge of patterns of injury attributed to specific modes of trauma can be used to predict associated injuries, since not all injuries are obvious at presentation. This knowledge also serves to develop or to improve safety features and equipment.

The magnitude, type and direction of forces, as well as material properties of bone and surrounding structures, dictate the fracture pattern to a certain degree. Severity of injury is determined by peak forces and moments resulting from the impact and the tissues' resistance to injury (DeGoede et al, 2003). The greater the energy absorbed by the bone, the more severe the fracture and the more likely that comminution and displacement will occur. Tissues surrounding bone, including muscle, tendons, ligaments, fat and skin, can affect fracture pattern by absorbing some of the load energy and also by creating additional load. The main factors that affect the load at which bone fails include bone geometry, bone material properties, load application point, load direction and the rate of load application (DeGoede et al, 2003). The main load bearing structure in bone is the cortex, which is denser, has greater volume and mass, and is in a location that makes it more capable of sustaining large loads. Trabecular bone largely functions to direct stresses to cortical bone. Multiple injuries can be caused by the same mechanism because forces can be transmitted along the entire length of a bone or through several bones, causing damage anywhere along the way.

5.1 Simple fracture patterns

There are a limited number of loading modes that bone can be subjected to, and these result in predictable fracture patterns. Complex fracture patterns occur when multiple loading modes and directions are applied during the same event. Loading modes include tensile loading, compressive loading, shear loading, bending load, and loading in torsion. Bone is weakest in tension and strongest in compression. When bone is loaded in tension it tends to fracture along a transverse plane that is approximately perpendicular to the direction of loading. When undergoing a compressive load, bone will fail secondary to shear stress since shear strength of bone is much less than compressive strength. During compressive loading, shear stresses develop at a plane that is approximately 45 degrees from the long axis of the bone, and it is along this oblique plan that bone fails. Max shear stress is approximately one half of the applied compressive stress. Bending is essentially a combination of tensile and compressive loading. When bone is undergoing bending, high tensile stresses develop on the convex side and high compressive stresses develop on the concave side. A transverse fracture is initiated on the tensile side, and two oblique fractures occur on the compressive side, creating what is referred to as a butterfly fragment. Fracture secondary to torsion usually begins at a small defect at the bone surface, and then the fracture follows a spiral pattern along planes of high tensile stress, since bone is weakest in tension (Browner et al, 2009; Bucholz et al, 2005; Canale, 2002). It is a worthwhile exercise for a traumatologist to carefully look at a radiograph after trauma and to recreate the mechanism of fracture based on the fracture pattern. More complex and comminuted fracture patterns are essentially a combination of these simple patterns (Browner et al, 2009; Bucholz et al, 2005; Canale, 2002). Materials properties of bone can be approximated as isotropic when load is delivered at a high rate.

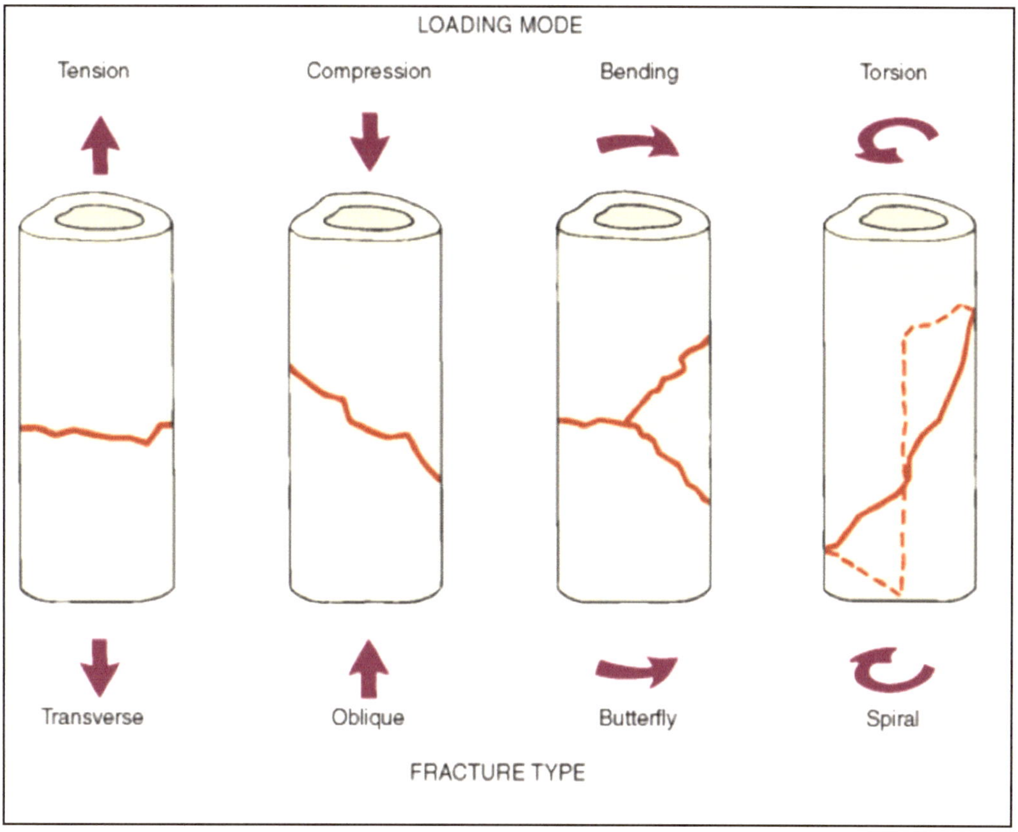

Fig. 4. Simple fracture patterns which occur as a result of loading mode. Figure from Browner et al, 2008, with permission from Elsevier Limited.

5.2 Fall

Fall is an important source of musculoskeletal injury and accounts for 87% of fracture in older adults (DeGoede et al, 2003). The two most common injuries secondary to fall are hip fractures and upper extremity fractures, and in some instances, they are related in that impacts at the wrist have been shown to modulate or lessen impacts at the pelvis during lateral and forward falls. This requires rapid reaction and movement times, as well as arm muscle strength, all of which decrease with age to some degree (DeGoede et al, 2003). One study measured reaction time of young and elderly women and found that the typical elderly female is able move her hands quickly enough to break a forward fall, but not a sideways fall, while young women are able to break both types of fall (Robinovitch et al, 2005).

5.3 Fall on outstretched hand

Fall on outstretched hand is a classic mechanism of injury leading to fracture of the scaphoid bone of the hand, fracture of the distal ulna and radius, fracture-dislocation of the elbow, fracture dislocation of the shoulder and fracture of the clavicle. This injury mechanism accounts for approximately 90% of fractures at the distal radius, humeral neck, and supracondylar elbow region (Robinovitch et al, 1998). During a fall on a stiff surface, hand contact force occurs in two stages: the first is a high-frequency peak load which corresponds to a large deceleration of arm mass, which occurs at the wrist at the moment of impact; the second is a low-frequency oscillation with a lower peak force, which is due to deformation of the shoulder spring (Figure 5) (Chiu & Robinovitch, 1998). Increases in body mass more strongly increase the peak magnitude of the low-frequency component, and increases in fall height more dramatically increase the high-frequency component (Chiu & Robinovitch, 1998).

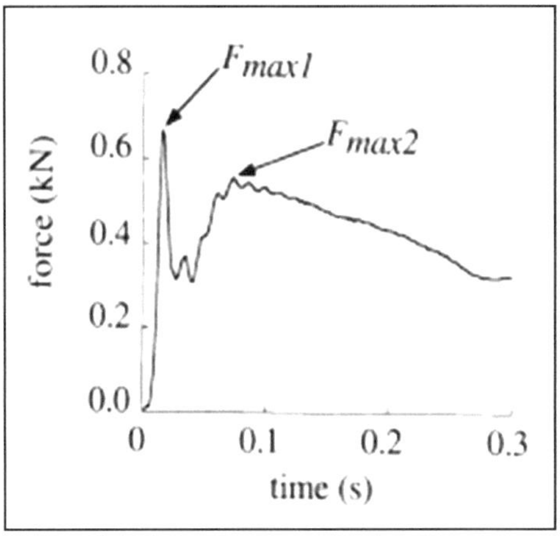

Fig. 5. Impact response of the body during a forward fall onto the outstretched hand. Measures of hand contact force during this event show a high-frequency transient (with associated peak force Fmax1) followed by a lower-frequency oscillation (with associated peak force Fmax2). Figure from Chiu et al, 1998 with permission from Elsevier Limited.

The fracture pattern depends on the force magnitude, on how force is distributed across the bones of the hand, and on how it is transmitted to other upper extremity structures. The magnitude and distribution of contact force during a fall also depends on the configuration of the body at impact and on the soft tissue thickness over the palm region (Choi & Robinovitch, 2010). The weakest area on the palm is over the scaphoid and lunate, which articulate directly with and transmit force to the distal radius. A fall with peak force localized to this area is most likely to result in fracture.

Understanding the mechanics of an injury helps to develop preventative measures. In one study patients were able to learn to reduce the impact force applied to the distal forearm by 27% by slightly flexing their elbows and reducing the velocity of the hands relative to the torso (DeGoede & Ashton-Miller, 2002). Another study showed that a 5mm foam pad reduced peak pressure and peak force by 83% and 13% respectively (Choi & Robinovitch, 2010), which can represent the difference between a fracture and isolated soft tissue damage. Additionally weight plays a role in degree of loading during a fall. Peak pressure was 77% higher in individuals with high body mass index (BMI) when compared to low BMI participants (Choi & Robinovitch, 2010). In contrast to what we see in the hip, having high BMI is not associated with increased thickness of soft tissue in the hand, and therefore the extra body mass contributed to the total force of the fall without providing extra tissue to absorb the energy.

5.4 Femoral neck fracture

Hip fracture or femoral neck fracture is a significant source of morbidity in the elderly population, and 90% of such fractures are due to fall from standing (Robinovitch et al, 1997; Parkkari et al, 1999). Hip fracture in the elderly is associated with a 20% chance of death and a 25% risk of long-term institutionalization (Parkkari et al, 1999). Changes that occur with aging in the material properties of bone play a significant role in femoral neck fracture; however, the mechanics of the fall (direction, location of impact) are critical as well. Although 90% of hip fractures are due to a fall, only 1% of falls actually result in hip fracture, which is surprising from a biomechanical perspective because the energy available during a fall from standing often exceeds that required to fracture both elderly and young proximal femurs (Robinovitch et al, 2000). Mitigating factors can be many.

The femoral neck undergoes constant bending loads during normal weight-bearing activities. Compressive force through the femoral head can range from 4-8 times the body weight during normal activities and this force acts through a significant moment arm (the length of the femoral neck), which causes large bending loads on the femoral neck (Browner et al, 2009). In normal gait the greatest stresses occur in the subcapital and mid-femoral neck regions. Within these regions maximum compressive stresses occur inferiorly where the cortex is thick and smaller tensile stresses occur superiorly where the cortex is thinner (de Baker et al, 2009). Sideways falls with impact to the greater trochanter are the events most directly related to hip fracture in older adults (Liang & Robinovitch, 2010; Parkkari et al, 1999; Courtney et al, 1994). The femoral neck is weakest when the posterolateral aspect of the greater trochanter is impacted. During a sideways fall on the greater trochanter, the stress state is reversed from normal ambulation and the greatest compressive stresses occur in the superior femoral neck while the smaller tensile stresses occur in the inferior region (Figure 6) (de Baker et al, 2004). Mayhew et al showed that the superior cortex of the femoral neck is significantly thinner in older than younger individuals, while the inferior cortex is significantly thicker in older than younger individuals (Mayhew et al, 2005). Therefore, during a sideways fall, which is more frequent in the elderly, the large compressive stress occurs in the superior cortex, which is thinner and more likely to fail in the elderly. Multiple studies have suggested that proximal femur fractures are typically initiated by a failure in the superior aspect of the femoral neck, followed by a failure in the inferior aspect of the femoral neck (de Baker et al, 2009; Lotz et al 1995; Mayhew et al, 2005). Wang et al showed that subjects with a longer moment arm in the context of a sideways fall increases the force applied to the hip and predisposes the subject to a hip fracture. Hip axis length and neck-shaft angle both contribute to the moment arm of the hip and both have been independently shown to predict hip fracture (Wang et al, 2008; Leslie et al, 2009; Patron et al, 2006; Crabtree et a, 2002). A fall onto the greater trochanter may also generate an axial force along the femoral neck, resulting in an impaction fracture. Additionally, investigators have reported that the lower extremity externally rotates during a fall and that, at the extremes of external rotation, the femoral neck impinges against the posterior acetabular rim. The acetabular rim then acts like a fulcrum to concentrate the stress experienced by that region at time of impact (Koval & Zuckerman, 1994).

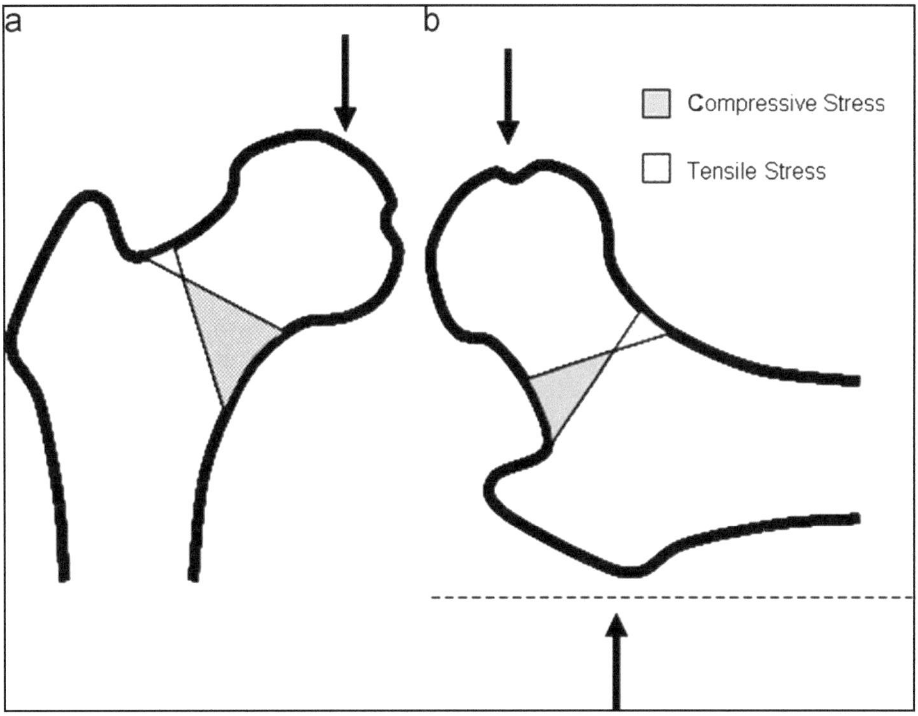

Fig. 6. The magnitude and nature of the stresses on the femoral neck differ depending on the applied load. For example in (a) walking: the inferior surface tends to be subjected to a large component of compressive stress, while the superior surface is subjected to a smaller tensile stress and (b) sideways fall on the greater trochanter: the inferior surface tends to be subjected to a small tensile stress, while the superior surface is subjected to a larger compressive stress. Figure from de Bakker et al, 2009 with permission from Elsevier Limited.

Since only a small fraction of falls actually result in fracture and the energy available in a fall is sufficient to fracture the proximal femur, there are mitigating factors that affect the actual impact forces. Some of these include soft tissue properties and body positioning at the time of impact. Energy of a fall can be dissipated by contracting muscles; this contraction is likely done more effectively in younger patients than older patients with slower, weaker muscles (Koval & Zuckerman, 1994). Substantial energy can also be absorbed by skin and fat overlying the hip region (Robinovitch et al, 2000). Peak femoral impact force actually decreases in a linear manner with increasing soft-tissue thickness at a rate of approximately 79 N per 1mm change in thickness (Robinovitch et al, 1995), and peak pressure over the greater trochanter averaged 266% higher in low BMI participants than in high BMI participants in another study (Choi & Robinovitch, 2010). Additionally, there are actions that fallers can take to moderate the force applied directly to the femur. Falling techniques can be taught to geriatric patients by physical therapists. In one study young subjects were able to impact the outstretched hand and pelvis near-simultaneously during an unexpected fall which distributed the body's impact energy (Robinovitch et al, 2000). Fallers can also produce "energy absorbing" work during descent, which occurs by eccentrically contracting lower extremity muscles, which increases the vertical component of foot reaction forces resulting in decreased downward acceleration (Robinovitch et al, 2000). Mats as thin as 1.5cm have been shown to decrease peak hip impact force by 8% and thicker mats have a greater effect (Liang et al, 2006). Ultimately, these modifiable factors, which diminish the peak impact force, are critical because they represent ways that hip fracture can be reduced or prevented.

5.5 Motor vehicle collision

Motor vehicle collision is a common source of polytrauma, injuring more than 5 million people every year (Peterson et al, 1998). Generally, injuries are sustained when the vehicle rapidly decelerates while the vehicle occupant continues to move at previous speeds. When the body absorbs energy beyond its tolerance fracture or injury occurs. Since bone and soft tissue resistance to injury decreases with age, elderly vehicle occupants are at increased risk of injury; this trend reaches statistical significance in the 7th decade (Moran et al, 2002; Peterson et al, 1998). The location of injury depends on which structures strike which car component and the severity depends on the speed and energy of the collision as well as timing of human contact to car structures. In a frontal collision an occupant continues to move forward as the vehicle stops. Forward motion of the occupant is arrested as the person connects either with the seatbelt or with anterior car structures, if unrestrained. Initial impact points are often lower extremities, resulting in fractures of the ankle, around the knee, or fracture of the femur. There are many factors that contribute to the amount of force transferred to specific anatomical structures including change in velocity at impact, timing of impact, degree of compartment intrusion, configuration of occupant and safety devices (Siegel et al, 2001; Bansal et al, 2009; Crandall et al, 1998; Nordhoff, 2004; Chong et al, 2007) Change in velocity at time of impact is closely associated with severity of injury as well as incidence of lower extremity injury (Figure 7) (Chong et al, 2007; Dischinger et al, 1998, Rupp & Scheider, 2004). The effect of timing is illustrated in the different degree of injury sustained when knee contact with instrument panel occurs during deceleration when the instrument panel may still be moving forward causing the localized contact velocity to be lower than impacts that occur once the car has stopped moving (Mackay, 1992). Occupant factors, such as age, gender, height and BMI also contribute to type and severity of injury. Height appears to be an important factor in pattern of injury; tall occupants (and males) sustain more knee, thigh or hip injuries while shorter (and female) occupants tend to sustain more foot and ankle injuries (Chong et al, 2007). Elderly occupants are at increased risk of injury (Moran et al, 2002; Peterson et al, 1998). There are studies that indicate that high BMI's are associated with increased severity of lower extremity injury (Arbabi et al, 2003; Boulanger e al, 1992).

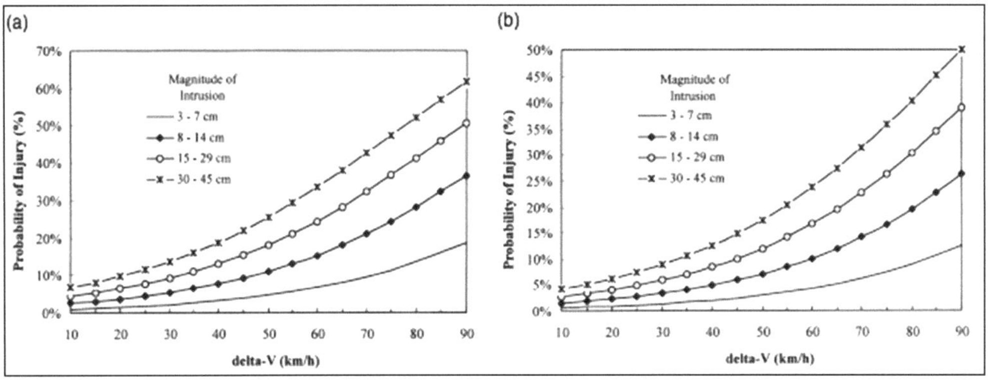

Fig. 7. Injury risk in a frontal MVC is related to magnitude of car intrusion and delta-V for both female (a) and male (b) occupants. Figure from Crandall et al (1998) with permission from Elsevier Limited

A typical dashboard injury pattern is often initiated by knee impact, usually on the instrument panel. This occurs most frequently in unrestrained occupants with or without airbag deployment. Force to the knee from the dashboard or instrument panel can result in knee laceration, patellar fracture, distal femur fracture, and proximal tibia fracture and forces can be transmitted through the femur to cause femoral shaft fractures, proximal femur fractures, acetabular or pelvic fractures, and posterior hip dislocation (Huelke, 1982; Rupp & Schneider, 2004). The risks for hip/pelvis injuries are generally greater than the risk for knee and thigh injuries at all crash severities and the right hip is more often injured than the left in forward-moving crashes, likely due to the effects of braking and bracing on occupant position and on muscle tension. Hip/pelvis fractures occur at lower impact force when the hip is flexed or adducted prior to impact; hip tolerance decreases approximately 1.8% for each degree of adduction from neutral and approximately 1% for each degree of flexion (Figure 8) (Rupp & Schneider, 2004). In an unrestrained driver, the body continues moving forward after the vehicle has stopped and the head, cervical spine and torso impact the windshield and steering wheel. During a lateral impact the occupant is accelerated away from the side of the vehicle that was struck and common injuries include lateral compression pelvic fracture, pulmonary contusion and intraabdominal solid organ injury (Mackay, 1992).

The other primary mechanism for lower extremity injury during a motor vehicle collision is impact caused by pedal interaction and toe pan intrusion (Crandall et al, 1998). One specific fracture that is well described is calcaneus or malleous fracture of the foot secondary to being forced against the brake pedal by the weight of the occupant or in combination with the floor pan of the car crushing into the space where the foot resides (Bucholz et al, 2005; Seipel et al, 2001). When the Achilles tendon resists dorsiflexion and the brake causes dorsiflexion, a three-point bending load occurs on the calcaneus with the posterior facet of the talus functioning as a fulcrum. This leads to a specific fracture pattern referred to as the tongue-toe calcaneous fracture pattern (Bucholz et al, 2005). Foot inversion or eversion in combination with compression force created by the brake pedal leads to malleolus fracture (Bucholz et al, 2005; Huelke, 1982; Crandall et al, 1998). High-heeled shoes have been shown to alter foot and ankle biomechanics leading to increased instability and injury during an MVC (Nordhoff, 2004). The effect of height on pattern of injury may be a reflection of leg position and may be related to the fact that shorter people sit closer to the steering wheel and reach for foot pedals, while taller people sit farther back with their knees closer to the level of the instrument panel (Chong et al, 2007).

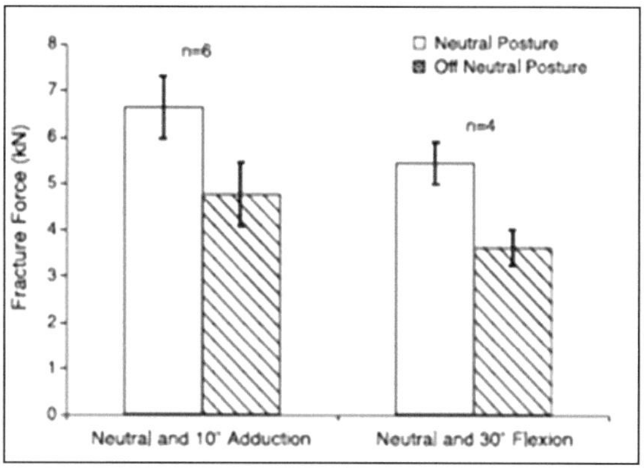

Fig. 8. Hip/pelvis fx occurs at lower impact forece when the hip is flexed or adducted prior to impact; Figure from Rupp & Schneider (2004) with permission from Elsevier Limited

Many safety systems, including seat belts, air bags, and vehicle deformation, take advantage of the fact that increasing time over which decelerations are applied to the passenger compartment decreases force experienced by the occupants (Peterson et al 1998). The concept of a "crumple zone" is based on this effect. Newer car designs provide an average of 2 ft of crushable car body, as well as steering mechanisms that collapse, which functions to increase deceleration time and also to dissipate a component of the energy by deformation (Peterson et al, 1998). Early goals of impact biomechanics and development of safety technology focused on decreasing mortality and head and thorax injuries to the extent that lower extremities are now the regions most likely to sustain injuries in frontal MVCs (Rupp & Schneider, 2004). These injuries are of substantial concern because they now account for up to 40% of treatment cost and nearly half of patients report significant long-term disability (Moran et al, 2002; MacKenzie et al, 2006).

Seat belts have had the single largest effect on reducing MVC-related mortality and injury, including extremity injury, decreasing fatalities by approximately 45-50% (Estrada et al, 2004; Cummins et al, 2008; Dihn-Zarr et al, 2001; McGwin et al, 2003). Seat belts increase deceleration time of the occupant via stretching of seat belt webbing and they distribute forces more uniformly on the body (Mackay, 1992; Peterson et al, 1998). There are multiple improvements in seatbelt technology that contribute to this effect. Pre-tensioners remove slack from the seatbelt upon detection of crash condition. Load limiters limits force imparted to the occupant by the seatbelt during the crash event by allowing the seatbelt webbing to yield when forces reach the set level. Web clamps lock the webbing to prevent or to minimize shoulder belt spool-out (Hinch et al, 2001).

Air bags are universally present in all new cars due to federal regulations, and it is well documented that they reduce risk of MVC-related mortality by 4-25% (Cummins et al, 2008; Dihn-Zarr et al, 2001; Estrada et al, 2004; McGwin et al, 2003). However, there is controversy regarding their effect on non-fatal injuries, particularly musculoskeletal injury. Air bag deployment without seat belt restraint is associated with increased incidence of lower extremity injury and some data suggests that air bag deployment together with seat belt restraint is also associated with increased incidence of lower extremity injury (Crandall et al, 1995; Cummins et al, 2008; Estrada et al, 2004; McGovern et al, 2000; Burgess et al, 1995; Chong et al, 2007). A possible contributing factor to the increased incidence of lower extremity injury is a "submarining" effect in which the pelvis and lower extremities are shifted under the airbag and down the seat into the knee bolster and floor of the car (Estrada et al, 2004; Crandall et al, 1998; Cummins et al, 2008). Lower extremity trauma leads to significant impairments in function, and may be the most frequent cause of permanent disability after motor vehicle collision (MacKenzie et al 1993; Sieple et al, 2001). Improvement in safety systems directed at preventing lower extremity injury will be critical in the future. There is now increased interest in "knee bolster airbags" which could reduce the negative impact of airbags on lower extremity injury and in "smart air bags". These would be able to accurately sense the crash pulse, deploy in a graded fashion depending on the occupant size and weight, and deploy only when truly necessary (Peterson et al, 1998).

5.6 Anterior Cruciate Ligament (ACL) tear

Nearly 75% of ACL injuries are non-contact and occur as a result of self-initiated movement usually during athletic activities. The mechanism of injury is based on the anatomy of the knee. The ACL is a fibrous connective tissue that attaches the posterior aspect of the femur to the anterior aspect of the tibia. It courses anteriorly, medially and distally as it runs from femur to tibia. The primary function of the ACL is to limit anterior translation of the tibia relative to the femur.

ACL injuries are usually associated with decelerating and changing direction; often ACL injuries are caused by an internal twisting of the tibia relative to the femur or combination of torque and compression during a landing (Meyer & Haut, 2008). Despite intense study of the ACL injury during the past three decades, the exact mechanism of injury is not known (Boden et al, 2009). ACL injury occurs when an excessive tension force is applied to the ACL (Yu & Garrett, 2007). It has also been noted that in 96% of ACL tears, an opposing player is within close proximity, which could cause an alteration in the players' coordination leading to dangerous leg positions (Boden et al, 2009). There is some controversy as to how this force occurs, but based on recent studies, it is likely that an axial compressive force acting on the posterior tibial slope contributes to many ACL tears. This axial force results in posterior displacement of the femoral condyle on the tibial plateau, which applies tension to the ACL (Boden et al, 2010; Boden et al, 2009; Meyer & Haut, 2008). Boden et al found that subjects who experienced an ACL tear initially came into contact with the ground with their hindfoot or with their foot flat (the "provocative" landing position), whereas control subjects landed on the forefoot. It appears that normally, during landing, the foot, ankle, knee and hip joints work to dampen ground reaction forces. However, when subjects come into contact with the ground with the hindfoot or with their foot flat, the foot, ankle, and calf muscles are not able to absorb ground reaction forces, and the leg is converted into a two-segment column (above and below the knee), and the knee ends up absorbing a large component of the loading force. Additionally, under normal circumstances, as the calf muscles contract during absorption of ground-reaction forces, they produce a flexion force on the knee, activating the normal knee absorption mechanics. In the absence of calf muscle contraction, the knee may abduct or internally rotate rather than flex (Boden et al, 2009). Additionally, higher hip flexion angle at landing places the torso farther posterior to the knee, requiring that the quadriceps muscle must be activating during landing. The quadriceps muscle force provides anterior shear force on the proximal tibia which increases ACL strain (Boden et al, 2009; Yu & Garrett, 2007). Knee abduction (or knee valgus) also may play a role, particularly in female athletes, by potentially reducing the compression force threshold needed to produce ACL injury (Boden et al, 2010). However, it may also be that valgus collapse is the result of the ACL being torn rather than a cause (Boden et al, 2010; Meyer & Haut, 2008).

6. Experimental methods for injury dynamics

Our understanding of the dynamics of injury has progressed as a result of biomechanical studies, which have evolved from cadaveric, and laboratory studies in which mechanical injury is artificially produced, to finite element analysis where it is modeled quantitatively. Obvious ethical considerations have made difficult the study of actual injuries as they occur in real trauma situations, but techniques using video analysis of live injuries obtained from video clips posted freely by individuals (such as YouTube) are now becoming increasingly available. YouTube and other video-sharing sites provide a means to study the mechanics of injury in real live situations, on living subjects undergoing true physiological loading.

Mechanical in vitro tests on cadaveric structures have been performed for over a century, and the resulting data are the foundation for our understanding of the biomechanics of injury. Physiologic loading is an interaction between anatomical geometry, material properties of bone and soft tissue, and complex loading conditions. In mechanical testing, investigators are able to isolate loading parameters and to examine each systematically, as well as apply actual complex physiologic loads to a specific sample. The only advantage of using cadaveric subjects is the ability to subject the cadaver to impact loads and energies believed to be representative of those occurring in real-life trauma. Cadaveric specimens have been used to evaluate basic biomechanical parameters like strength, elastic modulus, toughness, anisotropy, how these properties change, and how bone reacts to various loading parameters. However, the impact responses of a cadaver specimen may significantly differ from a living human due to lack of muscular tone and neuromuscular reflexes, which can generate substantial deforming forces or protective tensioning during a traumatic event. Post-mortem changes in skin and fat and changes in the passive properties of muscles spanning the joints due to rigor or other embalming processes or freezing can also affect experimental results in unrealistic ways. Also, preservation methods may induce tissue damage that could alter results, and long investigation times can induce changes in mechanical properties of cadaveric bone over the course of the study, particularly if the bones are fresh, stored in a freezer, and repeatedly refrozen and re-thawed. (Zdero & Bougherara, 2010; Robinovitch et al, 1997)

Investigation of dynamics of injury performed on living humans has also contributed to understanding of the biomechanics of injury. Unlike cadaveric studies, forces due to muscle contraction and reflexes are taken into account, as well as physiological soft tissue properties. Additionally real-life fall scenarios with their inherent complexity can be investigated. However, studies using living humans are limited because they can only be performed at safe loading levels. The effects of higher loads must be extrapolated from the results obtained with lower loading parameters, and it is difficult to prove that the extrapolation is accurate, particularly with regards to biological tissue which displays non-linear force-deflection and force-velocity properties. Additionally, study subjects are often young while the actual event under study is most common in the elderly with bones and soft tissue that have different material and geometric properties. Extrapolating from young subjects to older subjects may be more unpredictable than extrapolating from low loads to higher loads. Furthermore, unlike cadavers, it can be difficult to confirm that subjects were performing the experiment as instructed and often experimental falls are self-initiated rather than random, likely representing "best-case" falls. (Robinovitch et al, 1997; Robinovitch et al, 2000; Chiu & Robinovitch, 1998; Choi & Robinovitch, 2010; Liang & Robinovitch, 2010)

Finite element analysis (FEA) is an engineering tool that has been used extensively in the study of the biomechanics of injury. It can be utilized to investigate intricate structures subject to complex loads, including those that occur in true traumatic injury, and it can estimate, with accuracy, how an object (a whole bone or trabecular network) behaves when subject to external loads. The object of interest is represented as a collection of a finite number of elements. The investigator must specify the boundary conditions (applied loads and/or applied displacements) and material properties. In this era FEA geometry can be obtained from CT or MRI scans which are then converted into three-dimensional geometries. Investigators can examine various stress and strain distributions, material properties, and energy densities and failure properties. Finite element analysis can provide estimates of quantities that are commonly obtained through mechanical testing (like whole bone stiffness), as well as quantities that are difficult, if not impossible, to measure experimentally (like strain density distributions). The behavior of bone at both the material and structural levels can be investigated. This technique has been particularly useful for understanding and predicting fracture risk, especially in complex situations. Finite element analyses can be performed under conditions that are difficult to create experimentally. However, how well the finite element solution approximates the actual biomechanical phenomenon depends critically on the quality of the data used as input. Uncertainty in choice of material properties and boundary conditions can severely limit the value of the results. Early FEA assumed two-dimensional geometries and used homogenous, isotropic elastic properties. Advances in computer hardware, CT, and model design now permit the development of more representative geometries and material properties. Quality of data will continue to improve with the use of high-resolution CT scans of anatomy and the use of non-linear material properties for human tissue and other advances. Other problems in FEA include challenges inherent in simulating objects that also undergo biologic processes, such as osteolysis, bone resorption, growth, or remodeling. Ultimately, investigators must be mindful of the fact that computer models are only as good as the information entered and that FE simulations should be validated by actual biomechanical experimentation when possible. (Mackay, 1992; Zdero & Bougherara, 2010)

The above experimental methods, despite their disadvantages, have provided us with important data that have played a critical role in helping us to understand the biomechanics of injury. However, although they can be used to provide accurate data, they cannot provide information from actual injuries. Ultimately these experimental methods are simulations and have to be interpreted as such. Cadaveric, laboratory, and computer simulation studies have been useful because studying the actual biomechanics of injury is limited by the obvious ethical and practical problems associated with conducting injury studies at physiological loading levels in live participants. However, video analysis provides an excellent opportunity to analyze the mechanism of injury in living subjects under physiological loading conditions. This technique is gaining interest, and its use will likely increase due to improved access to videos via video sharing sites, like YouTube. Kwon et al used ankle fractures obtained from posted YouTube videos to create a database of live ankle fractures occurring during diverse activities (Kwon et al, 2010). They used this methodology to evaluate the validity of the Lauge-Hansen ankle fracture classification system, a system developed using cadaveric models in the early 1950's to describe ankle fractures mechanistically. The Lauge-Hansen system has been recently challenged by more modern cadaveric biomechanical study (Michelson) and an MRI imaging study (Gardner) revealing that the sequences of injures predicted from cadavers were not actually reproducible with modern techniques or visualized in the sequence described when MRIs were studied from true ankle fractures. YouTube searches generated videos of ankle trauma, and the individual posting the video was then offered participation in the study. Inclusion criteria required that the video demonstrated clear visualization of the mechanism of injury, that the subject sustained a fracture or dislocation, and that x-rays also revealed ankle fracture. Videos and radiographs were independently analyzed and categorized by mechanism of injury according the Launge-Hansen classification system. The radiographs and videos were then examined for consistency. The case series suggests that Launge-Hansens's mechanistic classification of radiographs does not correlate to the actual injury mechanism; the Lauge-Hansen system was only 58% overall accurate in predicting fracture patterns from the deforming injury mechanism. The classification system performed particularly poorly at predicting pronation external rotation type fracture patterns.

Other studies using video analysis to evaluate injury mechanism used athletic game footage. Giza et al evaluated game footage to determine the mechanism and weight-bearing status that placed soccer players at risk for foot and ankle injury (Giza et al, 2003). Kroshaug et al and Boden et al analyzed videos of athletic events to study the mechanism of ACL injury (Kroshaug et al, 2006; Boden et al, 2009). Andersen et al analyzed videos of game footage to describe injury mechanism for ankle injury in elite male football (soccer) (Andersen et al, 2004). There are disadvantages of this experimental methodology, which must be taken into account. Videos are collected as convenience samples, and therefore the camera angle is not always ideal for analysis, and clothing can make identifying anatomic landmarks difficult. Furthermore, it can be difficult to determine the exact moment at which the injury occurred; abnormal movements occurring after the injury could be confused for the mechanism of injury, as is clear from the controversy about abduction as either a cause or the result of ACL tear. The largest hurdle experienced by Kwon et al was their difficulty recruiting subjects from the internet-based video sharing site, YouTube.

7. Conclusion

Traumatic injuries in general, and fractures in particular, represent an important health concern and affect the majority of people at some point in their lives. There is an array of study techniques that take different approaches to studying the biomechanics of the musculoskeletal system, which have provided a basic understanding of bone properties and have helped to explore how they change with age. This has facilitated investigation of the mechanics of fracture and injury since the mechanical properties of the musculoskeletal system determine when and how structures will fail. In particular, the ability to study injury while it occurs under true physiologic loading conditions via video-sharing websites is an important tool that will likely continue to provide new insights into fracture mechanism. Strides have been made, based on this information, to develop means of decreasing or preventing injury. While a great deal is known about the biomechanics of injury and fracture healing, challenges remain, and areas of future study will be proposed.

8. References

Alexeeva L, Burkhardt P, Christiansen C, Cooper C, Delmas P, Johnell O, Johnson C, Kanis JA, Lips P, Melton LJ, Meunier P, Seeman E, Stepan J & Tosteson A. (1994).

Assessment of fracture risk and its application to screening for postmenopausal osteoporosis. WHO Technical Report Series. 843: 1-129.

Andersen TE, Floerenes TW, Arnason A, Bahr R. Video analysis of the mechanisms for ankle injuries in football. The American Journal of Sports Medicine; Jan 2004:32(1): 69S-79S

Arbabi S, Wahl WL, Hemmila MR< Kohoyda-Inglis C, Taheri PA & Wang SC. (2003). The cushion effect. Journal of Trauma. 54(6):1090-1093.

Arimoto HK, Forrester DM. (1980). Classification of ankle fractures: an algorithm. American Journal of Roentgenology. 135(5): 1057-63.

Armstrong DG, Newfield JT & Gillespie R. (1999). Orthopaedic management of osteopetrosis: results of a survey and review of the literature. Journal of Pediatric Orthopaedics. 19:122-132.

Bansal V, Conroy C, Lee J, Schwartz A, Tominaga G, Coimbra R. (2009). Is bigger better? The effect of obesity on pelvic fractures after side impact motor vehicle crashes. 67:709-714

Beck TJ, Looker AC, Ruff CB, Sievanen H & Wahner HW. (2000). Structural trends in the aging femoral neck and proximal shaft: analysis of the third national health and nutrition examination survey dual-energy X-ray absorptiometry data. Journal of Bone and Mineral Research. 15(12): 2297-2304.

Biffl W, Moore EE, Moore F & Peterson V. (1996). Interleukin-6 in the injured patient: marker of injury or mediator of inflammation? Annals of Surgery. 224(5): 647-664.

Black DM, Kelly MP, Genant HK, Palermo L, Eastell R, Bucci-Rechtweg C, Cauley J, Leung PC, Boonen S, Santora A, de Papp A, Bauer DC. (2010). Bisphosphonates and fractures of the subtrochanteric or diaphyseal femur. The New England Journal of Medicine. 363(19): 1761-71.

Boden BP, Sheehan FT, Torg JS & Hewett TE. (2010). Noncontact anterior cruciate ligament injuries: mechanisms and risk factors. Journal of the American Academy of Orthopaedic Surgery. 18:520-527.

Boden BP, Torg JS, Knowles SB & Hewett TE. (2009). Video analysis of anterior cruciate ligament injury: abnormalities in hip and ankle kinematics. American Journal of Sports Medicine. 37(2):252-259.

Bonaiuti D, 2004, Exercise for preventing and treating osteoporosis in postmenopausal women. Cochrane Database Syst Rev: issue 2

Bone LB & Giannoudis P. (2011). Femoral shaft fracture fixation and chest injury after polytrauma. The Journal of Bone and Joint Surgery Am. 93:311-317.

Bone LB, Johnson KD, Weigelt J & Scheinberg R. (1989) Early versus delayed stabilization of femoral fractures. A prospective randomized study. The Journal of Bone and Joint Surgery Am. 71:336-340.

Bonfield W. (1987). Advances in the fracture mechanics of cortical bone. Journal of Biomechanics. 20(11-12): 1071-1081.

Boulanger BR, Milzman D, Mitchel K & Rodriguez A. (1992). Body habitus as a predictor of injury pattern after blunt trauma. Journal of Trauma. 33(2): 228-232.

Bouxsein ML & Karasik D. (2006). Bone geometry and skeletal fragility. Current Osteoporosis Reports. 4:49-56.

Bouxsein ML & Jepsen KJ. (2003). Etiology and biomechanics of hip and vertebral fractures, In: Atlas of Osteoporosis. Eric Orwoll, 166-174. Current Medicine, ISBN 1-57340-198-6, Philadelphia, PA.

Bouxsein ML, Parker RA & Greenspan SL. (1999). Forearm bone mineral densitometry cannot be used to monitor response to alendronate therapy in postmenopausal women. Osteoporosis International. 10(6): 505-509.

Brockstedt H, Kassem M, Eriksen EF, Mosekilde L & Melsen F. (1993). Age- and sex-related changes in iliac cortical bone mass and remodeling. Bone. 14(4): 681-691.

Browner B, Jupiter J, Levine A & Trafton P. (2009). Skeletal Trauma: Basic Science, Management and Reconstruction (4th edition). Saunders, ISBN 978-1-4169-2220-6, Philadelphia, PA.

Bucholz RW, Heckman JD, Court-Brown CM & Tornetta P. (2005). Rockwood and Green's Fractures in Adults (6th edition). Lippincott Williams & Wilkins.

Burgess AR, Dischinger PC, O'Quinn TD & Schmidhauser CB. (1995). Lower extremity injuries in drivers of airbag-equipped automobiles: clinical and crash reconstruction correlations. Journal of Trauma. 39(4): 506-16.

Burr DB, Martin RB, Schaffler MB & Radin EL. (1985). Bone remodeling in response to in vivo fatigue microdamage. Journal of Biomechanics. 18(3):189-200

Canale ST. (2002). Campbell's Operative Orthopaedics (10th edition). Mosby, ISBN 978-0323012409. Philadelphia, PA.

Capeci CM & Tejwani NC. (2009). Bilateral low-energy simultaneous o sequential femoral fractures in patients on long-term Alendronate therapy. The Journal of Bone and Joint Surery Am. 91:2556-2561.

Carter DR, Beaupre GS, Giori NJ & Helms JA. (1998). Mechanobiology of skeletal regeneration. Clinical Orthopaedics and Related Research. 355S: S41-S55.

Carter DR, Blenman PR & Beaupre GS. (1988) Correlations between mechanical stress history and tissue differentiation in initial fracture healing. Journal of Orthopaedic Research. 6(5):736-748.

Chapuriat RD & Delmas PD. (2009). Bone microdamage: a clinical perspective. Osteoporosis International. 20:1299-1308.

Chavassioux P, Seeman E & Delmas PD. (2007). Insights into materials and structural basis of bone fragility from diseases associated with fractures: how determinants of the biomechanical properties of bone are compromised by disease. Endocrine Reviews. 28:151-164.

Chen JH, Liu C, YouL & Simmons CA. (2010). Boning up on Wolff's Law: mechanical regulation of the cells that make and maintain bone. Journal of Biomechanics. 43(1): 108-118.

Chiu J & Robinovitch SN. (1998). Prediction of upper extremity impact forces during falls on the outstretched hand. Journal of Biomechanics. 31:1169-1176.

Choi K, Kuhn JL, Ciarelli MJ & Goldstein SA. (1990). The elastic moduli of human subchondral, trabecularand cortical bone tissue and the size-dependency of cortical bone modulus. Journal of Biomechanics. 23(11): 1103-1113.

Choi WJ & Robinovitch SN. (2010). Pressure distribution over the palm region during forward falls on the outstretched hands. Journal of Biomechanics.

Chong M, Sochor M, Ipaktchi K, Brede C, Poster C & Wang S. (2007). The interaction of 'occupant factors' on the lower extremity fractures in frontal collision of motor vehicle crashes based on a level I trauma center. Journal of Trauma. 62(3): 720-729.
Ciarelli TE, Fyhrie DP, Schaffler MB & Goldstein SA. (2000). Variations in three-dimensional cancellous bone architecture of the proximal femur in female hip fractures and in controls. Journal of Bone and Mineral Research. 15(1):32-40
Clare MP. (2008). A rational approach to ankle fractures. Foot and Ankle Clinics. 13(4): 593-610.
Courtney AC, Wachtel EF, Myers ER & Hayes WC. (1994). Effects of loading rate on strength of the proximal femur. Calciied Tissue International. 55:53-58.
Crabtree NJ, Kroger H, Martin A, Pols HA, Lorenc R, Nijs J, Stepan JJ, Falch JA, Miazgowski T, Grazio S, Raptou P, Adams J, Collings A, Khaw T, Rushton N, Lunt M, Dixon AK & Reeve J. (2002). Improving risk assessment: hip geometry, bone mineral distribution and bone strength in hip fracture cases and controls. The EPOS study. European Prospective Osteoporosis Stuy. Osteoporosis International. 13(1): 48-54.
Crandall JR, Kuhlmann TP Pikley WD. (1995). Air and knee bolster restraint system: laboratory sled tests with human cadavers and the Hybrid III dummy. Journal of Trauma. 38(4): 517-20.
Crandall JR, Martin PG, Sieveka EM, Pikley WD, Dischinger PC, Burgess AR, O'Quinn TD & Schmidhauser CB. (1998). Lower limb response and injury in frontal crashes. Accident Analysis Prevention. 30(5):667-677.
Cummins JS, Koval KJ, Cantu RV & Spratt KF. (2008). Risk of injury associated with the use of seat belts and air bags in motor vehicle crashes. Bulletin of the NYU Hospital for Joint Diseases. 66(4):290-296.
Currey JD. (1988). The effect of porosity and mineral content on the Young's modulus of elasticity of compact bone. Journal of Biomechanics. 21(2): 131-139.
Currey, JD. (2002). Bones: Structure and Mechanics. Princeton University Press, ISBN 0-691-09096-3, Princeton, New Jersey 08540.
De Bakker PM, Mansek SL, Ebacher V, Oxland TR, Cripton PA & Guy P. (2009). During sideways falls proximal femur fractures initiate in the superolateral cortex: evidence from high-speed video of simulated fractures. Journal of Biomechanics. 42: 1917-1925.
DeGoede KM & Ashton-Miler JA. (2002). Fall arrest strategy affects peak hand impact force in a forward fall. Journal of Biomechanics. 35: 843-848.
Degoede KM, Ashton-Miller JA & Schultz AB. (2003). Fall-related upper body injuries in the older adult: a review of the biomechanical issues. Journal of Biomechanics. 36: 1043-1053.
Diegelmann RF & Evans MC. (2004). Wound healing: an overview of acute, fibrotic and delayed healing. Frontiers in Bioscience. 9:283-289.
Dihn-Zarr B, Sleet DA, Shults RA, Zaza S, Elder RW, Nichols JL, Thompson RS & Sosin DM. (2001). Reviews of evidence regarding interventions to increase the use of safety belts. American Journal of Preventative Medicine. 21(4S):48-65.
Dischinger PC, Kerns TJ & Kufera JA. (1995). Lower extremity fractures in motor vehicle collisions: the role of driver gender and height. Accident, Analysis and Prevention. 27(4): 601-606.

Dischinger PC, Siegel JH, Ho SM & Kufera JA. (1998). Effect of change in velocity on the development of medical complications in patients with multisystem trauma sustained in vehicular crashes. Accident, Analysis and Prevention. 30(6): 831-837.

Dong XN & Guo XE. (2004). The dependence of transversely isotropic elasticity of human femoral cortical bone on porosity. Journal of Biomechanics. 37:1281-1287.

Estrada LS, Alonso JE, McGwin G, Metzger J & Rue LW. (2004). Restraint use and lower extremity fractures in frontal motor vehicle collisions. The Journal of Trauma. 57(2):323-328.

Finkelstein EA, Corso PS & Miller TR. (2006). Incidence and Economic Burden of Injuries in the United States. Oxford University Press, ISBN 019517948X, New York.

Giannoudis PV, Giannoudi M & Stavlas P. (2009). Damage control orthopaedics: lessons learned. Injury. 40S4: S47-S52.

Giza E, Fuller C, Jung A & Dvorak J. (2003). Mechanisms of foot and ankle injuries in soccer. American Journal of Sports Medicine. 31(4): 550-554.

Glusti A, Hamdy NAT & Papapoulos SE. (2010). Atypical fractures of the femur and bisphosphonate therapy A systematic review of case/case series studies. Bone. 47:169-180.

Golden RD & Rodiriguez EK. (2010) Management of bilateral subtrochanteric femur fractures with internal fixation and rhBMP-7 in a patient with osteopetrosis. Journal of Medical Case Reports.

Hamilton BH & Best TM. (2011). Platelet-enriched plasma and muscle strain injuries: challenges imposed by the burden of proof. Clinical Journal of Sports Medicine. 21:31-36.

Hardwood PJ, Giannoudis PV, Criensven M, Krettek C & Pape H. (2005). Alterations in the systemic inflammatory response after early total care and damage control procedures for femoral shaft fracture in severely injured patients. The Journal of Trauma. 58:446-454.

Hauser CJ, Sursal T, Rodriguez EK, Appleton PT, Zhang Q & Itagaki K. (2010). Mitochondrial damage associated molecular patterns from femoral reamings activate neutrophils through formyl peptide receptors and P44/42 MAP Kinase. Journal of Orthopaedic Trauma. 24:534-538.

Hinch J, Hollowell WT, Kanianthra J, Evans WD, Klein T, Longthorne A, Ratchford S, Morris J & Subramanian R. (2001). Air Bag Technology in Light Passenger Vehicles. National Highway Traffic Safety Administration. June 27, 2001.

Huelke DF. (1982). Lower extremity injuries in automobile crashes. Accident Analysis and Prevention. 14(2): 95-106.

Hughes JM & Petit MA. (2010). Biological underpinnings of Frost's mechanostat thresholds: the important role of osteocytes. Journal of Musculoskeletal Neuronal Interaction. 10(2): 128-135.

Huiskes R. (2000). If bone is the answer, then what is the question? Journal of Anatomy. 197: 145-156.

Isaksson H, Wilson W, van Donkelaar CC, Huiskes R & Ito K. (2006). Journal of Biomechanics. 39:1507-1516.

Korpelainen R, Keinanen-Kiukaanniemi S, Keikkinen J, Vaananen K & Korpelainen. (2006). Effect of impact exercise on bone mineral density in elderly women with low BMD:

a population-based randomized controlled 30-month intervention. Osteoporosis International. 17:109-118.

Koval KJ & Zuckerman JD. (1994). Hip fractures: overview and evaluation and treatment of femoral neck fractures. Journal of the American Academy of Orthopaedic Surgery. 2:141-149.

Kreider JM & Goldstein SA. (2009). Trabecular bone mechanical properties in patients with fragility fractures. Clinical Orthopaedics and Related Research. 467:1955-1963.

Krosshaug T, Nakamae A, Boden BP, Engebretsen L, Smith G, Slauterbeck JR, Hewett TE & Bahr R. (2006). Mechanisms of anterior cruciate ligament injury in basketball: video analysis of 39 cases. The American Journal of Sports Medicine. 35: 359-367.

Kumar V, Abbas AK, Fausto N & Aster J. (2009). Robbins & Cotran Pathologic Basis of Disease (8th edition), Saunders, 1416031219, Philadelphia, PA.

Kwon JY, Chacko AT, Kadzielski JJ, Appleton PT & Rodriguez EK. (2010). Journal of Orthopaedic Trauma. 24: 499-482.

Laing AC, Tootoonchi I, Hulme PA & Robinovitch SN. (2006). Effect of compliant flooring on impact force during falls on the hip. Journal of Orthopaedic Research. 24:1405-1411.

Lenart BA, Neviaser AS, Lyman S, Chang CC, Edobor-Osula F, Steele B, van der Meulen MCH, Lorich DG & Lane JM. (2009). Osteoporosis International. 20:1353-1362.

Leslie WD, Pahlavan PS, Tsang JF & Lix LM. (2009). Prediction of hip and other osteoporotic fractures from hip geometry in a large clinical cohort. Osteoporosis International. 20(10): 1767-1774.

Liang AC & Robinovitch SN (2010). Characterizing the effective stiffness of the pelvis during sideways falls on the hip. Journal of Biomechanics. 43:1898-1904.

Linnau KF, Blackmore CC, Kaufman R, Nguyen TN, Routt ML, Stambaugh LE, Jurkovich GJ & Mock CN. (2007). Do initial radiographs agree with crash site mechanism of injury in pelvic ring disruptions? A pilot study. Journal of Orthopaedic Trauma. 21: 375-380.

Lotz JC, Cheal EJ & Hayes WC. (1995). Stress distributions within the proximal femur during gait and falls: implications for osteoporotic fracture. Osteoporosis International. 5: 252-261.\

Mackay M. (1992). Mechanisms of injury and biomechanics: vehicle design and crash performance. World Journal of Surgery. 16:420-427.

MacKenzie EJ, Bosse MJ, Kellam JF, Pollak, AN, Webb WX, Swiontkowski MF, Smith DG, Sanders RW, Jones AL, Starr AJ, McAndrew MP, Patterson BM, Burgess AR, Travison T & Castillo RC. (2006). Early predictors of long-term work disability after major limb trauma. Journal of Trauma. 61:688-694.

MacKenzie EJ, Cushing BM, Jurkovich GI, Morris JA, Burgess AR, deLatueur BJ, McAndrew MP & Swiontkowski MF. (1993). Physical impairment and functional outcomes six months after severe lower extremity fractures. Journal of Trauma. 34: 528-539.

McCreadie BR & Goldstein SA. (2000). Biomechanics of fracture: is bone mineral density sufficient to assess risk? Journal of Bone and Mineral Research. 15(12): 2305-2308.

McGovern MK, Murphy RX, Okunski WJ & Wasser TE. (2000). The influence of air bags and restraining devices on extremity injuries in motor vehicle collisions. 44(5): 481-485.

McGwin G, Metzger J, Alonso JE & Rue LW. (2003). The association between occupant restraint systems and risk of injury in frontal motor vehicle collisions. The Journal of Trauma. 54:1182-1187.

Mei-Dan O, Mann G & Maffulli N. (2010). Platelet-rich plasma: any substance into it? British Journal of Sports Medicine. 44(9) 618-619.

Meyer EG & Haut RC. (2008). Anterior cruciate ligament injury induced by internal tibial torsion or tibiofemoral compression. Journal of Biomechanics. 41: 3377-3383.

Moran SG, McGwin G, Metzger JS, Alonso JE & Rue LW. (2002). Relationship between age and lower extremity fractures in frontal motor vehicle collisions. Journal of Trauma. 54:261-265.

Morgan EF, Byraktar HH & Keaveny TM. (2003). Trabecular bone modulus-density relationship depend on anatomic site. Journal of Biomechanics. 36(7): 897-904.

Mori S, Burr DB. (1993). Increased intracortical remodeling following fatigue damage. Bone. 14(2): 103-109.

Mubarak SJ, Kim JR, Edmonds EW, Pring ME & Bastrom TP. (2009). Classification of proximal tibial fractures in children. Journal of Child ORthopaedics. 3(3): 191-197.

Nara-Ashizawa N, Liu LJ, Tokuyama HK, Hayashi K, Shirasaki Y, Amagai H & Saitoh S. (2002). Paradoxical adaptation of mature radius to unilateral use of tennis playing. Bone. 30(4): 619-623.

Nieves JW & Cosman F. (2010). Atypical subtrochanteric and femoral shaft fractures and possible association with bisphopshonates. Current Osteoporosis Reports. 8:34-39.

Nikander R, Sievanen H, Heinonen A, Daly RM, Kirsti UR & Kaunnus P. (2010). Targeted exercise against osteoprosis: a systematic review and meta-analysis for optimizing bone strength throughout life. BMC Medicine. 8:47

Nordhoff L. (2004). Motor Vehicle Collision Injuries (2nd edition). Jones & Bartlett Learning. ISBN 978-0763733353. Mississauga, ON.

Nyman JS, Roy A, Shen X, Acuna RL, Tyler JH & Wang X. The influence of water removal on the strength and toughness of cortical bone. Journal of Biomechanics. 39(5): 931-938.

O'Toole RV, O'Brient M, Scalea TM, Habashi N, Pollak AN & Turen CH. (2005). Resuscitation before stabilization of femoral fractures limits acute respiratory distress syndrome in patients with multiple traumatic injuries despite low use of damage control orthopedics. Journal of Trauma. 67: 1013-1021.

Olson SA. Pulmonary aspects of treatment of long bone fractures in the polytrauma patient. Clin Orthop Relat Res. 2004;422:66 -70.

Pape HC, Grimme K, Van Griensven M, Scott AH, Giannoudis P, Morley J, Roise O, Ellingsen E, Hildebrand F, Wiese B & Krettek C. (2003). Impact of intramedullary instrumentation versus damage control for femoral fractures on immunoinflammatory parameters: prospective randomized analysis by the EPOFF study group. Journal of Trauma. 55(1): 7-13.

Pape HC, Rixen D, Morley J, Husebye EE, Mueller M, Dumont C, Gruner A, Oestern HJ, Bayeff-Filoff M, Garving C, Pardini D, van Griensven M, Krettek C & Giannoudis P. Impact of the method of internal stabilization for femoral shaft fractures in patients with multiple injuries at risk for complications (borderline patients). (2007). Annals of Surgery. 246(3): 491-499.

Pape HC, Tornetta P, Tarkin I, Tziopis C, Sabeson V & Olson SA. (2009). Journal of the American Academy of Orthopaedic Surgery. 17: 541-549.

Pape HC, Tsukamoto T & Kobbe P. (2007). Assessment of the clinical course with inflammatory parameters. Injury. 38: 1358-1364

Pape HC, van Griensven M, Scott AH, Giannoudis P, Morley J, Roise O, Ellingsen E, Hildebrand F, Wiese B & Krettek C. (2003). Journal of Trauma. 55: 7-13.

Park SK, Stefanyshyn DJ, Ramage B, Hart DA & Ronsky JL. (2009). Alterations in knee joint laxity during the menstrual cycle in healthy women leads to increases in joint laods during selected athletic movements. The American Journal of Sports Medicine. 37: 1169-1177.

Parkkari J, Kannus P, Pavanen M, Natri A, Vainio J, Aho H, Vuori I & Jarvinen M. (1999). Calcified Tissue International. 65: 183-187.

Patron MS, Duthie RA & Sutherland AG. (2006). Proximal femoral geometry and hip fractures. Acta Orthopaedica Belgium. 72(1): 51-5.

Perren SM. (1979). Physiological and biological aspects of fracture healing with special reference to internal fixation. 138: 175-196.

Perren SM. (2002). Evolution of the internal fixation of long bone fractures. The Journal of Bone and Joint Surgery Br. 84B: 1093-1110.

Peterson TD, Jolly BT, Runge JW & Hunt RC. (1998). Motor vehicle safety: current concepts and challenges for emergency physicians. Annals of Emergency Medicine. 34: 394-393.

Petterlik H, Roschger P, Klaushofer K & Fratzl P. (2006). From brittle to ductile fracture of bone. Nature Materials. 5(1): 52-55.

Prendergast PJ, Huiskes R & Soballe K. (1997). Biophysical stimuli on cells during tissue differentiation at implant interfaces. 30(6): 539-548.

Reikeras O. (2010). Immune depression in musculoskeletal trauma. Inflammation Research. 59: 409-414.

Rho JY, Tsui TY & Pharr GM. (1997). Elastic properties of human cortical and trabecular lamellar bone measured by nanoindentation. Biomaterials. 18(20): 1325-1330.

Rizzoli R, Akesson K, Bouxsein M. Kanis JA, Napoli N, Papapoulos S, Reginster JY & Cooper C. (2010). Subtronchanteric fractures after long-term treatment with bisphosphonates: a European society on clinical and economic aspects of osteoprosis and osteoarthritis, and international osteoporosis foundation working group report. Osteoporosis International. 22(2): 373-390.

Robinovitch SN & Chiu J. (1998). Surface stiffness affects impact force during a fall on the outstretched hand. Journal of Orthopaedic Research. 16(3): 309-313.

Robinovitch SN, Chiu J, Sandler R & Liu Q. (2000). Impact severity in self-initiated sits and falls associates with center-of-gravity excursion during descent. Journal of Biomechanics. 33:863-870.

Robinovitch SN, Hayes WC & McMahon TA. (1997). Distribution of contact force during impact to the hip. Annals of Biomedical Engineering. 25: 499-508.

Robinovitch SN, McMahon TA & Hayes WC. (1995). Force attenuation in trochanteric soft tissues during impact from a fall. Journal of Orthopaedic Research. 13(6): 956-62.

Robinovitch SN, Normandin SC, Stotz P & Maurer JD. (2005). Time requirement for young and elderly women to move into a position for breaking a fall with outstretched hands. Journal of Gerontology A Biological Sciences and Medical Sciences. 60(12):1553-1557.

Ruppel ME, Miller LM & Burr DB. (2008). The effect of the microscopic and nanoscale structure on bone fragility. Osteoporosis International. 19: 1251-1265.

Sanchez M, Anitua E, Orive G, Mujika I & Andia I. (2009). Platelet-rich therapies in the treatment of orthopaedic sports injuries. Sports Medicine. 39(5): 345-354.

Scalea TM, Boswell SA, Scott JD, Mitchell KA, Kramer ME & Pollak AN. (2000). External fixation as a bridge to intramedullary nailing for patients with multiple injuries and with femur fractures: damage control orthopaedics. The Journal of Trauma. 48(4): 613-623.

Schaffler MD & Burr DB. (1988). Stiffness of compact bone: effects of porosity and density. Journal of Biomechanics. 21(1): 13-16.

Schroeder JE, Weiss YG & Mosheiff R. (2009). The current state in the evaluation and treatment of ARDS and SIRS. Injury. 40S4: S82-S89.

Sears BW, Strover MD & Callaci J. (2009). Pathoanatomy and clinical correlates of the immunoinflamatory response following orthopaedic trauma. Journal of the American Academy of Orthopaedic Surgery. 17(4): 255-265.

Seeman E & Delmas P. (2006). Bone quality—the material and structural basis of bone strength and fragility. The New England Journal of Medicine. 354: 2250-2261.

Seeman E. (2003). The structural and biomechanical basis of the gain and loss of bone strength in women and men. Endocrinology and Metabolism Clinics of North America. 32:25-38.

Seibel R, LaDuca J, Hassett JM, Babaikian G, Mills B, Border DO & Border JR. (1985). Blunt multiple trama, femur traction and the pulmonary failure-septic state. Annals of Surgery. 202(3): 283-295.

Seipel RC, Pintar FA, Yogananda N & Boynton MD. (2001). Biomechanics of calcaneal fractures: A model for the motor vehicle. Clinical Orthopaedics and Related Research. 388:218-224.

Siegel JH, Loo G, Dischinger PC, Burgess AR, Wang SC, Schneider LW, Grossman D, Rivara F, Mock C, Natarajan GA, Hutchins KD, Bents FD, McCammon L, Leibovich E & Tenenbaum N. (2001). Factors influencing the patterns of injuries and outcomes in car versus car crashes compared to sport utility, van or pick-up truck versus car crashes: crash injury research engineering network study. The Journal of Trauma. 51:975-990.

Silva MJ. (2007). Biomechanics of osteoporotic fractures. Injury. 3853: 569-576.

Singer FR. (2011). Metabolic bone disease: atypical femoral fractures. Journal of Biomechanics. 44: 244-247.

Smith C, Kruger MJ, Smith RM & Myburgh KH. (2008). The inflammatory response to skeletal muscle injury. Sports Medicine. 38(11): 947-969.

Tolar J, Teitelbaum SL & Orchard PJ. (2004). Osteoporosis. The New England Journal of Medicine. 351:2939-49.

Turner CH, Rho J, Takano Y, Tsui TY & Pharr GM. (1999). Journal of Biomechanics. 32(4): 437-441.

Ulstrup AK. (2008). Biomechanical concepts of fracture healing in weight-bearing long bones. Acta Orthopaedica Belgium. 74(3): 291-302.

Vestergaard P, Schwartz F, Rejnmark L & Mosekilde L. (2011). Risk of femoral shaft and subtrochanteric fractures among users of bisphosphonates and raloxifene. Oseoporosis International. 22: 993-1001.

Weninger P, Figi M, Spitaler R, Mauritz W & Hertz H. (2007). Early undreamed intremdullary nailing of femoral fractures is safe in patients with severe thoracic trauma. Journal of Trauam. 62(3): 629-696.

Wolff J. 1986. The law of bone remodeling [translated from the 1892 original, Das Gesetz der Transformation der Knochen, by P. Maquet and R. Furlong]. Berlin: Springer Verlag.

World Health Organization, Assessment of fracture risk and its application to screening for postmenopausal osteoporosis, 1994

Xiaodu W & Puram S. (2003). The toughness of cortical bone and its relationship with age. Annals of Biomedical Engineering. 32(1): 123-135.

Yu B & Garrett WE. (2007). Mechanisms of non-contact ACL injuries. British Journal of Sports Medicine. 41(Supp 1):i47-i51.

Zdero R & Bougherara H. (2010). Orthopaedic biomechanics: a practical approach to combining mechanical testing and finite element analysis, In: Finite Element Analysis. David Moratal, 171-194. InTech. http://www.intechopen.com/articles/show/title/orthopaedic-biomechanics-a-practical-approach-to-combining-mechanical-testing-and-finite-element-ana.

Zhang Q, Raoof M, Chen Y, Sumi Y, Sursal T, Junger W, Brohi K, Itagaki K & Hauser CJ. (2010). Circulating mitochondrial DAMPs cause inflammatory responses to injury. Nature. 464(7285): 104-107.

2

Assessment of Maxillary Distraction Forces in Cleft Lip and Palate Patients

Eduardo Yugo Suzuki and Boonsiva Suzuki
Faculty of Dentistry,
Chiang Mai University
Thailand

1. Introduction

Distraction osteogenesis is a process that depends on biomechanics, where the application of progressive traction forces leads to bone lengthening by gradual new bone formation. (Illizarov, 1989a, 1989b) Consequently, stretching of surrounding soft tissues occurs at different tissue depths, allowing correction of severe skeletal dysplasias in short periods of time. However, biomechanical data from the craniofacial distraction osteogenesis process is limited and the mechanical and biological nature of the traction forces involved is not fully understood (Gardner et al., 1997).

Assessment of distraction forces within the structure being distracted may provide current information about the mechanical response and therefore conditions in the distracted structure, including, premature consolidation, device failure, or the existence of incomplete osteotomies (Aarnes et al., 1994, Younger et al., 1994). This assessment may further lead to improved understanding of the nature and biology of distraction, and help determine optimum rates and rhythms (Samchukov, 1998).

Studies have been published on forces during distraction of the tibia and femur using instrumented external fixators in conjunction with micrometers or goniometers (Evans et al., 1988, Richardson et al., 1994, Aronson et al., 1994). Similar studies have been performed in animals (Gardner, 1998). However, the results obtained by these authors are extremely controversial. The great variability of distraction devices, complexity of methodology employed, site of distraction force application, and anatomical structure seem to dictate great influence.

In the craniofacial area, only few studies have examined the distraction forces required to lengthen the mandible during distraction, even though measurements were performed indirectly through the measurement of torque necessary to perform the activation of the distractor (Robinson et al., 2001, Burstain et al. 2008).

Recently, the authors have developed a simple mechanism to measure and adjust maxillary distraction forces during maxillary advancement (Suzuki & Suzuki, 2010). The mechanism was developed in order to allow direct assessment of distraction forces.

Therefore, the purpose of the present study is to monitor the distraction forces applied through maxillary distraction osteogenesis in cleft lip and palate patients with this simple mechamism.

2.1 Materials and methods

This clinical study was carried out on patients who underwent maxillary distraction osteogenesis through the use of the rigid external distraction (RED) device combined with a Twin-Track distractor in an attempt to optimize the distraction process and improve patient comfort during maxillary advancement. A simple mechanism to monitor the tension force on the traction wire was designed to obtain data, analyzing the behavior applied through maxillary distraction osteogenesis by means of a force gauge.

Twenty patients with a variety of dento-alveolar clefts and one non-cleft (asymmetric) patients that were selected for treatment by maxillary distraction osteogenesis were asked to take part in the study. Criteria for selection were based on the presence of a severe maxillary hypoplasia. There were 10 unilateral cleft lip and/or palate (UCLP) patients, 8 bilateral cleft lip and palate (BCLP) patients, and 2 non-cleft patients (Table 1). Maxillary advancement was performed at the mean age of 21.8 years (subjects ranged from 15.2 to 24.8 years of age). In none of these patients had alveolar bone grafting been previously performed.

			Distraction Protocol			Maximum
Case	Cleft Type	Age	Latency (days)	Activation (days)	Advancement (mm)	Force (N)
1	UCLP	15.6	5	10	16.0	35.6
2	UCLP	17.2	6	11	16.5	36.2
3	UCLP	22.6	5	9	14.6	35.0
4	UCLP	18.8	5	11	16.5	41.5
5	UCLP	19.2	5	10	15.6	42.0
6	UCLP	23.5	4	12	17.3	45.0
7	UCLP	18.6	4	13	21.2	46.0
8	UCLP	22.3	6	11	19.5	42.0
9	UCLP	26.0	6	10	18.6	40.0
10	UCLP	21.2	4	9	20.0	43.0
11	BCLP	23.4	5	11	13.0	29.0
12	BCLP	24.3	5	10	12.5	26.0
13	BCLP	21.6	5	9	12.6	24.3
14	BCLP	22.3	4	12	12.0	21.3
15	BCLP	24.2	4	14	11.3	24.0
16	BCLP	22.2	4	14	16.0	28.6
17	BCLP	25.3	4	16	15.0	27.0
18	BCLP	19.6	6	12	13.0	21.2
19	Non-Cleft	22.3	6	14	18.0	45.8
20	Non-Cleft	25.6	6	15	15.0	39.5
	Mean	**21.8**	**5.0**	**11.7**	**15.7**	**34.7**
	SD	2.8	0.8	2.1	2.8	8.7

Table 1. Patient characteristics and distraction protocol

All patients underwent a thorough history and clinical examination as well as complete dental and orthodontic examination. Clinical photographs, dental casts, lateral and postero-anterior cephalograms, panoramic radiographs, and three-dimensional computed tomography were taken preoperatively. Further lateral cephalograms were obtained after the latency period, during the distraction period, after completion of the active period of distraction, and at the completion of the consolidation period. The amount of distraction osteogenesis, the progression of osteogenesis and remodeling, and any relapse were evaluated on the radiographs.

2.1.1 Simple mechanism to measure distraction forces

A simple mechanism to measure and adjust the maxillary distraction forces was specially designed and assembled to the RED device in order to allow direct measurement of tension force during maxillary distraction osteogenesis (Figure 1). The mechanism was developed based on principles used in the US space programme and described by Iacomini in 1998. Iacomini proposed a simple mechanism to anchor and adjust tension force on cables in order to suspend a structure for thermal isolation. Unlike turnbuckles and other conventional cable-tensioning mechanisms, this mechanism facilitates direct measurement of the tension in the cable. Structural modification of Iacomini's method was performed in order to allow clinical assessment of the traction forces applied during the maxillary distraction osteogenesis. The near end of the cable was threaded through the mechanism and tied off in a loop at the crimp stopper. The tension was measured directly by simply pulling on the cable with an attached force gauge and reading the measurement when the stopper was unseated.

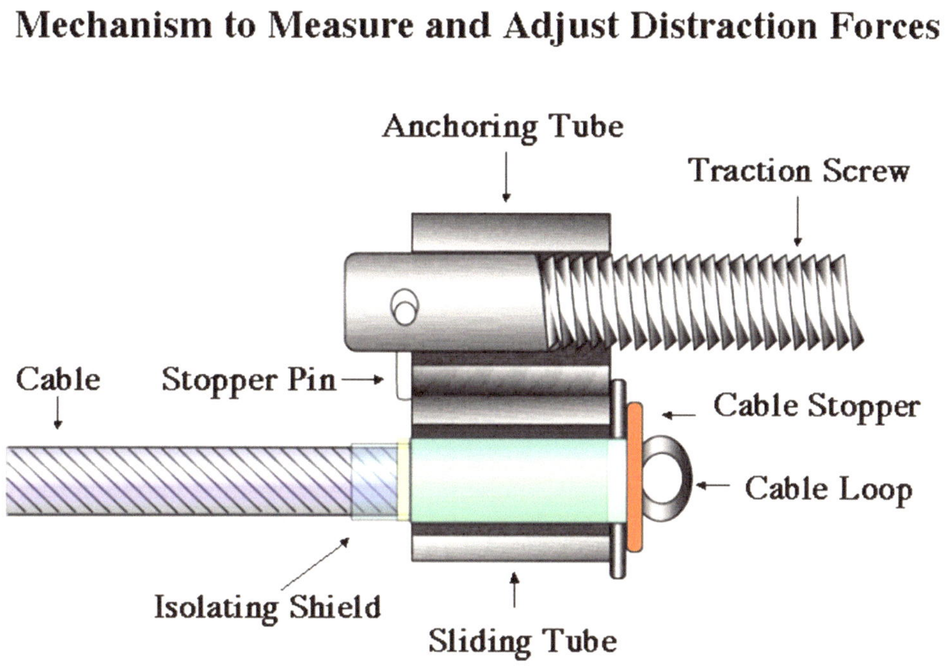

Fig. 1. Simple mechanism to measure and adjust distraction forces

2.1.2 Distraction protocol

2.1.2.1 Measurement

Maxillary distraction osteogenesis was performed after a complete Le Fort I osteotomy, under general anesthesia with orotracheal intubation, using an external distraction device (RED system, Martin L. P., Jacksonville, FL, USA) in combination with a Twin-track (Suzuki et al., 2006) and removable intraoral splint (Suzuki et al., 2006) for anchorage of distraction forces (Figure 2). A latency period of 4 to 6 days was preserved before initiating the distraction.

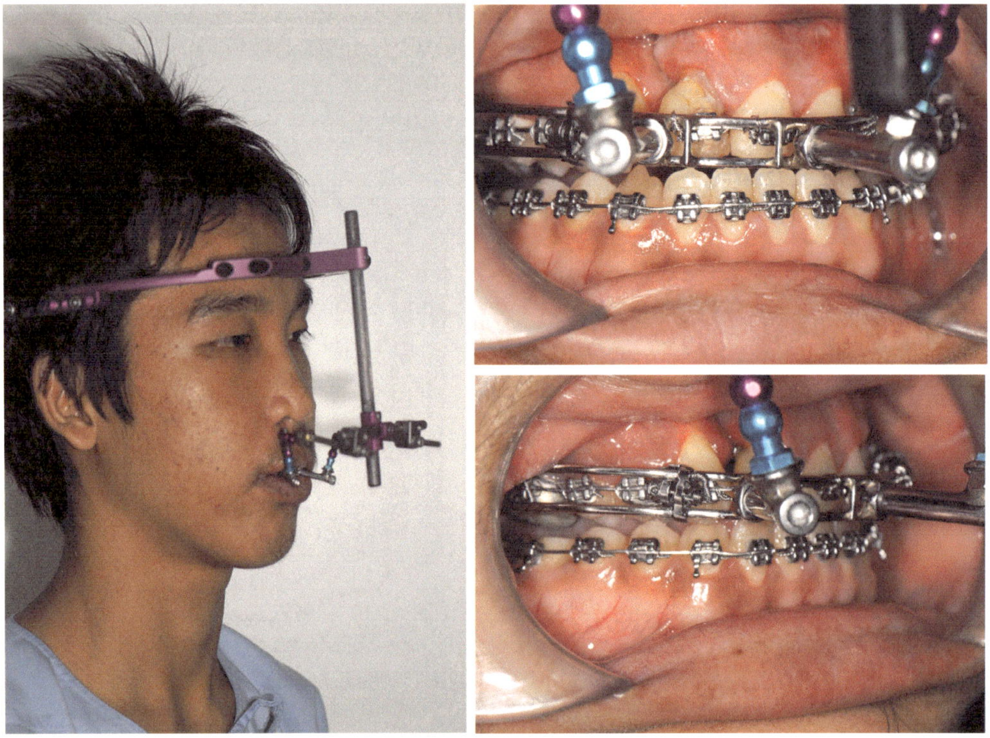

Fig. 2. RED system in combination with a Twin-Track distraction device.

The simple mechanism was connected bilaterally to the traction screws of a RED system in order to permit the assessment of distraction forces (Figure 3). In all cases, the maxilla was advanced parallel to the functional occlusal plane. The traction micro-cables replaced the conventional surgical wires in order to optimize the transference of traction forces to the maxillary bone, thereby avoiding the distortion that was observed in the traction wires.

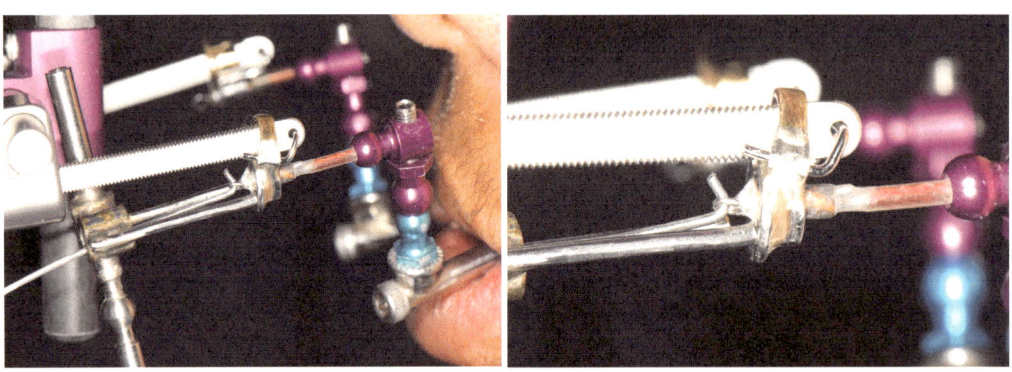

Fig. 3. The simple mechanism is connected bilaterally to the traction screws of a RED system in order to permit distraction force measurement.

Distraction force can be measured directly by simply pulling on the cable loop. An electronic light sensor was developed to identify the minimum distance necessary to unseat the stopper. Distraction force equals the measurement force that is just sufficient to unseat the stopper (Figure 4).

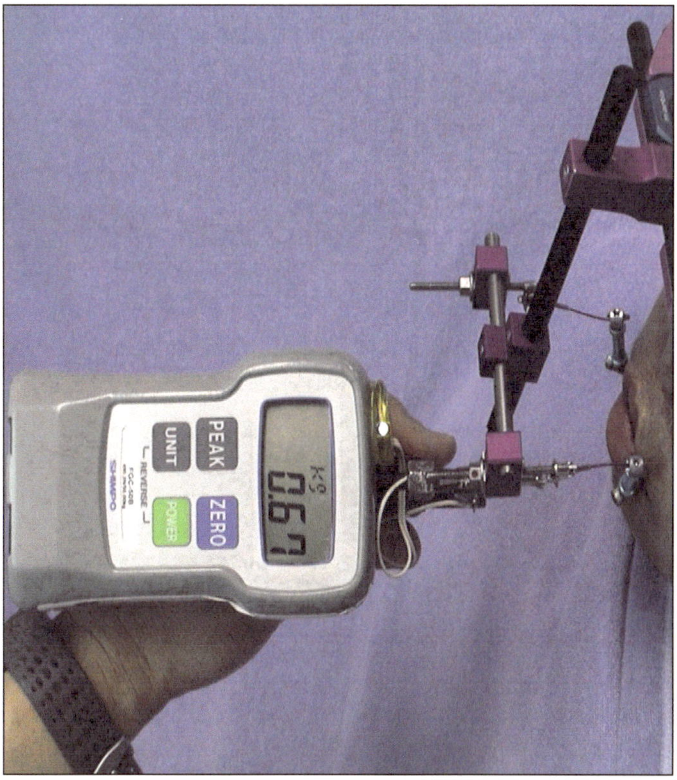

Fig. 4. A light sensor was developed to identify the minimum distance necessary to unseat the stopper

Distraction was performed at the rate of 1.0 mm/day in two increments, preserving a 12-hour interval between activations. Measurements were carried out before and after activation using a digital force gauge (Shimpo FGS-50S, Nidec-Shimpo America Corporation) during the distraction and consolidation periods. The amount of force being applied was monitored every day before the distraction was carried out. The duration of the maxillary distraction period was determined clinically and cephalometrically by the severity of the midface retrusion and anterior dental cross-bite. All patients remained in the hospital during the distraction period. Activation and distraction force measurements were performed by the same orthodontist (EYS). The patients were followed-up daily to assess progression of distraction until the proper overjet, overbite, and relatively stable occlusion were achieved. The device was maintained for three weeks for rigid retention after activation was completed. After this period, the patient was returned to the clinic for removal of the cranial portion of the RED device with a small amount of local anesthetic at the scalp pin sites. An additional 4 to 6 weeks of retention using facial mask elastics at night-time only was utilized.

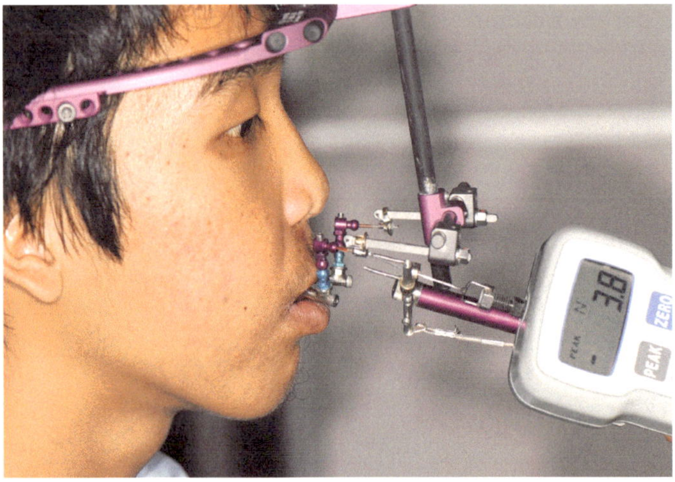

Fig. 5. Direct assessment of distraction forces in a patient. There were no complications, such as pain, discomfort, or procedural delays in measuring and adjusting the distraction forces.

3. Results

Distraction forces were monitored from the fourth to the sixth day following surgery. The typical patterns of the force registered immediately before and after distraction are shown in Figures 6 to 9. Forces recorded before and after each lengthening showed a progressive increase of distraction forces. Each distraction step resulted in an immediate increase in load followed by gradual but incomplete relaxation. As advancement progressed, distraction forces increased; on the other hand, the amount of maxillary movement decreased. Figures 6 to 9.

After distraction was discontinued the force decayed slowly and progressively. The amount of movement observed was inversely proportional to the increase of forces. Pain and discomfort were reported with high forces. In all patients, the intended amount of distraction was achieved. Figures 10 to 12.

The average maximum force applied throughout the distraction period was 34.7N (range 21.2 to 46.0N) with increments after activation averaging 6.7N (range 3.4 to 11.7 N). A significant correlation (0.738) was observed between the maximum forces and the amount of maxillary advancement.

In the UCLP patients, differential pattern of forces between the lateral segments were clearly observed. Distraction forces on the larger segment were aproximately 70% higher than on the lesser segment. The typical pattern of the force registered immediately before and after distraction in a UCLP patient is illustrated in the Figure 6.

The forces measured in both larger and lesser segments showed a cycle of instantaneous load increase after each distraction followed by a varying degree of stress relaxation. In both segments, the amount of movement observed was inversely proportional to the increase of forces.

The differential pattern of forces between segments (larger and lesser) was not observed in the BCLP patients. Figure 7 shows the typical pattern of the force registered immediately before and after distraction in a BCLP patient. As in UCLP patient, the forces measured in both segments showed a cycle of instantaneous load increase after each distraction followed by a varying degree of stress relaxation. In both segments, the amount of movement observed was inversely proportional to the increase of forces.

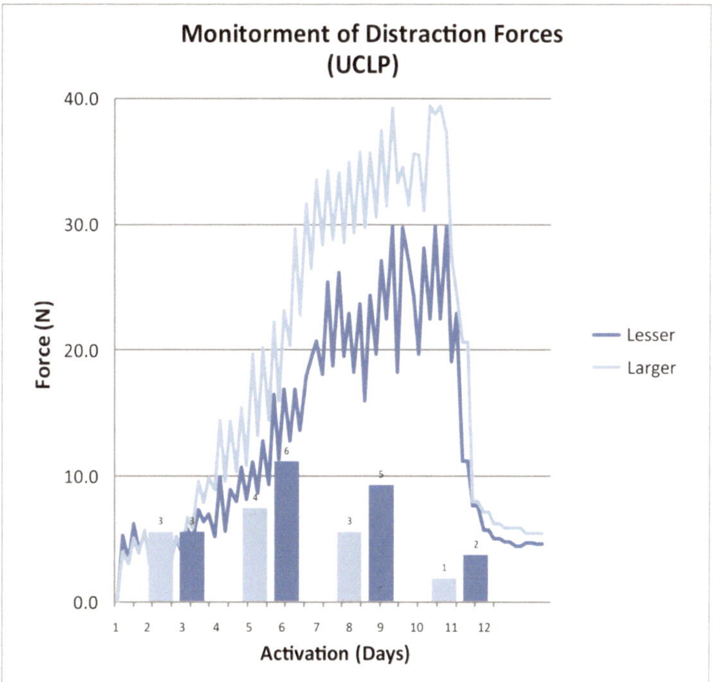

Fig. 6. Typical pattern of distraction forces observed in UCLP patients. As advancement progressed, distraction forces increased; on the other hand, the amount of maxillary movement decreased.

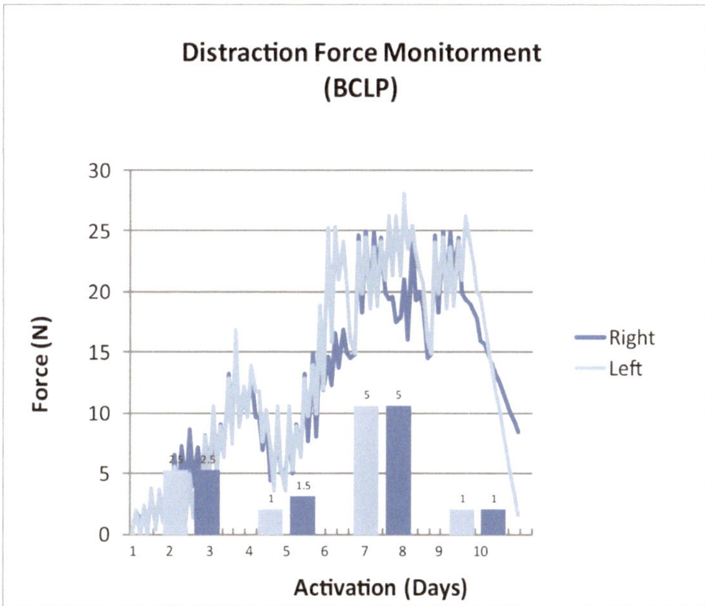

Fig. 7. Typical pattern of distraction forces observed in BCLP patients. Similar pattern of forces are observed in the right and left segments.

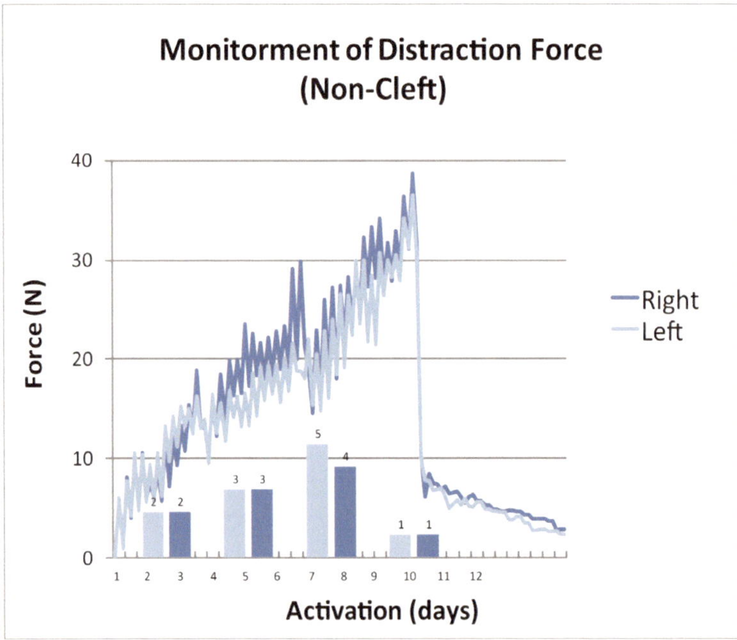

Fig. 8. Typical pattern of distraction forces observed in non-cleft patients. Similar pattern of forces are observed in the right and left segments.

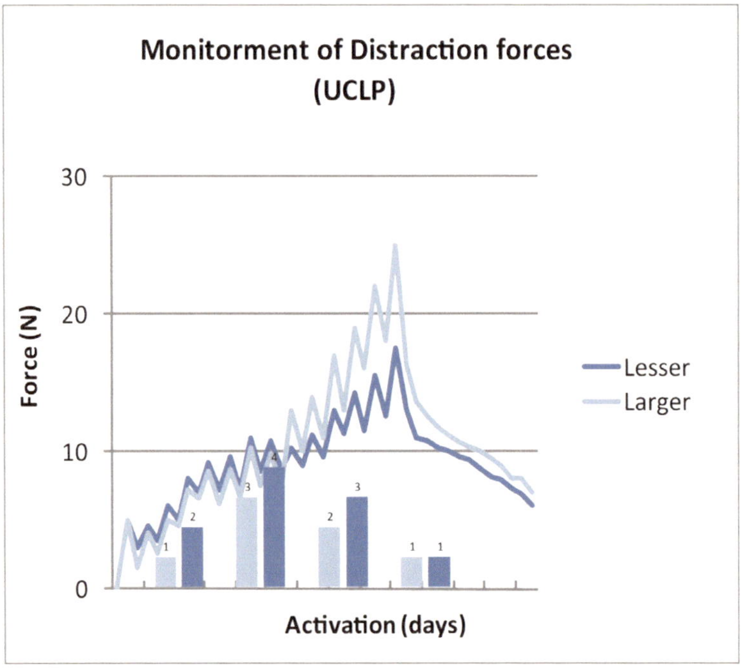

Fig. 9. Pattern of distraction forces observed in a young UCLP patient. Large amount of advancement was obtained in a short period of time.

No differential pattern of forces was observed in the non-cleft patients. Figure 8 shows the typical pattern of the force registered immediately before and after distraction in a non-cleft patient. The pattern of forces was similar to the BCLP patients.

Relatively short distraction period was necessary to complete the maxillary advancement in a young UCLP patient (Figure 9). Monitorment of distraction forces also demonstrated that the amount of force necessary to advance the maxilla in young patients is smaller than those applied in adult patients.

The most interesting aspect is the analysis of how forces varied during the course of maxillary distraction osteogenesis. We can thus see from the graphs how the force increases each day, rising dramatically after distraction, and then slowly falling until it reaches a value slightly greater than the final force on the previous days.

Monitorment of distraction forces was relatively easy and no time-consuming. There were no complications, such as pain, discomfort, or procedural delays in measuring and adjusting the distraction forces.

The mechanism remained intact in all patients through the active and retention phases. Distraction forces increased progressively with distraction.

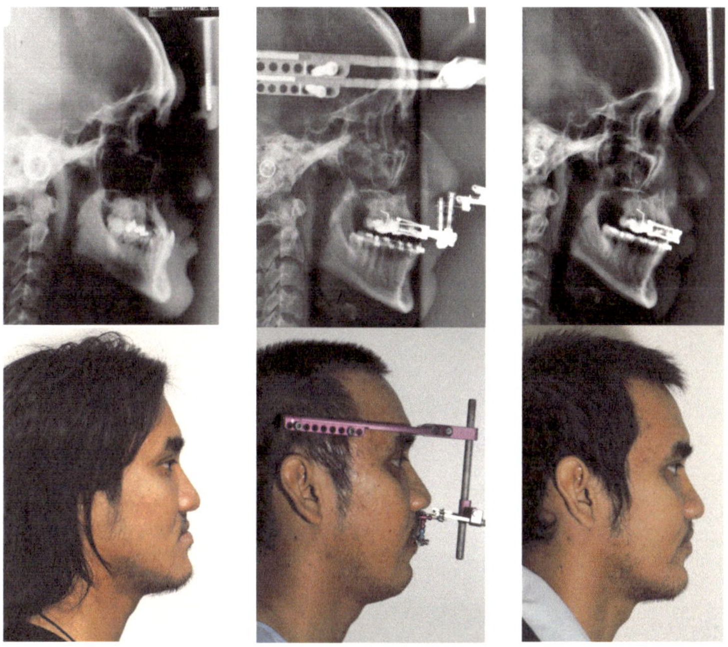

Fig. 10. Pre-surgical, distraction and post-distraction pictures. Significant improvement of the face and profile can be obtained with distraction osteogenesis.

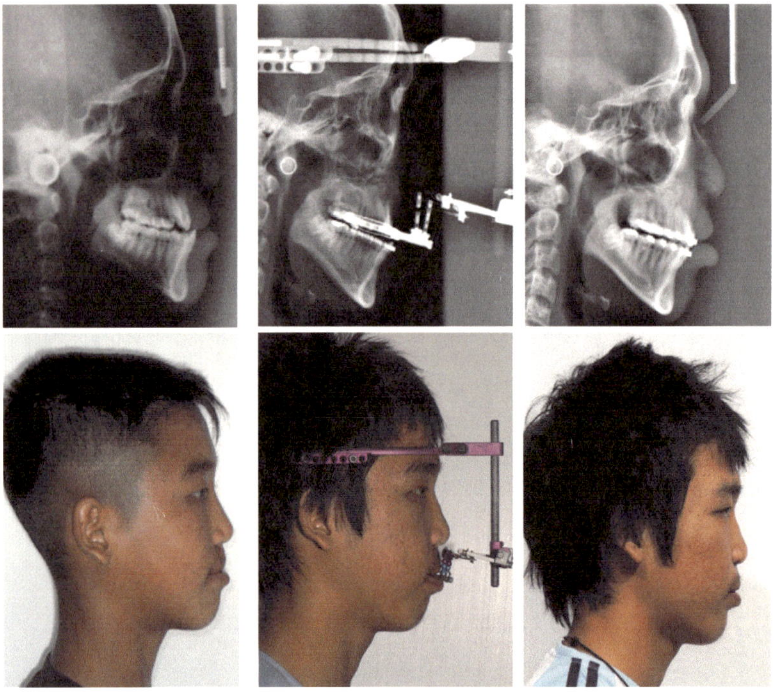

Fig. 11. Pre-surgical, distraction and post-distraction pictures. Significant improvement of the face and profile can be obtained with distraction osteogenesis.

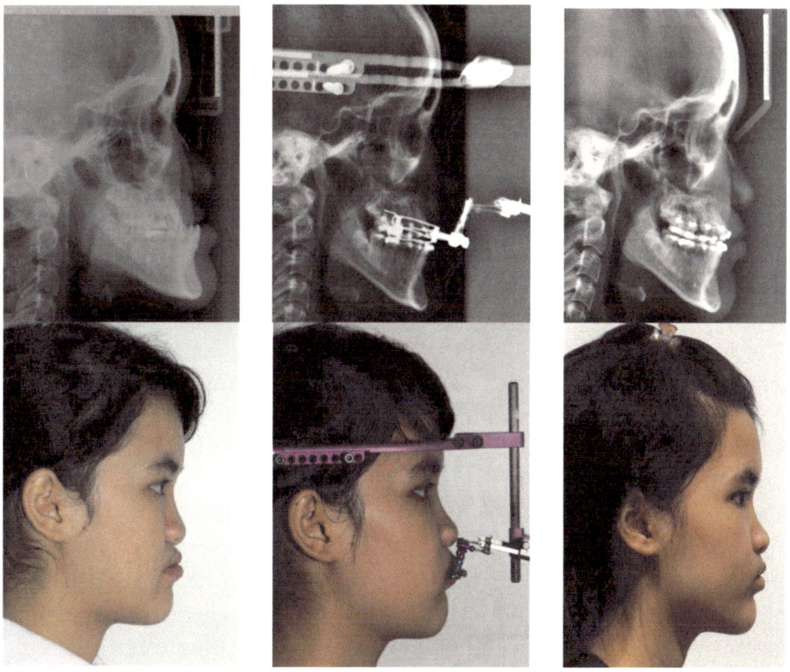

Fig. 12. Pre-surgical, distraction and post-distraction pictures. Large amount of advancement was obtained in a short period of time.

4. Discussion

The present study described the development of a simple method of adjusting and measuring tensile forces during maxillary distraction osteogenesis. Although distraction osteogenesis of the maxilla is well reported in the literature, no study has been published describing the monitorment of distraction forces necessary to advance the maxillary bone either in humans or in animals. It may be explained due to the difficulties encountered to measure the healing process accurately and for the complexity of monitoring techniques available today (Wiltfang *et al.*, 2001).

Several studies have been performed to assess the magnitude of traction forces applied on the distracted structure. However, most of measurements were performed in long bones or on experimental models basis. Moreover, the data obtained by these authors show great disparity. Forces exceeding 1500 N at the time of lyses were measured by Monticelli and Spinelli (1981) in two patients. Kenwright *et al.* (1990) recorded the force of 600 N, and Jones *et al.* (1989) a load of 400 N. Roermund *et al.* (1992) monitored continuously the traction forces during tibial lengthening in a patient and found that 800 N was required for complete lyses. Forriol *et al.*, (1997) measured the force required for distraction osteogenesis of the lamb tibia. The maximum force occurred after activation of force and attained values over 8 Kgf. In the craniofacial area, Wiltfang *et al.* (2001) using a micro hydraulic distractor device on the mandible of pigs observed that forces up to 2500kPa were necessary to move the cylinders` piston and 1200 -1300 kPa necessary for continuous distraction. Robinson *et al.* (2001) measured the mean force of 4.2 N-cm of torque or an equivalent force of 35.6 N to lengthen the human mandible. However, measurements were performed indirectly using laboratory data and clinical correlation. The great variability of distraction devices, complexity of measurement methodology applied, site of distraction force application, and anatomical structure seems to dictate great influence. All authors agreed that the assessment of distraction forces clinically is an important tool for the clinician to better understand the biomechanical response of the distracted structures and to manage the symptoms.

In the present study, the assessment of maxillary distraction forces was possible using the proposed mechanism. Distraction forces could be measured directly by simply pulling on the cable loop with a force gauge. The mean force observed in this group of patients was 34.7N. However, great variation of the maximum forces was observed in all patients, despite to the amount of maxillary advancement or cleft type suggesting that an individual adjustment of forces is highly desirable. During distraction, force measurement showed a gradual increase in the force needed to activate the device during the initial days. Force peaks were reached immediately after the activation of the distraction device. Twelve hours later the distraction force had fallen substantially and reaches a value slightly greater than the final force on the previous days. As the soft tissue has substantial viscoelastic behavior, these are just a transient peak force, and after distraction the force decrease exponentially (Leong et al., 1979) with an average rate of 2.3 N/h the first 3-5 h (Aarnes et al., 2002).

The main finding of this study was the differential pattern of forces between the lateral segments observed in unilateral cleft lip and palate subjects. Distraction forces measured on the larger segments were aproximately 70% higher than on the lesser segment, indicating differential force requirements to advance a cleft maxilla. On the other hand, the amount of advancement on the lesser segment was higher then on the larger segment, suggesting that the increase of distraction forces is inversely proportional to the amount of bone movement. Namely, the increased resistance to the movement causes the increase of forces. The magnitude and the pattern of forces are greatly determined by the biomechanical properties of the tissues to be lengthened. These biomechanical properties may vary between individuals, necessitating an individual adjustment of the distraction rate to prevent excessive traction forces. The explanation of the differential pattern of forces between the lesser and larger segments in unilateral cleft lip and palate patients should therefore be addressed to the cross-sectional area of the callus, modified by the rate, rhythm, and age of the patient rather than to the presence of scarring tissue.

In the present study, assessment of distraction forces did not allow differentiation between contribution from the soft tissue envelope and the regenerate. Previous investigations have suggested the soft tissue (Aarnes et al., 2002; Gardner et al., 1997), the regenerate (Aronson and Harp, 1994) or both (Gardner et al., 1998) to be the source of the tensile force. The force in the rigid external distractor is a result of the resistance in the composite tissue system, and the interpretation of the results depends on which structure provides the major resistance. If the force mainly originates from the regenerate, high forces suggest good bone mineralization and should be preferable. However, with the soft tissue being the major contributor a high tensile force indicates poor adaptation with risk for tissue damage, and lower forces are desired. Further studies are necessary to clarify the effects of distraction osteogenesis on the soft and hard tissues, and the influence of the scar tissue from both a clinical and an experimental point of view.

The process of distraction osteogenesis involves an interaction of mechanical and biological factors that influence each other. The mechanical factors are usually only defined in terms of distraction frequency and velocity, and in terms of rigidity of fixation.

In the present study, mini cables replaced the conventional surgical wires used to deliver the traction forces to the maxillary bone. It will optimize the traction forces applied to the maxillary bone avoid the lack of rigidity often observed on the traction wires that will result in an inadequate transmission of forces to the maxillary bone (Suzuki et al., 2004). Moreover, the ideal 1:1 ratio of bone to device movement will not be accomplished. As a result the recommended bone movement rate of 1mm/day will not be achieved (Block et al., 1995).

Complications arising from excessive forces are often severe and include pain and discomfort for the patient, traction injuries to the nerves and vessels, dental compensation and alteration in the mechanical conditions of the distraction device. To minimize the complications is necessary to optimize the procedure of lengthening biomechanically. The process of biomechanical optimization requires as examination of the constraints and continuous monitoring of forces. The measurement of distraction forces clinically using the innovated mechanism proved to be helpful to better adjust the distraction rate in the maxillary advancement and to reduce the risk of causing excessive tensile forces and associated complications. Moreover, the quantitative measure of bone loading capacity would allow an estimation of individual time requirements for healing, therefore permitting individual adjustments.

In the daily bone lengthening procedure, the greatest forces are produced in a short period of time immediately after lengthening. They could be reduced to decrease pain in the patient and loads on the device by performing lengthening over a greater number of steps or using dynamic equipment able to absorb these forces (Wiltfang *et al.*, 2001).

Aarnes et al. (2002) has shown that in the stepwise lengthening, a total lengthening of 1 mm cause less force accumulation than a 1.75 mm elongation. The present study indicates that this is valid for the maxillary distraction as well. Accordingly, there is a mutual dependency between the force increment and the amount of maxillary advancement. Lower rates seem to reduce the tensile force in the soft tissue during distraction osteogenesis. The reduction is assumed to be due to less tissue injury and increase of muscle growth, and thereby the increased adaptation of ability in the soft tissues.

To date, assessment of distraction forces during maxillary advancement have not been determined, consequently it has not been possible to examine optimum rates and rhythms for maxillary distraction. Knowledge of these forces can be used in the clinical setting to determine the safety margins for the device manufacturing and to give immediate clinical feedback regarding what may be happening in the distraction site, including, premature consolidation, device failure, or incomplete osteotomies. This information can be used to determine if the rate, rhythm, or distance of distraction should be modified.

The maximum mean force of 34.7N needed to distract the maxilla means that in designing a device, greater miniaturization is possible as long as a safety factor is incorporated into the design. At times, it is necessary to readjust the traction angle to permit the three-dimensional control over the maxillary bone (Polley and Figueroa, 1997). Assessments of distraction forces will permit the adjustment of forces delivered to the distraction process at the same levels, avoiding lose of forces. Another advantage of the force assessment is the possibility to adjust individually the amount of force delivered to the maxillary segments in cleft patients, therefore optimizing the distraction procedure and reducing the patient discomfort and symptoms.

5. Conclusion

We have developed a direct method for monitoring the distraction forces during maxillary distraction osteogenesis using a simple mechanism. Direct measurement of maxillary distraction forces provides current information about the mechanical response and, thereby, the condition in the distracted structures. Assessment of the forces within the maxillary bone during distraction osteogenesis may lead to a better understanding of the nature and biology of distraction, and help determine the most appropriate distraction protocol. The optimum distraction forces and a system to permit continuous distraction forces to the maxillary bone are to be determined by future studies.

6. Acknowledgment

The authors acknowledge the assistance of Dr. M. Kevin O Carroll, Professor Emeritus of the University of Mississippi School of Dentistry, USA, and Faculty Consultant, Chiang Mai University Faculty of Dentistry, Thailand, in the preparation of the manuscript.
Part of this study was supported by the Thailand Research Funding no. MRG5080347.

7. References

Aarnes, G.T.; Steen, H.; Kristiansen, L.P.; Ludvigsen, P. & Reikerås, O. (2002). *Tissue response during monofocal and bifocal leg lengthening in patients.* J Orthop Res. 2002 Jan;20(1):137-41.

Ahn, J.G.; Figueroa, A.A.; Braun, S. & Polley, J.W. (1999). *Biomechanical considerations in distraction of the osteotomized dentomaxillary complex.* Am J Orthod Dentofacial Orthop. 116: 264-70.

Aronson, J. & Harp, J.H. (1994). *Mechanical forces as predictors of healing during tibial lengthening by distraction osteogenesis.* Clin Orthop Relat Res. Apr;(301):73-9.

Block, M.S.; Cervini, D.; Chang, A. & Gottsegen, G.B. (1995). *Anterior maxillary advancement using a tooth-supported distraction osteogenesis.* J Oral Maxillofac Surg. May;53(5):561-5.

Burstein, F.D.; Lukas, S. & Forsthoffer, D. (2008). *Measurement of torque during mandibular distraction.* J Craniofac Surg. May;19(3):644-7.

Evans, M.; Kenwright, J. & Cunningham, J.L. (1988). *Design and performance of a fracture monitoring transducer.* J Biomed Eng. Jan;10(1):64-9.

Forriol, F.; Goenaga, I.; Mora, G.; Viñolas, J. & Canadell, J. (1997). *Measurement of bone lengthening forces; an experimental model in lamb.* Clin Biomech (Bristol, Avon). Jan;12(1):17-21.

Leong, J.C.; Ma, R.Y.; Clark, J.A.; Cornish, L.S. & Yau, A.C. (1979). *Viscoelastic behaviour of tissue in leg lengthening by distraction.* Clin Orthop Relat Res. Mar-Apr;(139):102-9.

Gardner, T.N.; Evans, M.; Simpson, A.H.; Kyberd, P.J. & Kenwright, J. (1997). *A method of examining the magnitude and origin of "soft" and "hard" tissue forces resisting limb lengthening.* Med Eng Phys. Jul;19(5):405-11.

Gardner, T.N.; Evans, M.; Simpson, H. & Kenwright, J. (1998). *Force-displacement behaviour of biological tissue during distraction osteogenesis.* Med Eng Phys. Nov-Dec;20(9):708-15.

Iacomini, R.G. (2001). *Mechanism for adjusting and measuring tension in a cable.* NASA Tech Briefs, engineering solutions for designs and manufacture. Lyndon B. Johnson Space Center, Huston, Texas. (www.nasatech.com)

Ilizarov, G.A. (1989). *The tension-stress effect on the genesis and growth of tissues. Part I. The influence of stability of fixation and soft-tissue preservation.* Clin Orthop Relat Res. Jan;(238):249-81.

Ilizarov, G.A. (1989). *The tension-stress effect on the genesis and growth of tissues: Part II. The influence of the rate and frequency of distraction.* Clin Orthop Relat Res. Feb;(239):263-85.

Jones, C.B.; Dewar, M.E.; Aichroth, P.M.; Crawfurd, E.J. & Emery, R. (1989). *Epiphyseal distraction monitored by strain gauges. Results in seven children.* J Bone Joint Surg Br. Aug;71(4):651-6.

Kenwright, J.; Spriggins, A.J. & Cunningham, J.L. (1990). *Response of the growth plate to distraction close to skeletal maturity. Is fracture necessary?* Clin Orthop Relat Res. Jan;(250):61-72.

Monticelli, G.; & Spinelli, R. (1981). *Distraction epiphysiolysis as a method of limb lengthening. III. Clinical applications.* Clin Orthop Relat Res. Jan-Feb;(154):274-85.

Polley, J.W. & Figueroa, A.A. (1997). *Management of severe maxillary deficiency in childhood and adolescence through distraction osteogenesis with an external, adjustable, rigid distraction device.* J Craniofac Surg.; 8: 181-185.

Richardson, J.B.; Cunningham, J.L.; Goodship, A.E.; O'Connor, B.T. & Kenwright, J. (1994). *Measuring stiffness can define healing of tibial fractures.* J Bone Joint Surg Br. May;76(3):389-94.

Robinson, R.C.; O'Neal, P.J. & Robinson, G.H. (2001). *Mandibular distraction force: laboratory data and clinical correlation.* J Oral Maxillofac Surg. May;59(5):539-44; discussion 544-5.

Samchukov, M.L.; Cherkashim, A.M. & Cope, J.B. (1998). *Distraction Osteogenesis: origins and evolution.* In: McNamara JA Jr, Trotman CA, eds. Advances in Craniofacial Orthopedics, Vol. 34, Craniofacial growth series. Ann Harbor: University of Michigan, Center for human growth and development,: 1-35.

Suzuki, E.Y.; Watanabe, M.; Buranastidporn, B.; Baba, Y. Ohyama, K. & Ishii, M. (2006). *Simultaneous maxillary distraction osteogenesis using a twin-track distraction device combined with alveolar bone grafting in cleft patients: preliminary report of a technique.* Angle Orthod. Jan;76(1):164-72.

Suzuki, E.Y.; Buranastidporn, B. & Ishii, M. (2006). *New fixation method for maxillary distraction osteogenesis using locking attachments.* J Oral Maxillofac Surg. Oct;64(10):1553-60.

Suzuki, E.Y. & Suzuki, B. (2007). *Removable splint with locking attachments for maxillary distraction osteogenesis with the RED system.* Int J Oral Maxillofac Surg. Dec;36(12):1153-7. Epub 2007 Jul 12.

Suzuki, E.Y.; Motohashi, N. & Ohyama, K. (2004). *Longitudinal dento-skeletal changes in UCLP patients following maxillary distraction osteogenesis using RED system.* J Med Sci. 51:27-33.

Suzuki, E.Y. & Suzuki, B. (2009). *A simple mechanism for measuring and adjusting distraction forces during maxillary advancement.* J Oral Maxillofac Surg. Oct;67(10):2245-53.

van Roermund, P.M.; Wijlens, R.A. & Renooij, W. (1992). *Continuous monitoring of forces during tibial lengthening by distraction epiphysiolysis.* Acta Orthop Belg.;58(1):63-8.

Wiltfang, J.; Kebler, P. Merten, H.A. & Neukam, F.W. (2001). *Continuous and intermittent bone distraction using a micro-hydraulic cylinder: an experimental study in mini-pigs.* Br J Oral and Maxillofac Surg.; 39; 2-7

Younger, A.S.; Mackenzie, W.G. & Morrison, J.B. (1994). *Femoral forces during limb lengthening in children.* Clin Orthop Relat Res. Apr;(301):55-63.

3

Drilling of Bone: Practicality, Limitations and Complications Associated with Surgical Drill-Bits

Nicky Bertollo and William Robert Walsh
Surgical and Orthopaedic Research Laboratories, Prince of Wales Clinical School, University of New South Wales, Prince of Wales Hospital, Sydney, Australia

1. Introduction

The drilling of bone is ubiquitous in many fields of surgery including orthopaedics, neurosurgery, plastics and reconstructive, craniomaxillofacial and ear nose and throat (ENT). A cylindrical tunnel is typically prepared in bone using a surgical drill-bit to accommodate a screw or other threaded device for rigid fixation which is provided by the integration of bone (cancellous and/or cortical) with the screw threads. In this configuration bone screws are resistant to axial and shear forces as well as bending moments and therefore suited to the load-bearing function of the skeleton during locomotion. Drill-bits are also used in the preparation of bony tunnels, such as in anterior cruciate ligament reconstruction.

Drilling is associated with the conversion of mechanical work energy into thermal energy causing a transient rise in temperature of adjacent bone and soft tissues to above normal physiological levels (Matthews and Hirsch 1972; Lavelle and Wedgwood 1980; Eriksson and Albrektsson 1984; Eriksson, Albrektsson *et al.* 1984b; Abouzgia and Symington 1996; Natali, Ingle *et al.* 1996; Toews, Bailey *et al.* 1999; Bachus, Rondina *et al.* 2000; Davidson and James 2003; Augustin, Davila *et al.* 2008; Franssen, van Diest *et al.* 2008; Bertollo, Milne *et al.* 2010). Primary sources of this thermal energy are plastic deformation and shear failure of bone and friction at the machining face. The magnitude of this temperature rise is determined by a number of factors, including drill geometry and diameter, rotational speed (rpm), feed-rate ($mm.s^{-1}$), axial thrust force (N), initial drill-bit temperature and internal or external cooling. The negative effect of elevated temperature on the viability of bone is well-acknowledged and measures to reduce them during surgery are frequently employed, such as manual irrigation with sterile saline (Matthews and Hirsch 1972; Jacob and Berry 1976; Lavelle and Wedgwood 1980; Camargo, Faria *et al.* 2007; Augustin, Davila et al. 2008). Viability (Eriksson, Albrektsson et al. 1984b) as well as the structure and mechanical properties (Bonfield and Li 1968) of bone are indeed compromised through exposure to elevated temperatures. Another important variable that can influence the biological response for drilled bone is the time which a temperature above a threshold value is maintained.

Excessive temperatures and durations at these elevated levels can result in the necrosis (death) of bone, a phenomenon termed osteonecrosis, or the impairment of osteogenic potential. Necrotic bone is resorbed through osteoclastic activity and this can have dire and catastrophic consequences for rigidity of bone screws and pins, ultimately resulting in the failure of fracture repair or implant fixation. Whilst there is no definitive consensus regarding critical values or their durations an increase in temperature of the cortical bone to above 50°C has been implicated with a reduced regenerative capacity (Eriksson and Albrektsson 1984; Eriksson, Albrektsson et al. 1984b) and above 56°C with osteonecrosis (Matthews and Hirsch 1972). Lundskog (Lundskog 1972) determined cellular necrosis to occur following a 30s duration at above 50°C whilst Eriksson and Albrektsson (Eriksson and Albrektsson 1983) demonstrated that a temperature elevation to above 47°C which is sustained for one minute has a potent osteonecrotic effect. Both *in vitro* and *in vivo* animal models have hitherto played a pivotal role in the determination of these threshold temperatures and critical durations.

The creation of a cylindrical hole or other defect in bone invokes a healing response characterised by the formation of bone reconstituting the defect. To illustrate this point, in the early to mid 20th century the random creation of holes in bone, 8 to 10 depending on the subjective assessment by the surgeon was advocated in the treatment of un-united fractures characterised by the presence of fibrous tissue (Easton and Prewitt 1937). In certain orthopaedic applications such as component fixation in uncemented joint arthroplasty this healing response is crucial in the formation and attainment of a biological and mechanical interlock through bone ongrowth and ingrowth into the porous domain of the implant (Svehla, Morberg *et al.* 2000; Svehla, Morberg *et al.* 2002; Bertollo, Matsubara *et al.* 2011). Excessive temperatures generated during the resection and preparation of bone could hinder postoperative outcome by affecting osteogenic potential. For example, oscillating saw blades used to resect bone in total knee arthroplasty have been shown to experience temperatures in excess of 100°C (Larsen and Ryd 1989), with progressively lower temperatures recorded in the bone moving away from the plane of the osteotomy. Similarly, it is not uncommon for temperatures of 100°C to be reached during Kirschner wire (k-wire) insertion and drilling of cortical bone. Temperature at the tool-bone interface is notoriously difficult to measure due to the complexities associated with placement of a temperature measurement device at this precise location. Thermocouples and infrared imaging are two measurement modalities used commonly in the experimental determination of temperature elevation in both the *in vivo* and *in vitro* settings (Matthews and Hirsch 1972; Augustin, Davila et al. 2008).

The operational environment for a surgical drill-bit is unique and very unlike that experienced by engineering drill-bits used in manufacturing, or traditional non-biological engineering (construction, building, etc). Bone is a complex anisotropic porous viscoelastic composite that is also non-homogenous both in material properties as well as geometry. The outer cortex of bone can be curved and irregular and holes drilled are rarely oriented perpendicular to this surface. In the absence of a pilot indentation to help guide the drill the drill-bit is susceptible to skiving, or wandering, along the cortex prior to purchase, thereby having implications for accuracy as well as final geometry of the cylindrical defect itself. To circumvent this problem the surgeon will often prepare a pilot indentation at a right-angle before positioning the hand-piece and drill-bit at the desired orientation. This is not always desirable as the unnecessary removal of bone stock can compromise screw fixation and pullout strength (Steeves, Stone *et al.* 2005). Skiving is particularly problematic in the case of bicortical drilling of long bones as the tip can skive along the endosteal surface of the far cortex, which induces a bending moment on the fluted portion of the drill-bit (Bertollo, Gothelf *et al.* 2008). If of sufficient magnitude this bending moment can increase the risk of breakage, with the broken portion sometimes becoming lodged in the medullary canal (Figure 1). The broken fragment is frequently left *in situ* due to complexities associated with extraction from this confined space (Fothi, Perren *et al.* 1992; Hirt, Auer *et al.* 1992). Anatomical constraints, including the presence of muscle as well as blood vessels and nerves also increases the complexity of the use of drills due to possible collateral damage of these structures and subsequent morbidities.

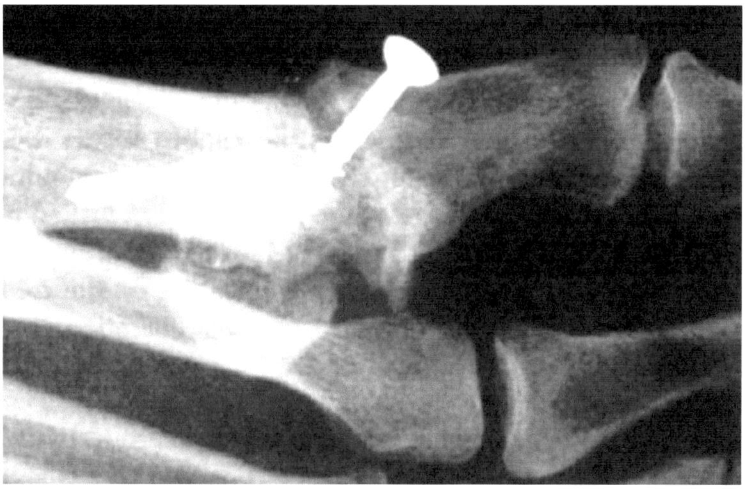

Fig. 1. A broken portion of a drill-bit left *in situ*. (Natali, Ingle et al. 1996)

Many geometrical and operational variables influence both the performance and maximal temperature elevation in bone as result of the use of drill-bits. Performance and maximal heat generation associated with a particular drill-bit are inevitably interrelated. As has been outlined above, prominent geometric variables include point angle, rake angle, diameter, chisel edge length and flute number. The maximal temperature attained during drilling and the performance of a drill-bit is highly dependent on the specific drill design (Harris and Kohles 2001; Ercoli, Funkenbusch *et al.* 2004; Chacon, Bower *et al.* 2006; Bertollo, Milne et al. 2010). Salient operational factors encompass axial thrust force, rotation speed, torque, orthotopic site, sharpness of the cutting edges, irrigation, cooling systems (closed or open loop), initial drill-bit temperature and cortical thickness. Conceivably, blood flow in the vessels and microvasculature contributes in the abatement of maximal temperature attained during drilling. There are very limited reports in the literature pertaining to quantification of this phenomenon. Similarly, bone quality (density as well as microstructure) is another parameter having an effect but which has not been extensively reported. The following sections will address these said operational and geometrical variables.

This chapter will present an overview of the bone cutting process, including heat arising from friction and breakage of molecular bonds and the potential effects which this may have on bone tissue. Factors influencing drill-bit performance and heat generation are also explored, including a review of experimental methods and animal models used hitherto in the determination of the maximal temperature rise and the response of tissue to this thermal insult.

2. Drill-bit types

Surgical twist drill-bits are available in a wide variety of configurations and sizes, with diameters typically ranging from 0.5mm to several millimetres. The diameter chosen is application specific but normally the diameter will rarely exceed 14mm, which would be a diameter required for the preparation and enlargement of medullary canals for intramedullary nails in osteosynthesis. These devices, referred to as reamers can also exhibit flexibility to account for the 'bow' or curvature of long bones, such as the femur which exhibits a slight anterior bow. The main difference between twist drills and reamers is the helix angle (Garcia, Mombiela *et al.* 2004).

Cannulated drill-bits are another permutation of the surgical drill-bit and are used in procedures such as anterior cruciate ligament reconstruction surgery of the knee, where the orientation of the prepared hole in three dimensions is critical not only for the drill hole but the screw used for fixation (Pinczewski, Lyman *et al.* 2007). These drills exhibit a hollow cylindrical recess along their length to accommodate smaller diameter pins or k-wires which are driven through the bone at the desired orientation in an intermediary step. The cannulated bit is then passed over this guide-wire and a cylindrical hole produced. The guidewire in this circumstance helps to limit deviation of the drill-bit from the desired orientation. Cannulated drills do not exhibit a chisel edge. A further variation of the cannulated drill is the olive-tipped drill-bit, where the lack of a traditional fluted portion is advantageous as it limits the infliction of damage to the cartilage on the medial condyle whilst allowing the surgeon to position the femoral tunnel at the desired orientation during anterior cruciate ligament reconstruction surgery. That is, the medial condyle is less of a physical obstruction to drilling.

K-wires are another permutation of the surgical drill and are typically used as an intermediary device during surgery to help stabilise or anatomically reduce a fracture, but they can equally be used as a more permanent structure in some cases. Popular k-wires points are the trochar and diamond, although there are others. Reports in the literature seem to suggest that the maximal temperature elevation associated with k-wires is markedly higher than that experienced with fluted drill-bits (Piska, Yang *et al.* 2002).

Burrs are another type of rotating bone cutting device, used primarily in orthodontic applications, but also occasionally used to decorticate bone in orthopaedic surgery. The design and function of surgical burrs falls outside the scope of this work. However, results in the literature pertaining to temperature rises encountered in the experimental setting during burring is presented and discussed.

3. Anatomy of a drill-bit

The medical profession has, with certain exceptions, tended to adapt commercially available instruments that have been developed for drilling other materials (Jackson, Ghosh *et al.* 1989). A drill-bit consists of a shank which is used to couple the piece to the chuck of the surgical hand-piece, flutes which channel bone chips and debris (swarf) away from the machining face and cutting edges (Figure 2).

The machining face can further be divided into the chisel edge and cutting edges, where the number of flutes exhibited by a drill-bit corresponds to the number of cutting edges. The length of the chisel edge is equivalent to the web thickness of a 2-fluted drill-bit and is also representative of the offset between cutting edges about the axis of rotation. Accordingly, the cutting edges produce/exert a slicing action through the material being machined (in this case, bone), thereby explaining why the oblique theory of cutting is applicable to drilling (to be elaborated on in a subsequent section).

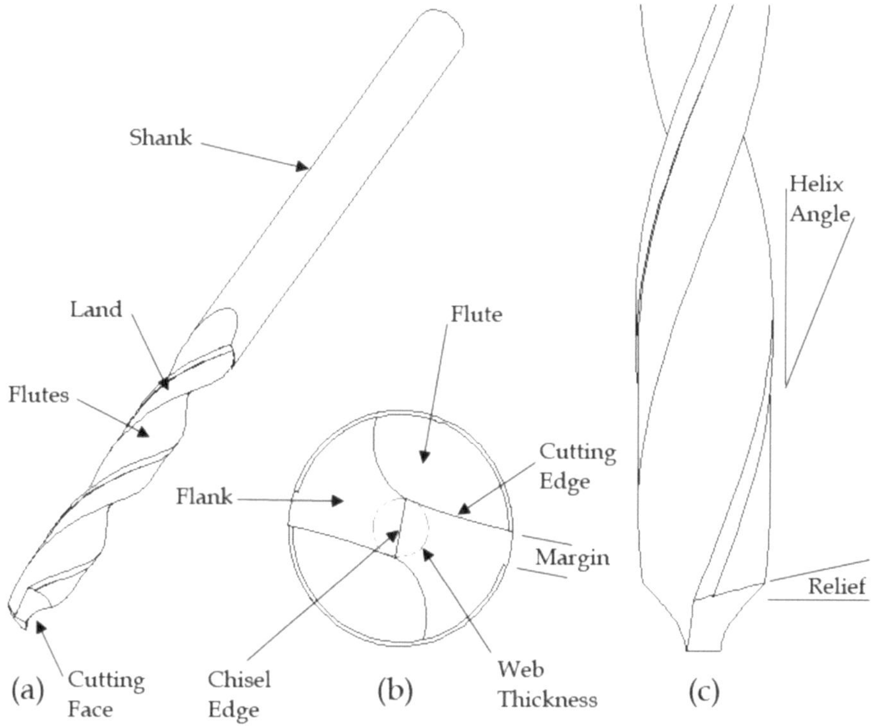

Fig. 2. Drill-bit geometry. (a) General geometry, (b) Point geometry, and (c) Relief and helix angles

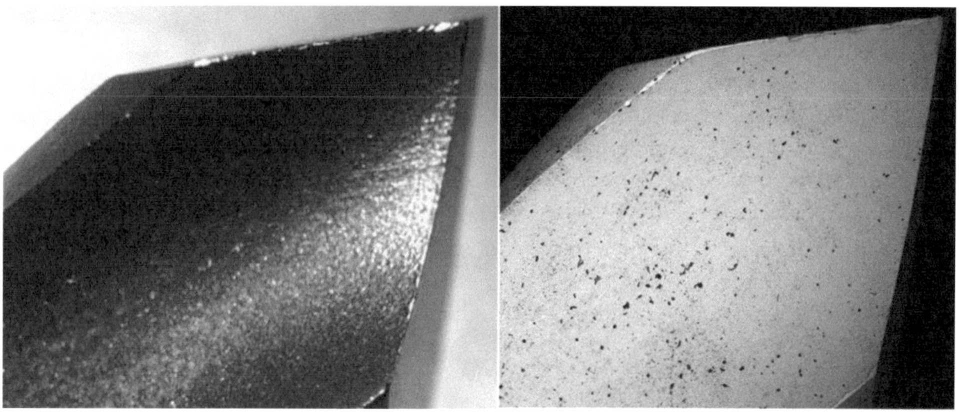

Fig. 3. Macroscopic (left) and scanning electron microscope (SEM) image (right) of a fresh Synthes 4.3mm diameter 2-fluted drill depicting the rake face, cutting edge and point. As an imaging modality SEM provides greater insight into the state and sharpness of cutting and chisel edges

The chisel edge contributes little to cutting and substantially to the axial thrust force, due to a relatively slow cutting velocity and a large negative rake angle. The extent of the contribution made by the chisel edge to the axial thrust force depends on the length ratio between the chisel and cutting edges. The chisel edge contributes roughly 50% of the thrust force for a typical drill with a web thickness (chisel edge length) equal to 20% of the diameter. Where the ratio increases to 30%, the contribution doubles and at 40% there is a quadrupling of the proportion attributed to the chisel edge length (Stephenson and Agapiou 1997). Several tip design strategies have been aimed at reducing the magnitude of the axial thrust force component attributed to the chisel edge length, one of which is web thinning (Ueda, Wada *et al.* 2010).

The point angle of a drill is the angle formed by the projection of the cutting edges onto a plane passing through the longitudinal axis of the drill-bit (Figure 4), and is especially relevant in orthopaedics as it prevents the walking of the drill point along the bony surface prior to purchase (Jacobs, Pope *et al.* 1974; Bertollo, Gothelf et al. 2008). Several optimal point angles for 2-fluted drill-bits have been advanced in the orthopaedic literature. Jacob and colleagues (Jacob and Berry 1976) recommended a point angle of 90°, whilst both Saha (Saha, Pal *et al.* 1982) and Natali (Natali, Ingle et al. 1996) advocated a value of 118°. This latter point angle is very common for general purpose 2-fluted drills, perhaps because thrust force varies parabolically with the point angle and reaches a minimum value at roughly 118° (Stephenson and Agapiou 1997).

Point angle has been shown to have little effect on the increase in temperature during drilling. Augustin and coworkers (Augustin, Davila et al. 2008) experimented with 80°, 100° and 120° point angles in a 2-fluted drill design in bovine bone showing negligible effect. Likewise, Hillery and Shauib (Hillery and Shuaib 1999) detected no significant difference in temperature elevation in bovine and cadaveric bone *in vitro* when testing point angles of 70°, 80° and 90°. Numerical models have also suggested point angle to have a negligible effect on the maximal temperature attained during drilling (Davidson and James 2003).

Ostensibly, a lower limit to the point angle which can be accommodated by 2-fluted drills without compromising the structural integrity of the point exists but which has not been described. Three-fluted drill-bits, on the other hand, are generally able to accommodate a more acute tip angle by virtue of the pyramidal shaped end. We have previously demonstrated that an acute point angle has positive implications for accuracy and targeting ability (Bertollo, Gothelf et al. 2008). In some respects, though, an acute point angle is undesirable as it may result in subsequent damage to muscles, blood vessels and nerves which could contribute to non-primary post-operative morbidity.

The helix angle of a surgical drill is the angle between a tangent to the leading edge of the land and the drill-bit long-axis. The material being machined is the primary variable which determines this parameter; brittle materials producing short chips (such as bone, brass, cast iron, etc) require slow spirals whilst more malleable materials producing longer chips are best handled by drills exhibiting quick spirals. Swarf produced by the cutting action consists of fragments of bone, but is inexorably contaminated with elements which interfere with passage along the flute, namely lipids, marrow, soft-connective tissue and blood, by markedly changing flow characteristics and viscosity. Surgical twist drill-bits are slow-spiral, meaning that the helix angle is quite small, making them ideal for the drilling of bone (Jacob and Berry 1976) as debris is ejected quickly. Although flutes are typically parabolic in cross-section, so as to maximise cross-sectional area, when the depth of the hole becomes appreciable in relation to its diameter the flutes tend to clog, having direct implications for driving torque and heat generation due to the effects of friction (Natali, Ingle et al. 1996). Cleaning of flutes between successive drilling episodes is therefore mandated. Natali and colleagues suggested the optimal helix angle for surgical drill-bits to be approximately 36° (Natali, Ingle et al. 1996), actually rendering it a fast helix.

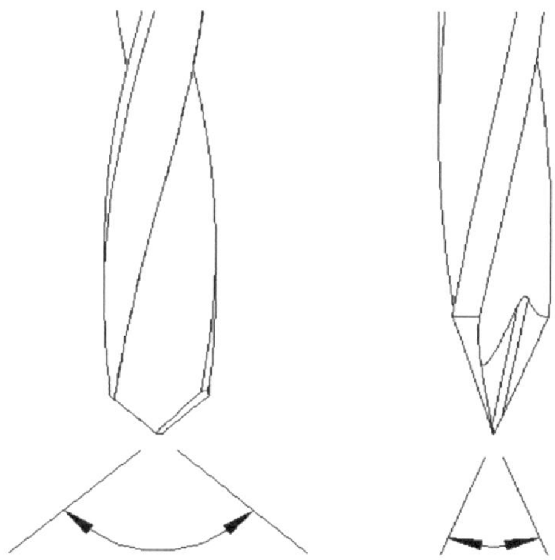

Fig. 4. Point angles of 2-fluted (left) drill-bits are generally less acute than for 3-fluted (right) surgical drill-bits. Web thickness at the tip of 2-fluted drill-bits limits the point angle which can be supported, as compared to the pyramidal shape of the 3-fluted tip

The helix angle of a drill-bit has implications for both rake angle and torsional rigidity (Narasimha, Osman *et al.* 1987) but has little effect on the maximal temperature elevation (Davidson and James 2003). Narasimha and co-workers (Narasimha, Osman et al. 1987) demonstrated that torsional rigidity varies parabolically with helix angle, reaching a maximum at approximately 28°. They suggested that this may be the reason for the choice of this angle across a wide range of drills used for a multitude of purposes.

Both 2-fluted and 3-fluted surgical drill-bits are in clinical use. Theoretically, 3-fluted drills are inherently more efficient due to the inclusion of an additional cutting face, which can potentially remove 50% more material per rotation than a diameter-matched 2-fluted drill-bit. Additionally, a more acute tip angle in general improves accuracy and targeting ability (Bertollo, Gothelf et al. 2008). Another fundamental difference is the chisel edge length. By virtue of symmetry of 3-fluted designs the cutting edges tend to converge at a single point, committing the chisel edge to a nominal value. As has been shown the ratio of the chisel edge length to the drill diameter is an important parameter in the determination of the effect which this length has on the axial thrust force and cutting efficiency. Despite these theoretical and perceived benefits there is little data in the literature in support of their use.

4. Cutting operation

Function of any drill-bit requires the application of rotational motion (rpm) and torque (N·m) which is normally provided by the drill, or hand-piece, and axial thrust force (N) which is applied by the operator manually or via a device such as drill-press. Translation of the machining face through the medium being drilled is defined as the feed-rate (mm.s^{-1}). In manufacturing processing and the like a constant feed-rate is normally applied mechatronically whereas in the clinical context a quasi-constant axial thrust force is applied to the hand-piece by the orthopaedic surgeon. This distinction is quite important as pertinent to surgical drill-bit research and the drilling of cortical bone. Appreciably, inter-surgeon variability in axial thrust force applied to a surgical handpiece is considerable. The literature seems to suggest that drill-bit diameter is an important variable affecting the magnitude of this force, although orthotopic drilling site and patient bone quality represent additional considerations. When drilling 3.2mm diameter holes in cortical bone we have previously found that the mean thrust force applied by the surgeon to be 110N (Bertollo, Milne et al. 2010), Natali and colleagues measured a maximum of between 10 and 20N whilst drilling 2.5mm diameter holes (Natali, Ingle et al. 1996) whilst Darvish *et al* (Darvish, Shafieian *et al.* 2009) applied 50N with a 2.5mm 2-fluted drill-bit. Using 2 to 3.25mm diameter burs Brisman (Brisman 1996) applied loads of 120 - 240N whilst Hobkirk and Rusiniak (Hobkirk and Rusiniak 1977) determined mean values applied during oral surgery to be in the order of 4 and 19N. The relationship between drill-bit diameter and axial thrust force producing a given feed rate is not constant but linear (Allotta, Belmonte *et al.* 1996).

Wear and dulling of the cutting face due to repeated use has also been shown to have a negative effect on axial thrust force, requiring the application of a higher thrust force to produce a hole in bone. This can have unintended complications, such as cortical breakthrough and uncontrolled plunging of the drill-tip. The effect of these variables on drill operation will be explored in detail in the following sections.

The cutting of bone is a dynamic shear failure process (Jacob, Pope *et al.* 1974). A primary source of heat in the drilling process is the release of energy through the mechanical overwhelming of intermolecular bonds. An idealised illustration of the oblique cutting process is shown in Figure 5.

The removal of bone at the machining face is achieved by the cutting edges which remove a finite thickness of material, t, with each rotation as they spiral through the bone, following a helical path. The material being machined is associated with a unique cutting force, and this determines the optimal rake angle, which for cortical bone is 25 to 35° (Jacob and Berry 1976). Unlike many engineering materials cortical bone is mechanically and structurally anisotropic, which has implications for the machining operation and cutting resistance. This is because as the drill-bit rotates the cutting resistance vector is constantly changing. Jacob and colleagues (Jacob, Pope et al. 1974) demonstrated the dependency of the cutting process on the osteon direction in cortical bone, where the cutting forces were greatest when cutting perpendicular to the osteon direction. Based on this work pertaining to orthogonal cutting it was established that a rake angle of 45° is associated with a markedly reduced cutting force, regardless of the osteon direction.

Jacob and Berry (Jacob and Berry 1976) went on to investigate the effect of drill geometry on axial thrust force and drilling torque. They essentially found an asymptotic relationship between both axial thrust force and torque with increasing rotation speed, providing that the feed rate remained constant. Based on their results they suggested that orthopaedic drill-bits should have an appreciable rake angle (25 to 35°), exhibit a point angle to prevent walking of the drill-bit tip prior to purchase, drilling should be done in the 750 to 1250rpm range and performed in the presence of a cooling agent. Further support for this rotation rate was provided by Hillery and Shuaib (Hillery and Shuaib 1999) who recommended a range of 800 to1400rpm.

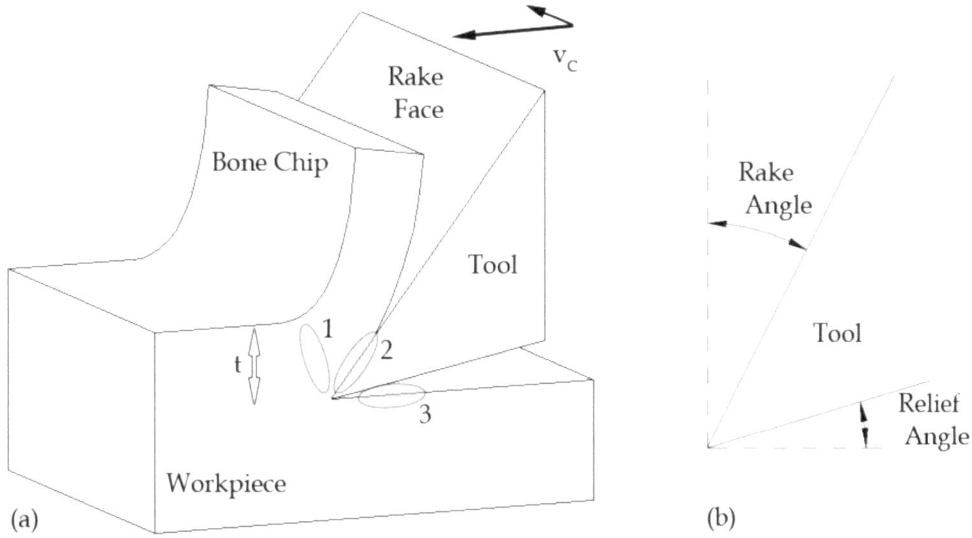

Fig. 5. (a) Mechanism of action of material removal at the rake face during oblique cutting. Regions of primary heat generation are also indicated; 1: shear deformation of the bone, 2: friction between the bone chip and tool and (3) friction between the tangential bone surface and tool. Note that in regions 2 and 3 slight deformation of bone is occurring, also. (b) Rake and relief angles

A relief angle in the design of drill-bits is optional but is often incorporated into the cutting process to relieve the thermal loading and mechanical inefficiencies arising from frictional drag between the surface tangential to the direction of cutting and tool. The *in vitro* work of Chacon *et al* (Chacon, Bower et al. 2006) suggests that relief angle has a significant effect on the magnitude of the maximal temperature rise during drilling of bone.

According to Allotta *et al* (Allotta, Belmonte et al. 1996) the relationship between thrust force and drill-bit diameter is approximately linear and not constant. Therefore, testing different diameter versions of the same drill-bit design at similar feed-rates may have a potentially confounding effect on the maximum temperature elevation. This is because at larger diameters a given feed-rate is associated with larger axial thrust forces. Many previous investigators have demonstrated that the maximum temperature elevation of bone is particularly sensitive to axial thrust force. To test multiple diameters of a single version of a drill at a particular feed rate has the potential to produce spurious results.

4.1 Heat generation and thermodynamics

The primary sources of thermal energy (heat) generation during drilling of bone are shear deformation of bone (1), friction between the bone chip and the rake face (2) as well as friction between cutting edge and underlying bone (3) (Figure 5). Secondary indirect heat sources are driven purely by friction, including that in occurrence between bone chips and flutes, bone chips and host bone and drill-bit webbing and host bone. It has been estimated that approximately 60% of the heat energy generated during drilling is dissipated by bone chips, which is substantially less than the 80% predicted to be removed by the chips during drilling of metals. The remainder of the heat is dissipated by the surrounding hard and soft tissues as well as by the drill-bit itself, causing a transient rise in temperature to above normal physiological levels. Numerical and mathematical models are best suited to the analysis of heat generation and transfer during the drilling operation.

Thermal conductivity is a thermodynamic parameter which describes a material's ability to conduct heat. Cortical bone, as a composite material consisting of organic (collagen) and inorganic (hydroxyapatite) phases, is a relatively poor conductor of heat. Davidson and James (Davidson and James 2000) demonstrated that bovine cortical bone is thermally isotropic, with thermal conductivity in the axial, radial and tangential directions being approximately 0.58 W/Km, which is in direct contrast to the anisotropic structural and mechanical properties. Thermal conductivity of surgical-grade stainless steel (316L), on the other hand, is of the order of 16.3 W/mK. Specific heat is another important material property (Chen and Gundjian 1976) in the determination of the maximal temperature attained by bone in the presence of a heat source. It has been demonstrated that the maximum temperature attained by cortical bone during drilling is more sensitive to changes in specific heat (heat capacity) than to thermal conductivity (Davidson and James 2003).

5. Mechanical properties

Surgical drills must be able to withstand the driving torques, axial thrust forces, shear forces and bending moments imparted to them during operation. The grinding of flutes into a solid rod (known in machining terms as a blank) to produce a drill-bit significantly alters both the rotational and bending stiffness properties. In the presence of excessive driving torques a drill bit can unravel (Narasimha, Osman et al. 1987), but this is rarely reported complication in the orthopaedic literature. Drill-bits are routinely subjected to bending loads, such as those depicted in Figure 6.

Three modes of bending are depicted in Figure 6; bending scenarios a and b relate to measures taken by the surgeon to counter the likelihood of the drill-tip to skive. Bending scenario c describes the situation where the drill-tip skives along the endosteal surface of the far cortex, inducing a bending moment. As the surgeon is blinded to activity at this location he or she cannot toggle the handpiece to compensate for this skiving and relieve the built-up bending moment. The idealised drill-bit depicted in the following figure responds to the moments and shear loads by deforming in the x-z plane of the global reference frame, the extent of which is governed by the flexural rigidity (EI_X), which is a function of the material properties (Young's modulus, E - MPa) and second (area) moment of inertia (I_X – mm^4) of the drill's cross section. Surgical drills are typically manufactured from surgical grade stainless steel (316L), although an alloy of titanium (Ti_6Al_4V) has also been used (Jochum and Reichart 2000). The physicochemical properties of these materials falls outside the scope of this work and will not be elaborated further.

5.1 Second (area) moment of inertia - I

The deformation profile in the y-z plane of a solid cylindrical bar subjected to the conditions depicted in the preceding figure would be, like the cross-sectional area uniform and therefore independent of drill-bit rotation. Conversely, the response of the fluted portion of a 2-fluted drill-bit is a function of both the cross-sectional area and rotation relative to a global reference frame. A cross-sectional view of the fluted portion of a 2-fluted drill-bit is shown in Figure 7.

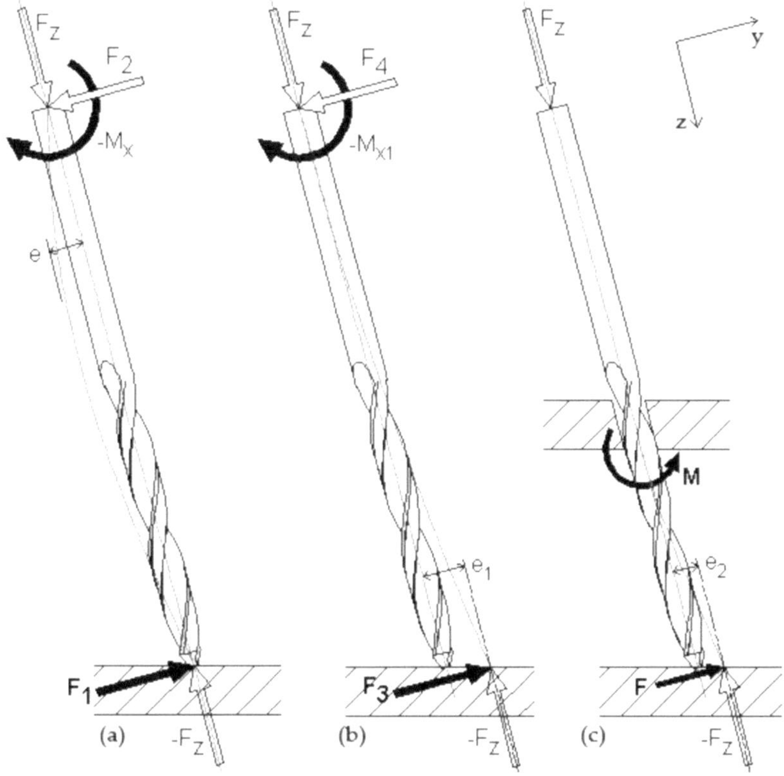

Fig. 6. Bending modes for a surgical drill. The deformation profile of the two-fluted drill-bit under each scenario is idealised and does not take into account the variation in second (area) moment of inertia properties along the length of the drill. (Bertollo, Gothelf et al. 2008)

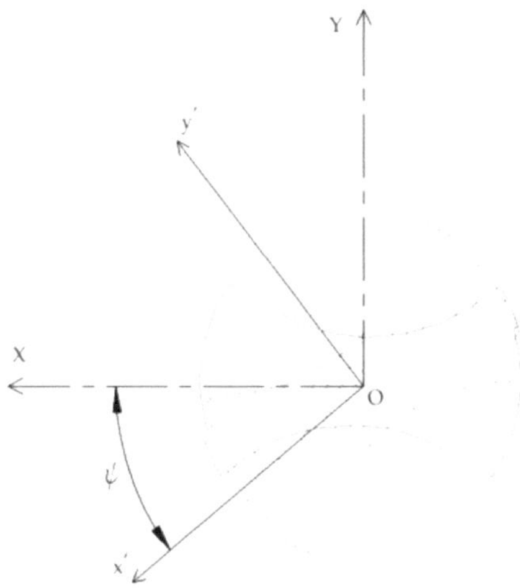

Fig. 7. Cross-section of a typical 2-fluted orthopaedic drill-bit. The second (area) moment of inertia of the fluted portion of the drill changes with rotation, ψ, of the cross-section relative to the global (x-y) coordinate system

In the above figure the x-y axes indicate orientation of the global reference frame, whilst the x′ and y′ axes are axes of symmetry of the cross-section. The second (area) moment of inertia, I_X, at any point along the length of the fluted portion of the drill as a function of drill rotation, ψ, is given by:

$$I_x=\int_A y^2 dA=\left[\frac{I_{max}+I_{min}}{2}+\frac{I_{max}-I_{min}}{2}\sin 2\theta - I_{xy}\sin 2\varphi\right] \quad (1)$$

where I_{max} and I_{min} is the moment of inertia taken about the x′ and y′ axes. As such, I_{max} and I_{min} are the principal moments of inertia. Furthermore, due to the symmetry inherent in the section the product of inertia, I_{xy}, tends to zero, such that the I_X of a 2-fluted drill-bit is therefore given by:

$$I_x=\left[\frac{I_{max}+I_{min}}{2}+\frac{I_{max}-I_{min}}{2}\sin 2\varphi\right] \quad (2)$$

The polar moment of inertia, I_Z, determines the torsional rigidity of the drill which is independent of rotation is given by:

$$I_z=I_{max}+I_{min} \quad 3$$

Where the torque applied to the drill overwhelms the polar moment of inertia the drill begins to unravel. There is anecdotal evidence to suggest that this type of failure mode does occur but is extremely rare.
In our previous work we have demonstrated that the I_X profile varies along the length of a 2-fluted drill-bit with rotation (Figure 8). Conversely, I_X of a 3-fluted drill does not vary as a

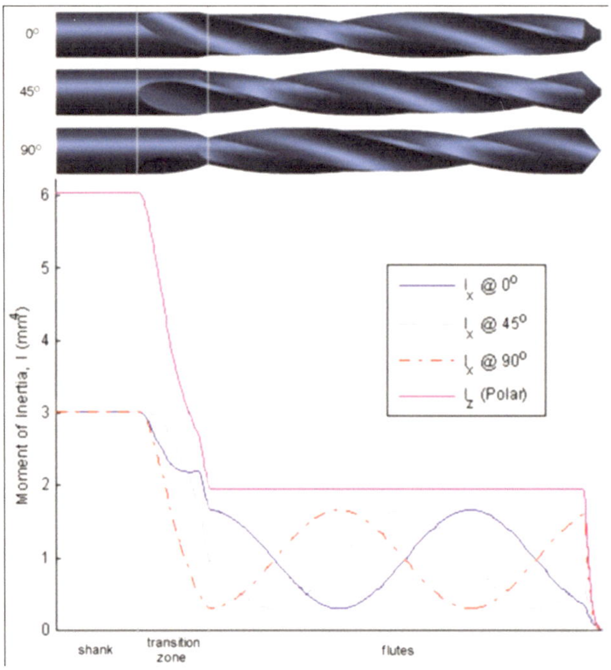

Fig. 8. I_X and I_Z profiles for a 2-fluted drill-bit. (Bertollo, Gothelf et al. 2008)

function of rotation (Figure 9). This property occurs as a result of the inherent symmterical arrangement of material about the prinical axes, such that the principal moments of inertia (I_{max} and I_{max}) are equal in magnitude and the relation in equation 2 becomes independent of rotation.

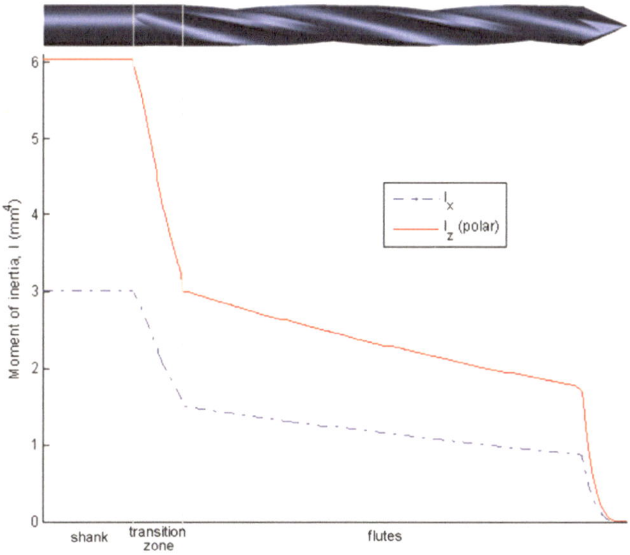

Fig. 9. I_X and I_Z profiles for a 3-fluted drill-bit. (Bertollo, Gothelf et al. 2008)

Two-fluted drills tend to deflect in the weaker principal direction under the action of a bending moment. Whilst the I_X and I_Y profiles for presented figures 8 and 9 are based on two different drill types the same general result applies to all drills. It follows that the flexural rigidity of 2-fluted and 3-fluted drill-bits are inherently different; this property varies as a function of rotation for 2-fluted drills but not 3-fluted drill-bits (Stephenson and Agapiou 1997; Bertollo, Gothelf et al. 2008). This has direct implications for the extent of skiving whilst drilling at oblique orientations as well as drill-bit breakage under the application of a bending moment (Bertollo, Gothelf et al. 2008). Generally, a diameter-matched three-fluted drill-bit is less likely to fail under the application of a bending moment.

6. Wear and dulling of the cutting face

Cutting edges of the drill-bit are mechanically and thermally loaded during machining. Cumulative wear at the cutting face has a deleterious effect on cutting efficiency of surgical drill-bits. This is manifest as a patent increase in the required axial thrust force, an increase in maximal temperature of bone and the initiation of vibration (due to an increase in surface roughness of the cutting edges). Scanning electron microscopy (SEM) is one imaging modality which can be used to analyse wear at the cutting edges. The primary types of wear seen at the cutting tip are abrasive wear and plastic deformation (Ercoli, Funkenbusch et al. 2004; Allan, Williams *et al.* 2005a; Marciniak, Z. Paszenda *et al.* 2007), which irreversibly modifies the dimensions and geometry of the chisel and cutting edges, as well as the rake face. Craters can also form on the rake face. Allan and colleagues (Allan, Williams *et al.*

2005b) investigated the effects of differing degrees of wear on maximum temperature elevation in cortical bone *in vitro*. Holes were drilled in porcine mandibles using drill-bits (1.5mm diameter, 2-fluted Leibinger) which were fresh, used in the preparation of 600 holes and taken directly from theatres and temperatures recorded. Six-hundred holes was the amount required to produce a statistically significant elevation in temperature compared to the fresh drill-bits (control). The extent of wear at the cutting face can be seen in Figure 10.

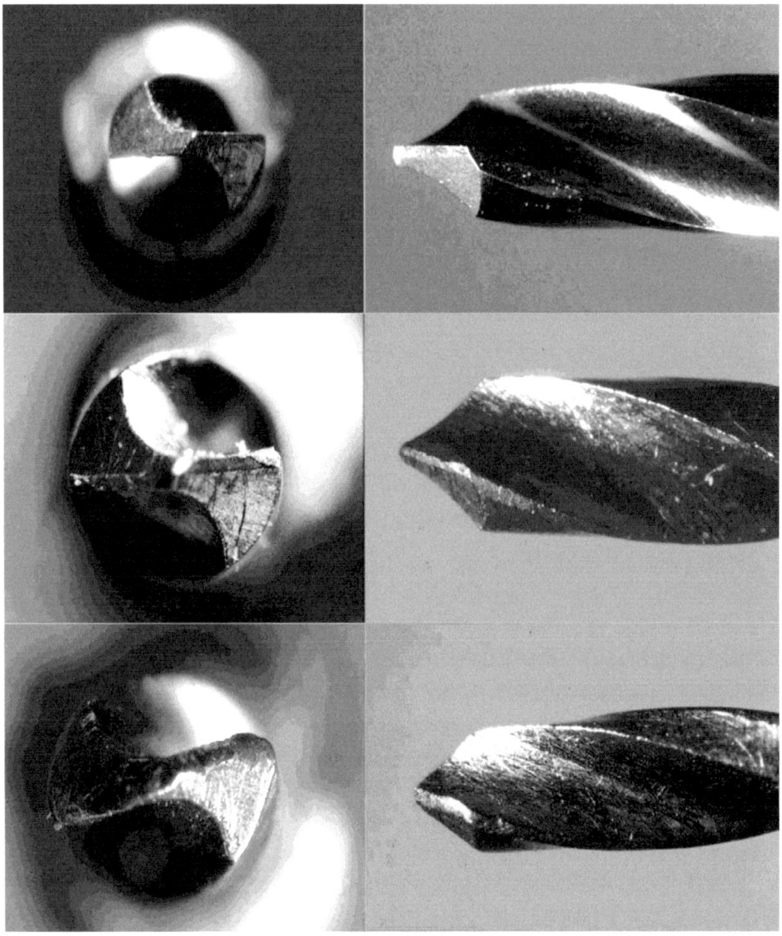

Fig. 10. End and side image taken of three 1.5mm diameter 2-fluted Leibinger drill-bits. Top: fresh. Middle: following the drilling of 600 holes. Bottom: Drill-bit taken directly from theatres. The drill-bit depicted has a split-point design. (Allan, Williams et al. 2005b)

In the above figure substantial wear of the chisel and cutting edges can be seen in the drill-bit following the preparation of 600 holes. In the case of the drill-bit taken from theatre wear is so extreme that both chisel and cutting edges are virtually indistinguishable. There was no indication given as to the estimated number of orthopaedic procedures this particular drill-bit was utilised in. It is not surprising that in their study a linear relationship between maximal temperature rise and wear was detected, with a maximum 54.5°C measured using the drill obtained directly from theatres.

Seventy-five percent of surveyed hospitals in the United Kingdom do not routinely monitor their surgical instruments for sharpness and wear (Singh, Davenport *et al.* 2010). Up to 45% of hospitals surveyed in the United Kingdom are utilising single-use drill-bits (Singh, Davenport et al. 2010), but for all intents and purposes orthopaedic surgical drill-bits are multiple-use items (Ashford, Pande *et al.* 2001). They are distinctly different from oscillating saw blades (another source of heat generation) and other cutting tools used in orthopaedic surgery in that they are not considered or treated as consumables.

Many researchers from both the maxillofacial and orthopaedic sub-specialities have demonstrated a positive correlation between repeated use and maximal temperature elevation. Jochum and Reichart (Jochum and Reichart 2000) demonstrated the effects of repeated drilling on the maximal temperature rise in bone, showing a positive correlation in the porcine mandible. In this study holes were created by a single operator whilst applying only minimal pressure. Harris and Kohles (Harris and Kohles 2001) employed a polymeric test bed to assess the effects of repeated use and sterilisation on drilling performance, concluding that there is a negative correlation with both. Chacon and co-workers (Chacon, Bower et al. 2006) also encountered increased temperature elevation and visual wear signs with successive drilling episodes using a combination of 2- and 3-fluted drills in bovine femurs *in vitro*. Earlier, Matthews and Hirsch (Matthews and Hirsch 1972) demonstrated a negative relationship between wear through repeated use and magnitude of the maximal temperature elevation in cadaveric femora. Garcia *et al* (Garcia, Mombiela et al. 2004) studied the effects of intramedullary reaming on cortical bone temperatures in an *in vivo* minipig model. Using the same instruments in all preparations the maximum temperatures encountered became progressively greater, reaching as high as 49.4°C, but was not associated with any histological evidence of osteonecrosis.

Considering the cost of a single drill-bit can be more than USD$100 a more economical alternative is reconditioning and reprocessing surgical drill-bits when they become blunt. Darvish *et al* (Darvish, Shafieian et al. 2009) investigated the ability of this process to restore the pristine geometry of the cutting tip, by measuring parameters such as lip length, chisel edge length and chisel edge angle and subsequently found that drilling efficiency was most sensitive to chisel edge length and angle.

Protective coatings have been applied to drills with the intention of improving durability but which have not been shown to be entirely effective (Ercoli, Funkenbusch et al. 2004). Another important consideration is delamination of these coatings during the cutting process as they may elicit a foreign body reaction when left *in situ*.

7. Complications

Intraoperative complications associated with the use of drill-bits includes drill-bit breakage (Fothi, Perren et al. 1992; Hirt, Auer et al. 1992; Benirschke, Melder *et al.* 1993; Miller 2002; Price, Molloy *et al.* 2002; Matthews, Landsmeer *et al.* 2006; Bodner, Woldenberg *et al.* 2007; Bassi, Pankaj *et al.* 2008; Pichler, Mazzurana *et al.* 2008; Gupta, Singh *et al.* 2009; Kosy and Standley 2010) and heat generation (Berning and Fowler). Another cause for concern, albeit a rarely reported complication, is microfracture of host bone adjacent to the drilled defect. This can occur as a consequence of the jarring action associated with cutting a structurally isotropic material that is bone, the severity of which can be exacerbated by a blunted drill-tip.

Excessively high temperatures may be generated at the orthotopic drilling site during the surgical procedure. The maximal rise in temperature during surgery is determined by a

number of operational variables including axial thrust force, drill-bit diameter, rotational speed, provision of irrigation and condition of the cutting tools .i.e. extent of fouling and blunting of the surgical drill-bit. Maximal temperatures in excess of 100˚C are not uncommon during the machining of bone with rotational cutting tools.
Whilst minimising the duration and magnitude of the maximum temperature elevation during the machining of bone during drilling and burring is of paramount importance and concern for the surgeon, consideration must also be given to the frictional heat and temperatures generated in the bearings of high-speed drills and drivers. At these speeds frictional heat within the tools themselves can produce temperatures in excess of 60˚C which can produce burns in the mouth of the patient or to tissue adjacent to the surgical site, as well to others handling the instrument (Anonymous 2008).

7.1 Intraoperative complications

7.1.1 Drill-bit breakage

It is reported that the drill-bit is the most frequently broken surgical instrument (Fothi, Perren et al. 1992; Hirt, Auer et al. 1992; Miller 2002; Price, Molloy et al. 2002; Pichler, Mazzurana et al. 2008) which represents a considerable dilemma for surgeons due to the complexities associated with removal of the broken portion from either the bone or medullary canal (Matthews, Landsmeer et al. 2006; Bassi, Pankaj et al. 2008). Actual breakage rates have been reported to vary between 0.14% (11/7,775 orthopaedic cases) (Price, Molloy et al. 2002), 0.194% (23/11,856 orthopaedic cases) (Pichler, Mazzurana et al. 2008) and 0.3% (3/1000 internal fixation procedures) (Hirt, Auer et al. 1992). It is generally agreed that actual rates are higher but that this complication is frequently under-reported. The primary reason for failure is the application of an excessive bending moment during operation, which overwhelms the bending strength (Flexural Rigidity, EI) of the drill-bit.

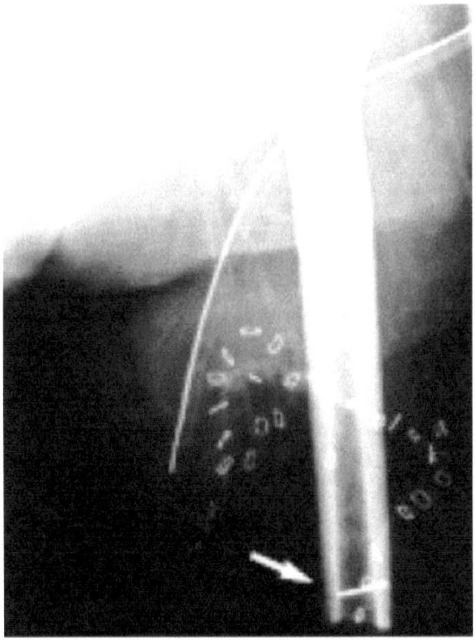

Fig. 11. Radiograph of a broken drill-bit embedded in a femur and left *in situ*. (Wolfson, Seeger *et al.* 2000)

Surgical drill-bits are manufactured from biologically inert materials and broken portions for this reason can be left *in situ* without any complications or concern. An important consideration for the surgeon, however, is whether a broken fragment is in contact with an implant as micromotion can generate wear particles and possibly metal ions. If sufficiently large these particles, whose physical size precludes them from being digested may elicit an inflammatory response resulting in osteolysis.

7.1.2 Heat generation

Drilling is also associated with the generation of thermal energy, causing a transient rise in temperature of bone and soft tissues as well as the drill-bit itself. Due to definite limitations imposed on intraoperative measurement of temperature the examination of bone drilling and heat generation has typically been performed in the *in vitro* laboratory setting by research groups from many surgical sub-specialities, including the orthopaedic, dental, maxillofacial and neurological fields. *In vivo* animal models (to be explored in a later section) have provided an additional biological endpoint in the determination of the reaction of cortical bone to heat exposure. Several seemingly subtle but fundamental differences between these studies, both in terms of the hardware (drills versus burs) as well as applied axial thrust force and drilling rotational speed exist. High speeds of 10,000 to 400,000rpm are routinely used for drilling and burring in dental applications, whilst considerably lower speeds (less then 1000rpm) are typically used in orthopaedic procedures. There seems to be little consensus in the literature, however, regarding the effects of these and other operational variables on the magnitude of the maximal temperature elevation in cortical bone. Furthermore, the reported range in maximal temperatures measured across these said experiments is also substantial.

Matthews and Hirsch (Matthews and Hirsch 1972) frequently measured maximum temperatures well in excess of 100°C whilst drilling holes in cadaveric femora with a 3.2mm diameter 2-fluted drill. They found increasing rotation speed from 345 to 2900prm to have little influence on the maximal temperature attained. Conversely, increasing axial thrust force from approximately 20 to 120N was associated with decreases in both maximum temperatures and their durations. Augustin *et al* (Augustin, Davila et al. 2008) likewise provided evidence for a reduction in peak temperature by increasing the feed rate. A limitation of their study is that the relationship between feed-rate and axial thrust force as a function of drill-bit diameter was not presented. In cadaveric femurs Bachus and colleagues (Bachus, Rondina et al. 2000) encountered both a reduction in magnitude and duration of the maximum temperature with increasing axial thrust force (53, 83, 93 and 130N) in the absence of irrigation using 3.2mm diameter drills at 820rpm. Hillery and Shauib (Hillery and Shuaib 1999) detected a significant decrease in the magnitude of the maximal temperature elevation with increasing drill speed (400 to 2000 rpm), also at a diameter level of 3.2mm.

Sharawy and co-workers (Sharawy, Misch *et al.* 2002) demonstrated a reduction in temperature elevation with increasing rotation rate (1225 to 2500 rpm) across a range of drill-bit diameters (1.5 to 4.2mm) during manual drilling of porcine mandibles. The drilling systems used in this study were both internally and externally irrigated. Iyer *et al* (Iyer, Weiss *et al.* 1997a) likewise found an inverse relationship between drill speed and the maximal temperature elevation in rabbit tibiae. Intraoperative measurements were made with the animal sedated whilst using burs to create cylindrical defects at low (2500rpm), intermediate (100,000rpm) and high (400,000rpm) rotation speeds. Intermittent pressure was applied by a single surgeon during drilling. Also using 2 to 3.25mm diameter burrs from the dental realm Brisman (Brisman 1996) demonstrated that increasing both axial thrust force and rotation speed independently from 120 to 240N and 1800 to 2400rpm, respectively, causes an increase in maximal temperature elevation. Conversely, increasing both rotation rate and axial thrust force concurrently had no effect on temperature and simultaneously increased drilling efficiency. Whilst this data was derived using burrs and is therefore not directly applicable to drill-bits these results do suggest that these operational variables can have a synergistic effect on temperature elevation.

Investigating burring speeds from 400 to 40,000rpm on temperature elevation in bovine cortical bone Reingewirt *et al* (Reingewirtz, Szmukler-Moncler *et al.* 1997) identified a pseudo-bimodal correlation between rotation speed and maximal temperature elevation, which correlated positively from 400 to 7,000 rpm, at which point the correlation became negative. At lower speeds (400 to 800rpm) enhanced axial thrust force (80 to 200N) had no effect on temperature. Using similar tissue and hardware, Krause (Krause, Bradbury *et al.* 1982) found that the effects of increased rotation speeds (20,000 to 100,000rpm) on temperature were dependent on the type of bur. In other words, the magnitude of the maximal temperature rise was more sensitive to geometric variables.

As has been shown there appears to be little agreement in the *in vitro* literature regarding the effects of rotational speed, feed-rate and thrust force on the maximal temperature attained during the drilling of bone, which may be indicative of the significant effects of drill-bit geometry on the maximal temperature elevation. Davidson and James (Davidson and James 2003) used a finite element (FE) model to demonstrate a positive relationship between maximum temperature and rotation speed, feed rate and axial thrust force, as well as a quasi-linear relationship between maximal temperature elevation and drill diameter. Their model, however, did not take into account the transfer of heat between bone chips and rake face of the tool nor friction between the cutting edge and new surface (regions 2 and 3 in Figure 5, respectively). Other FE models (Lee, Rabin *et al.* 2011) have taken these effects into account and demonstrated that the convection of heat at this interface and along the length of the fluted portion has a substantial effect on heat dissipation during drilling.

Toews and colleagues (Toews, Bailey et al. 1999) examined the effect of feed rate and drill speed on the maximal temperatures recorded in equine bone and found increasing feed rate was associated with decreased maximal temperature, whilst increasing rotation speed (317 to 1242rpm) increased mean maximal temperature. Increasing cortical thickness was also positively correlated with increasing mean maximal temperature. Cortical bone is of a finite thickness, which has definite implications for temperature elevation. One would reasonably surmise that increased axial force and feed rate would produce lower temperatures purely as a function of reduced drilling time. Cordioli and others (Cordioli and Majzoub 1997) demonstrated a clear relationship between drilling depth and maximum temperature in bovine femurs with 2 and 3mm diameter drills operating at 1500rpm with 200N applied axial load. Using cadaveric and bovine bone with markedly different cortical thicknesses Hillery and Shuaib (Hillery and Shuaib 1999) encountered significantly higher temperatures in bovine bone than in human bone whilst keeping the operational and geometric parameters constant. They attributed this result to the difference in mean cortical thickness between the cadaveric (3 to 5mm) and bovine (7 to 9 mm) samples. Eriksson *et al* (Eriksson, Albrektsson *et al.* 1984a) measured *in vivo* temperature elevations during drilling of rabbit, dog and human tibiae, encountering temperatures of 40°, 56° and 89°, respectively, under similar conditions. The differences in this study were also attributed to the difference in cortical thickness between species.

We recently tested the cutting efficiency and thermal profile of commercially available 2- and 3-fluted 3.2mm diameter surgical drill-bits in porcine bone *in vitro* (Bertollo, Milne et al. 2010). Characteristic feed rates for each drill-bit at the experimentally-determined upper and lower 95% CI bounds of axial thrust force were determined, with both 3-fluted drills requiring significantly higher feed rates to reproduce these forces. Despite the finding of improved cutting efficiency for the 3-fluted drills, this did not translate into a significant and parallel reduction in maximum cortical temperatures for both 3-fluted drills either in the presence or absence of external cooling.

Many investigators have examined the effects of operational drilling parameters on the maximal temperature experienced during drilling of bone. A large proportion of these studies have assumed that drilling speed remains constant during drilling and this may not be the case. Abouzgia and James (Abouzgia and James 1995) demonstrated that rotational speed decreases by as much as 50% during drilling.

7.1.2.1 Intraoperative temperature abatement strategies

In orthopaedic surgery external irrigation with sterile saline delivered via a syringe or other device is routinely applied during drilling, the efficacy of which has been demonstrated by several authors (Matthews and Hirsch 1972; Jacob and Berry 1976; Lavelle and Wedgwood 1980; Krause, Bradbury et al. 1982; Kondo, Okada *et al.* 2000; Camargo, Faria et al. 2007; Augustin, Davila et al. 2008; Sener, Dergin *et al.* 2009). Utilising a numerical model, Lee and co-workers (Lee, Rabin et al. 2011) modelled the effect of coolant applied to the shank and exposed fluted portion of the operational drill-bit, demonstrating that this application may have a significant effect on the maximum drill temperature, even in the advanced stages of drilling where the cutting face is embedded deep in the bone. This has important implications in the case of bi-cortical drilling as this result suggests that coolant applied to the shank may act to limit/reduce the maximal temperature experienced at the isolated far cortex, and is due to the relatively high thermal conductivity of surgical-grade stainless steel compared to bone.

Closed-loop and open internal cooling systems are available but are primarily limited to orthodontic and dental applications (Haider, Watzek *et al.* 1993; Sharawy, Misch et al. 2002; Silverstein 2007). Closed-loop cooling systems are those in which coolant courses through tubules and tunnels incorporated into the drill-bit or bur itself and back through a central heat exchanger. Thermal energy generated at the machining face heats the coolant through a mechanism of conduction, thereby preventing an increase in temperature of the bone to above a critical level. In open cooling systems fluid courses through tubules in the drill but exits through openings at the cutting tip, thereby absorbing heat but also providing some lubrication in the process of cutting. This, of course depends on the precise location of the outlet(s) in relation to the cutting edges. Strictly speaking, however, the application of coolants by external means does not lubricate the cutting process, as it is applied against the direction of swarf flow.

Using an ovine model, Haider and colleagues (Haider, Watzek et al. 1993) compared the biological response of compact (cortical) and spongy (cancellous) bone to implants placed into defects created in the presence of both internal and external manual cooling. Interestingly, on the basis of histological results at 4 weeks following implantation it was

found that externally applied manual cooling versus internal cooling was more beneficial to the biological response (implant bone ongrowth) at the cancellous site, but was only advantageous at superficial cortex depths. Internal cooling provided a distinct benefit at the deeper drill levels in compact bone. At later timepoints of 8 and 16 weeks no appreciable differences were observed between the sites as a function of irrigation type. The result obtained from the cancellous site adds strength to the argument that externally applied coolant may limit maximal temperature elevation even in the advanced stage of drilling (Lee, Rabin et al. 2011), such as at the far cortex in the case of bi-cortical drilling. Admittedly, little research has been directed at the temperature elevation in cancellous bone during drilling, with most if not all research having been conducted in a compact bone bed.
Pre-drilling and pilot hole creation are other methods which have been advocated to reduce the biological effects of heat generated during drilling (Matthews and Hirsch 1972). Using dental burs, however, Reinewirtz *et al* (Reingewirtz, Szmukler-Moncler et al. 1997) were unable to convey a benefit in terms of reduced temperature elevation but did observe a reduction in the drilling time. Sequential drilling at larger diameters is also performed to reduce maximal temperatures (Bubeck, Garcia-Lopez *et al.* 2009). Intermittent drilling/burring has also been advocated as a means to reduce maximal temperature elevation (Kondo, Okada et al. 2000).

7.2 Post-operative complications

7.2.1 Broken drill-bit portions

In today's medicolegal environment there have been several reported cases of compensation received by patients and fines issued to hospitals as a result of broken drill-bits left *in situ* without the patient's knowledge (Burruss 2010). Despite this there are still surgeons who do not routinely inform their patients of intraoperative drill bit failure. There are no reports in the literature of adverse reactions to portions of broken drill-bit which have been left *in situ* causing morbidities which have necessitated re-operation for removal, which is representative of the biologically inert nature of the materials used in drill-bit manufacture.

7.2.2 Thermonecrosis and failure of implant fixation

A by-product of the drilling process is the generation of heat energy, which causes a transient increase in temperature of the bone and soft tissues as well as the drill-bit itself. Whilst there is no consensus regarding critical values or their durations an increase above 47˚C of the cortical bone has been implicated with a reduced regenerative capacity and osteonecrosis (Lundskog 1972; Matthews and Hirsch 1972; Eriksson and Albrektsson 1983; Eriksson and Albrektsson 1984; Eriksson, Albrektsson et al. 1984b). Despite an acute awareness of the association between drilling and temperature rises in bone there are few reports in the clinical orthopaedic literature of complications or implant failures which could be attributed to this. One notable exception was a recent report by Berning *et al* (Berning and Fowler) presenting a case of a patient having osteomyelitis of the proximal tibia due to thermal necrosis following tracker pin placement in computer-navigated total knee arthroplasty. In fact, it appears that most of the evidence in the literature pertaining to thermonecrosis could most suitably be described as being anecdotal. A major limitation in determining thermonecrosis has occurred as a result of surgical intervention and drilling is a lack of hard evidence. Radiographic presentation of thermonecrosis is denoted by the presence of a phenomenon known as ring sequestrum around a drill hole (Figure 12).

Thermonecrosis remains a cause for concern for surgeons in the case of cemented fixation of components in joint arthroplasty also. The polymerisation of bone cement (Polymethylmethacrylate, PMMA) is an exothermic reaction in which a significant amount of heat energy is released. These excessive temperatures can lead to the resorption of bone adjacent to the cement mantle which can result in aseptic loosening of implants and failure of joint prostheses. Despite several research efforts there still remains a lack of consensus in the literature regarding critical temperature values and their durations. PMMA cement is also widely used to fill orthotopic defects which have arisen from the removal of tumours and compression fractures. One example is the utilisation of PMMA by spinal surgeons to stabilise osteoporotic compression fractures of the vertebral body, where temperatures in the cortex can reach 113°C (Belkoff and Molloy 2003).

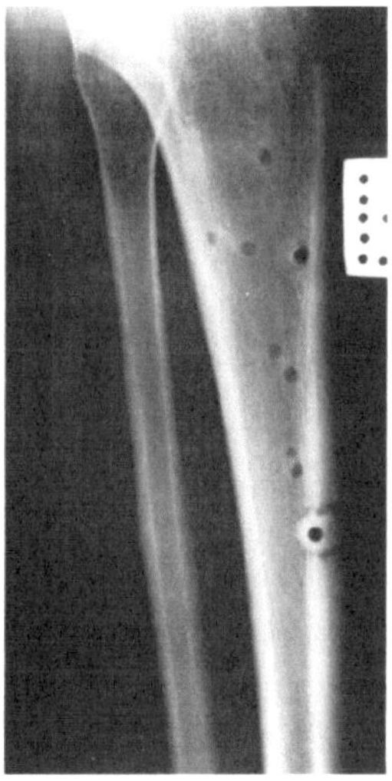

Fig. 12. Radiographic appearance of thermal necrosis as ring sequestrum. Image obtained following in vitro testing of human cadaveric tibiae (Matthews, Green *et al.* 1984)

8. Biological models in thermonecrosis research

Animal models have been heavily utilised to explore the effects of elevated temperatures on the viability of cells and bone. The obvious benefit to the use of animals in research is the availability of affected and control tissues for the experimental endpoints. Specifically, *in vivo* studies have been conducted in the ovine, laprine, porcine and canine models, and it appears that the extent of the effects which heat has on bone tissue depends on the maximal temperature attained and duration of the exposure. Of particular interest in these studies is viability of cortical bone following a thermal insult, with a histological hallmark of osteonecrosis being the presence of empty osteocyte lacunae (Eriksson, Albrektsson et al. 1984b; Franssen, van Diest et al. 2008) (Figure 13).

Using rabbits, Eriksson *et al* (Eriksson, Albrektsson et al. 1984b) created full-thickness defects in the femoral diaphysis using a 3mm diameter drill-bit at 20,000rpm with irrigation. In the same cohort of animals, fibulae were resected and excised and placed into heated saline baths maintained at 47°, 50°, 56° and 60° for 1 minute. Animals were sacrificed immediately following the procedure and cylindrical defect sites processed histologically where it was found that surrounding each of the defects was a 200µm radial zone of empty osteocyte lacunae. Immunohistological analysis of the tissue, however, painted a more severe picture of detrimental changes in the bone surrounding the defect. Using this method the necrotical border appeared to be radially dispersed at an average of 500µm, as determined by the absence of diaphorase enzyme activity. These intracellular enzymes are produced only by metabolically active cells. In an earlier study Eriksson and Albrektsson (Eriksson and Albrektsson 1983) performed a study in rabbits in which the cortical bone was heated to 47°C for varying durations and found the development of osteonecrosis with exposure for 1 minute. Lundskog (Lundskog 1972) observed that if bone is exposed to temperatures above 50°C for 30s cellular necrosis will occur.

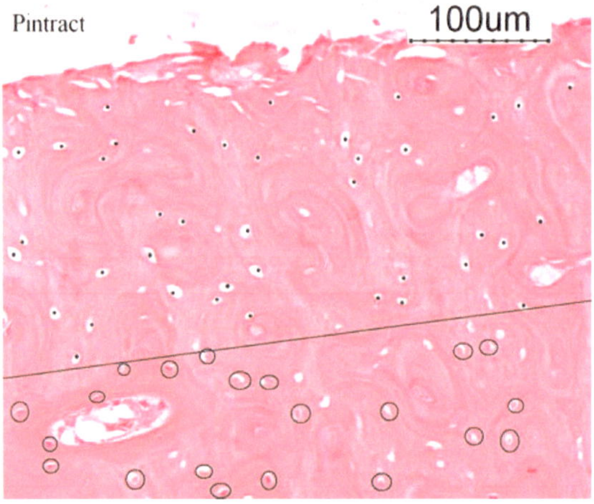

Fig. 13. Histological image (hematoxylin and eosin stain) depicting necrotic bone adjacent to a pintract denoted by the presence of empty osteocyte lacunae (dots). Healthy osetocytes (circled) are also evident. (Franssen, van Diest et al. 2008)

Franssen *et al* (Franssen, van Diest et al. 2008) investigated the biological effects of k-wire implantation on the viability of cortical bone in rabbits. Using a carefully constructed jig, trochar-tipped k-wires were drilled into the tibiae and femur under a constant load and speed of 1.5kg and 1200rpm, respectively. Evidence of osteonecrosis, denoted by the presence of empty osteocyte lacunae was evident immediately following recovery and at 4 weeks postoperatively (Figure 13). Ardan and co-workers (Ardan, Janes *et al.* 1957) heated surgically-created defects in canine femurs ultrasonically and detected delayed unions in addition to osteonecrosis.

The effect of exposure to heat on the osteogenic potential for healing and bone formation has also been explored using animal models. In rabbits, Ohashi and colleagues (Ohashi, Therin *et al.* 1994a) found bone formation in 4mm diameter defects prepared in the cortical bone of the tibia with a rotation speed of 5000rpm was significantly less that that associated with 500rpm. The authors attributed this result to the presence of thermonecrosis and vascular obstructions at the margin of the defect site. In a second cohort of animals cylindrical defects were created using the same conditions and drill type but which were subsequently filled with porous HA implant dowels (Ohashi, Therin *et al.* 1994c). The purpose of this study was to examine the effects of site preparation and osteotomy on the bony response to the implantation of an osteoconductive biomaterial, as would be the case for uncemented fixation of implants in joint arthroplasty. As their earlier result had intimated an increased amount of bone ingrowth associated with the HA dowels implanted into 3.3mm diameter defects created at 500rpm versus those prepared at 5000rpm was detected 4 weeks postoperatively. By 12 weeks, however, the differential in bone formation between sites, which was significant, had diminished, suggesting high speed drilling affects the short-term bony response to biomaterials. Ohashi's group (Ohashi, Therin *et al.* 1994b) also demonstrated a statistically significant dependence of the healing response on anatomical aspect, namely the radial direction, within the ovine metatarsal bone, with no difference observed in the longitudinal dimension of the bone.

Iyer *et al* (Iyer, Weiss et al. 1997a) measured intraoperative temperature elevation in the rabbit tibia during the preparation of 3mm diameter holes using a bur at low (2500rpm), intermediate (100,000rpm) and high (400,000rpm) rotation speeds. All drilling was performed by a single surgeon, with no additional provisions being made to control axial thrust force. No quantitative analysis of the histology was performed of the tibiae but a correlation between the maximal temperature and osteogenic potential was confirmed in a later study using the same hardware and methods, again in rabbits (Iyer, Weiss *et al.* 1997b). Specifically, as the speed of the osteotomies increased a greater rate and better quality of bone regeneration was observed 6 weeks postoperatively. In both these studies external irrigation was applied during burring.

Our group has previously investigated the effects of heat generation on the healing response and fixation of pedicle screws (pull-out strength) in the ovine model (Bertollo, Milne et al. 2010). We tested a novel 3-fluted drill-bit against commercially-available 2- and 3-fluted drill-bits. In part 1 of the study we detected significant differences between the drills in terms of the maximal heat generation in porcine bone *in vitro*. Based on these results we predicted that temperatures in excess of 60°C would be produced during the intraoperative creation of pilot holes in the ovine tibia into which the pedicle screws were implanted. Despite *in vitro* differences in maximal temperatures between the drills this did not translate into a marked improvement in either the fixation of pedicle screws as determined by a mechanical pullout test or histological appearance of the screw-bone interface following 2, 4 and 6 weeks *in situ*. No evidence of osteonecrosis was found at the drill sites at either timepoint. Hillery and Shuaib (Hillery and Shuaib 1999) conducted an *in vitro* screw pullout test in cadaveric and bovine bone to determine if the temperature rise during drilling of the pilot hole had implications for time zero fixation but found no differences, despite temperatures in the vicinity of the drilled defects reaching between 102 to 117.8°C.

Stubinger and others (Stubinger, Biermeier *et al.* 2010) employed an ovine model to evaluate the capabilities of alternatives to the mechanical machining of bone which have been introduced in the dental field, including Er:YAG lasers and piezoelectric devices. Defects were created in the pelvis using these methods as well as by conventional drilling. Histological and mechanical experimental endpoints confirmed that these methods were at least comparable to drill osteotomy in terms of bony response and implant fixation.

9. Measurement methods

Measurement of the temperature generated during drilling of bone has traditionally been performed using the classic thermocouple technique. More recently the decreased cost and increased availability of infrared thermal imaging cameras has resulted in their use for the experimental determination of temperature rises during drilling of bone (Udiljak, Ciglar *et al.* 2007; Augustin, Davila et al. 2008; Augustin, Davila *et al.* 2009; Bertollo, Milne et al. 2010; Yang, Wang *et al.* 2010). Both temporal methods of temperature measurement have their pros and cons. Infrared cameras are able to provide information regarding the distribution of temperature of the cortical bone surrounding the defect with greater resolution than is provided by a classic thermocouple nest (Augustin, Davila et al. 2009). Throughout the literature a total of three thermocouples are normally placed at increasing radial distances from the defect edge, with 0.5mm, 1mm and 3mm being normal values adopted. A major limitation of the thermocouple nest method is the time involved in preparing the pilot holes for the thermocouple probes, as well as an inability to measure the temperature at the tool-bone interface. Whilst this can theoretically be achieved using infrared imaging, a major limitation of this measurement method is a lack of depth perception in the data, that is, a complex three-dimensional field is simplified and reduced to a 2-dimensional planar dataset.

10. Future directions

Continual efforts are being directed at the improvement of drill-bit design to enhance performance for the surgeon and postoperative outcome for the patient. Ultrasonic assisted drilling is one such technology which applies ultrasonic vibrations along the longitudinal direction of the drill-bit to assist with the cutting process (Alam, Mitrofanov *et al.*). This technology has been shown to cause reductions in both axial thrust force and drilling torque. Feedback systems detecting real-time cortical break-through have also been developed (Allotta, Belmonte et al. 1996; Ong and Bouazza-Marouf 1998; Ong and Bouazza-Marouf 1999) with the intention of minimising the effect of break-through on hole geometry as well as minimising the damage inflicted to soft tissues by the drill-tip.

Alternatives to the mechanical machining of bone have been developed for dental operations, including Er:YAG lasers and piezoelectric devices (Stubinger, Biermeier et al. 2010). Piezoelectric osteotomy is based on ultrasonic vibration of an osteotomic device that permits precise cutting of bone structures without cutting adjacent soft tissues whilst lasers cause tissue ablation. These methods have the propensity to produce defects in an atraumatic manner which may have positive implications for healing.

11. Conclusion

The surgical drilling of bone is associated with the generation of heat which causes a transient rise in temperature of hard and soft tissues to above normal physiological levels. Depending on the magnitude of the maximal temperature attained and the duration for which the elevated temperature is maintained thermonecrosis of bone may ensue. Bone is particularly susceptible to high temperatures as it has a relatively low thermal conductivity, the implication being that heat is not easily dissipated. Coupled with a relatively low specific heat, the end result is that the inertial effect following a localised injection of heat can be considerable. The general consensus is that a temperature of 47°C is the critical threshold limit for thermonecrosis to occur in compact bone. This can have severe and dire implications for implant fixation as a result of osteoclastic resorption of necrotic bone. Osteogenic potential can also be compromised due to exposure to elevated temperatures which can hinder tissue infiltration and osseointegration required for biological fixation of implants, such as in uncemented joint arthroplasty.

The extent of the temperature rise during drilling in bone is affected by a number of operational and geometric variables, all of which have been studied extensively in the literature. Perhaps the most salient of the geometric variables, and certainly that which is reported consistently is dulling and wear of the cutting edges through repeated use which increases the axial thrust force required to propel the machining face through bone, causing a marked increase in maximal temperature elevation. Inevitably, imposing additional demand upon the surgeon compromises control which they are able to exert over the handpiece, that is, additional force increases the probability of uncontrolled plunging of the tip as well as cortical break-through. For all intents and purposes surgical drills are multiple use items, and a lack of routine monitoring in the hospital sterilisation departments may be the reason for blunted drill-bits remaining in circulation. Certainly, in our home country (Australia) a common complaint voiced by surgeons is the frequent encountering of dulled and blunted bits in clinical practice.

Operational variables affecting temperature elevation in bone are primarily axial thrust force and rotation speed. Many fundamental differences in the studies which have been performed regarding this rise during drilling exist. Firstly, they originate from many different surgical sub-specialities where there are subtle differences in hardware and protocol. Secondly, there is a considerable range in rotation speeds which have been investigated. High speed drilling and burring (2000 to 400,000rpm) is more pertinent to the dental and orthodontic applications whilst in orthopaedics speeds of typically less than 1000rpm are employed. Although the data which has been advanced in the literature is sometimes contradictory regarding the effects of these parameters, in general, increasing feed rate has been shown to decrease maximal temperature whilst increasing rotation speed has been shown to produce an increase. Intuitively, one would surmise that in the context of a finite cortical thickness a reduction in temperature would be realised based purely on a reduction in drilling time. If the transfer of heat during drilling is considered as time-dependent heat flux then it stands to reason that a reduction in drilling time reduces the heat energy injected into the system and, in turn, the maximum temperature attained.

There is definite agreement in the literature that temperatures well in excess of 100°C are possible during the surgical drilling of bone. Temperature abatement measures have been applied clinically, with the most effective strategy being the application of coolant. Sequential drilling has also been advocated to reduce temperatures, but which has the drawback of increased surgical time, and this can have considerable compounding effects. The heat generated during drilling in the absence of temperature abatement measures such as irrigation are comparable with those encountered during the curing of polymethylmethacrylate (bone cement). This material is heavily utilised in joint arthroplasty surgery for fixation of joint prostheses components to surgically-resected bone. Temperature abatement during the *in situ* polymerisation of PMMA bone cement is effectively an operational impossibility.

Both 2- and 3-fluted drills are in clinical use. Reports in the literature seem to suggest that diameter matched 3-fluted drills are more efficient than their 2-fluted counterparts. As has been demonstrated a reduction in drilling time due to increased feed rate can limit the magnitude of the temperature rise in bone. Three-fluted drills are also inherently stiffer and are less likely to fail under the application of a bending moment. Despite these potential benefits their use remains limited in surgical procedures entailing the cutting of bone.

12. References

Abouzgia, M. B. and D. F. James (1995). Measurements of shaft speed while drilling through bone. Journal of Oral and Maxillofacial Surgery 53(11): 1308-1315.

Abouzgia, M. B. and J. M. Symington (1996). Effect of drill speed on bone temperature. International Journal of Oral & Maxillofacial Surgery 25(5): 394-399.

Alam, K., A. V. Mitrofanov et al. Experimental investigations of forces and torque in conventional and ultrasonically-assisted drilling of cortical bone. Medical Engineering & Physics (In Press).

Allan, W., E. D. Williams et al. (2005a). Effects of repeated drill use on temperature of bone during preparation for osteosynthesis self-tapping screws. British Journal of Oral and Maxillofacial Surgery 43(4): 314-319.

Allan, W., E. D. Williams et al. (2005b). Effects of repeated drill use on temperature of bone during preparation for osteosynthesis self-tapping screws. British Journal of Oral & Maxillofacial Surgery 43(4): 314-319.

Allotta, B., F. Belmonte et al. (1996). Study on a mechatronic tool for drilling in the osteosynthesis of long bones: Tool/bone interaction, modeling and experiments. Mechatronics 6(4): 447-459.

Anonymous (2008). High-speed surgical drills may overheat and cause burns. Health Devices 37(7): 213-215.

Ardan, N. I. J., J. M. Janes et al. (1957). Ultrasonic energy and surgically produced defects in bone. J Bone Joint Surg Am 39-A(2): 394-402.

Ashford, R. U., K. C. Pande et al. (2001). Current practice regarding re-use of trauma instrumentation: results of a postal questionnaire survey. Injury 32: 37-40.

Augustin, G., S. Davila et al. (2008). Thermal osteonecrosis and bone drilling parameters revisited. Archives of Orthopaedic & Trauma Surgery 128(1): 71-77.

Augustin, G., S. Davila et al. (2009). Determination of spatial distribution of increase in bone temperature during drilling by infrared thermography: preliminary report. Archives of Orthopaedic & Trauma Surgery 129(5): 703-709.

Bachus, K. N., M. T. Rondina et al. (2000). The effects of drilling force on cortical temperatures and their duration: an in vitro study. Medical Engineering & Physics 22(10): 685-691.

Bassi, J. L., M. Pankaj et al. (2008). A technique for removal of broken cannulated drill bit: Bassi's method. Journal of Orthopaedic Trauma 22(1): 56-58.

Belkoff, S. M. and S. Molloy (2003). Temperature measurement during polymerization of polymethylmethacrylate cement used for vertebroplasty.[see comment]. Spine 28(14): 1555-1559.

Benirschke, S. K., I. Melder et al. (1993). Closed interlocking nailing of femoral shaft fractures: assessment of technical complications and functional outcomes by comparison of a prospective database with retrospective review. J Orthop Trauma 7(2): 118-122.

Berning, E. T. and R. M. Fowler Thermal Damage and Tracker-Pin Track Infection in Computer-Navigated Total Knee Arthroplasty. The Journal of Arthroplasty (Epub ahead of print)

Bertollo, N., T. K. Gothelf et al. (2008). 3-Fluted orthopaedic drills exhibit superior bending stiffness to their 2-fluted rivals: Clinical implications for targeting ability and the incidence of drill-bit failure. Injury 39(7): 734-741.

Bertollo, N., M. Matsubara et al. (2011). Effect of Surgical Fit on Integration of Cancellous Bone and Implant Cortical Bone Shear Strength for a Porous Titanium. Journal of Arthroplasty (In Press).

Bertollo, N., H. R. Milne et al. (2010). A Comparison of the Thermal Properties of 2- and 3-Fluted Drills and the Effects on Bone Cell Viability and Screw Pull-out Strength in an Ovine Model. Clinical Biomechanics 25(6): 613-617.

Bodner, L., Y. Woldenberg et al. (2007). Drill failure during ORIF of the mandible. Complication management. Med Oral Patol Oral Cir Bucal 12(8): E591-593.

Bonfield, W. and C. H. Li (1968). The temperature dependence of the deformation of bone. J Biomech 1(4): 323-329.

Brisman, D. L. (1996). The effect of speed, pressure, and time on bone temperature during the drilling of implant sites. International Journal of Oral & Maxillofacial Implants 11(1): 35-37.

Bubeck, K. A., J. Garcia-Lopez et al. (2009). In vitro comparison of cortical bone temperature generation between traditional sequential drilling and a newly designed step drill in the equine third metacarpal bone. Veterinary & Comparative Orthopaedics & Traumatology 22(6): 442-447.

Burruss, L. (2010). Hospital: Drill-bit piece accidentally left in patient's head: http://edition.cnn.com/2010/HEALTH/2010/2014/rhode.island.drill.bit/index.html.

Camargo, F. P., R. Faria et al. (2007). Poster #2780: Heat Production by Drilling Bone Tissue for Implant Procedures. Annual Meeting of the International Association for Dental Research, Ernest N. Morial Convention Cente, New Orleans, LA USA.

Chacon, G. E., D. L. Bower et al. (2006). Heat production by 3 implant drill systems after repeated drilling and sterilization. Journal of Oral & Maxillofacial Surgery 64(2): 265-269.

Chen, H. L. and A. A. Gundjian (1976). Specific heat of bone. Medical & Biological Engineering 14(5): 548-550.

Cordioli, G. and Z. Majzoub (1997). Heat generation during implant site preparation: an in vitro study. International Journal of Oral & Maxillofacial Implants 12(2): 186-193.

Darvish, K., M. Shafieian et al. (2009). The effect of tip geometry on the mechanical performance of unused and reprocessed orthopaedic drill bits Proceedings of the Institution of Mechanical Engineers, Part H: Journal of Engineering in Medicine 223(5): 625-635.

Davidson, S. R. and D. F. James (2003). Drilling in bone: modeling heat generation and temperature distribution. Journal of Biomechanical Engineering 125(3): 305-314.

Davidson, S. R. H. and D. F. James (2000). Measurement of thermal conductivity of bovine cortical bone. Medical Engineering & Physics 22(10): 741-747.

Easton, M. R. and P. V. Prewitt (1937). Ununited fracture treated by bone drilling. Journal of Bone & Joint Surgery - American Volume 19: 230-231.

Ercoli, C., P. D. Funkenbusch et al. (2004). The influence of drill wear on cutting efficiency and heat production during osteotomy preparation for dental implants: a study of drill durability. International Journal of Oral & Maxillofacial Implants 19(3): 335-349.

Eriksson, A. R. and T. Albrektsson (1983). Temperature threshold levels for heat-induced bone tissue injury: A vitalmicroscopic study in the rabbit. J Prosth Dent 50(1): 101-107.

Eriksson, A. R., T. Albrektsson et al. (1984a). Heat caused by drilling cortical bone. Temperature measured in vivo in patients and animals. Acta Orthop Scand. 55(6): 629-631.

Eriksson, R. A. and T. Albrektsson (1984). The effect of heat on bone regeneration: an experimental study in the rabbit using the bone growth chamber. Journal of Oral & Maxillofacial Surgery 42(11): 705-711.

Eriksson, R. A., T. Albrektsson et al. (1984b). Assessment of bone viability after heat trauma. A histological, histochemical and vital microscopic study in the rabbit. Scandinavian Journal of Plastic & Reconstructive Surgery 18(3): 261-268.

Fothi, U., S. M. Perren et al. (1992). Drill bit failure with implant involvement - an intraoperative complication in orthopaedic surgery. Injury 23(SUPPL. 2): S17-S29.

Franssen, B. B. G. M., P. J. van Diest et al. (2008). Drilling K-wires, what about the osteocytes? An experimental study in rabbits. Archives of Orthopaedic & Trauma Surgery 128(1): 83-87.

Garcia, O. G. R., F. L. Mombiela et al. (2004). The influence of the size and condition of the reamers on bone temperature during intramedullary reaming. Journal of Bone & Joint Surgery - American Volume 86-A(5): 994-999.

Gupta, R. K., H. Singh et al. (2009). Results of operative treatment of acetabular fractures from the Third World-how local factors affect the outcome. International Orthopaedics 33: 347-352.

Haider, R., G. Watzek et al. (1993). Effects of drill cooling and bone structure on IMZ implant fixation. Int J Oral Maxillofac Implants 8(1): 83-91.

Harris, B. H. and S. S. Kohles (2001). Effects of mechanical and thermal fatigue on dental drill performance. International Journal of Oral & Maxillofacial Implants 16(6): 819-826.

Hillery, M. T. and I. Shuaib (1999). Temperature Effects in the Drilling of Human and Bovine Bone. Journal of Materials Processing Technology 92-93: 302-308.

Hirt, U., J. A. Auer et al. (1992). Drill bit failure without implant involvement - an intraoperative complication in orthopaedic surgery. Injury 23(SUPPL. 2): S5-S16.

Hobkirk, J. A. and K. Rusiniak (1977). Investigation of variable factors in drilling bone. J Oral Surg. 35(12): 968-973.

Iyer, S., C. Weiss et al. (1997a). Effects of drill speed on heat production and the rate and quality of bone formation in dental implant osteotomies. Part I: Relationship between drill speed and heat production. International Journal of Prosthodontics 10(5): 411-414.

Iyer, S., C. Weiss et al. (1997b). Effects of drill speed on heat production and the rate and quality of bone formation in dental implant osteotomies. Part II: Relationship between drill speed and healing. International Journal of Prosthodontics 10(6): 536-540.

Jackson, C. J., S. K. Ghosh et al. (1989). On the evolution of drill-bit shapes. Journal of Mechanical Working Technology 18(2): 231-267.

Jacob, C. H. and J. T. Berry (1976). A study of the bone machining process--drilling. J Biomech: 343-349.

Jacob, C. H., M. H. Pope et al. (1974). A study of the bone machining process-orthogonal cutting. J Biomech 7(2): 131-136.

Jacobs, C. H., M. H. Pope et al. (1974). A study of the bone machining process-orthogonal cutting. J Biomech 7(2): 131-136.

Jochum, R. M. and P. A. Reichart (2000). Influence of multiple use of Timedur-titanium cannon drills: thermal response and scanning electron microscopic findings. Clin Oral Implants Res. 11(2): 139-143.

Kondo, S., Y. Okada et al. (2000). Thermological Study of Drilling Bone Tissue with a High-speed Drill. Neurosurgery 46(5): 1162-1168.

Kosy, J. D. and D. M. Standley (2010). Retrieval of a Broken Acutrack Drill Bit. Journal of Hand Surgery: European Volume 35: 683.

Krause, W. R., D. W. Bradbury et al. (1982). Temperature elevations in orthopaedic cutting operations. J Biomech 15(4): 267-275.

Larsen, S. T. and L. Ryd (1989). Temperature elevation during knee arthroplasty. Acta Orthopaedica Scandinavica 60(4): 439-442.

Lavelle, C. and D. Wedgwood (1980). Effect of internal irrigation on frictional heat generated from bone drilling. J Oral Surg 38: 499–503.

Lee, J., Y. Rabin et al. (2011). A New Thermal Model for Bone Drilling with Applications to Orthopaedic Surgery. Medical Engineering & Physics (Article in Press).

Lundskog, J. (1972). Heat and Bone Tissue. An Experimental Investigation of the Thermal Properties of Bone and Threshold Levels for Thermal Injury. Supplement 9. Scand J Plastic Reconst Surg.

Marciniak, J., Z. Z. Paszenda et al. (2007). Wear Investigation of Tools Used in Bone Surgery. Journal of Achievements in Materials and Manufacturing Engineering 20(1-2): 259-262.

Matthews, L. S., C. A. Green et al. (1984). The thermal effects of skeletal fixation-pin insertion in bone. Journal of Bone & Joint Surgery - American Volume 66(7): 1077-1083.

Matthews, L. S. and C. Hirsch (1972). Temperatures measured in human cortical bone when drilling. J Bone Joint Surg Am 54A: 297–308.

Matthews, S. J., R. E. Landsmeer et al. (2006). Removal of Broken Drill Bits and Locking Screws from an Intramedullary Nail. Annals of the Royal College of Surgeons of England 88(3): 316.

Miller, M. D. (2002). EndoButton drill bit failure. Arthroscopy 18(3): 322-324.

Narasimha, K., M. O. M. Osman et al. (1987). An investigation into the influence of helix angle on the torque-thrust coupling effect in twist drills. The International Journal of Advanced Manufacturing Technology 2(4): 91-105.

Natali, C., P. Ingle et al. (1996). Orthopaedic bone drills-can they be improved? Temperature changes near the drilling face. Journal of Bone and Joint Surgery 78-B(3): 357-362.

Ohashi, H., M. Therin et al. (1994a). The effect of drilling parameters on bone. Part I General healing response. Journal of Materials Science: Materials in Medicine 5(4): 225-231.

Ohashi, H., M. Therin et al. (1994b). The effect of drilling parameters on bone. Part II The influence of drilling site. Journal of Materials Science: Materials in Medicine 5(4): 232-236.

Ohashi, H., M. Therin et al. (1994c). The effect of drilling parameters on bone. Part III The response to porous hydroxyapatite implants. Journal of Materials Science: Materials in Medicine 5(4): 237-241.

Ong, F. R. and K. Bouazza-Marouf (1998). Drilling of bone: a robust automatic method for the detection of drill bit break-through. Proceedings of the Institution of Mechanical Engineers Part H - Journal of Engineering in Medicine 212(3): 209-221.

Ong, F. R. and K. Bouazza-Marouf (1999). The detection of drill bit break-through for the enhancement of safety in mechatronic assisted orthopaedic drilling. Mechatronics 9(6): 565-588.
Pichler, W., P. Mazzurana et al. (2008). Frequency of instrument breakage during orthopaedic procedures and its effects on patients. Journal of Bone & Joint Surgery - American Volume 90(12): 2652-2654.
Pinczewski, L. A., J. Lyman et al. (2007). A 10-Year Comparison of Anterior Cruciate Ligament Reconstructions With Hamstring Tendon and Patellar Tendon Autograft: A Controlled, Prospective Trial. American Journal of Sports Medicine 35: 564-574.
Piska, M., L. Yang et al. (2002). Drilling efficiency and temperature elevation of three types of Kirschner-wire point. Journal of Bone & Joint Surgery - British Volume 84(1): 137-140.
Price, M. V., S. Molloy et al. (2002). The rate of instrument breakage during orthopaedic procedures. Int Orthop 26(3): 185-187.
Reingewirtz, Y., S. Szmukler-Moncler et al. (1997). Influence of different parameters on bone heating and drilling time in implantology. Clin Oral Implants Res. 8(3): 189-197.
Saha, S., S. Pal et al. (1982). Surgical drilling: design and performance of an improved drill. Journal of Biomechanical Engineering 104(3): 245-252.
Sener, B. C., G. Dergin et al. (2009). Effects of irrigation temperature on heat control in vitro at different drilling depths. Clin Oral Implants Res. 20(3): 294-298.
Sharawy, M., C. E. Misch et al. (2002). Heat generation during implant drilling: the significance of motor speed. Journal of Oral & Maxillofacial Surgery 60(10): 1160-1169.
Silverstein, C. C. (2007). Self-Cooling Cavity Burs for Surgical Drills. Journal of Medical Devices 1(4): 293-296.
Singh, J., J. H. Davenport et al. (2010). A national survey of instrument sharpening guidelines. The Surgeon 8(3): 136-139.
Steeves, M., C. Stone et al. (2005). How pilot-hole size affects bone-screw pullout strength in human cadaveric cancellous bone. Canadian Journal of Surgery 48(3): 207-212.
Stephenson, D. A. and J. S. Agapiou (1997). Metal Cutting Theory and Practice.
Stubinger, S., K. Biermeier et al. (2010). Comparison of Er:YAG laser, piezoelectric, and drill osteotomy for dental implant site preparation: a biomechanical and histological analysis in sheep. Lasers Surg Med 42(7): 652-661.
Svehla, M., P. Morberg et al. (2002). The effect of substrate roughness and hydroxyapatite coating thickness on implant shear strength. The Journal of Arthroplasty 17(3): 304-311.
Svehla, M., P. Morberg et al. (2000). Morphometric and mechanical evaluation of titanium implant integration: comparison of five surface structures. J Biomed Mater Res 51(1): 15-22.
Toews, A. R., J. V. Bailey et al. (1999). Effect of feed rate and drill speed on temperatures in equine cortical bone. American Journal of Veterinary Research 60(8): 942-944.
Udiljak, T., D. Ciglar et al. (2007). Investigation into Bone Drilling and Thermal Bone Necrosis. Advances in Production Engineering and Management 2(3): 103-112.
Ueda, T., A. Wada et al. (2010). The Effect of Drill Design Elements on Drilling Characteristics when Drilling Bone. Journal of Biomechanical Science and Engineering 5(4): 399-407.
Wolfson, K. A., L. L. Seeger et al. (2000). Imaging of Surgical Paraphernalia: What Belongs in the Patient and What Does Not. Radiographics 20(6).
Yang, Y., C. Wang et al. (2010). Drilling Force and Temperature of Bone by Surgical Drill. Advanced Materials Research 126-128: 779-784.

4

Application of Growth Factors for Enhancement of Mechanical Strength of Grafted Tendon Following Anterior Cruciate Ligament Reconstruction

Harukazu Tohyama and Kazunori Yasuda
Department of Sports Medicine, Hokkaido University School of Medicine, Sapporo, Japan

1. Introduction

Anterior cruciate ligament (ACL) injury is a relatively common knee injury during sports activities (Uhorchak, 2003). A torn ACL usually occurs through a twisting force being applied to the knee whilst the foot is firmly planted on the ground or upon landing (Boden, 2000). The traditional surgical treatment for ACL rupture is ACL reconstruction by an autogenous tendon graft. However, fibroblasts of the tendon graft are necrotized immediately after transplantation of an autogenous tendon graft, and, then, extrinsic fibroblasts infiltrate in the graft (Amiel, 1986; Arnoczky, 1982; Kleiner 1986). During this process, the grafted tendon weakens in the early phase after ACL reconstruction surgery, even if the grafted tendon is subjected in the mechanically physiological condition (Jackson 1991). In addition, a case report of histology of patellar tendon graft 18 months after ACL reconstruction suggested that the cell infiltration into a core portion of the graft occurs very slowly after ligament reconstruction (Delay, 2002). The slow graft maturation may result in graft failure during the postoperative rehabilitation period. It has been known that growth factors enhance proliferation, migration, and matrix synthesis of cells in vitro (Deie, 1997; DesRosiers, 1996; Kobayashi, 2000; Marui, 1997; Scherping, 1997; Schmidt, 1995). The authors conducted a series of animal experimental studies for the application of growth factors to ligament reconstruction. We will review our recent experimental studies that intended to enhance mechanical strength of grafted tendon after ligament reconstruction using growth factors.

2. Biological characteristics of infiltrative fibroblasts into the necrotized tendon

Previous studies have demonstrated that, in the grafted tendon for ligament reconstruction, fibroblast repopulation from an extrinsic origin occurs with revascularization after intrinsic fibroblasts in the tendon are necrotized (Kleiner 1986). The authors have reported that infiltration of the extrinsic fibroblasts results in mechanical deterioration of the extracellular matrix of the grafted tendon (Tohyama 2000, Tohyama 2006). Thus, the infiltrative fibroblasts play an important role in remodeling of the autogenous tendon graft. Infiltrative fibroblasts repopulating in the skin wound are phenotypically distinct from normal dermal fibroblasts. Amiel et al. (1995) and Hannafin et al. (1999) reported that proliferation and migration characteristics of the ligament fibroblasts depended on their origin. Therefore, there is a high possibility that extrinsic fibroblasts infiltrating in the necrotized tendon have significantly different biological characteristics, compared with the intrinsic fibroblasts in the normal tendon. To understand the remodeling of the tendon autograft in ligament reconstruction, it is necessary to clarify differences in biological characteristics between the infiltrative and intrinsic fibroblasts.

We have compared the biological characteristics of infiltrative fibroblasts into the patellar tendon after fibroblast necrosis using an in situ freeze-thaw procedure to normal patellar tendon fibroblasts (Ikema, 2005; Tohyama, 2007). The in situ frozen-thawed patellar tendon simulates ligament reconstruction with the patellar tendon graft under ideal condition. To obtain the infiltrative fibroblasts, we performed an in situ freeze-thaw treatment on the patellar tendon to kill the intrinsic fibroblasts (Fig. 1). In this in situ freeze-thaw treatment, the patellar tendon was frozen with liquid nitrogen for 1 minute. The frozen patellar tendon was then thawed by physiological saline solution. We confirmed that this procedure killed 97% to 100% of intrinsic fibroblasts in the rabbit patellar tendon. After this treatment, only the extrinsic fibroblasts were available to repopulate in the patellar tendon (Tohyama, 2000). Six weeks later, the patellar tendons were harvested and placed in Dulbecco's modified Eagle's medium (DMEM) containing 10% FBS. A confluent monolayer formed in 2 weeks. Thus, infiltrative cells, >95% fibroblast-like as confirmed by microscopic analysis, were obtained from the right patellar tendon. For comparison, the untreated patellar tendon was similarly incubated and normal fibroblasts were isolated in the same manner.

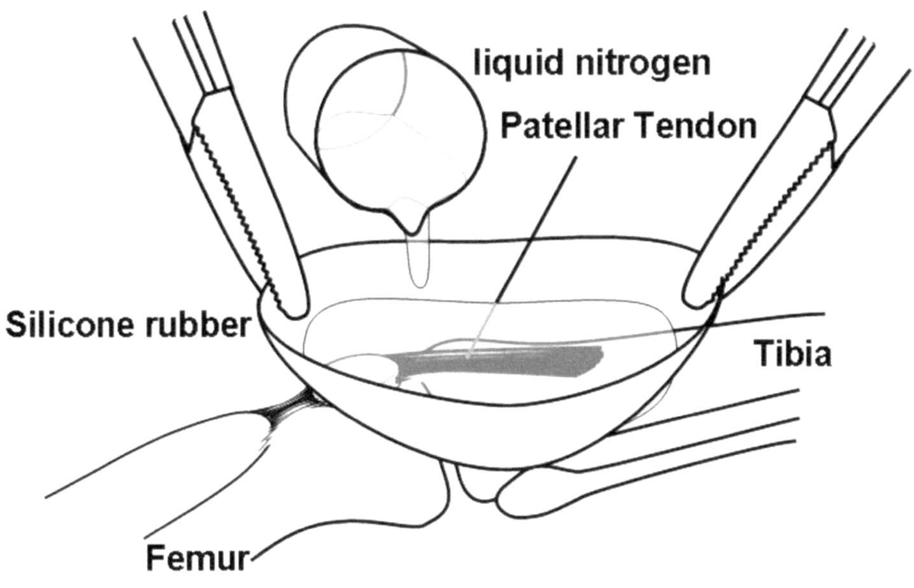

Fig. 1. The in situ freeze-thaw treatment for necrotizing intrinsic fibroblasts in the patellar tendon (From ref. Ikema (2005))

a.

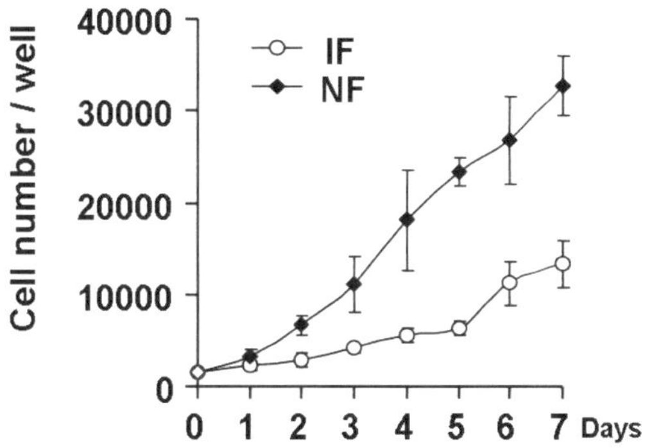

b.

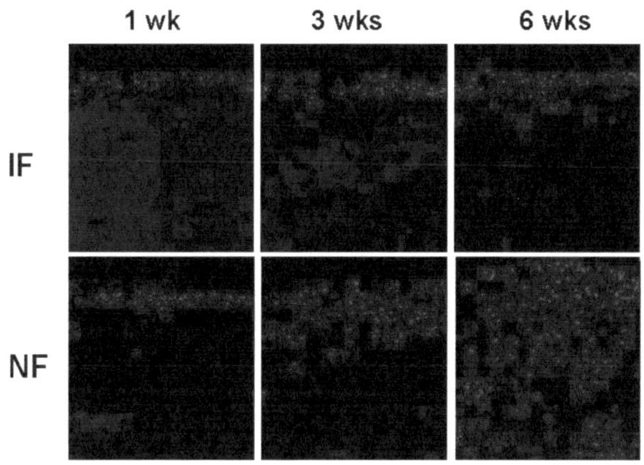

c.

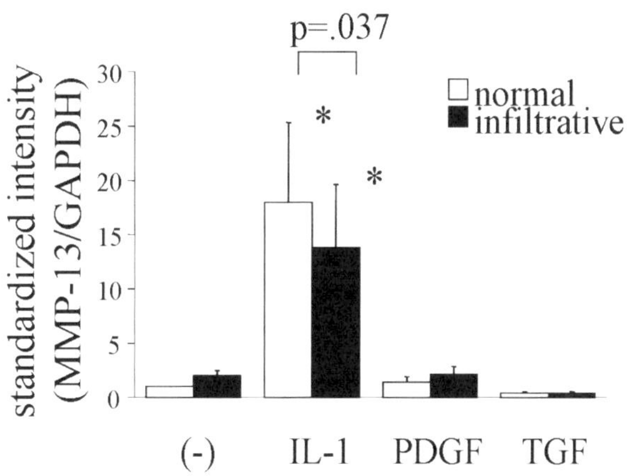

Fig. 2. Cellular proliferation (a), migration (b) and responsiveness to IL-1beta (c) of infiltrative fibroblasts (IFs) and normal fibroblasts (NFs) (From ref. Ikema (2005) and ref. Tohyama (2007)).

The authors then found that the cellular proliferation, migration, and responsiveness of infiltrative fibroblasts to IL-1beta, which is one of the major inflammatory cytocine, are quite inferior to those of normal fibroblasts (Fig. 2)(Ikema, 2005; Tohyama, 2007). The slow remodeling process in the tendon graft may be attributed to these inferior potentials of infiltrative fibroblasts. Therefore, we may be able to accelerate the remodeling process of the grafted tendon after ligament reconstruction if we restore the potentials of infiltrative fibroblasts to the levels of normal tendon fibroblasts with regard to cellular proliferation, migration, and responsiveness to cytokines.

3. Growth factor application to the graft after ACL reconstruction

As described above, previous studies have demonstrated that intrinsic fibroblasts in the tendon grafted across the knee joint to reconstruct the ACL are necrotized immediately after transplantation, and that cellular repopulation from an extrinsic origin and revascularization sequentially occur (Arnoczky, 1982; Kleiner, 1986). In this process, the mechanical properties of tendon autografts deteriorated after ligament reconstruction surgery, and they remain inferior even at 8 months after surgery (Beynnon, 1997). Also, the cell infiltration into the grafted tendon occurs very slowly after ACL reconstruction (Delay, 2002). Recently, a number of studies have shown that application of various growth factors stimulates cellular proliferation, angiogenesis, and synthesis of extra-cellular matrix in tendon and ligament tissues (Deie, 1997; DesRosiers, 1996; Kobayashi, 2000; Marui, 1997; Scherping, 1997; Schmidt, 1995; Zachary, 1998). Therefore, there are two approaches in the application of growth factor to the graft after ACL reconstruction. The first approach is to enhance angiogenesis and cellular repopulation in the grafted tendon after the necrosis. The second one is to improve tissue quality of the grafted tendon via remodelling of the collagen matrix after ACL reconstruction.

3.1 Growth factor application for enhancement of angiogenesis

Angiogenesis is a biological mechanism of new capillary formation and involves the activation, migration, and proliferation of endothelial cells from preexisting venules. Angiogenesis can be influenced by many factors including hypoxia, growth factors, and matrix components. The angiogenic activation of endothelial cells probably plays a role in promoting and regulating other biological events, such as inflammation, fibroblast proliferation, and extracellular matrix synthesis in the remodeling process of the grafted tendon after ACL reconstruction. Vascular endothelial growth factor (VEGF) is considered to be a potent mediator of angiogenesis in various pathological conditions (Ferrara and Davis-Smyth, 1997). Recently, our study in the rabbit ACL reconstruction model clarified that infiltrative cells produced VEGF before revascularization in the grafted tendon (Fig. 3) (Yoshikawa, 2006a). This has suggested that VEGF mediates angiogenesis in the intra-articular tendon graft for the ACL reconstruction.

Based on our finding, an administration of VEGF may significantly enhance angiogenesis in the grafted tendon after ACL reconstruction and then may accelerate the remodeling process of the grafted tendon after necrosis. On the other hand, there is also a possibility that the revascularization induced by VEGF deteriorates the mechanical strength of the grafted tendon. Newly formed vessels in the graft may weaken the grafted tendon as soft-tissue "flaws" (Shrive, 1995). Therefore, we examined the effect of an application of VEGF in

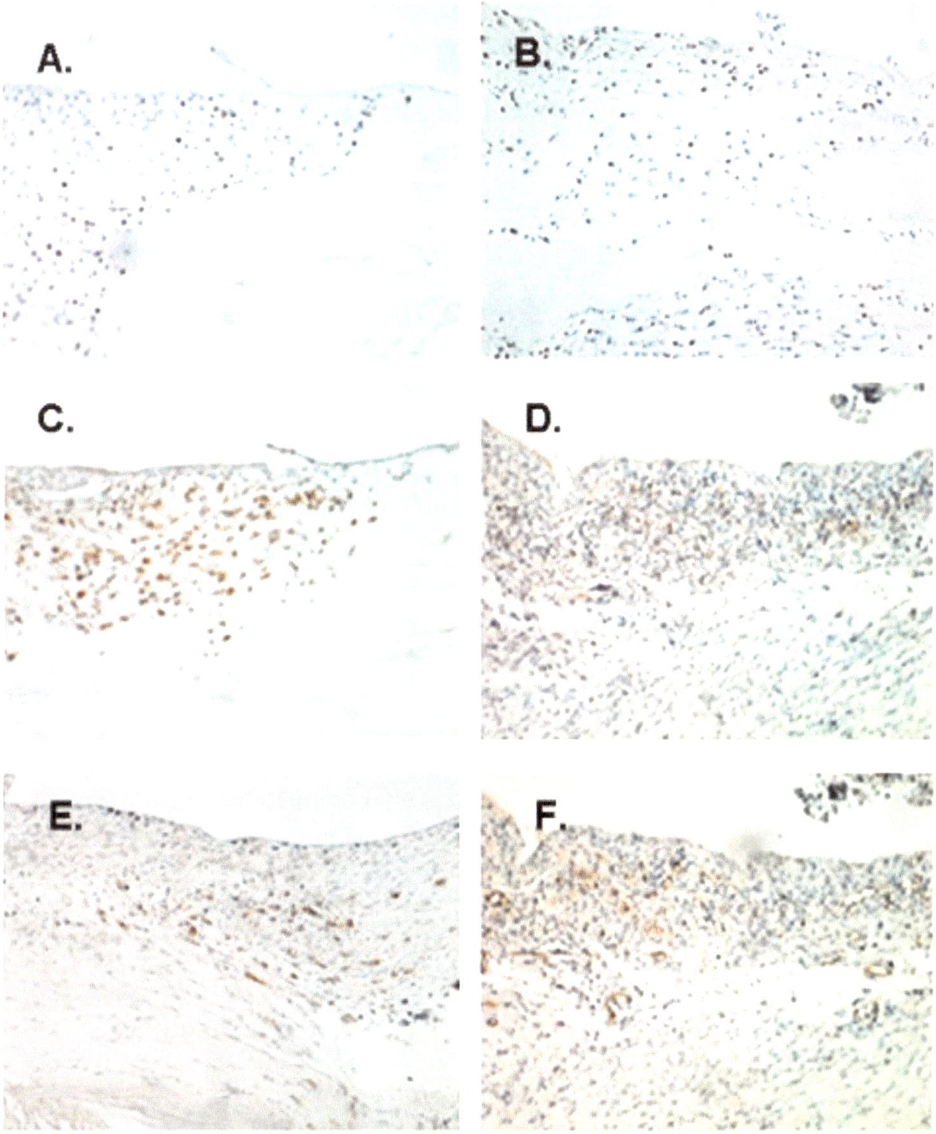

Fig. 3. Immunohistologies for proliferative cells (PCNA stain)(A: 2 weeks, B: 8 weeks), VEGF (C: 2 weeks, D: 8 weeks), and vascular endothelial cells (CD31 stain) (E: 3 weeks, F: 8 weeks) of the patellar tendon graft after ACL reconstruction in the rabbit model. A: Proliferative cells were frequently found at the superficial portion of the tendon graft at 2 weeks. B: At 8 weeks, few proliferative cells were observed in the patellar tendon graft. C: At 2 weeks, VEGF-positive cells scattered at the similar area where proliferative cells existed. D: At 8 weeks, VEGF-positive cells were seldom observed in the patellar tendon graft. E: At 3 weeks, vascular endothelial cells appeared at the midsubstance portion apart from the surface area of the graft tendon in spite of lack of vessel formation at this time. F: At 8 weeks, a number of vessel formations were observed in the tendon graft (From ref. Yoshikawa (2006a)).

the rabbit in situ frozen-thawed ACL and the sheep ACL reconstruction models. The in situ frozen-thawed ACL, which is anatomical but acellular, has been established as an idealized ACL graft model (Jackson, 1991; Katsuragi, 2000; Sakai, 2002). In the rabbit model, we performed the freeze–thaw treatment for the right ACL (Fig. 4) and then injected 30-μg VEGF with 0.2-ml phosphate-buffered saline in the right knee joint. Several vessels formed by endothelial cells were observed at the superficial portion of the ACL 3 weeks after the in situ freeze-thaw treatment and VEGF injection, while few vascular endothelial cells were found in the ACL at 3 weeks after the in situ freeze-thaw treatment alone (Fig. 5)(Ju, 2006). The number of vessels with endothelial cells was significantly higher in the ACLs after the in situ freeze-thaw treatment and VEGF injection than in the ACLs after the in situ freeze-thaw treatment alone (Fig. 5). This finding implied that recombinant VEGF therapy may be used to enhance graft remodeling in ACL reconstruction. However, the in situ frozen–thawed ACL was not a true model of ACL reconstruction by use of a free tendon graft. Biological differences must exist between the frozen-thawed ACL and the intra-articular grafted tendon after ACL reconstruction, since bone marrow-derived cells contribute to a graft that is placed in a bone tunnel. Therefore, we conducted a following large animal model study to clarify if recombinant VEGF application affects the mechanical properties of the grafted tendon after ACL reconstruction before its clinical application of recombinant VEGF therapy to ACL reconstruction.

In this experiment, we used mature female Suffolk sheep (Yoshikawa, 2006b) . We harvested the semitendinosus tendon from the right leg and then soaked the tendon in recombinant human VEGF with 10-ml phosphate buffered saline (PBS) for 15 minutes and then perfrmed ACL reconstruction using this semitendinosus tendon in the same leg (Fig. 6). These animals were killed 12 weeks after ACL reconstruction for the histological and biomechanical evaluations. Conserning mechanical evaluation, the antero-posterior (A-P) drawer tests were performed in 30°, 60°, and 90° of flexion and neutral rotation with load application. The knee was mounted to a custom-made adjusting device with 3 degrees of freedom (translations in the anterior-posterior, medial-lateral, and proximal-distal directions) in a materials testing machine. An A-P force of ±100 N was applied 15 times with a load displacement rate of 50 mm/min and the A-P displacement between ±100-N A-P forces was quantified. After A-P drawer testing, all soft tissue including the menisci was removed, leaving only the grafted tendon. The cross-sectional area of the graft was measured at the middle level of intra-articular portion of the graft by a non-contact optical method with video dimension analyzer. The femur-graft-tibia (FGT) complex underwent tensile testing at the cross head speed of 50 mm/min until the FGT complex failed.

The A-P translation of the tibia relative to the femur in the experimental group was significantly larger than that in the control group, in which the knee underwent identical procedures to those of the experimental group except that the harvested tendon was soaked in 10-ml PBS instead of recombinant VEGF with 10-ml PBS (Fig. 7) (Yoshikawa, 2006). At the failure tests to determine the structural properties of the femur-graft-tibia complex, all grafts failed at the midsubstance portion in the graft during tensile testing, while normal ACL specimens had avulsion fractures at the tibial insertion sites to the ACLs. The linear stiffness of the femur-graft-tibia complex in the experimental group was significantly lower than that in the control group, while there were no significant differences in the ultimate failure load or the energy absorbed at failure between the experimental and the control group (Fig. 8).

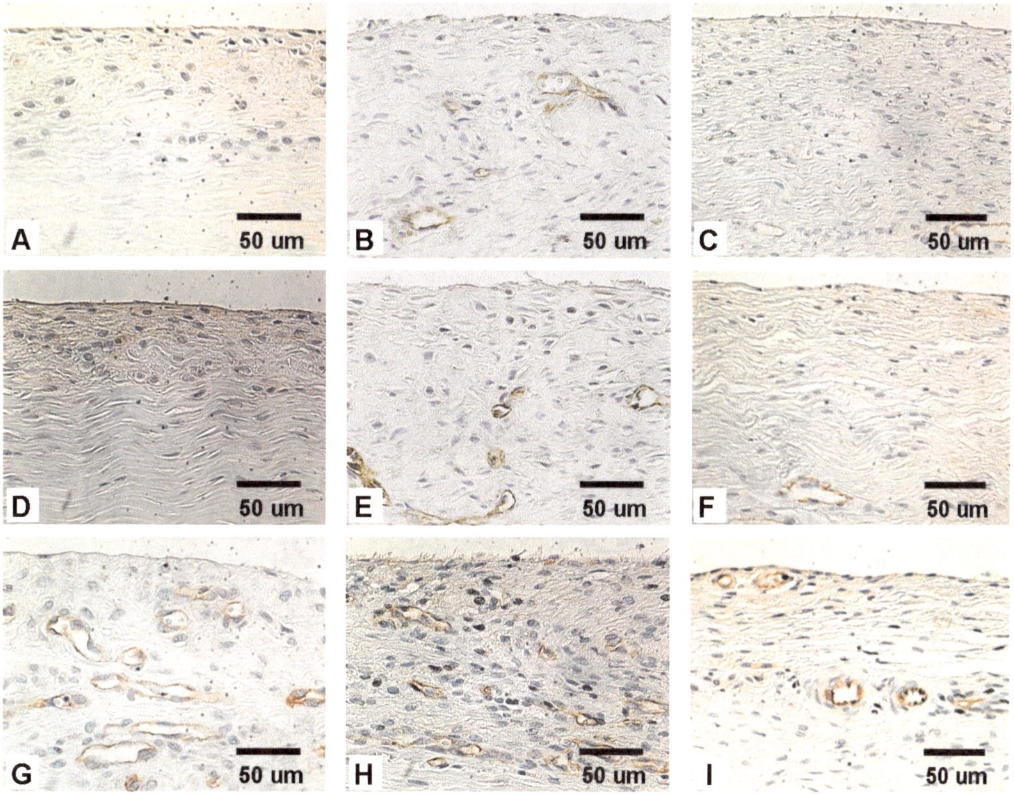

Fig. 4. Immunohistologies for vascular endothelial cells to evaluate the effects of local VEGF application on vessel formation in the ACL at 3 weeks (A,B,C), 6 weeks (D,E,F), and 12 weeks (G,H,I) after the in situ freeze-thaw treatment in the rabbit model (CD31 stain). At 3, 6, and 12 weeks after surgery, we did not find any obvious differences in angiogenesis between the ACLs with (C,F, and I) and without intra-articular injection of.2-ml phosphate-buffered saline (A, D, G). On the other hand, several vessels formed by endothelial cells were observed at the superficial portion of the ACL 3 weeks after the in situ freeze-thaw treatment and VEGF injection (B) (Ju, 2006). The number of vessels with endothelial cells was significantly higher in the ACLs after the in situ freeze-thaw treatment and VEGF injection (B,E,H) than in the ACLs after the in situ freeze-thaw treatment alone (B,E,H)(Fig. 5).(From ref. Ju (2006)).

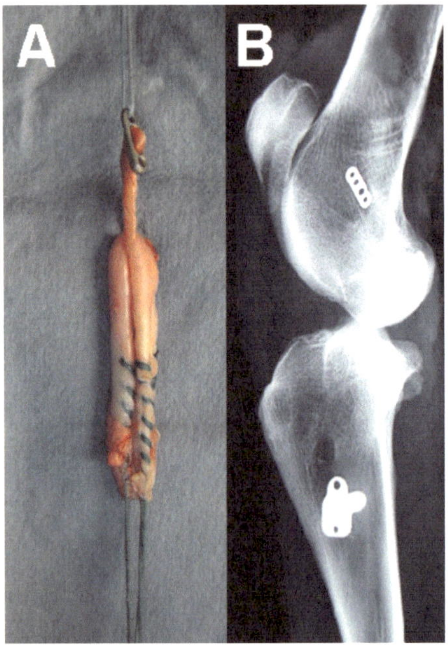

Fig. 6. Anterior cruciate ligament reconstruction procedure in the sheep model. A: semitendinosus tendon graft, B: a radiographic lateral view immediately after the surgery (From ref. Kondo (2011)).

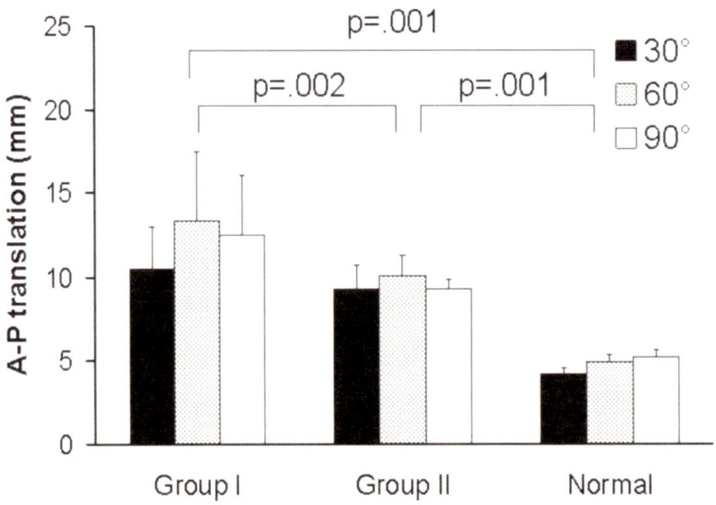

Fig. 7. The effects of VEGF application on A-P displacement between ±100-N A-P forces (From ref. Yoshikawa (2006b)) . Group I: the knee 12 weeks after ACL reconstruction with semitendinosus tendon graft soaked in phosphate buffered saline, Group II: the knee 12 weeks after ACL reconstruction with semitendinosus tendon graft soaked in VEGF solution, Normal: normal knee with no treatment.

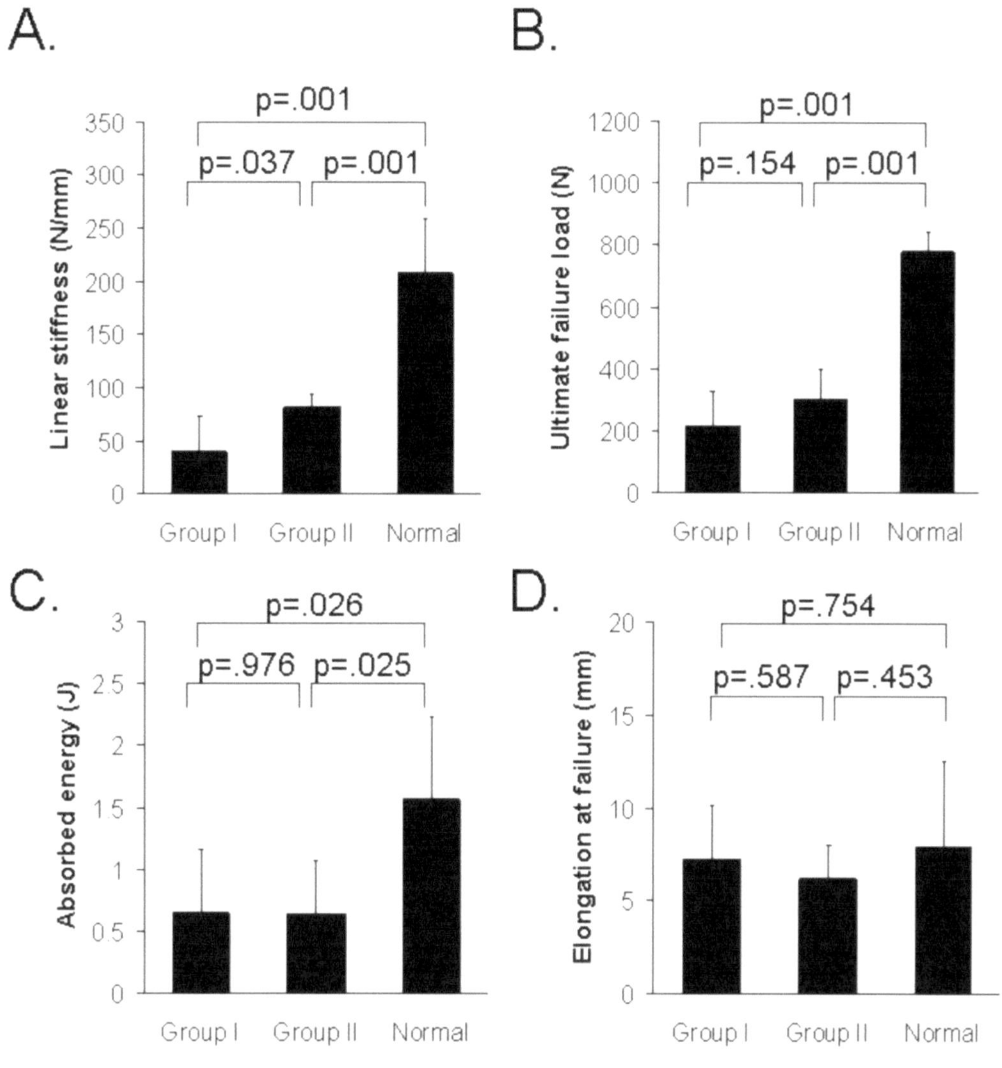

Fig. 8. The effects of VEGF application on structural properies of the femur-graft-tibia complex after ACL reconstruction (A: The linear stiffness; B: The ultimate failure load; C: The absorbed energy; D: Elongation at failure) (From ref. Yoshikawa (2006b)). Group I: the femur-graft-tibia complex 12 weeks after ACL reconstruction with semitendinosus tendon graft soaked in phosphate buffered saline, Group II: the femur-graft-tibia complex 12 weeks after ACL reconstruction with semitendinosus tendon graft soaked in VEGF solution, Normal: normal the femur-graft-tibia complex with no treatment.

We did not know exactly why our VEGF application reduced the stiffness of the grafted tendon after ACL reconstruction. Shrive et al. (1995) reported that in the medial collateral ligament injury model in the rabbit, the area of newly formed vessels, infiltrative cells and disorderly arranged collagen fibers in the scar tissue was reversely correlated with mechanical strength of the scar tissue and that a number of newly formed vessels and infiltrative cells might act as "flaws" and enhance the deterioration of the mechanical property of the grafted tendon. Therefore, a number of newly formed vessels and infiltrative cells which VEGF administration induced in the ACL graft might deteriorate mechanical properties of the ACL graft as soft tissue flaws. In addition, it was reported that VEGF promotes collagenese production by some types of cells (Ferrara, 1997; Munaut, 2003; Pufe, 2004; Zachary, 1998). Therefore, VEGF-induced collagenese directly might digest the matrix of the graft. VEGF was widely used for patients with extensive tissue ischemia in whom primary vascular reconstruction procedures were not feasible or had previously failed in clinical trials (Kusumanto, 2003). Early clinical data provide evidence that the VEGF application can achieve beneficial angiogenesis, with minimal side-effects. Our findings imply that an application of the recombinant VEGF therapy can supposedly enhance revascularization in the graft as well as cellular infiltration after ACL reconstruction. On the other hand, our biomechanical results have indicated that exogenous VEGF application decreases the stiffness of the grafted tendon at least temporarily after ACL reconstruction. Therefore, if we intend to apply exogenous VEGF as a treatment to accelerate angiogenesis and cellular infiltration in the tendon graft for ACL reconstruction, we should take into account this adverse effect of exogenous VEGF application on the mechanical characteristics of the grafted tendon.

3.2 Growth factor application for collagen synthesis in fibroblasts

Numerous studies have shown that various types of cells can over-expressed growth factors such as transforming growth factor-beta (TGF-beta), basic fibroblast growth factor (b-FGF), and platelet-derived growth factor (PDGF), epidermal growth factor (EGF) during healing process of the tissue. In addition, these factors regulate the synthesis and degradation of collagen by the fibroblasts of tendons and ligaments. Therefore, the effects of growth factors on mRNA expression of MMP-13, which is main collagenase in the rat, were evaluated in the rat model using Northern blot analysis. At 6 hours after the challenge with PDGF-BB, up-regulation of MMP-13 mRNA became apparent at the dose of 100 ng/ml, while slight up-regulation of MMP-13 mRNA was observed at the dose of 10 ng/ml (Fig. 9A). In contrast, down-regulation of MMP-13 mRNA was found at 6 hours after the stimulation with TGF-beta1. The suppression of MMP-13 mRNA by TGF-beta1 was dose-dependent in the range less than 10 ng/ml (Fig. 9A). We also found that TGF-beta1 significantly increases the ratio of type I collagen mRNA to type III collagen mRNA in extrinsic fibroblasts infiltrative fibroblasts (Fig. 9-B). It is well known that EGF stimulates fibroblast proliferation in vitro (Schmidt, 1995). A combined application of these two growth factors enhances these effects (DesRosiers, 1996). Therefore, we conducted following animal experimental studies for the application of TGF-beta1 and EGF to ligament reconstruction.

First, we investigated the effects of a combined application of TGF-beta and EGF on the rabbit in situ frozen-thawed ACL (Sakai, 2002). In this study, a low and a high doses of combinations (low dose: 4-ng TGF-beta1 and 100-ng EGF, high dose: 2-microgram TGF-beta1 and 50-microgram EGF) mixed with the fibrin sealant were applied to rabbit ACLs after the in situ freeze-thaw treatment, compared with in situ frozen-thawed ACLs without any other treatment and with fibrin sealant alone. These ACLs were evaluated at 12 weeks

A.

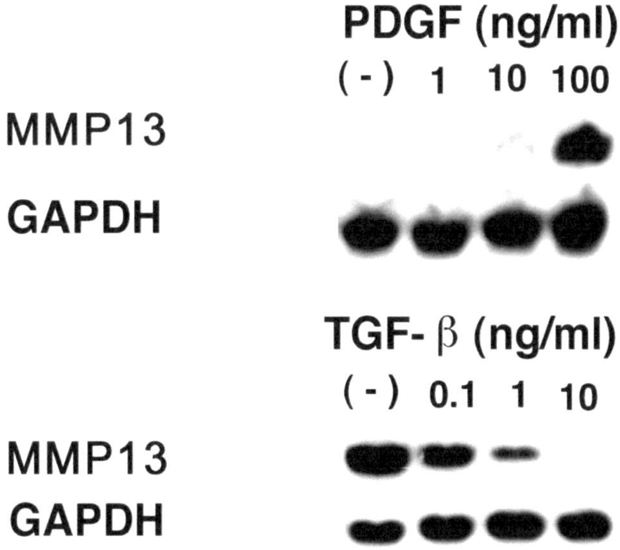

B.

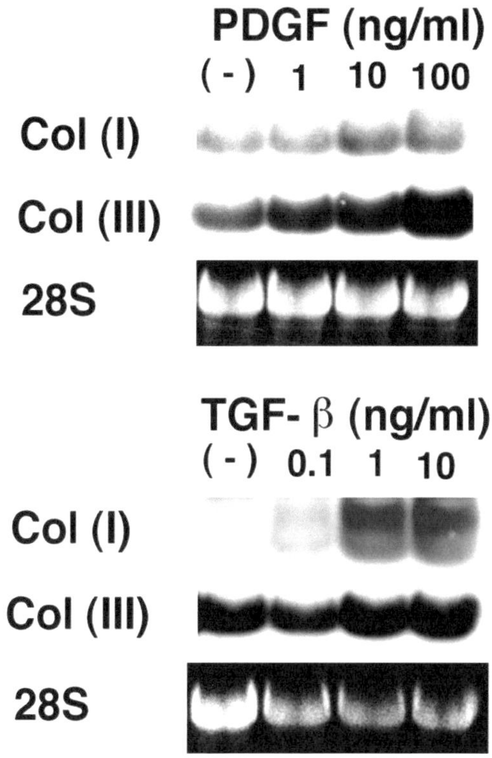

Fig. 9. The effects of growth factors on gene expression of extrinsic infiltrating fibroblasts into the patellar tendon after the necrosis (A. MMP-13 mRNA; B. type-I and type-II collagens mRNAs).

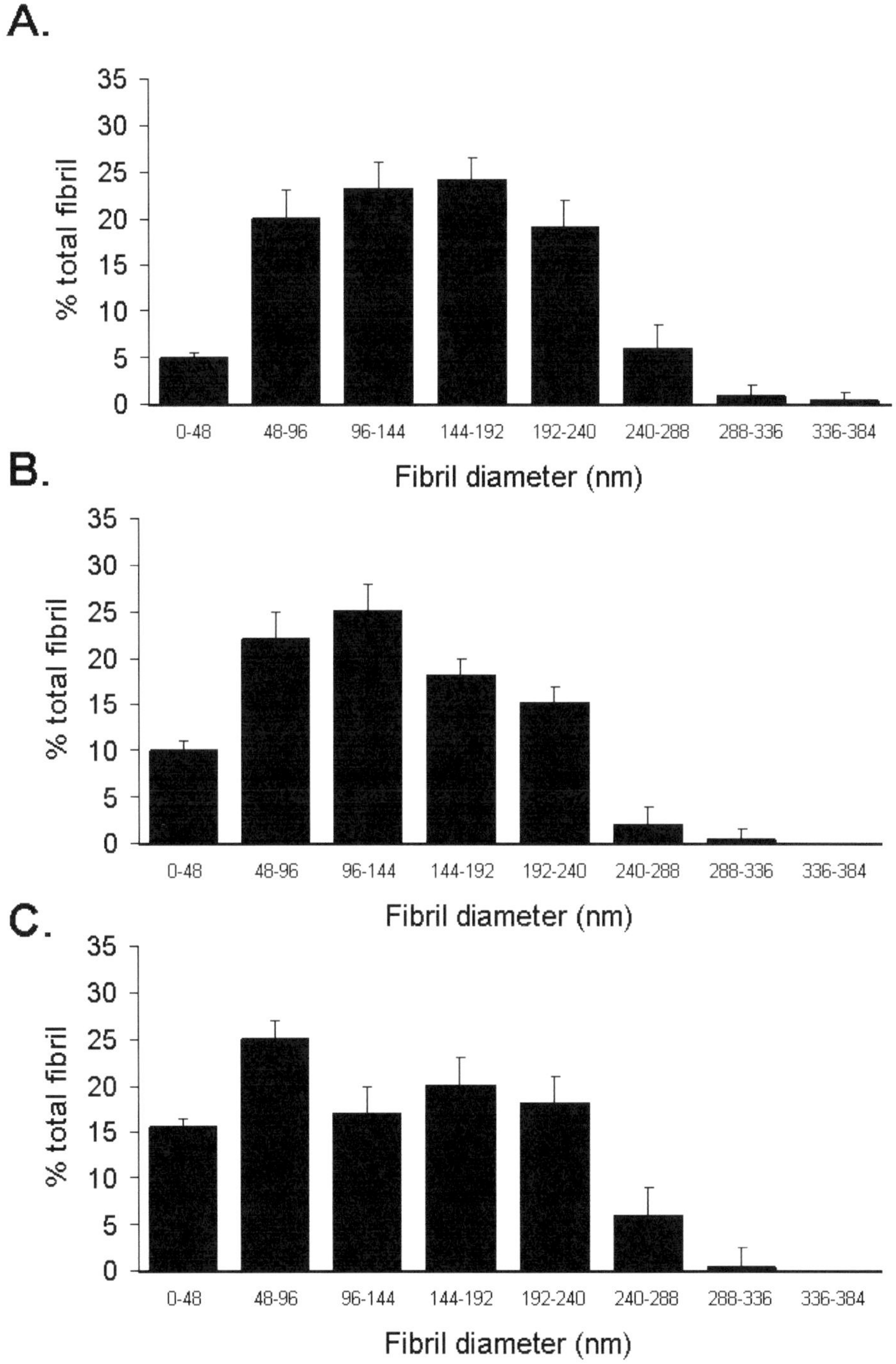

Fig. 10. Histograms of the collagen fibril diameter in the normal control ACL (A) and the ACL after the in situ freeze-thaw treatment without TGF-beta/EGF application (B) and with a high dose of TGF-beta and EGF ((From ref. Sakai (2002)).

A.

B.

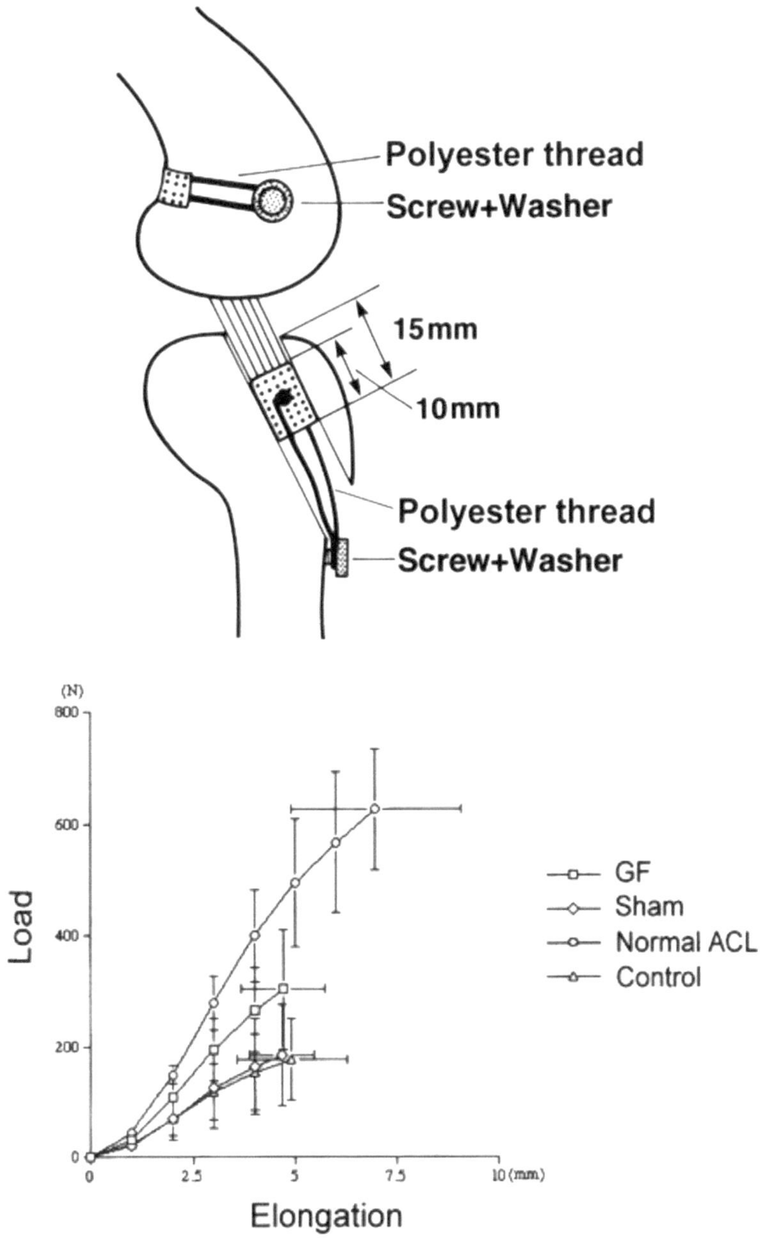

Fig. 11. The effects of low-dose application of TGF-beta and EGF on structural properties of the femur-graft-tibia complex after ACL reconstruction (From ref. Yasuda (2004)). A. ACL reconstruction procedure with the bone–patellar tendon–bone graft, B. The load-elongation curves of the femur-graft-tibia complexes in the knees with growth factor application (GF), with fibrin sealant alone (Sham), and without growth factor or fibrin sealant (Control) groups and the normal femur-ACL-tibia complex (Normal ACL).

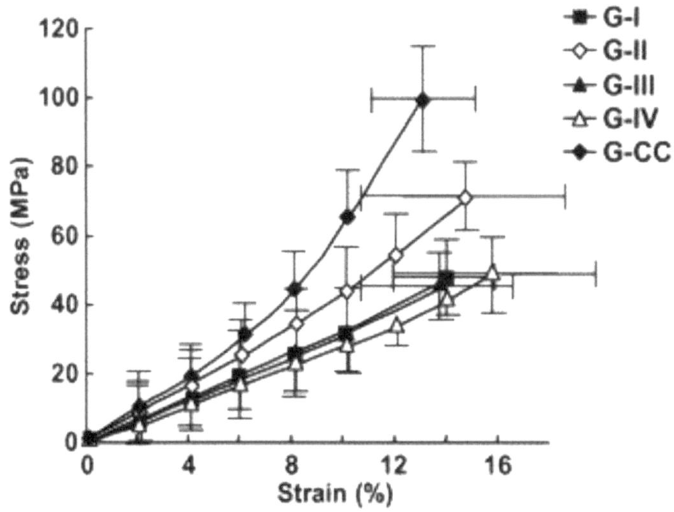

Fig. 12. The effects of a separate application of TGF-beta, EGF, and PDGF-BB on the material properties of the ACL 12 weeks after the in situ freeze-thaw treatment (From ref. Nagumo (2005)). The stress–strain curves of the anteromedial bundle of the ACL in Group I (G-I, only 0.2 ml fibrin sealant was applied), Group II (G-II, 4 ng TGF-beta1 mixed with 0.2 ml fibrin sealant was applied), Groups III (G-III, 100 ng EGF mixed 0.2 ml fibrin sealant was applied) Group IV (G-IV, 4 μg PDGF-BB mixed with 0.2 ml fibrin sealant was applied) and Group "contralateral control" (G-CC).

on the basis of mechanical properties, water content, and histological and ultrastructural observations. As a result, the cross-sectional area and the water content of ACLs with a low dose of TGF-beta1 and EGF were significantly less than those of ACLs with other treatments at 12 weeks. The tensile strength of ACLs with a low dose of TGF-beta1 and EGF was significantly greater than those of ACLs with other treatments at 12 weeks. In addition, the average tangent modulus of with a low dose of TGF-beta and EGF was 96% of the average value in the normal ACLs, while that with a low dose of TGF-beta and EGF was 68% of the normal ACLS. A unimodal distribution of collagen fibril diameters was noted in ACLs without TGF-beta/EGF application, while a bimodal pattern was found in ACLs with a low dose of TGF-beta1 and EGF (Fig. 10). These findings revealed that low-dose application of TGF-beta and EGF significantly inhibited not only the increased water content and cross-sectional area, but also the decreased tensile strength caused by the freeze-thaw treatment, while a high dose of TGF-beta and EGF does not have the same beneficial effects.

Second, we conducted a canine model study to clarify if low-dose application of TGF-beta and EGF enhances the mechanical properties of the grafted tendon after ACL reconstruction (Yasuda, 2004). In this study, 20 dogs underwent ACL reconstruction with the autogenous bone-patellar tendon-bone graft, which is a standard graft for ACL reconstruction, in bilateral knees. A combination of 12 ng TGF -beta and 300 ng EGF mixed with fibrin sealant was applied to the left knee and compared to the right knee without any treatment after identical ACL reconstruction procedure to the left side. In the remaining 10 dogs, fibrin sealant alone was applied to the left knee. We then found that combined application of TGF-beta and EGF increased the stiffness and maximum failure load of the femur-graft-tibia complex at 12 weeks, while the application of fibrin sealant alone did not significantly affect

them (Fig.11). Our findings suggest that application of transforming growth factor-beta and epidermal growth factor improves the structural properties of the femur-graft-graft complex after ACL reconstruction. Therefore, application of growth factors is a possible strategy to prevent graft deterioration in ACL reconstruction.
Third, we evaluated effects of a separate application of TGF-beta, EGF, and PDGF-BB on the material properties of the in situ frozen-thawed ACL (Nagumo, 2005). In this study, we applied 4 ng TGF-beta, 20 ng EGF, and 4 microgram PDGF-BB to the ACL after the in situ freeze-thaw treatment, separately. We also applied only fibrin sealant to the ACL after the in situ freeze-thaw treatment as a control. At 12 weeks after growth factor application, the tensile strength and the tangent modulus of the ACL with TGF-beta application was significantly higher than in the control group (Fig. 12). On the other hand, there were no significant differences in the strength and the modulus among the ACLs with EGF application, PDGF-BB application and the controls. These findings suggests that that the effect of TGF-beta was significant, but the effect of EGF not. Therefore, there is the possibility that the application of TGF-beta enhances maturation of the graft after ligament reconstruction.

4. Conclusion

After ligament reconstruction, the cell infiltration into a core portion of the graft is considered to occur very slowly (Delay, 2002). The slow graft maturation may result in graft failure during the postoperative rehabilitation period. In this chapter, the authors showed the recent experimental findings suggesting that an administration of growth factors, in particular, TGF-beta can inhibit the deterioration of mechanical properties of the grafted tendon after ACL reconstruction. Therefore, application of growth factors, in particular TGF-beta, is a possible strategy to enhance maturation of the graft after ligament reconstruction. However, a few recent studies reported that TGF-beta induced arthritic changes of the articular cartilage in the knee joint (Hulth, 1996; van Beuningen, 1994). Therefore, intraarticular administration of TGF-beta may be unsuitable for clinical application with an ACL reconstruction procedure. The cell-based therapy with cellular activation by growth factors may be a potential solution against this problem (Kondo, 2011; Okuizumi, 2004). The recent advancement in biology about ligament reconstruction can bring new strategies in additional therapeutic options to accelerate the remodeling of the graft and enhance mechanical strength of the grafted tendon after ACL reconstruction.

5. Acknowledgment

The authors acknowledge Yasunari Ikema, M.D., Ph.D., Young-Jin Ju M.D., Ph.D., Toshikazu Yoshikawa M.D., Ph.D., Fumihisa Tomita, M.D., Ph.D., and Akira Nagumo, M.D., Ph.D. for their contribution as primary investigators of the studies which were introduced in this chapter.

6. References

Amiel, D., Kleiner, J.B., & Akeson, W.H. (1986). The natural history of the anterior cruciate ligament autograft of patellar tendon origin. Am J Sports Med, 14, pp.449-462

Amiel, D., Nagineni, C.N., Choi, S.H., & Lee, D. (1995). Intrinsic properties of ACL and MCL cells and their responses to growth factors. Med Sci Sports Exerc, 27, pp. 844-851

Arnoczky, S.P., Tarvin, G.B., & Marshall, J.L. (1982). Anterior cruciate ligament replacement using patellar tendons. J Bone and Joint Surg Am, 64, pp.217-24

Beynnon, B.D., Risberg, M.A., Tjormsland, O., Ekeland, A., Fleming, B.C., Peura, G.D., & Johnson, R.J. (1997). Evaluation of knee joint laxity and the strucural properties of the anterior cruciate ligament graft in the human. A case report. Am J Sports Med, 25: pp.203-206

Boden, B., Dean, G., Feagin, J. Jr., & Garrett, W. Jr. (2000). Mechanisms of anterior cruciate ligament injury. Orthopedics, 2000, 23(6), pp.573-578.

Deie, M., Marui, T., Allen, C.R., Hildebrand, K.A., Georgescu, H.I., Niyibizi, C., & Woo, S.L. (1997). The effects of age on rabbit MCL fibroblast matrix synthesis in response to TGF-beta 1 or EGF. Mech Ageing Dev, 97, pp. 121-130

Delay, B.S., McGrath, B.E., & Mindell, E.R. (2002). Observations on a retrieved patellar tendon autograft used to reconstruct the anterior cruciate ligament. A case report. J Bone Joint Surg Am, 84-A, pp.1433-438

DesRosiers, E.A., Yahia, L., & Rivard, C.H. (1996). Proliferative and matrix synthesis response of canine anterior cruciate ligament fibroblasts submitted to combined growth factors. J Orthop Res, 14, pp.200-208

Ferrara, N., & Davis-Smyth, T. (1997). The biology of vascular endothelial growth factor. Endocr Rev, 18, pp.4-25

Hannafin, J.A., Attia, E.T., Warren, R.F., & Bhargava, M.M. (1999). Characterization of chemotactic migration and growth kinetics of canine knee ligament fibroblasts. J Orthop Res, 17, pp. 398-404.

Hulth, A., Johnell, O., Miyazono, K., Lindberg, L., Heinegard, D., & Heldin, C.H. (1996). Effect of transforming growth factor-beta and platelet-derived growth factor-BB on articular cartilage in rats. J Orthop Res, 14, pp.547-553

Ikema, Y., Tohyama, H., Nakamura, H., Kanaya, F., & Yasuda, K. (2005). Growth kinetics and integrin expression of fibroblasts infiltrating devitalised patellar tendons are different from those of intrinsic fibroblasts. J Bone Joint Surg Br, 87(12), pp. 1689-1693.

Jackson, D.W., Grood, E.S., Cohn, B.T., Arnoczky, S.P., Simon, T.M., & Cummings, J.F. (1991) The effects of in situ freezing on the anterior cruciate ligament. An experimental study in goats. J Bone Joint Surg Am, 73, pp.201-213

Ju, Y.J., Tohyama, H., Kondo, E., Yoshikawa, T., Muneta, T., Shinomiya, K., & Yasuda, K. (2006). Effects of local administration of vascular endothelial growth factor on properties of the in situ frozen-thawed anterior cruciate ligament in rabbits. Am J Sports Med, 34(1), pp.84-91

Katsuragi, R., Yasuda, K., Tsujino, J., Keira, M., & Kaneda, K. (2000) The effect of nonphysiologically high initial tension on the mechanical properties of in situ frozen anterior cruciate ligament in a canine model. Am J Sports Med, 28, pp.47–56

Kleiner, J.B., Amiel, D., Roux, R.D., & Akeson, W.,H. (1986). Origin of replacement cells for the anterior cruciate ligament autograft. J Orthop Res, 4, pp.466-474

Kobayashi K, Healey RM, Sah, R.L., Clark, J.J., Tu, B.P., Goomer, R.S., Akeson, W.H., Moriya, H., & Amiel, D. (2000). Novel method for the quantitative assessment of cell migration: a study on the motility of rabbit anterior cruciate (ACL) and medial collateral ligament (MCL) cells. Tissue Eng, 6, pp.29-38

Kondo, E., Yasuda, K., Katsura, T., Hayashi, R., Azuma, C., & Tohyama H. (2011) Local Administration of Autologous Synovium-Derived Cells Improve the Structural Properties of Anterior Cruciate Ligament Autograft Reconstruction in Sheep. Am J Sports Med, 39(5), pp.999-1007.

Kusumanto, Y.H., Hospers, G.A., Mulder, N.H., & Tio, R.A. (2003). Therapeutic angiogenesis with vascular endothelial growth factor in peripheral and coronary artery disease: a review. Int J Cardiovasc Intervent, 5, pp.27-34

Marui, T., Niyibizi, C., Georgescu, H.I., Cao, M., Kavalkovich, K.W., Levine, R.E., & Woo, S.L. (1997). Effect of growth factors on matrix synthesis by ligament fibroblasts. J Orthop Res, 15, pp.18-23

Munaut, C., Noel, A., Hougrand, O., Foidart, J.M., Boniver, J., & Deprez, M. (2003). Vascular endothelial growth factor expression correlates with matrix metalloproteinases MT1-MMP, MMP-2 and MMP-9 in human glioblastomas. Int J Cancer, 106, pp.848-855

Nagumo, A., Yasuda, K., Numazaki, H., Azuma, H., Tanabe, Y., Kikuchi, S., Harata, S., & Tohyama, H. (2005). Effects of separate application of three growth factors (TGF-beta1, EGF, and PDGF-BB) on mechanical properties of the in situ frozen-thawed anterior cruciate ligament. Clin Biomech (Bristol, Avon), 20(3), pp.283-290.

Okuizumi, T., Tohyama, H., Kondo, E., & Yasuda, K. (2004). The effect of cell-based therapy with autologous synovial fibroblasts activated by exogenous TGF-beta1 on the in situ frozen-thawed anterior cruciate ligament. J Orthop Sci, 9(5), pp.488-494

Pufe, T., Harde, V., Petersen, W., Goldring, M.B., Tillmann, B., & Mentlein, R. (2004). Vascular endothelial growth factor (VEGF) induces matrix metalloproteinase expression in immortalized chondrocytes. J Pathol, 202, pp.367-374

Sakai, T., Yasuda, K., Tohyama, H., Azuma, H., Nagumo, A., Majima, T., & Frank, C.B. (2002). Effects of combined administration of transforming growth factor-beta1 and epidermal growth factor on properties of the in situ frozen anterior cruciate ligament in rabbits. J Orthop Res, 20(6), pp.1345-1351

Scherping, S.C. Jr., Schmidt, C.C., Georgescu, H.I., Kwoh, C.K., Evans, C.H., & Woo, S.L. (1997). Effect of growth factors on the proliferation of ligament fibroblasts from skeletally mature rabbits. Connect Tissue Res, 36, pp.1-8

Schmidt, C.C., Georgescu, H.I., Kwoh, C.K., Blomstrom, G.L., Engle, C.P., Larkin, L.A., Evans, C.H., & Woo, S.L. (1995). Effect of growth factors on the proliferation of fibroblasts from the medial collateral and anterior cruciate ligaments. J Orthop Res, 13, pp.184-190

Shrive, N., Chimich, D., Marchuk, L., Wilson, J., Brant, R., & Frank, C. (1995). Soft-tissue "flaws" are associated with the material properties of the healing rabbit medial collateral ligament. J Orthop Res, 13, pp.923-929

Tohyama, H., & Yasuda, K. (2000). Extrinsic cell infiltration and revascularization accelerate mechanical deterioration of the patellar tendon after fibroblast necrosis. J Biomech Eng, 122(6), pp.594-599

Tohyama, H., Yasuda, K., & Uchida, H. (2006). Is the increase in type III collagen of the patellar tendon graft after ligament reconstruction really caused by "ligamentization" of the graft? Knee Surg Sports Traumatol Arthrosc, 14(12), pp.1270-1277.

Tohyama, H., Yasuda, K., Uchida, H., & Nishihira, J. (2007). The responses of extrinsic fibroblasts infiltrating the devitalised patellar tendon to IL-1beta are different from those of normal tendon fibroblasts. J Bone Joint Surg Br, 89(9), pp.1261-1267

Uhorchak, M., Scoville, R., Williams, G., Arciero, R., St Pierre, P., & Taylor, D. (2003). Risk factors associated with noncontact injury of the anterior cruciate ligament: A prospective four-year evaluation of 859 West Point cadets. Am J Sports Med, 31(6), pp. 831-842

van Beuningen, H.M., van der Kraan, P.M., Arntz, O.J., & van den Berg, W.B. (1994). Transforming growth factor-beta 1 stimulates chondrocyte proteoglycan synthesis and induces osteophyte formation in the murine knee joint. Lab Invest, 71, pp.279-290

Yasuda,K., Tomita, F., Yamazaki, S., Minami, A., Tohyama, H. (2004). The effect of growth factors on biomechanical properties of the bone-patellar tendon-bone graft after anterior cruciate ligament reconstruction: a canine model study. Am J Sports Med, 32(4), pp.870-880

Yoshikawa, T., Tohyama, H., Enomoto, H., Matsumoto, H., Toyama, Y., & Yasuda, K. (2006a) Expression of vascular endothelial growth factor and angiogenesis in patellar tendon grafts in the early phase after anterior cruciate ligament reconstruction. Knee Surg Sports Traumatol Arthrosc, 14(9), pp.804-810

Yoshikawa, T., Tohyama, H., Katsura, T., Kondo, E., Kotani, Y., Matsumoto, H., Toyama, Y., & Yasuda, K. (2006b). Effects of local administration of vascular endothelial growth factor on mechanical characteristics of the semitendinosus tendon graft after anterior cruciate ligament reconstruction in sheep. Am J Sports Med, 34(12), pp.1918-1925

Zachary, I. (1998). Vascular endothelial growth factor. Int J Biochem Cell Biol, 30, pp.1169-1174

5

Minimally Invasive Plate Osteosynthesis (MIPO) in Long Bone Fractures – Biomechanics – Design – Clinical Results

Paul Dan Sirbu, Tudor Petreus, Razvan Asaftei, Grigore Berea and Paul Botez
"Gr.T.Popa" University of Medicine and Pharmacy Iasi
Romania

1. Introduction

Complex periarticular fractures of the long bones are difficult to treat. Classic intramedullary osteosynthesis do not provide a stable fixation (Wiss et al., 1986), while open reduction and rigid fixation by classic plates (recommended in the 60s-70s) is requiring large incisions with important deperiostation. Potential complications as infections, consolidation delays and construct damage due to nonunions undergo frequently (Bucholz et al., 1996). At that time, standard operative procedures considered that in epiphyseal-metaphyseal fractures, each fragment either from the articular or metaphyseal area should be subject for anatomical reduction and stabilization. There were obtained superior biomechanical results (absolute stability) but poor long-term biological effects (Baumgaertel et al., 1998). The main disadvantages of the anatomic reduction and rigid fixation by plates led to the development of the "biological plate osteosynthesis" concept. By the development of new plates (bridging plates, Limited Contact-Dynamic Compression Plate / LC-DCP, Point-Contact fixator / PC-Fix, plates with angular stability) and new surgical techniques (indirect reduction and Minimally Invasive Plate Osteosynthesis / MIPO) , biological plate osteosynthesis is important to preserve bone vascularization, to improve consolidation, to decrease infection rate, to avoid iterative fractures or bone grafting. While indirect reduction techniques (using a distractor) are limiting the medial dissection and avoid bone grafting, MIPO techniques are limiting both the medial and lateral dissection in complex extraarticular fractures of the proximal and distal femur (Krettek et al, 1997a). MIPO techniques avoid direct exposure of the fracture site and transforms the implants in an internal extramedullary splint. Furthermore, MIPO was successfully extended to complex tibial fractures, being actually indicated in all long bones complex fractures that are not suitable for intramedullary osteosynthesis.

MIPO can be structured in 4 steps or techniques:

a. MIPO technique with proximal and distal incisions. It was described by Wenda (Wenda et al., 1997) that have used a femoral limited lateral approach, proximally and distally from the fracture site, with plate insertion beneath the vastus lateralis;

b. Minimally Invasive Percutaneous Plate Osteosynthesis (MIPPO) procedure was developed for extraarticular fractures of the distal and proximal femur; the key for this technique is represented by the usage of a two-part implant, the Dynamic Condylar Screw (DCS) (Krettek et al, 1997a);
c. Transarticular Approach and Retrograde Plate Osteosynthesis (TARPO) procedure was developed by Krettek (Krettek et al, 1997b), for the osteosynthesis of the distal femoral intraarticular fractures.
d. Procedures that uses specific implants for MIPO procedures (Plates with angular stability and tools for percutaneous insertion).

MIPO special characteristics are represented by:

1. The treatment purpose in minimally invasive plate osteosynthesis consists in anatomic reconstruction of the articular area, axis, rotation and length reestablishment for the metaphyseal-diaphyseal area, long plates osteosynthesis with screws fixed only distally and proximally from the fracture, bridging the comminution and with early functional rehabilitation.
2. Various studies results demonstrate that MIPO and TARPO have undeniable advantages over classic techniques: fast healing, reduced complication rate, reduced primary or secondary grafting requirements, and shortening of the operative time. Moreover, TARPO procedure provides a good exposure of the knee joint.
3. Good results obtained by minimally invasive plate osteosynthesis are due to a fast healing by vascularization protection and also to an increased resilience to mechanical stress.
4. Fixation with long plates only distally and proximally from the fracture site maintains a certain instability degree that is useful for an accurate and fast healing (relative instability).
5. Minimally invasive plate osteosynthesis is a demanding technique, requiring a cautious intraoperative clinical and fluoroscopic control in order to reestablish limb axis, rotation and length.

2. MIPO techniques in complex humeral shaft fractures

The treatment of complex humeral shaft fractures is a challenge due to the fact that open reduction and internal fixation with plates by anterolateral or posterior approach (the gold standard) is associated with a high morbidity (Livani et al., 2004; Sirbu et al., 2008) while locked intramedullary nails (the best option) do not offer a sufficient control of rotational movements in unstable and distal fractures (Rommens et al., 2000; Changulani et al., 2006; Sirbu et al., 2008).

In a recent study on plastic bones (Asaftei et al., 2010) we have evaluated the mechanical behavior of three different types of implants used in the osteosynthesis of comminuted humeral shaft fractures. We instrumented the fractures with 3 types of implants: an intramedullary nail, two types of locked plates and a "classic" DCP. All of them were submitted to torsion essays in external and internal rotation as to obtain the same amount of torque. The loading-deforming diagrams were compared and statistically analyzed for each type of implant.

The shorter locked compression plate (LCP- Synthes®) seems to be the most rigid implant for each type of loading essay, the mean values of the loading forces being the highest in the entire group. The intramedullary nail proved to be the most elastic implant on all types of loading. In external rotation, the Dynamic Compression Plate - DCP gives surprisingly values of torsion forces relatively close to the longer locked plate (AxSOS - Stryker®). This seems to be related to the different "working length" of the different plates and also to the different total length of the implants. Regarding the advantages of indirect reduction and biological plate osteosyntesis, Livani and Belangero (Livani et al., 2004) developed MIPO technique by anterior approach in humeral shaft fractures. This MIPO technique avoids the problems related to the neural vascular structures of the arm and especially to the radial nerve. For proximal and middle shaft fractures they have used a proximal limited approach (between biceps - medially and deltoid muscle - laterally) and a distal approach between biceps and brahialis muscle (Fig. 1).

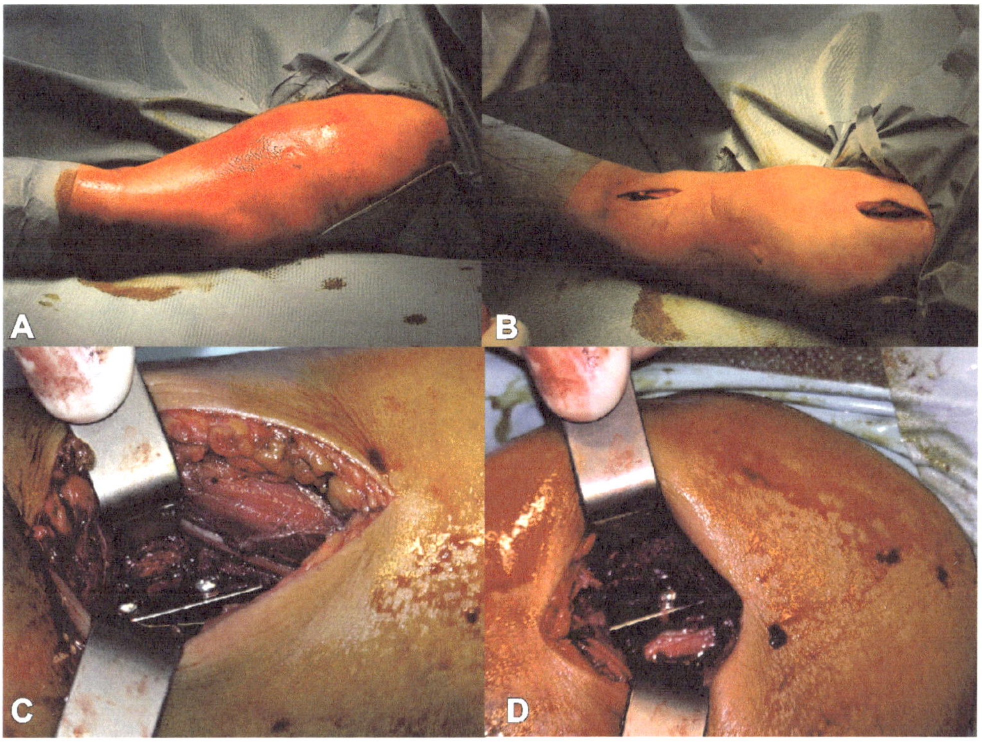

Fig. 1. (A-D) MIPO by anterior approach in a mid-shaft humeral fracture: (A) Arm positioning; (B) Proximal and distal approach; (C,D) Plate fixation

A DCP narrow plate with 12 holes and no previous molding was inserted from proximal to distal, placed on the anterior humeral face and fixed onto the shaft with at least 2 proximal and 2 distal screws. For distal fractures, they have used the same proximal approach and a distal limited approach performed by subperiosteal dissection of the lateral supracondylar ridge of the humerus, with retraction of brachioradialis and long carpal extensor muscle, as well as the radial nerve (even though unseen). A narrow DCP plate of 4.5 mm with 12 holes was molded and twisted medially to adapt to the anterior face of the humeral lateral column and diaphysis, thus avoiding occlusion of the coronoid or of the olecranon fossae. The plate was inserted from distal to proximal and fixed onto the shaft with at least 2 proximal and 2 distal screws, after reestablishing the humeral axis, length and rotation. The radial nerve may be endangered in the lateral column approach but even in such circumstances its identification is not required. This technique can be used for fractures of the distal humerus with paralysis of the radial nerve. Following identification and restoration of the radial nerve through a separate approach, the molded plate is inserted from distal to proximal and fixed as previously described.

We have just finished a prospective study including 34 humeral shaft fractures (6 type 12-A, 8 type 12-B and 20 type 12-C/AO classification) treated with MIPO technique by anterior approach (using Livani and Belangero technique). We have used classic or narrow large fragment DCP plates of 10-14 holes, according to the fracture type. After a short immobilization (1-2 weeks) the patients started rehabilitation. All fractures healed within a mean time of 9 weeks following surgery, with good functional results regarding elbow and shoulder mobility (Fig. 2). There were no vascular or nerve complications, except 2 postoperative temporary paresthesia for the radial nerve in distal fractures.

The following tips and tricks are crucial in this technique : last distal screw - first inserted - relatively loose; arm abduction 60°; slide traction of the distal fragment, first proximal screw inserted, tightening the distal screw; clinical and radiological assessment; two more screws placed in each fragment; tightening the screws for pulling to the bone to the plate and reduction completion.

At the end of this study we can emphasize the advantages of this technique regarding safety and feasibility, without requiring special tools and demanding implants or excessive radiographic control. The plate stability allows a fast rehabilitation with superior functional results comparing with the conservative techniques. MIPO seems to be the best option for distal third humeral fractures and a viable solution for distal fractures with radial nerve palsy.

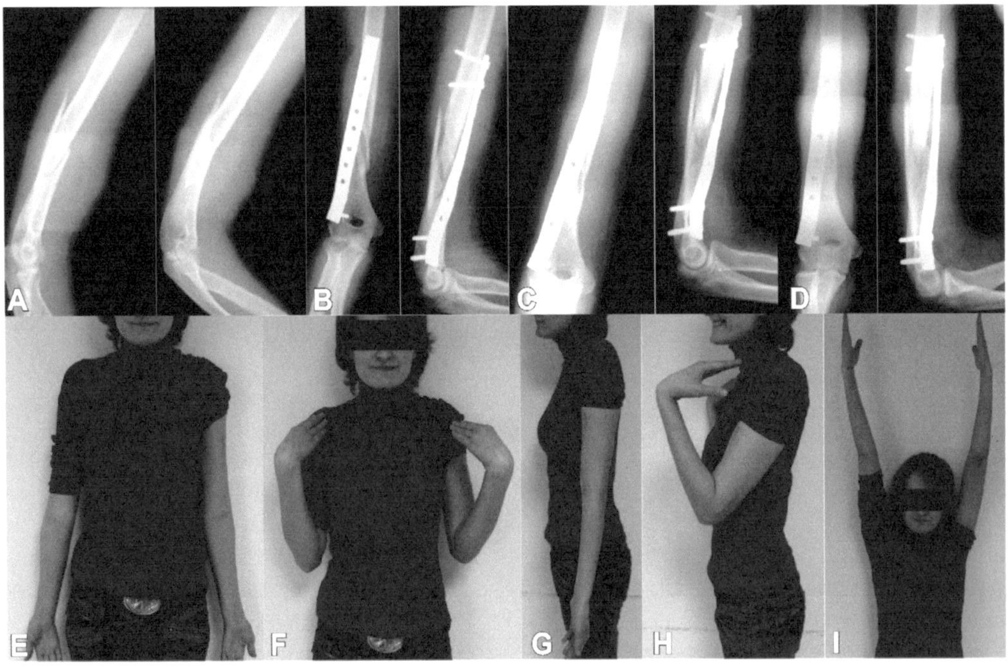

Fig. 2. Clinical case. Female, 23 Yrs, Distal Shaft Fracture type 12C / AO, luge incident; MIPO by anterior approach: (A) Preoperative aspect; (B) Postoperative aspect; (C) At 3 weeks; (D) Callus formation at 8 weeks; (E-I) Excellent functional recovery at 8 weeks.

3. MIPO techniques in complex subtrochanteric fractures

Subtrochanteric area is submitted to an eccentric biomechanical stress, and compression forces in the medial cortex are overwhelming compression forces in lateral cortical area (Hoffmann et al., 1999). Medial cortex comminution in high energy trauma involves major problems regarding reconstruction and internal fixation. Closed intramedullary osteosynthesis protects fragments vascularization better than plate osteosynthesis, giving special biomechanical improvements. The accurate implantation of these intramedullary constructs in subtrochanteric fractures is not an easy task, its difficulty being frequently underestimated.

MIPO by proximal and distal incisions was imagined by Wenda (Wenda et al., 1997) who used first a Condylar Blade Plate - CBP (Fig. 3), a single-unit construct that is difficult to be inserted in three plans at the same time, even with large incisions and femur visualization.

While the CBP was initially inserted with the blade pointing towards the surgeon, the MIPO technique was simplified by the use of the two-part and two-plane alignment achieved by Dynamic Condylar Screw (DCS) (Krettek et al., 2001). The technique consisted in 5 major steps (Fig. 4): 1. condylar screw insertion using minimal incision; 2. DCS-plate selection by fluoroscopy; 3. DCS-plate insertion beneath the vastus lateralis; 4. an additional minimal distal incision allows plate positioning and its slipping onto the condylar screw; 5. after the restoration of limb axis, length and rotation, the plate was fixed to the shaft with 3 or 4 screws placed divergently.

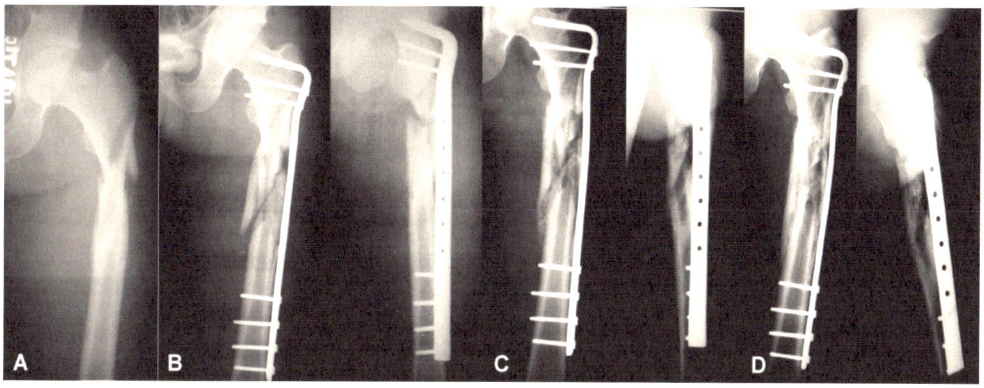

Fig. 3. (A-G): (A) Type IV (Seinsheimer) subtrochanteric fracture, with diaphyseal extension; (B) CBP minimally invasive osteosynthesis- postoperative control; (C) Callus presence at 2 months postoperatively; (D) Abundant callus at 6 months postoperatively.

Using special instruments, Krettek imagined MIPPO technique, implanting the DCS construct in a percutaneous and submuscular way (Krettek et al., 1997a).

We have performed a prospective study (Sirbu et al., 2008) in order to evaluate the outcome of 38 subtrochanteric femoral fractures treated by MIPO technique, using a 95° CBP in 7 cases, a DCS in 19 cases, a titanium-made Limited Contact-DCS (LC-DCS) (Fig. 5) in 11 cases and 1 reverse titanium-made Limited Contact - Condylar Butress Plate (LC-CBtP). For reverse LC-CBtP the anterograde insertion under vastus lateralis was easily accomplished (Fig. 6).

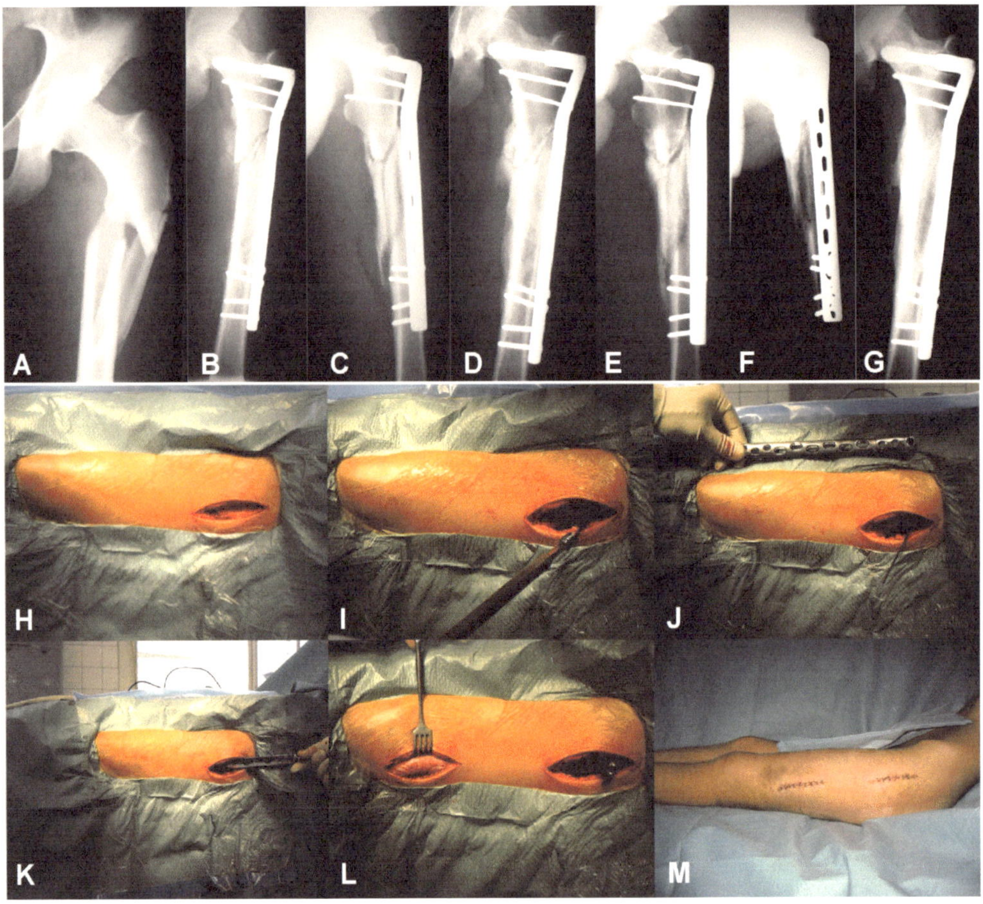

Fig. 4. (A-J). (A) Complex subtrochanteric fracture; (B,C) MIPO with DCS, incipient callus at 2 months postoperatively; (D,E) Fracture healing at 4.5 months postoperatively; (F,G) Xray aspect at 1 year postoperatively; (H) Proximal incision; (I) DCS screw insertion; (J) Plate selection under RX control; (K) Plate insertion beneath the vastus lateralis; (L) Additional distal incision; (F) Final aspect of the operative wound.

The fractures were classified according to Seinsheimer (2 type IIB, 3 type IIC, 5 type IIIA, 4 type IIIB, 14 type IV and 10 type V). The crucial steps are represented by the reestablishment of axis, length and rotation of the femur, using Krettek techniques (Krettek et al., 1998): cable technique (in frontal plane), lateral fluoroscopic projection (in sagittal plane), the lesser trochanter shape sign - if intact (for rotational alignment) and meterstick technique (for length).
All fractures healed, within a mean time of 10.2 weeks (range 8-22 weeks).There were no infections or serious implant failure. One patient that fallen after operation undergone distal screw breakage with secondary displacement in varus, requiring re-intervention. At follow-up, there were 5 varus/valgus deformities above 5°, 4 leg length discrepancies over 15 mm and 1 malrotation of 20°. The final outcome (according to the Neer scale) was excellent in 24 cases, satisfactory in 13 cases and unsatisfactory in 1 case.
The conclusion was that this demanding technique has the advantages of a faster rate of union, with no need for bone grafting. Adjustment of adequate axial and rotational alignment is an essential aspect requiring careful attention.

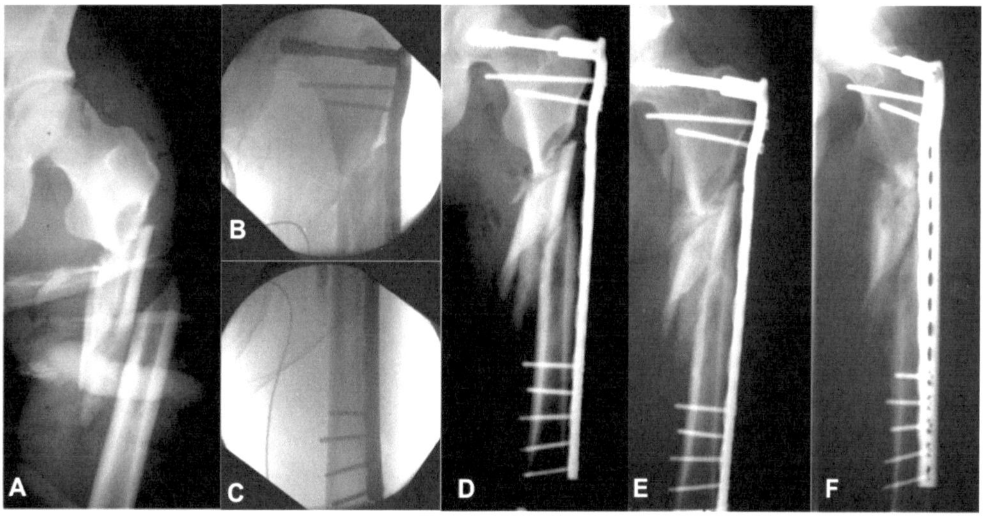

Fig. 5. (A-F): MIPO with LC-DCS in a complex subtrohanteric fracture; (A) Preoperative Xray; (B,C) Intraoperative fluoroscopic control MIPO with LC-DCS; (D) Postoperatively Xray, with main fragments alignment; (E,F) Fracture healing at 4 months postoperatively

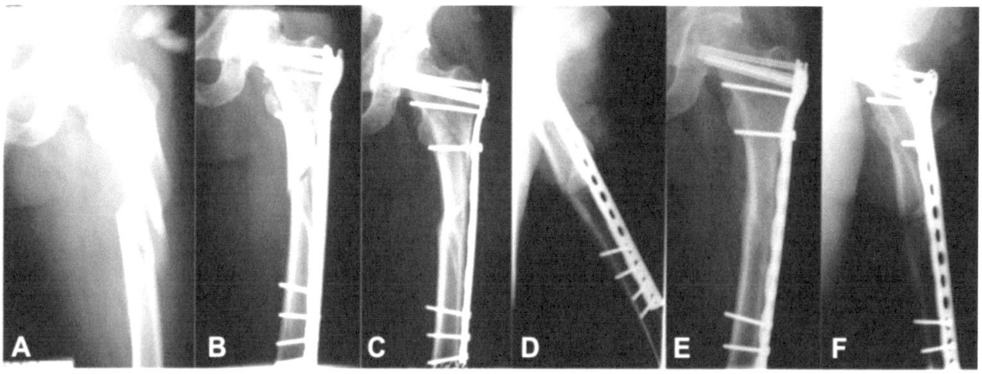

Fig. 6. (A-F): MIPO with LC-CBP in a subtrochanteric fracture. (A) Complex subtrochanteric fracture; (B) MIPO with LC-CBP, postoperatively Xray; (C,D) 1 month postoperatively, incipient callus in fracture site; (E,F) Fracture healing at 3 months postoperatively.

Even if the last generation of intramedullary nails and the locked proximal femoral plates represents the best alternative due to their biomechanical advantages, the elevated costs of these implants, the demanding technique of nailing in fractures with short proximal fragment and trochanteric extension, as well as our good results with a thorough biological technique using cheap classic implants led to the conclusion that MIPO with DCS is still a reasonable alternative in these difficult lesions.

4. MIPO techniques in distal femoral fractures

Complex distal femoral fractures represent a challenge for orthopaedic surgeons due to the comminution, soft tissue damage and complex intra-articular tracts (Wiss et al., 1999).

Open reduction and internal fixation - ORIF (early principles of the "Arbeitgemeinschaft für Osteosynthesefragen" - AO) through a standard lateral approach was associated with large dissections, ligature of the perforating arteries and fragment devitalization, followed by a high incidence of infections, nonunions, iterative fractures and a need for bone grafting (Schatzker et al., 1979; Sirbu, 2007). The idea of splinting with intramedullary implants in diaphyseal fractures of femur and tibia and the associated biological response despite non-anatomical reduction prompted the usage of plates in a similar manner and the concept of biological plate osteosynthesis have radically improved the treatment of complex meta- and epiphyseal fractures (Krettek et al., 2001). New types of surgical techniques, starting with indirect reduction and continuing with MIPO (Krettek et al., 2001), MIPPO (Krettek et al., 1997a) and TARPO (Krettek et al., 1997b) for intraarticular distal femoral fractures have the advantages of a faster rate of union, with no need for bone grafting (Krettek et al., 2001).
We have evaluated the outcome of 25 extraarticular fractures of the distal femur (type A2-A3/AO) treated by MIPO technique, using a CBtP (8 cases from which 4 cases LC-CBtP) (Fig. 7), DCS (13 cases from which LC-DCS - 5 cases)(Fig. 8), premolded Dynamic Compression Plate - DCP (3 cases) and Chiron Utheza plate - 1 case (Sirbu et al., 2008). The plates were carefully inserted through limited distal and proximal incisions only, beneath the vastus lateralis. They were fixed with screws after establishing the adequate limb alignment, length and rotation. All fractures healed within a mean time of 11.4 weeks. The functional outcome was excellent in 15 cases, satisfactory in 9 cases and unsatisfactory in one case. The authors concluded that MIPO technique is safe and has the biological advantage of a faster rate of union, with low complication rate.

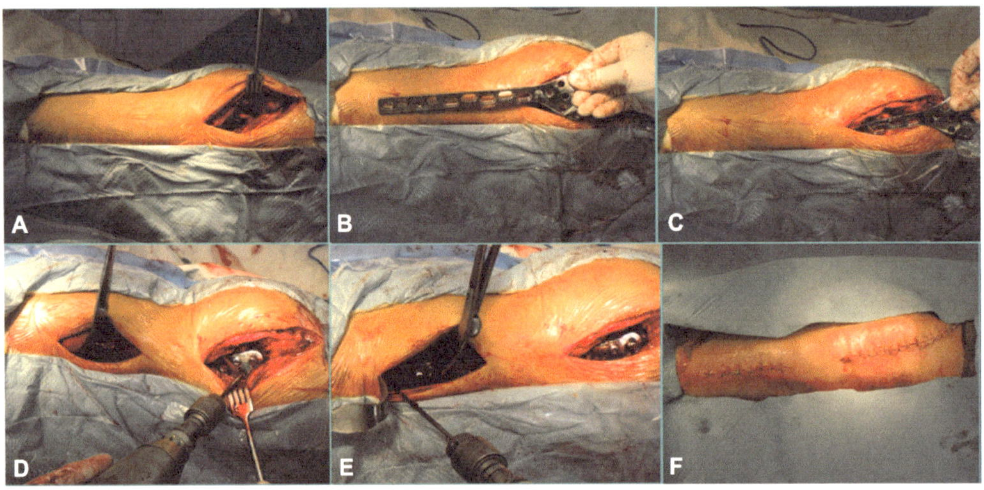

Fig. 7. (A-F) MIPO with limited proximal and distal incisions only, in a distal femoral fracture. (A) Antero-lateral approach; (B) Plate selection under fluoroscopic control; (C) Retrograde plate insertion beneath the vastus lateralis; (D) Plate distal fixation; (E) Plate proximal fixation, by additional incision; (F) Final operative wound aspect.

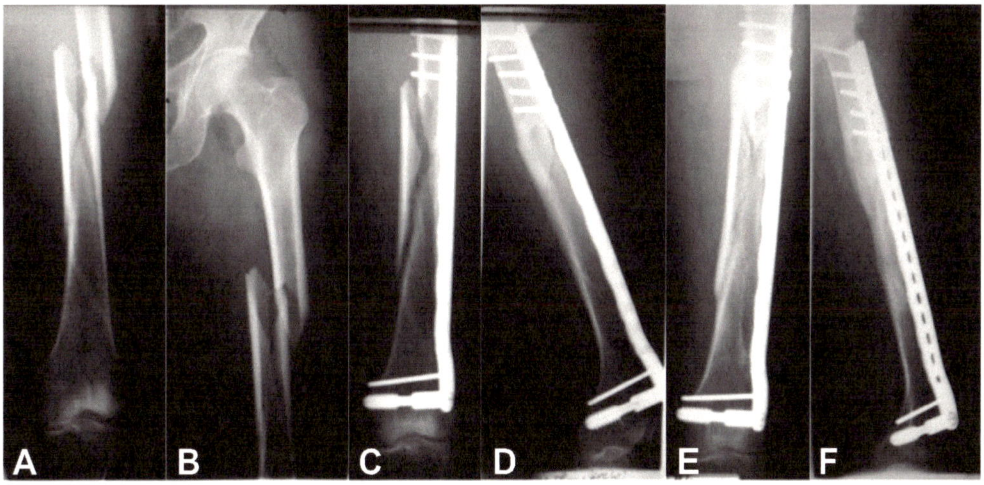

Fig. 8. (A-F). Supracondylar fracture of the left femur, with diaphyseal extension; MIPO with LC-DCS: (A,B) Preoperatively aspect; (C,D) Postoperatively aspect; (E,F) Callus formation at 6 months postoperatively

The ideal implant for the distal femur fractures is controversial. However, while plates with angular stability (types LISS and LCP) and retrograde interlocking nail seem to be the best choice for treatment, CBP and DCS still represent the most used implants, due to their biomechanical and financial advantages. In a biomechanical study we have performed a comparative study on plastic bones regarding the mechanical stiffness of the bone/osteosynthesis material (DCS or CBP) construct in complex supracondylar femur fractures (Sirbu et al., 2009a). These complexes were tested for 7 load types.
Compression force and loading force were measured by a force transducer and linear deformation values for the compression (Fig. 9) were measured by two inductive transducers applied in frontal axis (TD1) and sagittal axis (TD2).

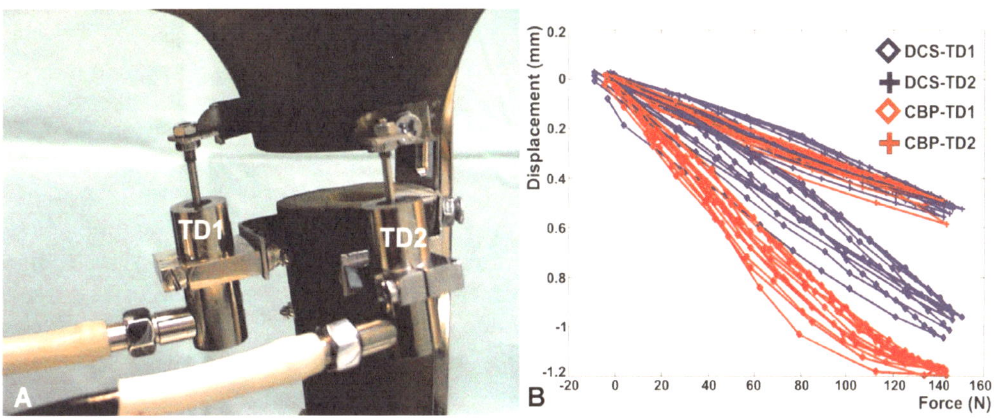

Fig. 9. (A) Deformation measuring methods. Transducers: TD1 - frontal axis; TD2 - sagittal axis; (B) Internal compression (DCS/CBP). Six loading tests. TD1 deformations, 12-16% higher for CBP than DCS; TD2 deformations, comparable for CBP vs DCS. Negative values (osteotomy closure). Mechanical hysteresis (both implants)

The femur-DCS complex is more stable in all compression types except the posterior and axial one, where CBP appear to be more resistant for TD2 transducer.
By changing the instruments required to insert the DCS construct, Krettek (Krettek et al., 1997a) has imagined the MIPPO technique for the proximal and distal femur (fig. 10). The key for this procedure is the usage of a two-part DCS implant.

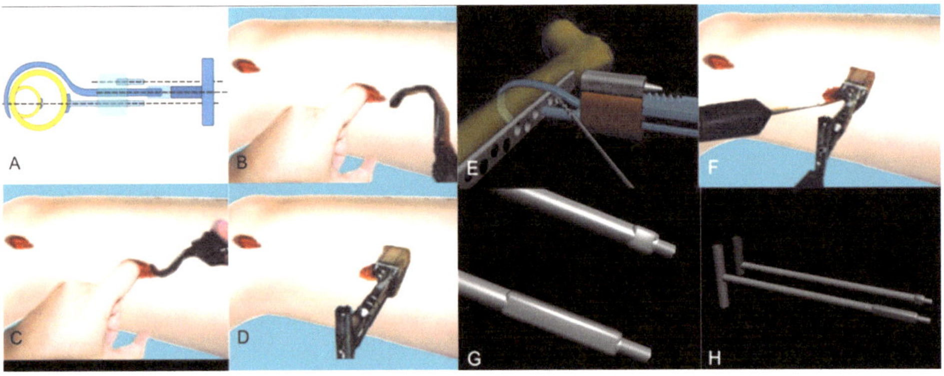

Fig. 10. Special instruments used in MIPPO of the distal femur

In complex supra- and intercondylar fractures, the exposure and direct reconstruction of the joint surface helped by the maintenance of a minimally invasive technique for the metaphyseal-diaphyseal part are procedures difficult to be performed by classic lateral approach; this requires a medial placement for the retractors in order to visualize the articular comminution (mainly posteromedial), with consecutive metaphyseal deperiostation and healing delay. Moreover, the knee flexion determines the patella pressure in the medial condyle associated with its secondary displacement.
For a complete joint visualization and to limit soft tissue dissection in the metaphyseal-diaphyseal areas, Krettek (Krettek et al., 1997b) introduced TARPO.
A very strict external parapatellar arthrotomy if extended proximally (by separating the rectus femoris from vastus lateralis) and distally (up to the tibial tuberosity), allow medial patella displacement with direct and anatomic reduction of the articular surface (Fig. 11). The articular condylar area is then indirectly reduced to diaphysis by a retrograde inserted plate, beneath the vastus lateralis (without the exposure of the metaphyseal-diaplhyseal area and without tempting an anatomical reduction). The plate is fixed proximally to diaphysis by screws that are inserted percutaneously or by minimal incisions (Fig. 12).
We have performed a prospective study in order to evaluate the outcome of 27 displaced complex AO type C2–C3 distal femoral fractures treated by TARPO procedure (Sirbu et al., 2008). There were 20 closed and 7 open fractures (3 grade I, 3 grade II and 1 grade IIIA, according to Gustilo classification). All fractures healed, within a mean time of 12,2 weeks (range 8-20 weeks). We have recorded 1 infection, 1 delayed union, 2 distal implant failures with secondary varus (1 case with infection). We have to reoperate in 3 cases. The results (using the Neer scale) were excellent in 14 cases, satisfactory in 8 cases, unsatisfactory in 4 cases with 1 failure. At follow-up there were 5 varus–valgus deformities exceeding 5°, two leg length discrepancies over 1,5 cm and one malrotation of 15°.
The conclusion was that this demanding technique has the advantage of a faster rate of union, no need for bone grafting and improved exposure of the knee joint. Care should be taken to ensure adequate axial and rotational alignment.

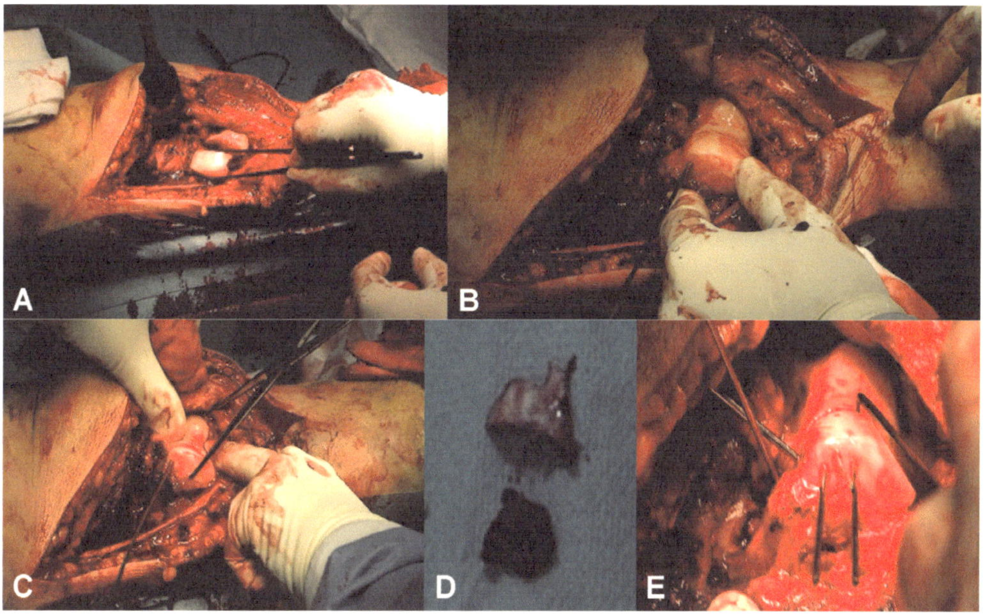

Fig. 11. (A-E) TARPO technique: (A) lateral parapatellar arthrotomy and fracture site inspection; (B-E) anatomical reduction of the articular block and fixation with Kirschner wire with (D) removal of shattered bone fragments.

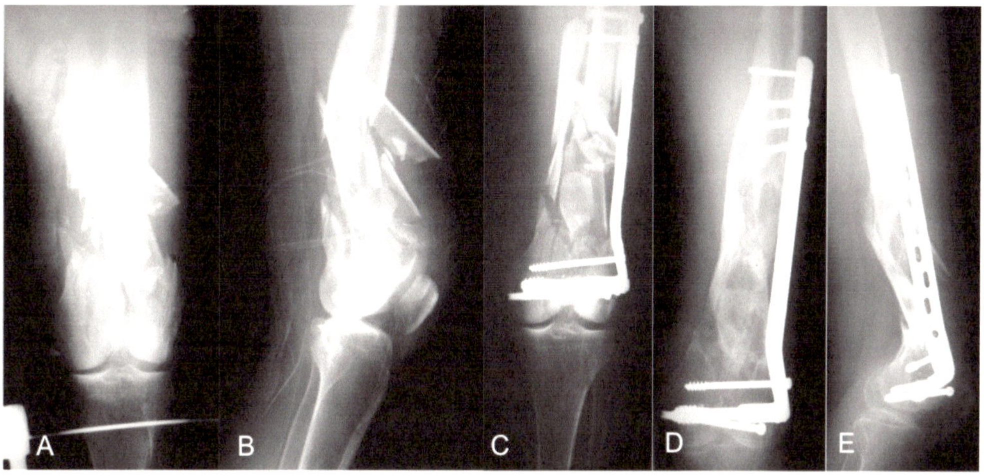

Fig. 12. (A,B) Fracture type C2/AO with diaphyseal extension; (C) TARPO with classic DCS, postoperatively aspect with perfect fracture fragments alignment; (D,E) Fracture healing at 5 months postoperatively, with an abundant callus in the fracture site. Uneventful healing at 5 months, despite extreme comminution of the metaphyseal area.

A major problem of the minimally invasive surgical techniques is that the classic implants (CBP, CBtP and DCS) are not specially conceived for the percutaneous implantation, and so the procedures are demanding (Krettek et al., 1997b; Sirbu, 2007; Sirbu et al., 2008). On the other side, Frigg (Frigg et al., 2001a, 2001b) have emphasized three problems during internal fixation with classic plates and screws: primary displacement of the fragments, secondary displacement and periosteal compression that determine the reduction of the blood flow (fig. 13).

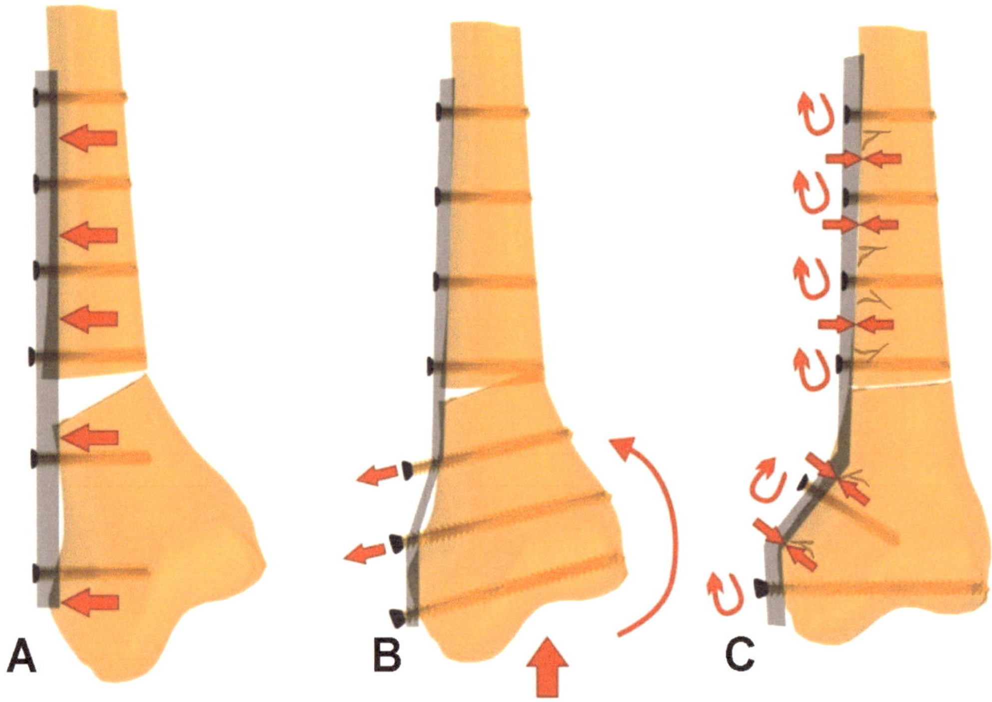

Fig. 13. (A-C) Complications for the fixation with classical plates: (A) Immediate fragment displacement; (B) Secondary displacement; (C) Periosteal compression.

The combination of three imperative criteria (biomechanical aspect of the stiffness bone-implant, anatomical reduction of the articular surfaces, axis, length and rotation reestablishment with minimal devascularization for the femur and percutaneous insertion of the implant) have led to the development of a new generation of locked plates and instruments for meta- and epiphyseal fractures. They were denominated Less Invasive Stabilization Systems - LISS (fig. 14A) and have been initially destined for the distal femur (LISS-DF) and then for proximal tibia (LISS-PLT) (Krettek et al., 2001; Frigg et al., 2001a). The next improvement for this type of plates with angular stability was represented by the Locked Compression Plates - LCP (Frigg et al., 2001b).

The high performance LISS-DF combines perfectly the aspects of a CBtP with the advantages of a fixed angle of a DCS system and with the characteristics of a Point-Contact Fixator (PC-Fix). LISS-DF system is formed by a titanium plate with an anatomical contour with round threaded holes in which the threaded head of the monocortical self-taping self-drilling screws are locked. Even if it does not participate to axis reestablishment due to multiple fixed angle screws, the LISS system behaves like an internal fixator (Sirbu, 2007; Sirbu et al., 2008; Frigg et al., 2001a, 2001b). While in classic plates (Fig. 15A) the system stability results from the frictional forces between bone and implant (requiring bicortical screws), for the internal fixator the forces that act on the bone are being transferred to the fixator by the connection between the screws threaded head and the holes in the plate (Fig. 15B).

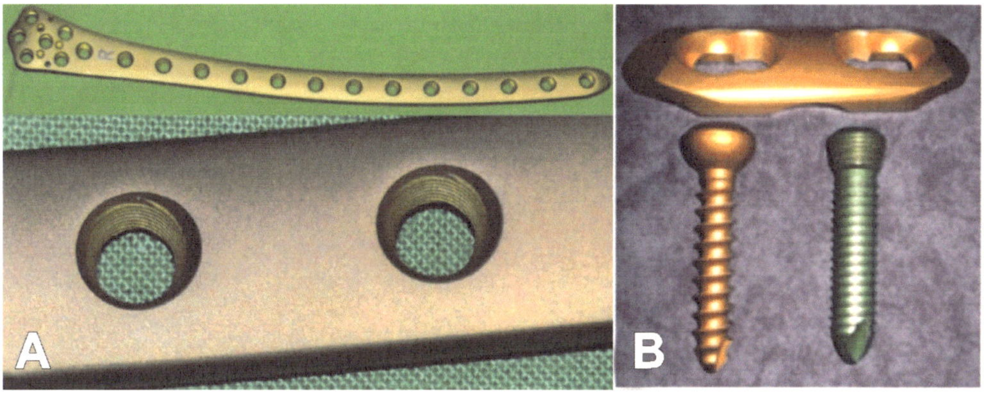

Fig. 14. Plates with angular stability. (A) LISS-DF; (B) LCP.

The screw lock in the implant holes determines the stability increase and eliminates the risk of the reduction loss due to eventual screws lag in the plate. Moreover, the periosteal blood supply is conserved due to the absence of the contact between the bone and the fixator (Frigg et al., 2001a)

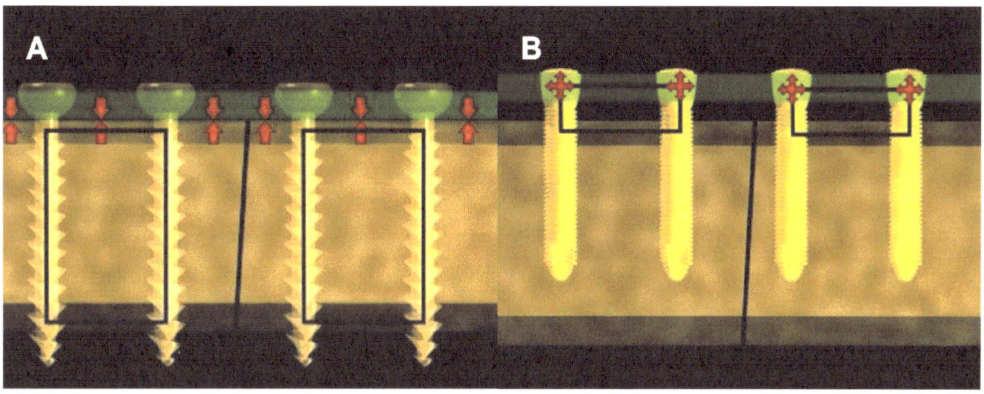

Fig. 15. Differences between distribution of the biomechanical load for standard plates (A) by comparison with LISS (B) and the bone implant interface.

The restriction of the round hole of LISS-DF led to the development of LCP-DF with combi-hole. Half of the hole is formed by a "dynamic compression unit" whose purpose is to allow the usage of standard screws; the other half is conical and threaded, allowing the usage of the special threaded head screws (Locking Head Screw-LHS). This leaves the decision of which screw to use after having chosen the plate (Mayo, 2005); the combi-hole confer the opportunity of variation without changing the implant.
In a recent study (Sirbu et al, 2009b) we have shown the biomechanics of the internal fixators as well as an evaluation of the results in treating the complex distal femoral fractures using these systems. The clinical study included 15 fractures (3 type A2, 5 type A3, 4 type C2 and 3 type C3/AO).

Two fractures were above total knee prosthesis. Three patients presented open fractures: 1 type I, 1 type II and 1 type IIIA, according to Gustilo classification. We have used 10 LISS-DF and for the other 5 cases, LCP-DF system. For extraarticular fractures we have performed a 6-8 cm distal anterolateral approach (Fig. 16, 17) while for intraarticular fractures we used an anterior approach with lateral parapatellar arthrotomy (Fig. 18, 19).

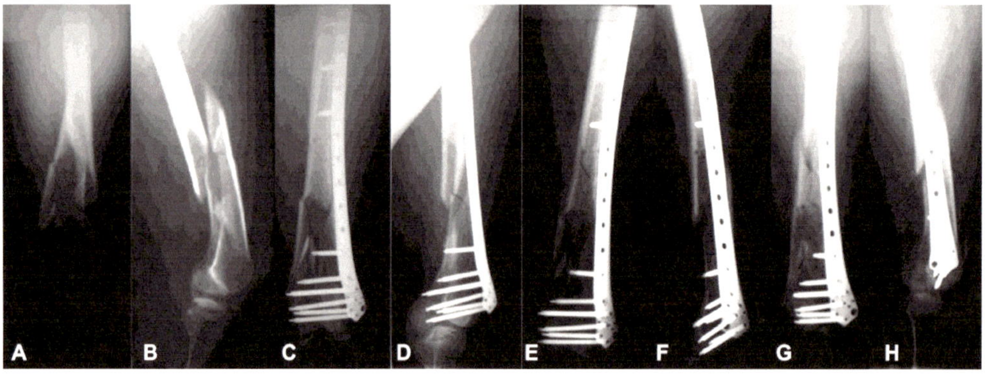

Fig. 16. A3/AO distal femoral fracture; 39 years old patient with systemic scleroderma; MIPO with LISS-DF; (A,B) Preoperative; (C,D) Postoperative; (E,F) 1 month postoperatively with slight callus; (G,H) 4 months postoperatively with fracture healing

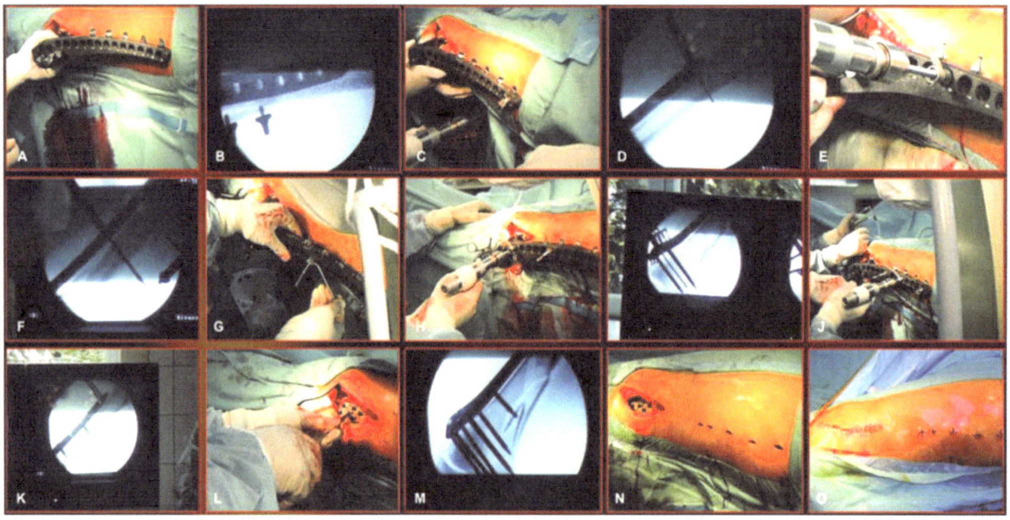

Fig. 17. (A) Limited antero-lateral incision, insertion of LISS; (B) Fluoroscopic check of the proper plate position; (C,D) Proximal fixation with a wire; (E,F,G) Whirly-bird insertion and reduction improvement; (H,I) Distal fixation with locked self drilling and self taping screws, using cooling system; (J,K) Proximal fixation with unicortical LHS; (L,M) Insertion of the last distal screw through hole A (after removing the insertion guide); (N,O) Final aspect.

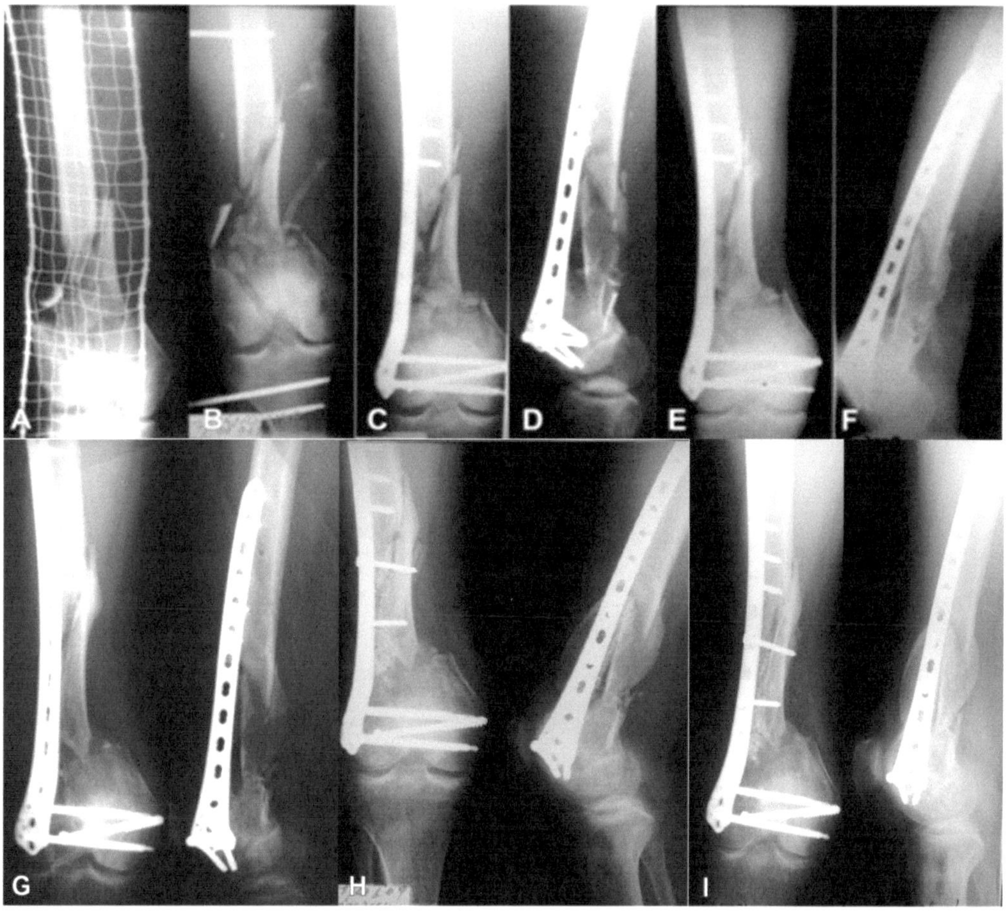

Fig. 18. (A) Distal femoral fracture C3/AO open type IIIA with bone loss; (B) Damage control with external fixation; (C,D) TARPO with LCP-DF; (E,F) Xray aspects at 6 weeks; (G) Xray aspects at 10 weeks; (H) Bone grafting and bone substitute; (I) Healing at 2 months from bone graft.

The steps for the surgical technique using LISS-DF (Fig. 17) or LCP-DF (fig.18) are: 1. anatomical reduction of the condyle using special instruments (collinear reduction clamp) in order to achieve interfragmentary compaction with lag screws (fig.19); 2. Close reduction of the metaphyseal and diaphyseal fracture with restoring of the length, rotation and alignment, keeping in mind that the LISS and LCP plate are not meant to aid in reduction and they only hold fragments in place; 3. the plate insertion between the periosteum and the muscle with the aiming device; 4. fluoroscopic control of the alignment and the position of the plate on the diaphysis; 5. provisional plate fixation with proximal and distal Kirschner wires; 6. whirly bird special tool insertion which bring the diaphysis to the plate, revise the reduction in frontal plan and prevent the medial diaphyseal displacement by self drilling/self-taping screws insertion; 7. insertion of the distal locked screws using the distal holes of the aiming device; the length of the screws can be found on a table according to the width of the femoral condyle that have been measured preoperatively; 8. the insertion of the self-drilling/self-taping monocortical diaphyseal screw, using stab incisions; 9. Continuous check of the axis and rotation; 10. Removal of the aiming device and eventual insertion of a distal LHS in the hole A.

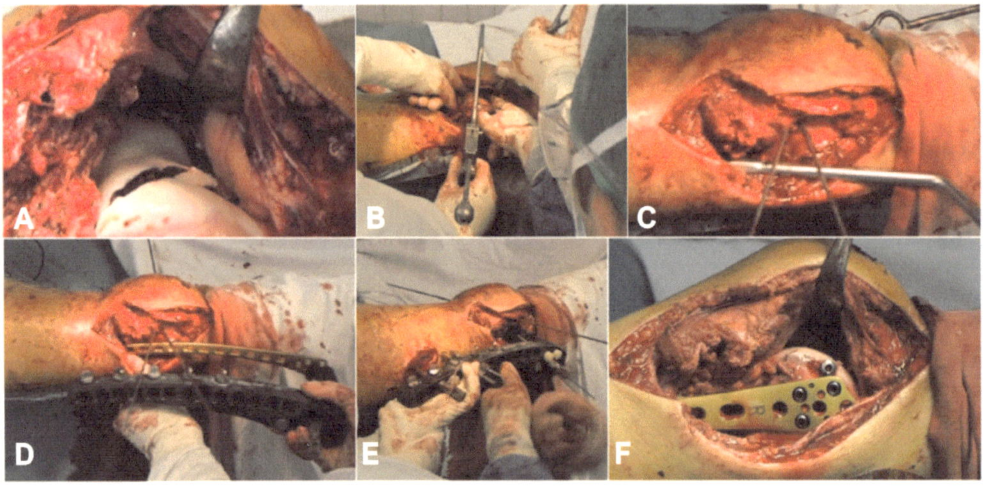

Fig. 19. (A) Parapatellar arthrotomy; (B) Reconstruction of the articular block using a collinear reduction clamp; (C) Tunneling with special instruments; (D) LCP-DF insertion with aiming device; (E) Diaphyseal fixation with monocortical screws (tightening with torque limited screwdriver); (F) Final aspect.

All patients were followed for at least 1 year. The fractures healed within a mean time of 12,4 weeks (with limits of 7-20 weeks) without primary or secondary bone grafting in 14 cases. For 1 case with open type 3A and bone loss, we have performed, at 3 months postoperatively, secondary bone grafting combined with osteoconductive bone substitution with uneventful healing at 5 months (Fig. 18). There were no infections or implant failures. According to the Neer scale, 10 patients had excellent results, while the other 5 had satisfactory results.

Our experience based also on literature data (Kregor, 2005) led to some tips and tricks gathering: 1. The usage of longer plates with spaced screws instead of short plates; 2. Perfect positioning of the plate on diaphysis (misplacement determines the fixation failure of the monocortical screws and the poor anchorage); for these reasons, a limited incision on the last holes in the plate (with visualization and manual palpation) is recommended for the obese patient or for plates with 11-13 holes; 3. Usage of bicortical screws for severe osteoporosis; 4. Perfect knowledge on the operative technique and instruments and of the anatomy of the distal femur; 5. Position of the distal region of the implant very close to the lateral condyle in order to avoid the irritation of the ilio-tibial tract.

In conclusion, these preliminary results showed that LISS-DF and LCP-DF represent an improvement of percutaneous techniques. With a good knowledge of the operative technique and careful preoperative planning, these systems represent an excellent, safe procedure, for the treatment of almost all distal femoral fractures. Care should be taken to insure a proper closed reduction before stabilization by locked plates. Even if the authors prefer the LCP system due to its versatility and combi-holes, LISS-DF and LCP-DF provide a unique answer in complex fractures type C3/AO with distal short fragments, fractures on osteoporotic bone, fractures above knee prosthesis and even open fractures.

One of the disadvantages of the monoaxial angular stability plates is represented by the preformed angle of the threaded holes; thus, the locking screw orientation is dictated by the plate design. Poliaxially locked plates allow the adjustment of screw trajectory, their placement being adapted to the fracture type (Richter at al, 2006; Sirbu et al., 2009b, 2010). The screw position can be changed with 15° in any direction inside a solid cone (with a 30° allowance)(Fig. 20).

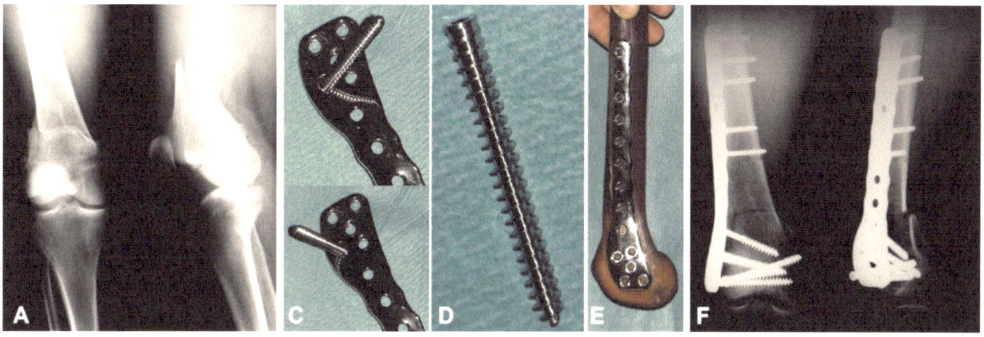

Fig. 20. TARPO with Numelock polyaxial locked plate in a distal femoral fracture type C3/AO.

However, the best option for screw locking is controversial and insufficient investigated. The authors present in a recent study (Sirbu et al., 2010) their personal experience regarding angular stability plate osteosynthesis for the fractures of the proximal humerus, distal radius, distal femur, proximal tibia. Results for the treatment with internal fixator plates are much better than the results for classic implants osteosynthesis (mainly in fractures on osteoporotic bones), accounting for construct stability, lack of secondary displacements, early rehabilitation. The authors experience show that LCP plates is to be preferred and the newer polyaxial locked plate face to the internal fixator with round thread holes due to the ability to choose the screw type and its trajectory.

5. MIPO techniques in proximal tibial fractures

Complex fractures of the proximal tibial represent severe lesions that raise treatment problems. In displaced or unstable complex fractures (with/without articular involvement) the main indication is represented by the plate osteosynthesis (White et al., 2000) The incidence of tegumentary necrosis, nonunions and infections is increased especially for the extended external and medial approach. These complications induce a decrease of the local blood flow due to excessive deperiostation and fragment devitalization. The disadvantages of the external placed plates determined authors as Krettek (Krettek et al., 2001b) to introduce MIPPO technique by medial approach. The main advantages are represented by the ease of molding technique and the subcutaneous placement, without deperiostation or blood flow limitations (Sirbu et al., 2006)(Fig. 21).

In a prospective study (Sirbu et al., 2008) we have presented the preliminary results using a medial approach and MIPO for complex proximal extraarticular fracture of tibia. 12 fractures in 12 patients (9 males, 3 female) were investigated. The fractures were classified according to AO/ASIF (4 cases with 42-C1 type, 3 case with 42-C2 type and 4 cases with 42-C3 type). There were 5 open fractures (3 of Grade I, and 2 of Grade II, Gustilo).

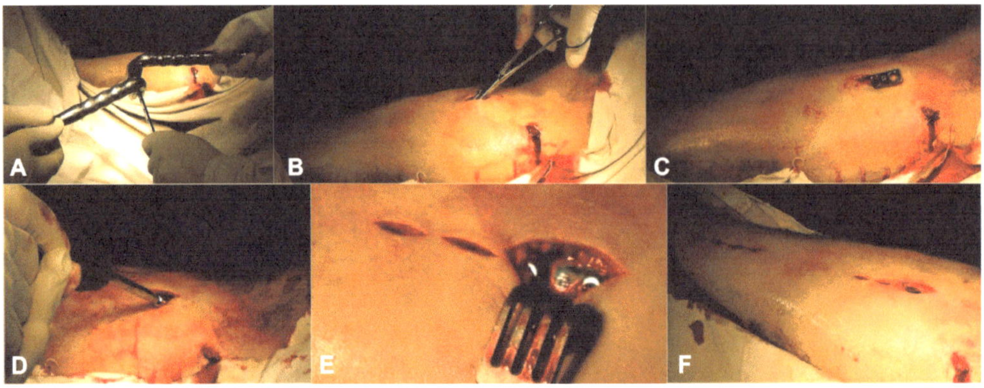

Fig. 21. (A-F) MIPO proximal tibia - medial approach: (A) Plate premold and torsion; (B) Limited proximal incision and tunneling by clamp; (C) Plate insertion; (D,E) Plate proximal fixation by screws; (F) Proximal and distal incisions for percutaneous plate fixation

After alignment of the fracture by indirect reduction, the plate is introduced through a short incision beneath the skin, and pushed distally on the medial aspect of tibia. The bridging plate is initially fixed proximally, the alignment is checked using fluoroscopy and finally, the plate is fixed distally (with percutaneous divergent screws) (Fig. 22).

11 fractures healed, within a mean time of 15 weeks, while we have registered only 1 "tight" nonunion; there were no infections, skin troubles or implant failures. Two fractures healed with larger than 5° of varus, 2 with valgus over 5°, 1 with more than 10° recurvatum but the other 7 achieved an acceptable alignment. For nonunion we have performed plate removal and Ilizarov external fixation. In 6 cases we have removed the plates. All patients had a satisfactory knee movement range. The conclusion was that this demanding technique represents a reasonable alternative to the lateral approach in proximal fractures of tibia but it requires practice and experience in indirect reduction techniques.

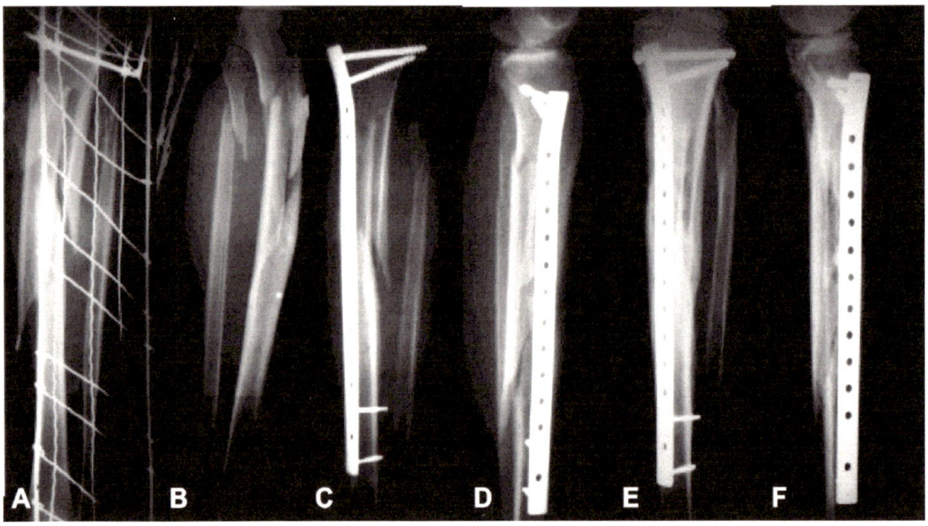

Fig. 22. Diaphyseal tibial fracture type 42-C with proximal extension; internal fixation by MIPO technique; (A,B) preoperative radiographs; (C,D) postoperative radiographs; (E,F) 1 year postoperatively

While MIPO with classic plates has determined the result improvement, the angular stability plate type Less Invasive Stabilization System - proximal lateral tibia (LISS-PLT) or Locked Compression plate (LCP-PLT) were specially designed for this kind of fractures.

In a published study from 2009 (Sirbu et al 2009c) the authors emphasize the design of the plate, the concept of the internal fixator and the importance of the aiming device for percutaneous insertion. There were investigated 8 fractures of the proximal tibia in 8 patients, with a mean age of 39.5 years. Fractures were classified according to AO/ASIF in 2 type A3, 2 type C1, 2 type C2 and 2 type C3). There were three open fractures (1 type I and 2 type II) according to Gustilo. In all 8 cases we have performed minimally invasive plate osteosynthesis, using a LISS-PLT system in 5 cases (Fig. 23) or a LCP-PLT in 3 cases.

We have used either a curved incision or a strait incision from the Gerdy tubercle about 50 mm in distal direction. The anterior tibial muscle was detached 1 cm from the tibial ridge, allowing the LISS plate insertion between periosteum and bone. For complex intraarticular fractures we have performed first an indirect reduction and the bone defect was filled with bone substitute (Fig. 24). The postoperative X-rays and the follow-up showed an excellent reestablishment of the axis with a good stability of the bone-device complex, despite the monocortical screws in the diaphysis.

All fractures healed after a mean time of 13 weeks (range 8-22 weeks) without bone grafting. At the most recent follow-up, all patients were fully weight bearing without crutches with good knee mobility (mean knee flex-ion 105°; range 95-140°). There were no infections or implant failures. Even if there is a correlation between fractures type C3/AO and a moderate functional result, it seems that the age does not influence the functional outcome.

Even if the study was limited, the authors experience with MIPO with classic plates in proximal tibia and the present results with MIPPO with LISS-PLT and LCP-PLT allow them to consider the internal fixators as "ideal" for these difficult lesions.

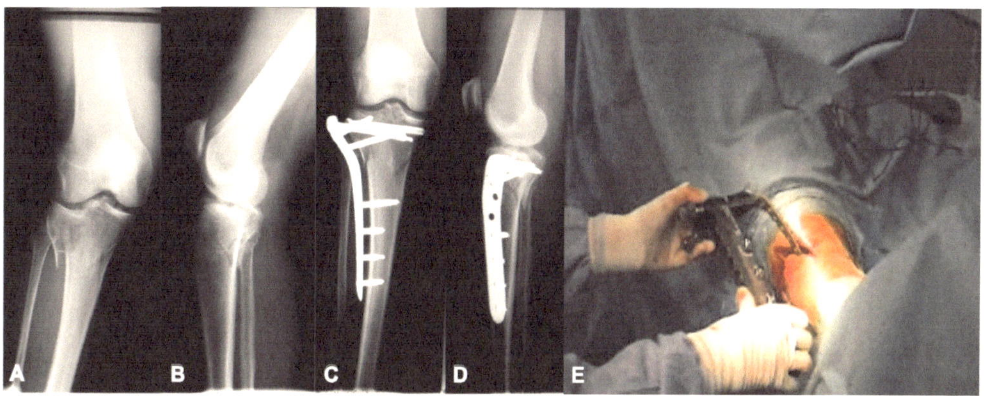

Fig. 23. (A,B) Proximal tibia fracture C1/AO (C,D) MIPPO with LISS PLT.(E) LISS-PLT with aiming device, made of carbon reinforced PEEK; LISS insertion through a limited curved approach, beneath the anterior tibial muscle.

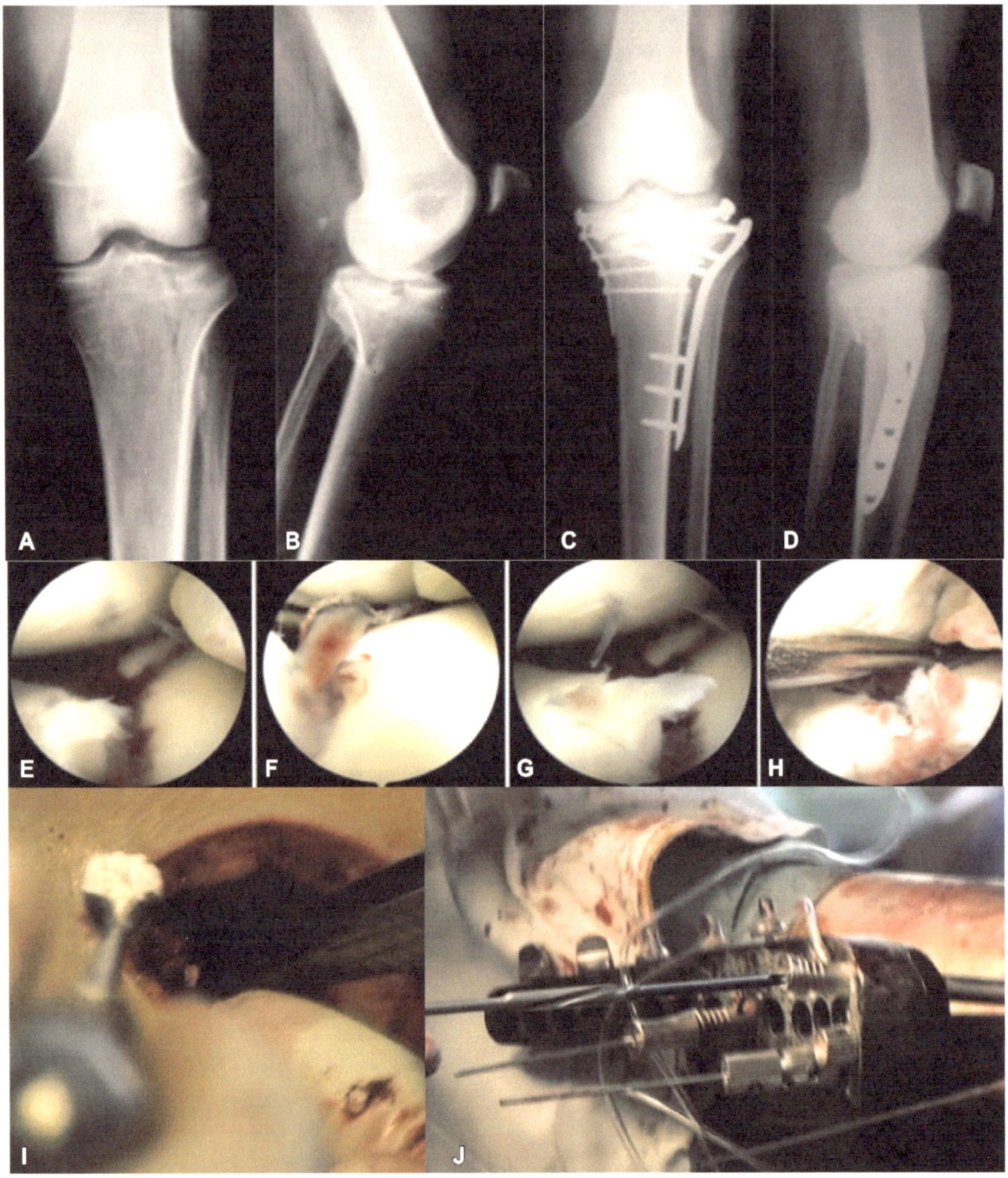

Fig. 24. (A-J) Proximal tibia fracture (type C3/AO): (A,B) preoperative aspect; (C,D) medial approach, reduction of the articular surface, small T-plate, lateral approach, close reduction, LCP-PLT, bilateral filling with Eurocer - postoperative aspects; (E,H) arthroscopic reduction control; (I) defect filled with Eurocer granules; (J) internal fixation with LCP-PLT on the lateral side.

6. MIPO techniques in distal tibial fractures

Distal tibial fractures show some characteristics as: hardship regarding reduction and stabilization, an increased local complication rate following classic osteosynthesis by

metallic plates (nonunions, infections, tegumentary necrosis) and also consecutively to intramedullary osteosynthesis (malalignment) or to external fixation (healing delay).
On one side, MIPO shows the advantage of periosteal circulation preservation with positive effect on bone healing (Baumgaertel et al., 1998; Farouk et al., 1997), and on the other side, it provides a good stability for the fracture site. Promising results for MIPPO procedure in proximal and distal femur recommended this technique for distal tibia too (Helfet et al., 1997). According to Helfet, the standard protocol that precedes MIPO procedure includes: a. tibial fracture alignment with external triangular temporary fixation, extended from heelbone to tibia; b. reduction of the fibular fracture and plate fixation by a precontoured third tubular plate or by a DCP 3.5 mm. MIPO by medial approach is recommended at 5-7 days from accident; type 1 and 2 (Gustilo) open fractures does not represent contraindications. As implants, we may use 4.5 mm DCP plates, LC-DCP, LCP or semi-tubular plates. Preoperatively, these plates are molded on the plastic tibia, a copy of the anatomical tibia. Patients can be operated on a radiolucent operative table or on orthopaedic table (with transcalcanean nail). A medial approach is performed, by two limited incisions, distal and proximal from the fracture. To maintain reduction we recommend a sharp autostatic nipper that provides the transcutaneous fracture contention (Fig. 25). Percutaneous insertion of the pre-molded plate is performed only from the distal to the proximal wound, either directly, or following a subcutaneous tunneling with blunt scissors. Subcutaneous plate progress is performed by a Kocker clamp or by other devices (Fig. 25). The plate is fixed with 4.5 mm cortical screws, usually with 3 proximal and 3 distal screws (Fig. 26). During surgery, clinical and fluoroscopic control should be performed to check axis, rotation and length of the tibia.

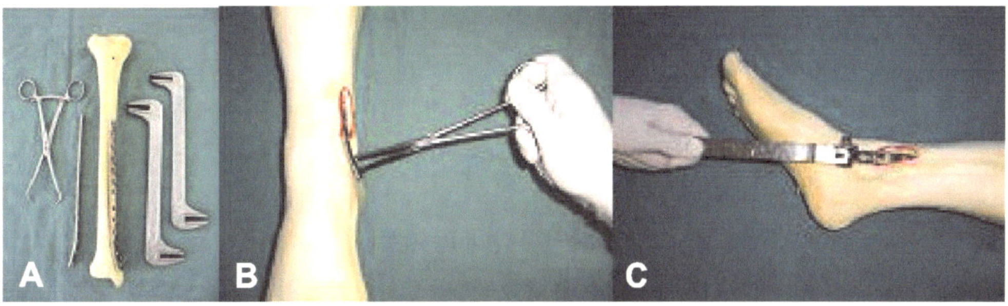

Fig. 25. (A) Devices for MIPO technique: reduction clamp and plate bent device (B) Plate pushing by a Kocher clamp or (C) With a condylar blade plate holder.

In 2006, we have published the preliminary results (Sirbu et al., 2006) using a medial approach and MIPO technique for unstable proximal and distal fractures of tibia. 22 fractures (2 A-type, 4 B-type and 16 C-type fractures/ AO) were investigated. Under clinic and fluoroscopic control for axis and rotation, the plate is inserted beneath the skin by a limited medial approach and fixed by screws. All fractures healed, within a mean time of 13 weeks (no bone grafting); there were no infections, nonunions, skins troubles or implant failures. 4 fractures healed with more than 5° of varus/valgus alignment, and 1 fracture healed with more than 10° recurvatum. All patients had a satisfactory knee and ankle range of motion. The conclusion was that this demanding technique represents a reasonable alternative to the standard methods of internal or external fixation in these fractures.

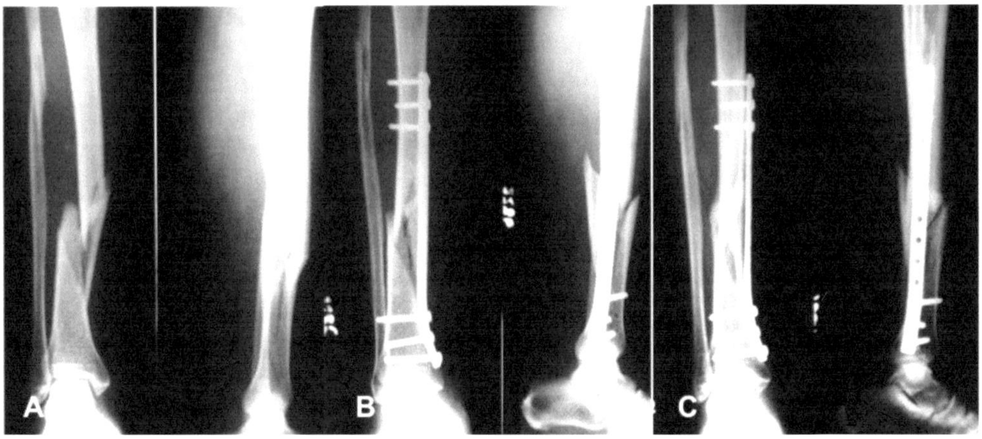

Fig. 26. (A-C). MIPO of distal tibia by medial approach with fracture healing at 4 months;

7. Conclusions

The results obtained by the authors in different services of trauma and orthopaedics showed that plates with angular stability represents an improvement of the internal fixation of the complex periarticular fracture of the long bones as well as an improvement of a percutaneous technique.
With a good knowledge of the operative technique and careful preoperative planning, these plates represent excellent and safe procedures for difficult articular fractures. Internal fixators can be expected to maintain, but not obtain fracture reduction, so care should be taken to insure a proper close reduction before insertion of the locked screws.
In the future, the real time photogrammetry and triangulation techniques by top-performance software will allow the trauma surgeon to obtain accurate images in order to reestablish the length, axis and rotation during minimally invasive techniques (Ip, 2006)
Close cooperation between orthopedic surgeon, biomechanics and robotics specialist, and the departments of cell biology and pathology will contribute to the creation of the ideal internal fixator and will represent the premises for experimental investigations required to elucidate the dynamic and coherent process of callus formation.

8. References

Wiss, D.A.; Fleming, C.H.; Matta, J.M. & Clark, D (1986). Comminuted and rotationally unstable fractures of the femur treated with an interlocking nail. *Clin Orthop Relat Res.*, No.212, pp. 35-47, ISSN 0009-921X

Bucholz, R.W. & Brumback, R.J (1996) Fractures of the Shaft of the Femur, In: *Rockwood and Green's Fractures in Adults,* C.A. Rockwood Jr, D.P. Green, R.W. Bucholz, J.D. Heckman (Ed.), 1827-1910, Lippincott-Raven Publishers, ISBN 978-0397515097, Philadelphia, New York

Baumgartel, F.; Buhl, M. & Rahn, B.A. (1998). Fracture healing in biological plate osteosynthesis. *Injury*, Vol.29, Suppl.3, pp. C3-6, ISSN 0020-1383

Krettek, C.; Schandelmaier, P.; Miclau, T. & Tscherne, H (1997). Minimally invasive percutaneous plate osteosynthesis (MIPPO) using the DCS in proximal and distal femoral fractures. *Injury,* Vol.28, Suppl.1, pp. A20-30, ISSN 0020-1383

Wenda, K.; Runkel, M.; Degreif, J. & Rudig, L (1997). Minimally invasive plate fixation in femoral shaft fractures. *Injury,* Vol.28, Suppl.1, pp. A13-9, ISSN 0020-1383

Krettek, C.; Schandelmaier, P.; Miclau, T.; Bertram, R.; Holmes, W. & Tscherne, H (1997). Transarticular joint reconstruction and indirect plate osteosynthesis for complex distal supracondylar femoral fractures. *Injury,* Vol.28, Suppl.1, pp. A31-41, ISSN 0020-1383

Livani, B. & Belangero, WD (2004). Bridging plate osteosynthesis of humeral shaft fractures. *Injury,* Vol.35, No.6, pp. 587-595, ISSN 0020-1383

Sirbu, P.D.; Schwarz, N.; Belangero, W.D.; Livani, B.; Margrit, L., Botez, P. & Mihăilă R.I. (2008). *Minimally invasive plate osteosynthesis in long bone fractures,* Casa de editura Venus, ISBN 978-973-756-083-4, Iasi, Romania

Rommens, P.M.; Kuechle, R.; Bord, T.; Lewens, T.; Engelmann, R. & Blum, J. (2008) Humeral nailing revisited. *Injury,* Vol.39, No.12, pp. 1319-1328, ISSN 0020-1383

Changulani, M.; Jain, U.K. & Keswani, T. (2007). Comparison of the use of the humerus intramedullary nail and dynamic compression plate for the management of diaphyseal fractures of the humerus. A randomised controlled study. *Int Orthop,* Vol.31, No.3, pp. 391-395, ISSN 0341-2695

Asaftei, R.; Sirbu, P.D.; Carata, E.; Bar, M. & Botez, P. (2010). Biomechanical Analysis of Three Different Types of Implants in Humeral Diaphysis Fractures, *Advanced Technologies for Enhancing Quality of Life (AT-EQUAL), 2010,* pp. 14-17, ISBN 978-1-4244-8842-1

Hoffmann, R.; Kolbeck, S.; Schiitz, M. & Haas, N.P. (1999). Treatment of proximal fractures of the femur. *Injury,* Vol.30, pp. 21-30, ISSN 0020-1383

Krettek, C.; Müller, M. & Miclau, T. (2001). Evolution of minimally invasive plate osteosynthesis (MIPO) in the femur. *Injury,* Vol.32, Suppl.3, pp. SC14-23, ISSN 0020-1383

Krettek, C.; Miclau, T.; Grün, O.; Schandelmaier, P. & Tscherne, H. (1998). Intraoperative control of axes, rotation and length in femoral and tibial fractures. *Injury,* Vol.29, Suppl.3, pp. 29-39, ISSN 0020-1383

Wiss, D.A.; Watson, J.T.; & Johnson, E.E. (1996). Fractures of the Knee, In: *Rockwood and Green's Fractures in Adults,* C.A. Rockwood Jr, D.P. Green, R.W. Bucholz, J.D. Heckman (Ed.), 1972-1994, Lippincott-Raven Publishers, ISBN 978-0397515097, Philadelphia, New York

Schatzker, J. & Lambert, D.C. (1979). Supracondylar fractures of the femur, *Clin. Orthop.,* 1979, No.138, pp. 77 - 83, ISSN 0009-921X

Sîrbu, P.D. (2007). *Osteosinteza minim invazivă cu plăci în fracturile femurului distal,* Casa de editura Venus, ISBN 978-973-756-057-5, Iasi, Romania

Sirbu, P.D.; Carata, E.; Petreus, T.; Munteanu, F.; Popescu, C.; Asaftei, R. & Botez, P. (2009). Dynamic Condylar Screw (DCS) versus Condylar Blade Plate (CBP) in Complex Supracondylar Femoral Fractures - A Biomechanical Study, *IFMBE Proceedings,* Vol.26, pp. 409-412, ISBN 978-3-642-04292-8, Cluj-Napoca, Romania, September 29, 2009

Frigg, R.; Appenzeller, A.; Christensen, R.; Frenk, A.; Gilbert, S. & Schavan, R. (2001). The development of the distal femur. Less Invasive Stabilization System (LISS), *Injury*, Vol.32, pp. 24-31, ISSN 0020-1383

Frigg, R.; Frenk, A.; Haas, N.P. & Regazzoni P. (2001). The Locking Compression Plate System, *AO Dialogue*, Vol.14, No.I, pp. 8-9

Mayo, K. (2005). Why I use the LCP for distal femoral fractures?", *AO Dialogue*, Vol.18, No.3, pp. 17-18

Sirbu, P.D.; Carata, E.; Petreus, T.; Asaftei, R. & Botez, P. (2009). Minimally Invasive Plate Osteosynthesis with Systems with Angular Stability in Complex Distal Femoral Fractures. Design, Biomechanics and Clinical Results, AT-EQUAL, pp. 36-41, ISBN 978-0-7695-3753-5, Iasi Romania, June 22, 2009

Kregor, F.J. (2005). Why I use LISS for distal femoral fractures?, *AO Dialogue*, 2005, Vol.18, No.3, pp. 14-16

Richter, M.; Droste, P.; Goesling, T.; Zech, S. & Krettek, C. (2006). Polyaxially-locked plate screws increase stability of fracture fixation in an experimental model of calcaneal fracture. *J Bone Joint Surg Br.*, Vol.88, No.9, pp.1257-63, ISSN 0301-620X

Sîrbu, P.D; Friedl, W.; Schwarz, N.; Asaftei, R.; Bar, M.; Berea, G.; Petreus, T. & Botez, P. (2010). Polyaxial vs. Monoaxial Angular Stability in Osteosynthesis with Internal Fixators for Complex Periarticular Fractures, AT-EQUAL, AT-EQUAL 2010, pp. 23-26, ISBN 978-1-4244-8842-1, Iasi Romania, June 22, 2010

White, R.R. & Babikian GM (2000). Tibia: shaft, in *AO Principles of Fractures Management*, Rüedi T.P., Murphy W.M., Dell'Oca A.F., Holz U., Kellam J.F., Ochsner P.E (Eds.), 519-536, Thieme, ISBN 978-1-58890-556-7, Stuttgart., New York, USA

Krettek, C.; Gerich, F.T. & Miclau, T.H. (2001). A minimally invasive medial approach for proximal tibia. *Injury*, Vol.32, No.1, pp. 4-13, ISSN 0020-1383

Sirbu P., Mihaila R., Ghionoiu G., Bruja R., Asaftei R. (2006). Minimally invasive plate osteosynthesis (MIPO) in proximal and distal fractures of tibia. *Proceedings of 7th European Trauma Congress*, pp. 349-354, ISBN 978-88-7587-242-7, Medimond Italy, May 14-17, 2006

Sirbu, P.D.; Carata, E.; Petreus, T.; Munteanu, F.; Popescu, C.; Asaftei, R. & Botez, P. (2009). Minimally Invasive Surgery by Angular Stability Systems in Proximal Tibia Fractures - Biomechanical Characteristics and Preliminary Results, *IFMBE Proceedings*, pp. 413-416, 2009, ISBN 978-3-642-04292-8, Cluj-Napoca, Romania, September 29, 2009

Farouk, O.; Krettek, C.; Miclau, T.; Schandelmaier, P.; Guy, P. & Tscherne, H. (1997). Minimally invasive plate osteosynthesis and vascularity: preliminary results of a cadaver infection study. *Injury*, Vol.28, Suppl.1, pp. 7-12, ISSN 0020-1383

Helfet, D.L.; Shonnard P.Y.; Levine, D. & Borrelli, J. (1997). Minimally invasive plate osteosynthesis of distal fractures of the tibia. *Injury*, Vol.28, Suppl.1, pp. 42-48, ISSN 0020-1383

Ip, D. (2008). *Orthopedic Traumatology – A Resident's Guide*; Springer, ISBN 978-3-540-75860-0, Berlin-Heidelberg, Germany

Part 2

Spine Biomechanics

6

Applications of Upper Limb Biomechanical Models in Spinal Cord Injury Patients

Angel Gil-Agudo[1], Antonio del Ama-Espinosa[1],
Ana de los Reyes-Guzmán[1], Alberto Bernal-Sahún[2] and Eduardo Rocón[3]
[1]*Biomechanics and Technical Aids Department. National Hospital for Spinal Cord Injury, SESCAM.*
[2]*INDRA Sistemas S.A.*
[3]*Bioingeneering Group. CSIC,*
Spain

1. Introduction

Impaired upper limb function is one of the most common sequelae in central nervous system. In spinal cord injury (SCI) patients, upper limbs are affected in more than 50% of cases (Wyndaele and Wyndaele 2006). Upper limb strength is impaired to some extent in people who have suffered cervical SCI making it difficult for them to perform many activities of daily living (ADL) essential for their autonomy such as wheelchair manual propulsion, eating, drinking, and personal hygiene (Parker et al. 1986; Nakayama et al. 1994). In contrast with lower limbs, upper limbs have extensive functionally due to the mobility of numerous joints that can execute fine movements thanks to complex neuromuscular control. Lower limbs movements have been broadly analyzed in biomechanical studies specially regarding gait analysis. Gait analysis has evolved over the last decades as an important technique to assist in the clinical assessment of patients with mobility dysfunction. These techniques are useful for evaluation, treatment, and surgical planning; in addition, sequential assessments help to provide a functional outcome evaluation. Motion analysis offers an objective method for quantifying movement and is considered a gold standard for evaluating lower limb function during gait in different types of patients.

Therapeutic and surgical interventions to improve upper limb function primarily focus on muscle balance and joint position to maximize hand function; however, the methods for characterizing specific upper limb motion deficits and measuring the functional outcome are varied and mostly subjective. Upper limb function has traditionally been evaluated by different scales that only assess the quality of upper limb movement based on observational analysis, e.g. Fugl-Meyer Assessment, Frenchay Arm Test, Motor Assessment Scale, Action Research Arm Test, Box and Block Test, Nine Hole Peg Test (Wade 1992; Finch 2002). These outcome measures are reliable and sensitive for measuring gross changes in functional performance but have less sensitivity to smaller specific changes. These tools provide information concerning the quality of movement and a quantifiable score of performance, yet they are lengthy, require the subjects to perform numerous tasks and are based on subjective and observational analysis.

A better understanding of upper limb movements requires more objective testing and accurate analysis of motion. Similarly to gait analysis, objective measurement elements and exact systems of movement analysis are necessary to be able to describe upper limb activities. Kinematic analysis is one such method. Kinematic describes movements of the body through space and time, including linear and angular displacements, velocities and accelerations, but without reference to the forces involved (van Anden et al. 2008). Three-dimensional motion capture systems have turned out to be a powerful tool for a quantitative assessment of movement in all degrees of freedom. Up to now, upper limb biomechanical analysis is not so often presented in the literature and in clinical practice, probably because motion analysis of the upper limb is more technically challenging. The models for lower extremity movements and gait analysis have been well established in biomechanical and clinical research and are now applied to the diagnosis and treatment planning of patients. However, the variety, complexity and range of upper limb movements is a challenge to assessment and interpretation of data and the clinical routines for 3-D analysis in upper limbs are not fully established (Murphy et al. 2006). The kinematic and kinetic equipments are ready to register, collect and analyze lower limb data from gait, but when considering upper limb movement it can be necessary to define and implement a biomechanical upper limb model that make more complex the analysis. On the other hand, gait analysis is a cyclic movement clearly defined and mainly in saggital plane but upper limb can perform a great variety of non-cyclic movements difficult to categorize in all planes. Finally, another point is the increased range and complexity of motion at the shoulder joint. As a result, few researchers have used motion analysis to characterize upper limb kinematics until recently, and there remains no generally accepted evaluation protocol.

Taking into account that most of population with SCI can not walk, upper limb biomechanical analysis of functional tasks becomes a very important issue. New applications of such studies are now continuously appearing. Data obtained from upper limb biomechanical analysis can be used not only for evaluation and treatment planning but also to give support to new research lines such as robot-assisted therapy or virtual reality applications in upper limb rehabilitation disorders (de los Reyes-Guzmán et al. 2010). In present chapter they are presented several different clinical applications of upper limb biomechanical studies in patients with SCI including biomechanical model description. First, it will be presented an upper limb model to study manual wheelchair propulsion in different levels of SCI; the second example is related to the biomechanical analysis of ADL such as drinking from a glass; it will also be described a clinical application of motor rehabilitation based on a virtual reality system with an upper limb biomechanical model developed and finally a model will be described to analyze tremor in upper limbs.

2. Clinical applications of upper limb biomechanical models in spinal cord injury patients

2.1 Manual wheelchair propulsion

Interest in the biomechanical analysis of manual wheelchair propulsion has increased as previous studies have reported an increasing age population of persons with SCI and a high incidence of upper extremity pathology. Although there is little research into the cause of repetitive strain injuries in manual wheelchair users there is abundance of reports discussing the prevalence of this condition. The majority of the articles are surveys or interviews with the wheelchair users. Shoulder pain prevalence has been reported in 36% patients with paraplegia (Sie et al., 1992). It has been found 100% of the subjects more than 15 years out from SCI had shoulder pain as compared to 20% of those less than 15 years out from injury (Gellman et al. 1988). The most common neurologic cause of upper extremity pain in wheelchair users is carpal tunnel syndrome (CTS). The prevalence of CTS in this group is between 49% and 73% (Boninger et al. 1999).

Biomechanical analysis of wheelchair propulsion yields pertinent information to identify the factors that predispose to such injuries. The high prevalence of complaints is a clear indication that the mechanical load of wheelchair propulsion must be unfavorably high. One of the reasons for the high mechanical load can most likely be found in the fact that much muscular effort is needed for stabilization of the shoulder mechanism and especially for prevention of shoulder luxations. These extra muscular forces would then lead to overload of one or more of those muscles, but also to high compression forces in the gleno-humeral joint, which in turn might lead to damage to joint cartilage (van der Woude et al. 2001).

To date, most researchers have investigated many aspects of manual wheelchair propulsion predominantly in persons with paraplegia (Collinger et al. 2008). Only a few investigations focusing the biomechanical pattern of manual wheelchair propulsion have taken into account persons with tetraplegia (Newman et al. 1996; Newman et al. 1999; Dallmeijer et al. 1994; Dallmeijer et al. 1998; Kulig et al. 2001; van Drongelen et al. 2005) although it has been found a greater proportion of individuals with tetraplegia experienced shoulder pain as compared with paraplegic subjects (Curtis et al., 1999). Specific topics such as hand-rim force application (Dallmeijer et al. 1998) or shoulder joint kinetics (Kulig et al., 2001) and global aspects such as wheelchair propulsion temporal characteristics (Newman et al., 1996) or upper-limb kinematics (Newman et al. 1999) have been studied in wheelchair users with different levels of SCI including those with cervical level injuries. These studies suggested that the subject´s level of SCI could influence the biomechanics of wheelchair propulsion. But little information has been reported on global upper limb kinetics pattern. Only one study was found of the upper extremity kinetics during wheelchair propulsion in a group with upper limb impairment (Finley et al. 2004). In another previous report, two populations of patients with SCI were compared (Bednarczyk and Sanderson 1994). With the help of kinematic analysis, these authors found that children propelled their wheelchair in the same manner as adults. Information regarding the kinetics approach of manual wheelchair propulsion in population with paraplegia and tetraplegia will increase the overall knowledge base about performance of the task in each group of wheelchair users. It may provide insight into mechanisms of secondary pathologies and criteria for specific ergonomic wheelchair design for each group of users.

The ability of an individual to push a wheelchair efficiently and without injury is related to the way in which the users apply force to the pushrim during propulsion. A number of factors influence the interaction between user and wheelchair, including level of SCI, design of the wheelchair, fit between user and chair, stroke mechanics, user fitness levels and history of upper-extremity injury. Understanding how forces generated by the individual are applied to the pushrim will provide insight into how these forces are related to optimizing efficiency, improving performance, identifying mechanisms of injuries, developing injury prevention techniques and implementing changes in wheelchair design (Cooper 1995). So, first of all, it is necessary to measure pushrim forces and then try to calculate joint kinetic data.

The complexity of developing a system for measuring pushrim forces is evident. A number of researchers have attempted to develop a force-sensing system with varying degrees of success. The wheelchair kinetic data reported in the literature can be divided into three catergories: (1) static force measurements using, for instance, a system of springs to restrain a pushrim (Brauer and Hertig 1981), (2) external devices for measuring forces and torques like a force plate to measure the force generated during the initiation of wheelchair propulsion for the grab and start technique (Tupling et al. 1986) or a wheelchair with a gear attached to the hub connected by a chain and gear to an isokinectic dynamometer (Samuelson et al. 1989) and (3) measurement of force components at the pushrim (indirectly or directly) using a system based upon a special wheel with a slotted disk mounted to the hub with three beams instrumented with strain gauges like SmartWheel system. This system allows measurement of puhsrim forces in the plane of the wheel and the turning moment about the hub axis when mounted on everyday chairs. (Cooper 1995).

To get an impression of the mechanical load, joint kinetic data and the underlying mechanisms, a biomechanical model is a prerequisite. For calculation of the extra forces that would be necessary to stabilize the shoulder, a model would be required that is not only able to calculate net joint torque, but also to calculate individual muscle forces (van der Woude et al. 2001)

In biomechanics, the inverse-dynamic modeling approach is often used. The inverse-dynamic modeling approach takes its starting point, contrary to the direct-dynamic approach, in the resulting movement and external forces. This approach has been widely used in robotics to estimate robot joint torque and forces needed to move the robot. The robot is modelled as an articulated chain and, starting from the last segment, joint forces and moments are estimated by using the Newton's second and third laws (Figure 1). This procedure can be used to estimate net joint torques and forces in the human members, but introducing some modifications into the equations. Newton's second law for linear and angular movement is expressed by:

$$\sum \mathbf{F}_i = m_i \cdot \mathbf{a}_i \quad \sum \mathbf{M}_i = \frac{d\mathbf{H}_i}{dt}$$

If those equations are developed for an arbitrary segment of the upper extremity (Figure 1), we get the following expressions

$$\sum \mathbf{F}_{i,p} = m_i \cdot \mathbf{a}_i + m_i \cdot g\mathbf{j} + \sum \mathbf{F}_{i,d}$$

$$\sum \mathbf{M}_{i,p} = \left([I]_i \cdot \frac{d\boldsymbol{\omega}_i}{dt} + \boldsymbol{\omega}_i \times \left([I]_i \times \boldsymbol{\omega}_i \right) \right) - \sum \mathbf{M}_{i,d} - \left(\cdot \mathbf{c}_i \times m_i \cdot g\mathbf{j} \right) - \sum \left(\mathbf{d}_i \times \mathbf{F}_{i,d} \right)$$

Those equations give the proximal net force and torque from the distal net force and torque, as well as the movement and the inertial characteristics of the segment. Therefore, the input of the inverse-dynamic model comprises anthropometry, the movements and the torques and forces resulting from the interaction of the segments with the environment. This implies, of course, that they have to be measured.

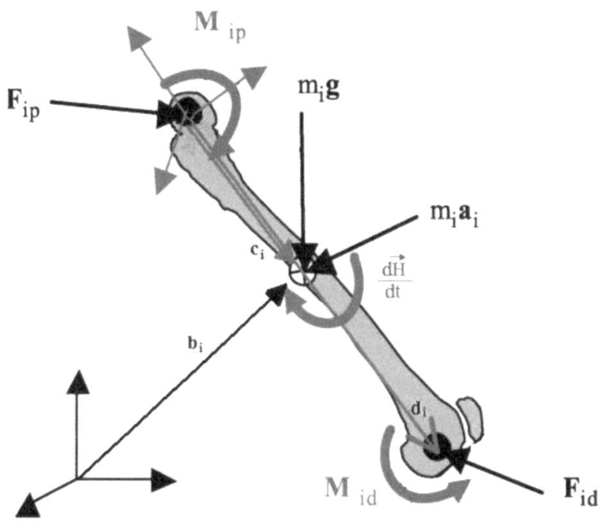

Fig. 1. Arbitrary body segment.

The anthropometric model represents the inertial and mass characteristics of the segments. The anthropometric model of the upper limb presented in this chapter follows the mathematical model of the human segments developed previously (Hannavan 1966). This model assumes the human limbs as rigid solids which shape is assumed to be revolute segments. Then, this model is corrected with Clausser's density coefficients (Clauser et al. 1969). As result, center of mass position and magnitude, segment geometry and inertial characteristics are easily linked to the anthropometric measures over the subject.
Kinematic model refers to the mathematical manipulation of the movement data acquired by the kinematics equipment (usually marker positions but there is a growing interest in using inertial measurement units) in order to match the angular velocity and acceleration of the above equations. Also, the kinematic model is used to report segment and joint kinematic. There are several mathematical approaches to solve and represent the relative kinematic of a segments chain, i.e. the helical axis, quaternion or the Euler angles are among the most used in the literature. However, in clinics the limb movements are usually described with respect to the anatomical planes of the body, projecting the segment or joint movement into the saggital, coronal and frontal plane of the body or the segment. Therefore, the use of Euler angles has been taken as the basis to solve the segment kinematics in the model developed to analyze manual wheelchair propulsion. However, one of the disadvantages of Euler angles with respect to other methods is that Euler angles are dependent on the order of rotations chosen to solve the 3D segment rotation, so care must be taken in order to define the rotation sequence to accomplish main objectives: first is to avoid indeterminations while calculating the Euler angles, whereas the second objective is to guarantee that the results can be easily compared with the literature, which only can be guaranteed if the same rotation sequence is used. In this respect, the kinematic model of the upper limb presented in this chapter has been developed taking into account the International Society of Biomechanics recommendations to define both the local reference systems for the upper limb segments as well as the order of rotations (Wu et al , 2005). Kinematic data can be measured with sophisticated high-speed automatic systems based upon active or passive markers technology, in which the absolute position of the markers is

measured. In some type of movements a two-dimensional system usually suffices because it can be assumed that movements in other planes are small and also of lesser importance. For wheelchair propulsion this obviously is not the case as movements do not occur in one plane. There is a growing interest on the use of the inertial measurement technology, which gives the absolute pose of the body (assumed rigid) in which the unit is attached.
Both anthropometric and kinematic model are joined in the dynamic model given by the above equations to form the general dynamic model of a segment (Fig. 2). As mentioned above, net proximal joint moment and forces are solved with respect to the distal ones, so a recursive procedure can be easily implemented to solve the whole segment dynamics. This recursive algorithm begins at the contact point of the segment with the environment, the handrim in the case of manual wheelchair propulsion, where it is necessary to record the externally applied forces and moments. These forces can only be measured with highly specialized equipment such as wheelchair simulator (Niesing et al. 1990) or instrumented wheels like Smart-Wheels (Cooper et al. 1997) or Opti-Push (Max-Mobility, 5425 Mount View Parkway, Antioch, TN).

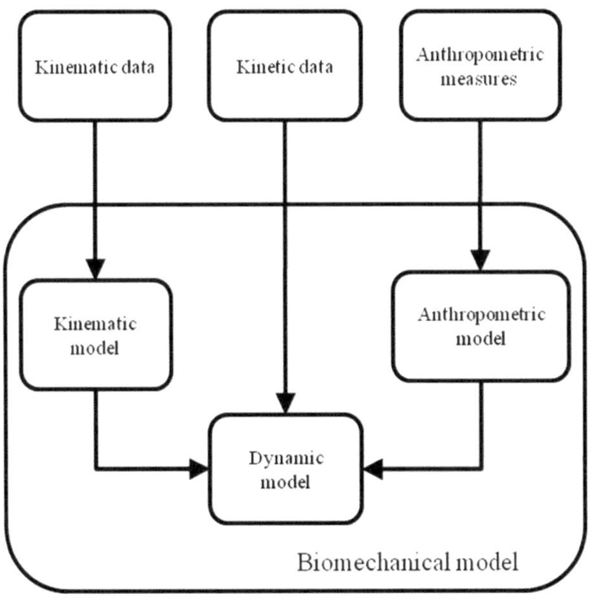

Fig. 2. Biomechanical model composition.

Most inverse-dynamic models are capable of calculating the net joint torque and power (Cooper et al. 1996; Cooper et al. 1997; Rodgers and Tummarakota 1998; Rodgers et al. 2000; Boninger et al. 1997, Boninger et al. 1999). Net torque values give a good indication of the net muscular forces that are needed around a joint. However, these torques are net values, which implies that they are the sum of all muscle force around that joint. Net torque values are thus likely to be underestimations of the actual muscle forces. If, for instance, two antagonists produce the same force against the same torque arm, the resulting force will be zero, while the sum of muscle forces is not. In the shoulder, it is likely that, because of the need for sufficient joint stability, antagonists will be active at the same time. In analyses of muscle function in the shoulder, a biomechanical model will therefore be needed that estimates the contribution of

muscles to net torques and resulting movements. A biomechanical model has been developed which includes muscles of the arm and shoulder. This model can now also be applied to manual wheelchair propulsion (van der Helm and Veeger 1999).
In a previous report, the influence has been analyzed of different levels of SCI in upper limb kinetics during wheelchair propulsion taking into account a biomechanical model using inverse-dynamic model (Gil-Agudo et al. 2000). Therefore, the purpose was to compare the forces and moments at shoulder, elbow and wrist during wheelchair manual propulsion of persons with four different levels of SCI (two tetraplegic and two paraplegic) on a treadmill. It was intended that the findings from this study will provide a baseline for future comparisons with data from wheelchair users with any upper limb impairment.
Fifty-one persons were enrolled in this study. The inclusion criteria required that subjects have a SCI with neurological level between C6 and L3, with severity classified by American Spinal Injury Association as ASIA A or B (Maynard et al., 1997), age over 18 and under 65 years, duration of the injury of at least of 6 months, no history of shoulder pain conditions and no regular participation in sports activities. Subjects were categorized into four groups according to the neurological level of their lesion: C6 tetraplegia (G1, n=12), C7 tetraplegia (G2, n= 8), paraplegia between D1-D10, also known as "high paraplegia" (G3, n=17) and paraplegia between D11 and L3, or "low paraplegia" (G4, n=14). A standard adjustable wheelchair, the Action3 Invacare (Invacare Corp, Elyria OH, USA), was properly fitted to each subject and placed on a treadmill (Bonte Zwolle B.V., BO Systems, Netherlands). Power output was determined in the form of a drag test in which the drag force of the wheelchair-user system was measured (van de Woude et al. 1986) with a force transducer (Revere ALC 0,5. Vishay Revere Transducers BV. Breda, The Netherlands). After a two-minute adaptation period, participants propelled the wheelchair at 3 km/h during one minute. We used a digital slope meter (Solatronic EN 17, Fisco Tools Limited. Brook Road, Rayleigh, Essex, UK) to verify that the treadmill surface remained parallel to the floor at all times. Propulsion trials on the treadmill were conducted with a safety system. A spotter at the front of the treadmill controlled the safety tether.
The biomechanical model is focused on the shoulder and did not consider the movements of the scapula, clavicle and thoracic spine. The net forces and moments were transformed to the local coordinate system of the proximal segment of the shoulder joint, i.e., the trunk. All shoulder joint net forces and moments were referenced to the trunk local coordinate system (Cooper et al. 1999; Mercer et al. 2006). Segment kinematics was recorded from right upper limb, where reflective markers were positioned following ISB recommendations (Wu et al., 2005) to define local reference systems on the hand, forearm and arm (Figure 3). Trunk local reference system was modified and defined using markers placed on the seventh cervical vertebra (C7) and on the right (ACRR) and left (ACRL) acromio-clavicular joints (Figure 3). The axes of this reference system were calculated as follows:
The Z-axis (+extension/-flexion) was formed with the right and left acromio-clavicular markers:

$$\vec{z}_{trunk} = \frac{\vec{ACR}_R - \vec{ACR}_L}{\left\| \vec{ACR}_R - \vec{ACR}_L \right\|}$$

The y-axis (+rotation toward the left/-rotation toward the right) was defined as the cross product of the z-axis and the vector formed by the markers on the seventh cervical vertebra and left acromio-clavicular joint:

$$\vec{y}_{trunk} = \frac{\left(\overrightarrow{C7 - ACR_L}\right) \times \vec{z}_{trunk}}{\left\| \left(\overrightarrow{C7 - ACR_L}\right) \times \vec{z}_{trunk} \right\|}$$

The x-axis (+ right tilt/- left tilt) was defined as the cross product of the y-axis and the z-axis:

$$\vec{x}_{trunk} = \frac{\vec{y}_{trunk} \times \vec{z}_{trunk}}{\left\| \vec{y}_{trunk} \times \vec{z}_{trunk} \right\|}$$

Finally, to ensure the orthogonality of the reference system of the trunk, the definitive z-axis was calculated as the cross product of the x and y vectors:

$$\vec{z}_{trunk} = \frac{\vec{x}_{trunk} \times \vec{y}_{trunk}}{\left\| \vec{x}_{trunk} \times \vec{y}_{trunk} \right\|}$$

Photogrametric data was collected at 50 Hz with four camcorders (Kinescan-IBV, Instituto de Biomecánica de Valencia, Valencia, Spain). Once digitalized, spatial marker coordinates were smoothed out using a procedure of mobile means. The kinetic data were collected by replacing the wheels of the chair by two SMARTWheels (Three Rivers Holdings, LLC, Mesa, AZ, USA). It was assumed that the force was applied on the third metacarpal as the point of hand contact (Cooper et al., 1997). However, in the case of the tetraplegic subjects, the point of contact with the pushrim was assumed to be the proximal part of the palmar face of the hand, due to the weaker grip of these subjects. A synchronization pulse from the Kinescan-IBV was used to trigger the start of kinetic and kinematic collection. Kinetic data were recorded at a frequency of 240 Hz and filtered using a Butterworth, fourth-order, low-pass filter with a cutoff frequency of 20Hz and a zero phase lag. Spatial marker coordinates were interpolated by cubic spline to synchronize with the kinetic data. All subjects were right-hand dominant. The data recorded with the right wheel were used for the kinetic analysis. The left wheel also was replaced to balance the inertial characteristics of both axes and thus ensure symmetrical propulsion.

Once solved the dynamic model with anthropometric, kinematic and kinetic data from the trials, joint net forces and moments were transformed to the local coordinate system of the proximal segment of the joint. The forces reported constituted the reaction forces on the joint, expressed on the proximal reference system of the joint. Moments were reported as the action moments and also expressed on the proximal reference system of the joint.

In this comprehensive analysis of the upper limb kinetics during manual wheelchair propulsion of persons with levels of SCI from C6 tetraplegia to low paraplegia, our initial hypothesis was confirmed: differences were found between persons with paraplegia and tetraplegia. Most of the differences were found in vertical axe and were related to wrist kinetics. They could be attributed to absence of intrinsic hand musculature in persons with tetraplegia.

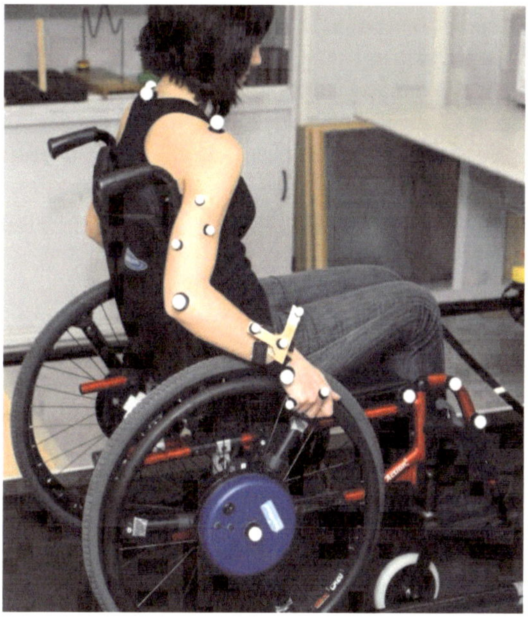

Fig. 3. Reflective marker placement.

The presence or absence of abdominal musculature in the two paraplegic groups did not alter any of the kinetics recorded in the upper limb, as previously reported in kinematic upper limb analysis (Newman et al. 1999). Two different manual wheelchair propulsion patterns of upper limb kinetics in persons with upper limb impairment have been proposed. In an earlier study, individuals with altered upper limb strength generated increased medial forces on the pushrim to provide the necessary friction to maintain grip (Dalmeijer et al. 1998). The other wheelchair propulsion pattern described involves the reduction of joint excursion and contact time with the pushrim, which constrains the user-wheelchair interface and may allow a larger percentage of tangential force to be applied (Finley et al. 2004). However, medial forces on the pushrim were not increased and hand contact time was not reduced in our current study.

The most noteworthy findings in both tetraplegic groups were an increase on upward joint forces in the shoulder, elbow and wrist and an increased adduction moment in the shoulder. Comparisons between studies are often difficult because of different testing procedures, units of measurement, equipment employed and characteristics of the sample studied (Finley et al. 2004). In this study, propulsion analysis was carried out using a wheelchair placed on a treadmill, which some authors have characterized as the ideal mechanical situation (Richter et al. 2007). Other investigators have used dynamometers (Kulig et al. 1998; Newman et al. 1999; DiGiovine et al. 2001) or ergometers (Niesing et al. 1990). Another differential aspect between studies is the testing velocity. Most studies report that net forces and moments depend strongly on the propulsion speed (Koontz et al. 2002; Veeger et al. 2002; van Drongelen et al. 2005; Collinger et al. 2008). A uniform velocity (3 km/h) for all subjects was chosen in this study to optimize test performance in the tetraplegic group and to provide a control within the testing protocol. This allowed group differences to be determined (Finley et al., 2004) and ensured a submaximal exercise level for all subjects (van Drongelen et al., 2005). The characteristics of our four SCI groups were the same as in studies by other investigators (Kulig et al. 2001; Newman et al. 1996; Newman et al. 1999).

Due to their limited physical capacity, subjects with tetraplegia applied force to the pushrim ineffectively. They propelled the wheelchair with an increased push/recovery time, but achieved less distance with each stroke. The predominance of the adductor moments of the shoulder forces during the push phase is due to similar mechanisms as the increased lateromedial forces on the pushrim reported in other studies (Djalmeijer et al. 1998). Both mechanisms allow people incapable of actively extending the elbow and with impaired hand strength to bring the upper limb closer to the pushrim.

The upper limb joint kinetics pattern identified in the present study provides some insight into why people with SCI have a high prevalence of shoulder and wrist pain (Sie et al. 1992; Gellman et al. 1988; Subbarao et al. 1995), especially in the case of tetraplegia (Curtis et al. 1999). The predominant force in people with tetraplegia is applied to the pushrim abruptly and downward on the vertical axis. This force of action on contact with the pushrim elicits an opposite force of reaction that is transmitted to all the upper limb joints, so that there is a clear predominance of upward vertical forces during the push phase in every joint. This situation predisposes to the compression of structures like the median nerve in the carpal tunnel or the rotator cuff in the subacromial space due to elevation of the humeral head. In an earlier study no increase in the joint compression forces was found in people with upper limb impairment, probably because the propulsion conditions were not uniform for all the groups (Finley et al. 2004). The net joint moments of the glenohumeral joint correlate closely with the glenohumeral joint compression forces (Praagman et al. 2000, Mercer et al. 2006) and pushrim forces have been related to carpal tunnel syndrome (Gellman et al. 1998; Boninger et al. 1999).

Most kinetic differences between people with tetraplegia and paraplegia can be attributed to the point of force application of the hand on the pushrim, which influences the calculation of hand torque (Linden et al. 1996). In the case of people with paraplegia, the point of application of force is located at the head of the third metacarpal. However, people with tetraplegia lack full hand muscle function and it is more difficult for them to grasp the pushrim. Consequently, the point of application of the force is shifted to the proximal part of the hand. This involves a change in the model with backward displacement of the point of application of force, which originates relevant differences in the moments of force on the carpus. In the tetraplegic groups, the joint moments remained practically constant throughout the cycle. The value of the joint moments depends on inertia and muscular action. Since the muscular action is practically nonexistent in people with tetraplegia, the final result depends on inertia alone, which in turn depends mainly on weight, making it an almost constant value.

2.2 Biomechanical analysis of activities of daily living

Upper limb functionality is fundamental for the execution of basic (ADL) like drinking, eating and personal hygiene. Upper limb strength is impaired to some extent in people who have suffered cervical SCI. They may require technical assistance. Therefore, these patients experience sharp limitations in their level of activity and participation in the social setting, as people who have suffered another central nervous system injury, such as stroke (Broeks et al. 1999).

Until now, upper limb function in ADLs has been evaluated mainly using a serie of functional scales. These tools are sensitive to gross functional changes, but less sensitive in measuring small and more specific changes (Murphy et al. 2006). Moreover, the use of these scales is not exempt from a degree of subjectivity.

Biomechanical analysis and, specifically, kinematic analysis techniques are interesting tools for obtaining objective data. Complex systems of kinematic analysis allow movement analysis in three dimensions. In order to analyze the upper limb movement it is necessary to define and to develop the biomechanical model based on the activity to be analyzed.

Kinematic studies have considered upper limb in which reaching/grasping movements on a horizontal plane as a free movement without arm support (van Anden et al. 2008) and with arm support (McCrea et al. 2002; Dwan and McIntosh 2006) have been analyzed. However, the analysis of purpose-oriented movements must be proposed because the musculoskeletal system has potentially a larger number of ways to achieve the motor task, permitting the organism to adapt to different environmental conditions. So, the musculoskeletal system takes advantage of this feature of the motor apparatus by selecting a desired trajectory and an interjoint coordination among many possible strategies to make goal-oriented movements (Roby-Brami et al. 2003). Studies have been published on kinetic analysis of the shoulder and elbow in healthy subjects performing a set of ADLs (Murray and Johnson 2004; Murgia et al. 2004) and on complete kinematic analysis of the upper limb during the movement of drinking from a glass (Murphy et al. 2006).

It has been confirmed that movement characteristics can vary depending on the objective to be completed. For example, upper limb kinematics is not the same in pointing to an object as when a grasping function is added (Dwan and McIntosh 2006; Safaee-Rad et al. 1990). Several studies have been published recently on the three-dimensional analysis of ADLs in healthy subjects (Murphy et al. 2006; van Anden et al. 2008; Petuskey et al. 2007). Similar studies have been made in patients with different neurological conditions (Mosqueda et al. 2004; Fitoussi et al. 2006). Although there have been few reports in patients with SCI, the results of the kinematics of grasping and the movements of pointing toward an object in patients with C6 tetraplegia have been described (Laffont et al. 2000). However, recently, it has been reported a methodology to analyze the kinematic data of the upper limb when performing a functional activity like drinking from a glass in patients with different levels of cervical SCI (de los Reyes-Guzmán et al. 2010) which is going to be developed here.

Twenty-four subjects divided into three groups were included in this study: a control group (CG), subjects with metameric level C6 tetraplegia (C6 group) and subjects with metameric level C7 tetraplegia (C7 group). Each group contained 8 subjects. All subjects were right-handed. In the case of subjects with C6 and C7 tetraplegia, the etiology of injury was trauma in every case. The patients screened had to fulfill the following criteria to be included in the study: age 16 to 65 years, injury of at least 6 months' duration and level of injury C6 or C7 classified according to the American Spinal Injury Association (ASIA) scale into grades A or B (Maynard et al. 1997). Patients who presented any vertebral deformity, joint restriction, surgery on any of the upper limbs, balance disorders, dysmetria due to associated neurologic disorders, visual acuity defects, cognitive deficit, or head injury associated with the SCI were excluded. The subjects were classified into C6 or C7 tetraplegia by a physical examination.

Three-dimensional movement capture was recorded with CodaMotion equipment (Charnwood Dynamics, Ltd, UK). This equipment has active markers that emit infrared light, which was recorded by two scanning units in this study. The marker images are displayed on a computer screen and projected as X, Y, and Z coordinate values.
One of the cameras was placed in front of the table, slightly to one side with respect to midline and contralateral to the study side of the subject. The other camera positioned laterally in the same side of experimentation (Figure 4). The system was calibrated by placing three active markers on the floor to serve as the laboratory reference system. The coordinate system was defined with the X-axis directed forward (anterior), the Y-axis upward (superior) and the Z-axis to the side (lateral) (Wu et al. 2005). The location of the cameras and markers was validated with a person sitting in the measurement area to ensure that the markers were recorded at least by one of the cameras throughout the drinking activity.

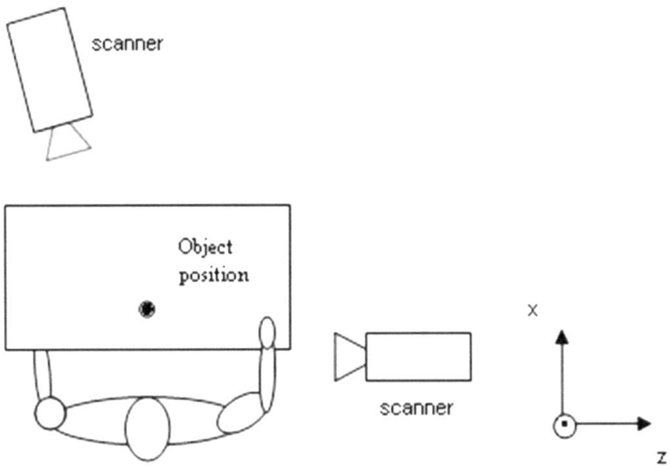

Fig. 4. View from above of the set-up for the activity of drinking from a glass. The XYZ coordinate system is visible. The subject has the arm at the starting point.

Eighteen markers were used. Following the recommendations of earlier studies, the body segments were defined by placing 8 markers on the superficial bony prominences of the right upper limb, which were easily positioned in the different analyses (Cirstea and Levin 2000; Michaelsen et al. 2001; Murphy et al. 2006; Dwan and McIntosh 2006). These markers were placed on the head of the third metacarpal, radial and ulnar styloid processes of the wrist, lateral and medial epicondyles of the elbow, right and left acromion and right iliac crest. The biomechanical model of upper limb movement was completed with another 10 markers mounted on rigid pieces that were placed on each body segment. These pieces were used with the aim of minimizing any error created by possible marker displacement on the skin. These pieces had to be light, comfortable for the subject to wear, and had to be fixed onto points where the least amount of movement was possible (Fitoussi et al. 2006). Four markers were placed on the chest, three mounted on a support and one directly on the skin; three markers mounted on a support placed on the arm, and the last three markers mounted on a support placed on the forearm (Figure 5). The final position of the last 10 markers and the position of the cameras was the position that yielded the best marker visibility to the scanning cameras during the movement of drinking from a glass and the best measurement results in the processed recordings.

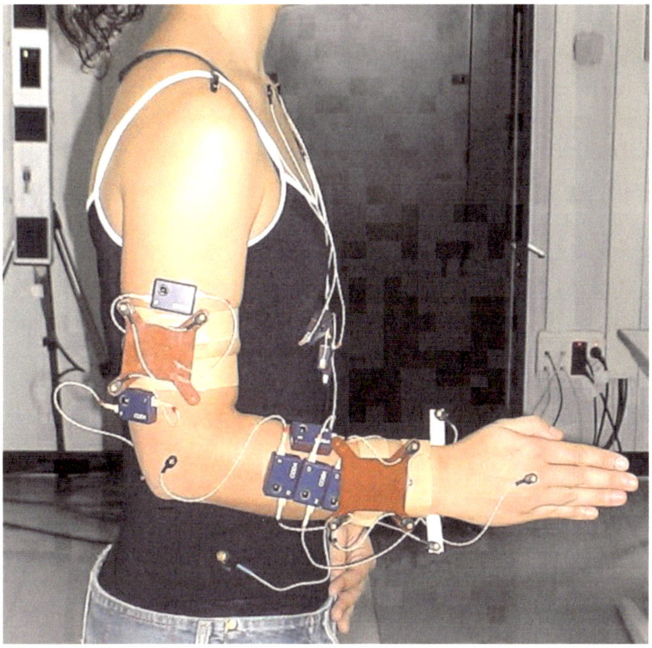

Fig. 5. Actual markers position on the subject. Figure show a sagittal plane view (X-Y).

All subjects were right-handed and performed the drinking task with the right arm. Subjects with C6 or C7 tetraplegia sat in their own wheelchairs and the control subjects sat in a conventional wheelchair, Action3 Invacare (Invacare Corp, Elyria OH, USA) with a configuration similar to that of the wheelchair of the subjects with tetraplegia. The chair was placed before a table measuring 120x60x72 cm. In every case, the subject-to-table distance was 18-20 cm and the angle between the seat and back was 90-100°. The starting position (position of calibration) for all the subjects was defined as a position in which the subject's trunk rested firmly against the back of the chair. All subjects put their feet on the footrests with a foot-leg angle of 90°. The right upper arm was placed against the trunk and the elbow was flexed 90° flexion and in a neutral pronation-supination, i.e., with the palm of the hand perpendicular to the table surface and facing inward (medial). The ulnar side of the wrist rested close to the surface of the table. In every case, the sitting and table heights could be adapted with the aim of obtaining the same starting position for all the subjects. The subject rested the left hand on the lap. A hard plastic glass measuring 6.5 cm in diameter by 17.5 cm high was used. It was filled with 1 dl of water and placed 18 cm from the edge of the table where the subject was seated, in the area marked on the table (Figure 4).

Each subject received an explanation about how to perform the drinking task, which consisted of reaching out for the glass from the starting position and grasping it, raising the glass to the mouth, drinking, lowering the glass to the pickup point, and returning the hand to the starting position. All the subjects practiced the activity twice to find a comfortable sitting position before the movement exercise was recorded. This test confirmed that the subjects could carry out the activity. Once this phase was completed, a static calibration recording was made. Using the static calibration recording, it was checked that each marker was visible at least by one of the scanning cameras at all times. Movement recordings were made as the subject executed the drinking task at a comfortable, self-selected speed. Before a recording was accepted as validated, it was checked it to ensure that the markers were visible at all times. Five valid recordings of each subject were obtained for analysis and processing.

The consistency and repeatability of the test protocol were assessed by conducting a test-retest sequence with four randomly selected control subjects. Test-retest involved recording the action of the drinking task and then removing the markers. The entire procedure was repeated fifteen minutes later.

The recordings were processed with Visual 3D software (C-Motion, Inc., USA), which involved using a signal processing program to obtain signals of the movement of different joints at a sampling frequency of 200 Hz, the maximum allowed for the 18 markers used with the two scanning units. Signals were filtered using a low-pass Butterworth filter with a cutoff frequency of 1.5Hz. The three best recordings were selected from the five recordings made on the basis of best marker visibility in each recording. The mean of these three recordings yielded the final measurement value for each subject. The human arm was modelled for three-dimensional kinematic analysis in three segments, the arm, forearm and hand, which were considered as rigid solids (Biryukova et al. 2000). A local coordinate system was defined for each segment following the recommendations of the International Society of Biomechanics (Wu et al. 2005). In the arm, the origin of the reference system was at the center of the glenohumeral joint, 2 cm below the acromion. Also, the Y-axis corresponded to the line that joined the midpoint between the lateral and medial epicondyles and the center of the glenohumeral joint in proximal direction and the Z-axis was the mediolateral axis pointing to the right. In the forearm, the origin was at the midpoint between both epicondyles of the elbow, the Y-axis was formed by the line that joined the midpoint between the radial and ulnar styloid processes with the midpoint between the lateral and medial epicondyles proximally and the Z-axis was the line that joined both epicondyles in the lateral direction. In the hand, the origin was at the midpoint between radial and ulnar styloid of the wrist, the Y-axis was the line joining the head of the third metacarpal with the midpoint between the radial and ulnar styloid processes proximally and the Z-axis joined both styloid processes laterally. We obtained trunk movement with respect to the laboratory coordinate system, arm movement with respect to the trunk, forearm movement with respect to the arm, and hand movement with respect to the forearm using Euler angle notation and a sequence of ZXY rotations of the trunk, arm and hand, and ZYX rotations of the forearm.

In each recording, a complete cycle of the drinking task was identified. The beginning of the cycle was the onset of displacement of the marker on the head of the third metacarpal and the end of the cycle was the return of the marker to the starting point after completing the drinking task. As it happens with other cyclical movements, such as walking, several phases were established in the drinking task to facilitate task analysis. Phases and events delimiting the phases have been previously described: reaching, forward transport, drinking, back transport and return (Murphy et al. 2006).

Once the recordings were made and analyzed, the results were described in terms of analysis of the following variables:

- Movement times: the duration of each phase and the complete cycle.
- Peak velocities: the velocities were obtained by calculating the linear velocity with which the hand moves in the phases of the cycle of reaching, forward transport, back transport and return to start position.

- Joint angles: flexion-extension and lateral inclination of the trunk; flexion-extension, abduction-adduction and external-internal rotation of the shoulder joint; flexion-extension and pronation-supination of the elbow joint; and dorsal-palmar flexion of the wrist. For each joint angle, we calculated the maximum, minimum, range of motion (ROM) and moment in the complete drinking cycle in which these values were reached.
- Coordination between the shoulder and elbow joints, particularly between the shoulder flexion angle and the elbow flexion angle, in the reaching phase.

In order to compare the three groups analyzed, the duration of the cycles was adjusted for time and expressed as percentages. Consequently, data were expressed in relation to the percentage of the drinking task cycle that had lapsed (0-100% of the drinking task cycle) when the movement was recorded.

The goal of this study was to analyze the three-dimensional kinematic differences between two groups of people with tetraplegia and a control group during the ADL of drinking from a glass. The most relevant findings of this study suggest that subjects with C6 tetraplegia perform the drinking task at a slower velocity and with more prolonged phases. The greatest differences between the two tetraplegia groups and controls were in the wrist.

However, more functional movements should be studied. Previous studies of upper limb kinematics have been made of control subjects performing ADLs such as feeding, grooming and drinking (Cooper et al. 1993; Magermans et al. 2005; Murphy et al. 2006). These movements are complex tasks in terms of kinematics because they consist of several discrete movements.

Much of the methodology reported here followed the recommendations of a previous one of healthy subjects in which five sequential phases of drinking task were identified (Murphy et al. 2006). However, the current experience has resolved previous limitations and provides a full and detailed three-dimensional kinematic analysis of the drinking task in control subjects and two groups of patients with tetraplegia, analyzing the shoulder, elbow and wrist at all possible joint angles except for lateral wrist inclination.

Using the upper limb model developed, we were able to estimate the location of the center of the joints involved, which made it possible to measure all the joint angles described. Likewise, the use of markers mounted on rigid pieces to position some of the markers helped to reduce tissue artifacts. These artifacts appear with limb displacement when markers are placed on the skin surface.

The duration of the drinking activity was longer in subjects with C6 tetraplegia compared to controls and the duration of the reaching phase was longer in subjects with C6 and C7 tetraplegia. As mentioned, the reaching phase includes grasping. In order to grasp, both groups of patients with tetraplegia developed a compensatory strategy called "tenodesis," in which these patients extend the wrist to close the fingers passively. This pattern suggests that in subjects with tetraplegia reaching and grasping are executed sequentially compared to controls, who prepare for grasping during the reaching phase (Jaennerod 1984).

The absence of triceps brachialis muscle activity in subjects with C6 tetraplegia slows the velocity of the forward transport and back transport phases, in which this muscle controls the eccentric or concentric displacement of the elbow in flexion-extension. As in an earlier study, the peak velocity of the reaching phase was similar in patients with tetraplegia and controls (Laffont et al. 2000). Another factor that could condition the velocity of movements is performing the movement with a load. Upper limbs weakness becomes more evident

when raising an object with a certain weight. In the absence of any additional load, peak velocity in the reaching phase is reached earlier in groups of patients with tetraplegia. However, in the forward transport phase, the glass of water is raised to the mouth and the peak velocity is notably faster in controls. It is difficult to compare the velocities obtained in other pathologies because they have not been studied using the phases defined in our study (Rönnqvist and Rösbled 2007).
In a reaching movement, as shoulder flexion increases, elbow extension also increases. So it was interesting to know the index of coordination between both movements (de los Reyes-Guzmán et al. 2010). This coordination is shown in Figure 6 and the trajectory is continuous describing an almost linear relation between shoulder and elbow flexion movements. The result was that, as in healthy subjects, but in contrast with subjects who have experienced stroke and have a hemiparetic arm, there was a strong coordination between shoulder and elbow joint excursion in the reaching phase, indicating good interjoint coordination in C6 and C7 tetraplegic people (Levin 1996) (Figure 6).

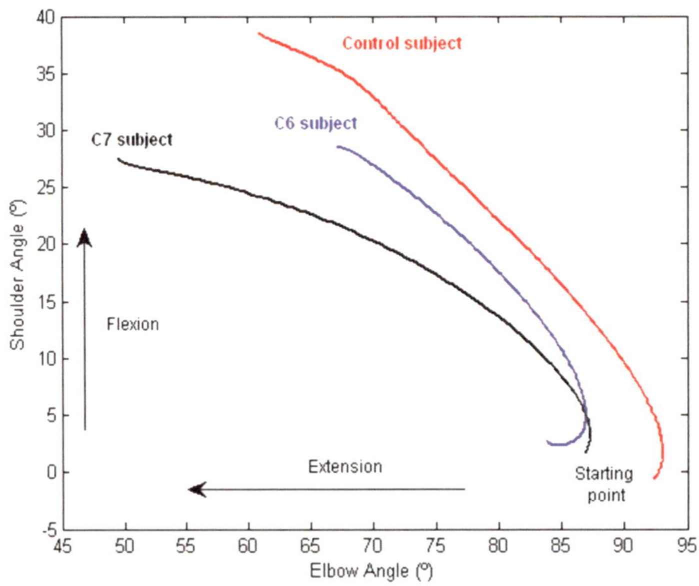

Fig. 6. Shoulder-elbow joint coordination in the reaching phase for one randomly selected subject in the control group (red), C6 group (blue) and C7 group (black).

The wrist was the joint with the most relevant differences between the three groups. Wrist palmar flexion angles were greater in both groups of subjects with tetraplegia and the maximum wrist palmar flexion in both cases was observed in the back transport phase, probably because no eccentric resistance is offered by wrist extensor muscles as the glass is lowered from the mouth to the table; passive wrist palmar flexion occurred in both tetraplegia groups. The minimum wrist palmar flexion angle was found in subjects with C6 or C7 tetraplegia in the forward transport phase. This is probably because at this time the subject required maximum wrist dorsal flexion to grasp a glass that has some weight, which optimized the tenodesis effect and the ability to pick up an object. The elbow extension was greater in both tetraplegia groups and occurred in the back transport phase, perhaps also because elbow extension favored the tenodesis effect in the wrist (Figure 7).

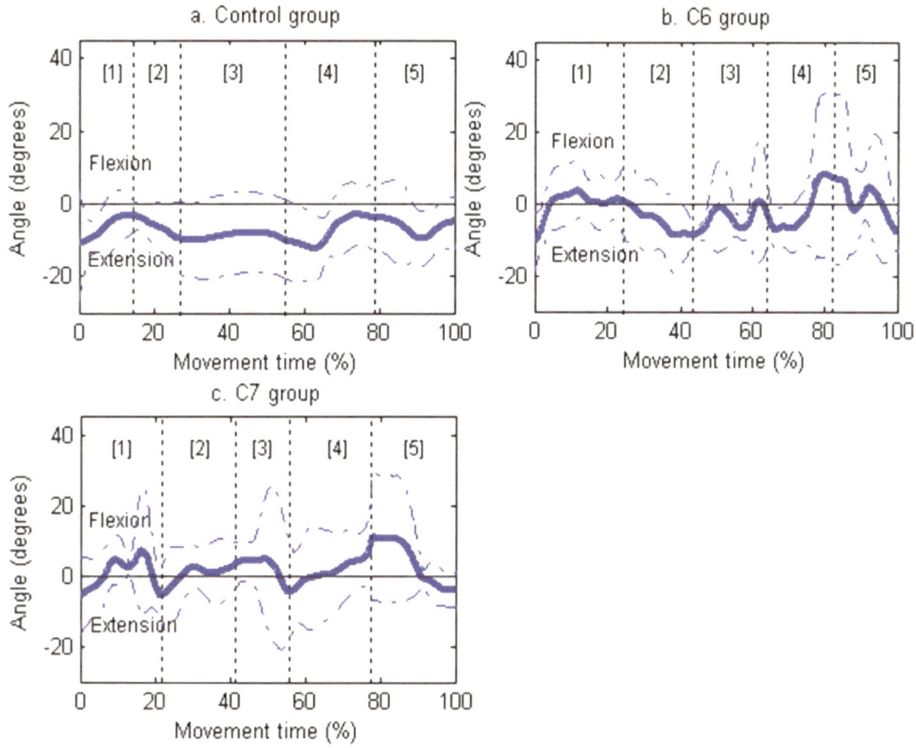

Fig. 7. Wrist dorsal-palmar flexion. Joint angles for wrist (dorsal flexion-downward, palmar flexion-upward). Figures 9a, 9b and 9c show the mean (continue thick line) and standard deviation (dashed line) of the CG, subjects with C6 tetraplegia and subjects with C7 tetraplegia, respectively. The vertical lines delimit the duration of the phases for each group. [1] reaching, [2] forward transport, [3] drinking, [4] back transport, and [5] return to beginning.

Mean retest values were within for the 95% confidence interval of the first test. Based on this data, it can be concluded that there were not differences between the test and retest with a probability of 95%. However, for measurements as maximum shoulder flexion, maximum external rotation, maximum elbow flexion, maximum pronation, even maximum wrist palmar flexion, wide confidence intervals were obtained. It could be probably due to the natural large variation between the subjects in those measurements. It is necessary to take into account that people can perform a goal-oriented task with many different combinations of individual joint movements.

2.3 Upper limb biomechanical model for virtual reality application

Human body movement is developed in a 4 dimensional space (3 spatial dimensions and time dimension). Each body segment takes orientations in the spatial space as long as movement is performed. This added to the well known articulated chain setup of the arm, causes that each segment takes several interrelated positions during movement, drawing their own trajectory in space in a complex manner. This complexity makes more difficult the comprehension of movement and the integration of movement information into clinical application. Therefore, a new model of movement representation that facilitates its application is presented next and an application of this new biomechanical model as part of a virtual reality and motion capture rehabilitation system called TOYRA.

To reduce this complexity, movement is traditionally analysed in 2 dimensions, projecting or enclosing movement into an adequate plane. Positions and trajectories are drown in cartesian planes, referenced to the gravity centre of body and frequently orientations are described against anatomical planes (saggital, coronal and transverse planes) (Villalba 2003). This kind of representations are very appropriate to describe movements like human walking, that are almost always enclosed into one plane. Although they are not enough clean while trying to describe mentioned complex movements in space, most of the times due to the inconsistencies that those representations have.

In upper limb particular case, the references of the orientations and movements are defined at one arbitrary pose. Anatomic pose is very commonly used but not the only one. This pose consists in a body standing position, with the arm falling down resting and the hand palm looking to the front (Rau 2000). Motion-capture applications commonly use the t-pose. This pose consists in a body standing position, with the arm in lateral horizontal position, perpendicularly to body, and hand palm looking towards front or facing down.

Rodriguez et al (Rodriguez 2005) proposed to reference to anatomic pose with a small modification (hand palm in resting position towards the body) and tried to establish a comprehensive mathematical representation of 3D orientations for arm body segments. They opened the way of representing complex 3D movements of the upper limbs in a more precise & comprehensive manner (Rau, et al., 2002).

Present work identifies some inconvenient of those upper limb movement representations and completes Rodriguez et al formulation to a really univoque representation model. In first place, some simplifications will be described from the real human body model assumed in this work. After that, relevant clinical angles will be identified. Then, for each body segment former angle definitions (traditional and Rodriguez et al) will be analysed and new definitions will be proposed and discussed.

Then some simplifications from the real human body model are assumed to facilitate the analysis:

1. Each joint is defined through one articular centre, considered fixed to both joined segments. Specially, the shoulder joint, is considered as a simple spherical joint that follows same movement functionality of shoulders but not their real configuration.
2. The clavicle will be considered as part of thorax and its movements are not included (Ray and Schmidt, 2000).
3. The forearm is considered as a rigid body. Therefore pronation-supination movements must be reallocated in elbow joint.
4. The whole hand is modelled as one rigid-body. It will be considered as open hand.

Taking into account this simplifications, just seven elemental movements are required to describe the movement of upper limbs: three rotations on shoulder, flexo-extension of elbow, fore-arm rotation and two wrist rotations from fore-arm are considered to complete the description. These elemental movements are defined independently using planes and reference axis of the human body.

To analyse those 7 elemental movements, it is presented in next paragraphs a new definition proposal for poses & movements of upper limb based in previous proposals of Rodriguez et al and Rau et al., 2000. A vectorial model is used to measure and describe movements of upper limb, formalizing the definitions of each of the mentioned elemental movements. To measure movements of one segment from previous segment of the chain is needed to define a local reference system for each segment. This reference system includes three unitarian and orthogonal vectors.

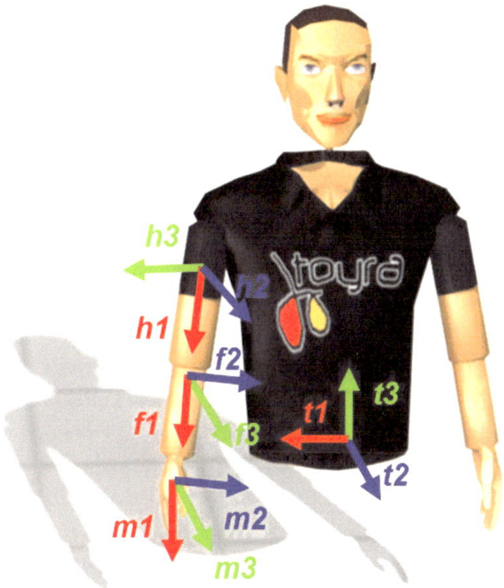

Fig. 8. Thorax, Humerus, Forearm and Hand reference system.

As global reference, it is defined a reference system fixed to the thorax (t1, t2, t3), as shown in Figure 8. Vector t1 follows transversal axis from one shoulder to another, vector t2 follows frontal axis from back to front of thorax and vector t3 follows vertical axis completing orthogonal base (t3 = t1 x t2). This reference system will be placed centred in the base of the thorax.
Local reference system of humerus movements **(h1, h2, h3)** may be defined as follows (Figure 8):

- Vector **h1** follows longitudinal axis of arm, fixed to humerus, from shoulder to elbow.
- Vector **h2** follows frontal axis (A) from back to front of thorax when arm rests vertically downwards.
- Vector **h3** follows transverse axis (T) from other shoulder to actual shoulder when arm rests vertically downwards, completing orthogonal base (**h3 = h1 x h2**).

This reference system will be placed in the centre of the shoulder joint. Then, Rodriguez et al. defined the humerus (or shoulder) movements as:
Humerus Flexion: represented by the angle formed between upper arm and coronal plane, it can be calculated as PI/2 radians less the angle formed between **h1** & **t2** vectors.
Humerus Abduction: represented by the angle formed between upper arm and saggital plane, it can be calculated as PI/2 les the angle formed between **h1** & **t1** vectors.
Humerus Rotation: is defined as the angular movement of humerus over its own longitudinal axis (over vector h1). To measure this angle is needed to move arm in a vertical downward just reducing flexion and abduction without longitudinal rotation. Therefore humerus will be aligned as **h1 = -t3** and rotation angle will be the angle formed by **h2** and **t2**.

They also established as reference for these movements (the anatomical pose): vertically downward extended arm without rotation. But these definitions do not establish a really univoque relation between arm positions and values of those three magnitudes (humerus flexion, abduction and rotation). To demonstrate this idea, we can analyze the elevation movement of the extended arm in the saggital plane for instance. According to Rodriguez definition, abduction will point to 0 radians all the time, and flexion will range from 0 to PI/2 (when arm gets perpendicular to the body) and again 0 radians (when arm gets upwards). Then zero values of flexion abduction angles may represent two different poses of the arm: vertically downwards or upwards. This also happens to every two symmetric positions of the arm to horizontal plane. It happens also in movements inside coronal plane with flexion = 0 and abduction varying from 0 to PI/2 and to 0 again. Another problem of Rodriguez's proposal is the lack of definition of humerus rotation angle. As long as reference system rotation is not a commutative operation, the humerus rotation angle result may vary as the alignment path is defined. For example, humerus rotation angle will be different if you first reduce humerus flexion or humerus abduction (as the first step to align **h1** and **t3** for instance). To avoid these problems, it is now proposed:

- To apply a differentiating criteria for angles below and over the transverse plane located at shoulder height. Humerus flexion when arm is located vertically downwards should value 0 radians, when arm is located horizontally perpendicular to body should value PI/2 radians and when is located vertically upwards should value PI radians. Same ranges for humerus abduction.
- To choose arbitrarily one path of alignment of **h1** and **t3** and always apply the same path. As long as many combinations may be established, the simpler one is selected: to rotate humerus through a single rotation to reach the alignment desired. Always it is possible to find appropriate rotation for any vector pairs, except when they are parallel. In this case, should be applied a symmetry transformation.

Therefore, humerus (or shoulder) movement definitions are reformulated as follows:

Humerus Flexion: represented by the angle formed between upper arm and coronal plane. It can be calculated as PI/2 radians less the angle formed between **h1** and **t2** vectors when **h1** is below transverse plane and as PI/2 plus the angle formed between **h1** and **t2** when **h1** is over transverse plane.

Humerus Abduction: represented by the angle formed between upper arm and saggital plane. It can be calculated as PI/2 less the angle formed between **h1** and **t1** vectors when **h1** is below transverse plane and as PI/2 plus the angle formed between **h1** and **t1** when **h1** is over transverse plane.

Humerus Rotation: is defined as the angular movement of humerus over its own longitudinal axis (over vector **h1**). To measure this angle is needed to rotate arm to a vertical downward pose just with one single rotation. Then humerus will be aligned as **h1 = -t3** and humerus rotation angle will be the angle formed by **h2** (rotated) and **t2**. If initial **h1** is parallel to **t3**, humerus rotation angle will be the angle formed by **–h2** and **t2**.

Applying this definitions, one pose is represented by only one combination of humerus flexion, abduction and rotation values and viceversa. It is established a really univoque relation. As it will be exposed in the examples included in next parragraphs.

Forearm movements are defined respect previous segment (the humerus), not from global reference system (Figure 10). It is defined a local reference system fixed to forearm (**f1, f2, f3**), following next considerations:

- Vector **f1** vector follows the longitudinal direction of the forearm from the elbow to the wrist.
- Vector **f3** vector is perpendicular to f1 and parallel to the wrist from ulna eminence to radius eminence.
- Vector **f2** completes the reference system to build a dextro-rotatory system.

Rodriguez et al defined then forearm movements as the humerus case referencing traditional concept to facilitate its comprehension:

Elbow Flexion: is the angle between **f1** and **h1** vectors plus PI/2.

Pronation-Supination: this movement occurs when the line formed by ulna eminence and radius eminence of the wrist rotate over forearm axis. In the arm model this would be considered as a rotation of forearm over its longitudinal axis not really possible. To measure this angle it is needed to align forearm and humerus in a way that **h1** = **f1**. Then pronation-supination angle is formed between **h2** and **f3**.

And zero position of the forearm is defined respect to humerus position, when arm is completely extended (**h1** is parallel to **f1**) and hand palm looks toward leg. But again, as it happened for humerus, these definitions do not establish a really univoque relation between arm positions and values of elbow flexion and pronation-supination. Again there is a problem with the lack of definition of rotation angle, pronation-supination. Also the proposed forearm flexion origin does not fit with the proposed definition.

To avoid these problems, it is proposed:

- To reformulate flexion definition, eliminating constant term of PI/2.
- To arbitrary choose one path of alignment of **h2** and **f3**. Again to rotate forearm with a single rotation to reach the wanted alignment.

Therefore the forearm movement description is proposed as:

Elbow Flexion: is the angle between **f1** and **h1** vectors (according to zero position definition when arm is completely extended).

Pronation-Supination: is defined as the angular movement of forearm over its own longitudinal axis (over vector **f1**). To measure this angle is needed to extend arm completely. Then humerus will be aligned with forearm and **f1** = **h1**. Then Pronation-Supination angle is formed by **h2** (once is rotated) and **f3**.

Applying this definitions, one pose is represented by only one combination of forearm flexion and rotation values and viceversa. As it will be exposed in next examples.

Last analyzed are hand movements. It is defined a local reference system fixed to hand (**m1, m2, m3**) describing its movements respect to forearm. In the proposed model hand is represented by only one rigid body. It will be considered that hand is open because this assumption will facilitate definition of vectors:

- Vector **m1** goes over hand palm from centre of wrist to the extreme of the fingers.
- Vector **m2** is perpendicular to hand palm.
- Vector **m3** is **m1 x m2**

Again Rodriguez et al defined then hand movements as before referencing traditional concept to facilitate its comprehension:

Radio-Ulnar deviation: it is the angle formed by vector **m1** and the plane that includes **f1 and f2** vectors. Then this angle can be measured as PI/2 less de angle between **m1** and **f3.**

Wrist flexion: it is the angle formed by vector **m1** and the plane that includes **f1 and f3** vectors. Then this angle can be measured as PI/2 less de angle between **m1** and **f2.**

Zero pose of the hand is defined when **m1** & **f1**, **m2** & **f2** and **m3** & **f3** are parallel.

These definitions have the same problems as the definitions of humerus flexion and abduction when angles are greater than PI/2, but as long as the hand cannot normally flex or deviate beyond that limit, the definitions by Rodríguez will be accepted without changes by now. As already mentioned, the proposed mathematical model is implemented in a new virtual reality and motion capture application for upper limb rehabilitation called TOYRA. It acquires segment orientations and reports clinical angle evolution to clinicians. TOYRA covers the whole process from patient assessment, therapy configuration and planning, treatment development and registration to exposition of relevant clinical information to physicians. Stroke, SCI or upper limb orthopedic pathology patients benefit from this system.
The main objectives for TOYRA system are:

- Increase patient motivation through inserting his rehabilitation activity in a virtual world and involving social interaction thanks to comparative performance scores table.
- Introduce objective information to facilitate proper assessment, treatment and supervision of patient's clinical process.
- Improve professional performance through offering objective information reports on patient evolution and configuring proper therapy plans and exercises for their patients.

The system was developed and validated by an integrated team with clinicians specialized in the field of SCI and engineers from top ITS company (National Hospital for Spinal Cord Injury at Toledo and Indra Sistemas S.A., Madrid, Spain). So far, 13 patients have been subjected to several interactive sessions with the system, in order to validate it and obtain enough information for building a normalized movement data base. The system has two fundamental parts: centralized therapy managing/information subsystem (TMIS) and interactive therapy subsystem (ITS) (Figure 9). The first subsystem is deployed in a network server and uses a relational data base to work. It exposes its functionality to users with a web application through the local area network. Every PC station on the network would have access to the application through a web browser. The second subsystem includes a wearable motion capture system and two graphical user interfaces in a specific PC work station (in the hospital version). It is possible to connect as much as work stations as wanted to the same server. The integration between both subsystems is built with web services. The server exposes the required operations that will be invoked by the work stations when needed.

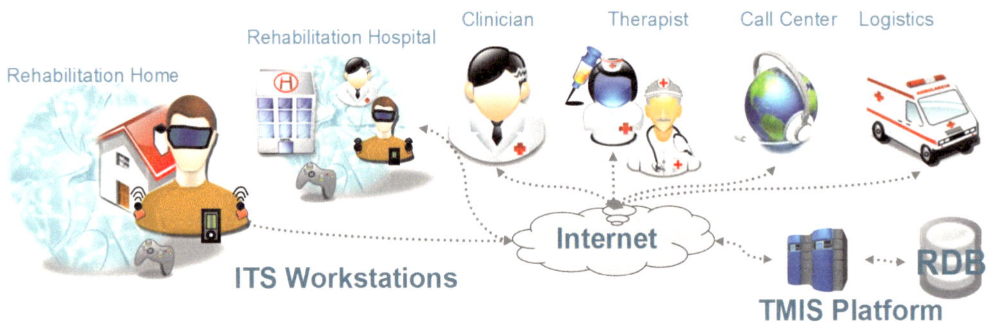

Fig. 9. TMIS and ITS subsystems.

From the functional perspective, the first subsystem includes the programming and planning of the patient's therapy, patient information managing, registry and access to the information gathered from the second subsystem related to the therapy sessions, etc. From a functional point of view, the second subsystem has two orientations by user type - one on each graphical user interface. One of the user interfaces provides the information for the therapist to manage rehabilitation and interactive evaluation sessions. The other interface shows the patient for the patient a virtual reality environment with a specular avatar inside which mirrors the patient's every movement and displays visual cues for therapeutic exercises (as defined by clinicians).

Each subsystem has its own architecture scheme (Figure 10). The TMIS is based on Sun Microsystems Java 2 Enterprise Edition architecture, using Hibernate for persistent information, Apache Spring Framework for service layer construction, Adobe Flex for user web interface and Sun JAX-WS for web service interface. The ITS follows a very different architectural approach because it is a virtual reality system. It is developed in Microsoft C/C++ following the Indra's simulators architecture: several modules in form of Dynamic Libraries (DLLs) managed, coordinated and communicated through a host application developed under Windows platform. The modules covers every aspect from motion-capture to visualization, from calculations and information elaboration to reporting information to TMIS, from controlling therapy exercise logic to therapist graphical user interface.

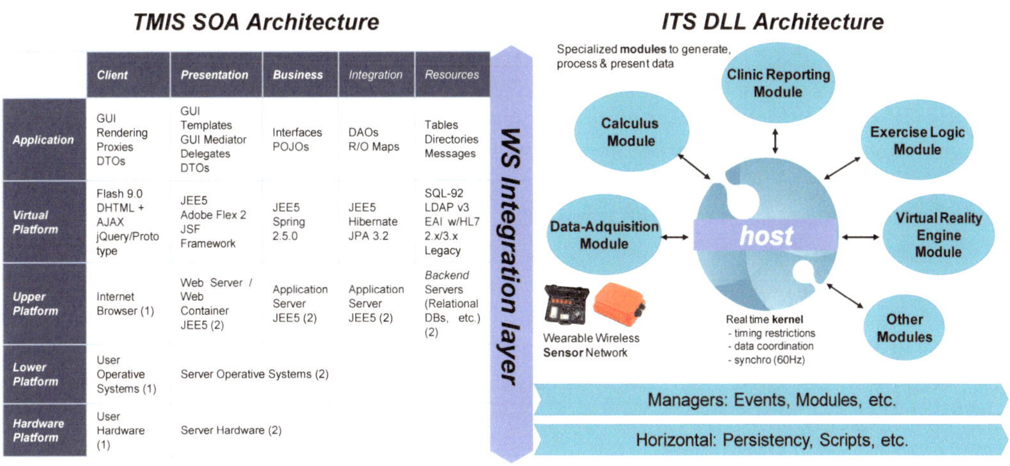

Fig. 10. TMIS and ITS architectures.

A very important component of the system is the motion capture sensors. After studying different solutions and technologies in this field, it was decided to use inertial sensors by Xsens Inc, an European manufacturer. Xsens has strong expertise in biomechanics and inertial sensor technology. The combination of expertise in human motion analysis and innovative inertial motion sensors makes Xsens a leader in inertial human motion capture solutions. There are several Xsens sensors models but in this case, the MTx model was the most appropriate for human motion capture as recommended by the manufacturer, and also because of their size and other features.

The MTx is a small and accurate 3DOF Orientation Tracker. It provides drift-free 3D orientation as well as kinematic data: 3D acceleration, 3D rate of turn and 3D earth-magnetic field. The MTx is an excellent measurement unit for orientation measurement of human body segments. The standard version MTx has a full scale acceleration of 5g, full scales of 18g are available as well. The MTx uses 3 rate gyroscopes to track rapidly changing orientations in 3D and it measures the directions of gravity and magnetic north to provide a stable reference. The system's real-time algorithm fuses all sensor information to calculate accurate 3D orientation, with a highly dynamic response, which remains stable over time. Also an MT_X Development Kit is provided that allows users to take full advantage of the possibilities and the integration of the MTx with your own system. Pre-set user scenarios are available optimizing the Extended Kalman Filter routine for different applications. Based on the chosen scenario the MT_X will apply appropriate filter settings recommended for the application. The MTx is available as a stand-alone unit or as an Xbus version. On the Xbus (Xsens' digital data bus) multiple MTx's can easily be used simultaneously, enabling ambulatory and cost-effective measurement of human motion.

Then a DLL module was developed to capture body segment orientation in real-time. This data is captured from the sensor subsystem, through its driver which offers different formats for orientation data as rotation angles, quaternion, orientation matrix, etc. For this the orientation matrix format was chosen as it facilitates later calculations and avoids confusion about the order of arbitrary rotation angles.

Once the orientation data are available, another DLL module is responsible to insert it into a human body model, scaled to patient's anthropometric measurements (which are provided from TMIS). The avatar's movement as well as relevant clinical information are obtained from the human body model thanks to new algorithms developed specifically for this system (according to the model exposed in previous paragraphs). This clinical information includes flexion, abduction and rotation angles of each body segment, their maximums and minimums values, their velocities, etc. Therefore these algorithms convert from orientation matrix information from the body model to clinic angle information of each body segment under measurement. Then other DLL modules insert the avatar's movement into the virtual reality scenario and report relevant clinical information to TMIS through the web service interface. In Figure 11 examples are provided of virtual scenarios and avatars used for the system implementation.

In the near future the system scope will be extended to home care scenarios. It will also be validated with stroke patients as well as including more interactive virtual scenarios, emotional tagging and affective interface capabilities to increase patient motivation. Also sensor systems will be improved (miniaturization, wireless, cost, etc.) to make them more wearable and easily usable and accessibility and usability of the entire system will be revised. Finally based in the system described, some simple exercises will be showed below in order to demonstrate the proposed model coherence. For each exercise, description and angle graphs are provided. These graphs have in horizontal axis the percentage of movement (from start at 0% till end at 100%) and in vertical axis measured angle in radians.

Humerus frontal elevation – lateral descent: With humerus flexion and abduction fixed to zero, arm extended (vertically downward) and palm facing the leg, the patient raises their arm inside saggital plane until maximum angle is reached. Then the patient moves down their extended arm laterally (inside coronal plane). In the beginning of the downward movement, patient performs a humerus rotation until hand palm is facing outside to facilitate the descent. Movement is maintained until initial position (arm extended vertically downward) is reached (Figure 12). Humerus flexion, abduction and rotation are represented. Rest of measured angles are almost constantly zero except the of pronation-supination angle, which has a peak of approximately PI/2 over 55% of movement reasons why they will not be represented.

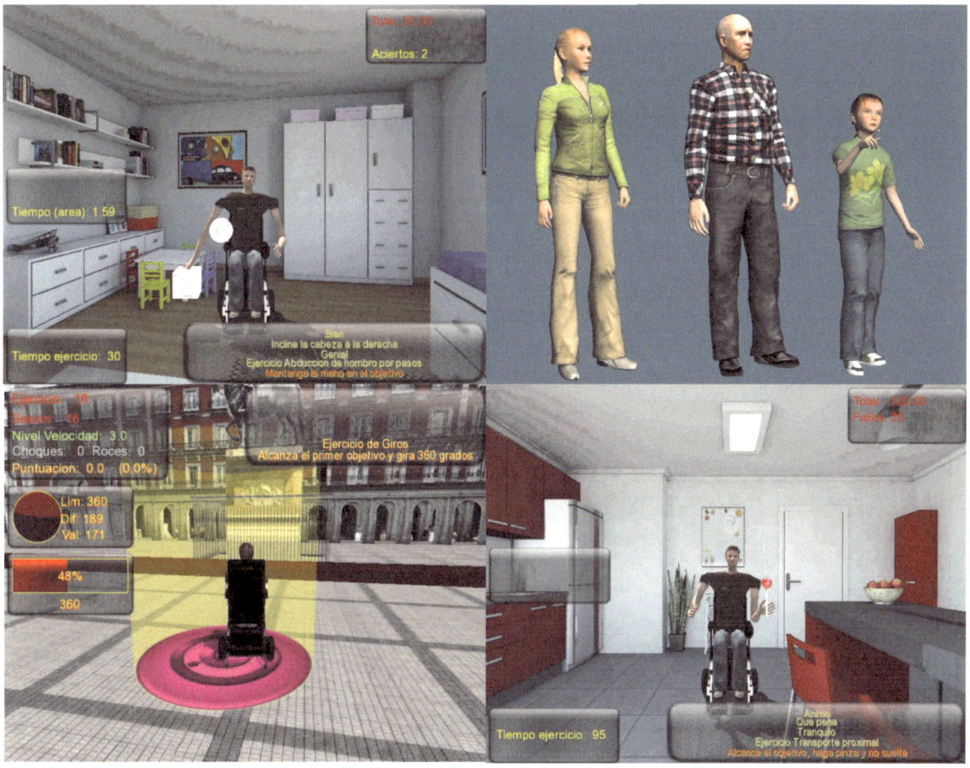

Fig. 11. Virtual scenarios and avatar´s used in the virtual reality environment. Evaluation exercises for patient assessment are performed in the bedroom scenario. Activities for daily living exercises are performed in the kitchen scenario. Wheelchair driving simulation takes place in the street (big open square). Other avatars used are also included.

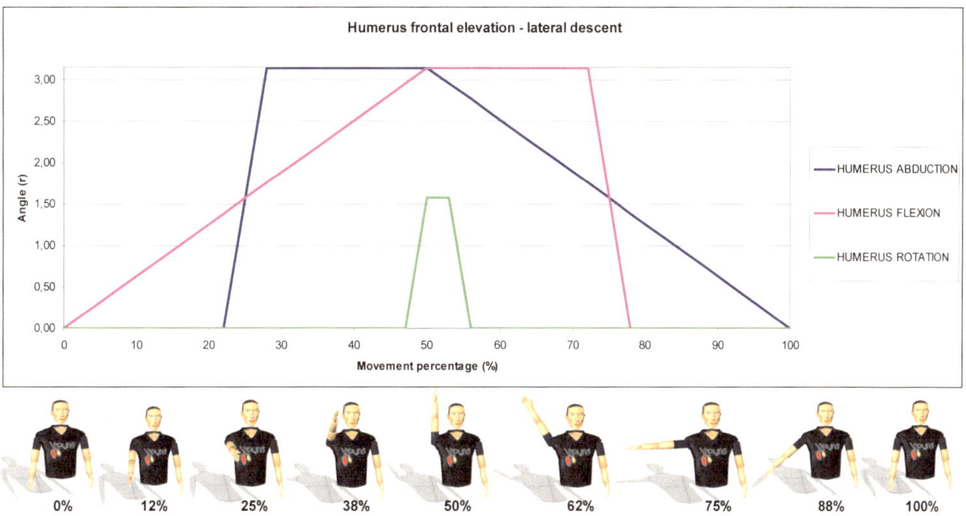

Fig. 12. Humerus frontal elevation – lateral descent

Note that the humerus abduction angle jumps from 0 to PI when the transverse plane is crossed on the way up (at 25% of the movement) while humerus flexion raises continuously. In the way down, humerus flexion angle jumps from PI to 0 when crossing transverse plane (at 75% of the movement) and humerus abduction angle descents continuously until 0 is reached. This is consequence of new definition and helps to differentiate when movement takes place in lower or upper spaces. This way coherence is achieved in the expected values of flexion and abduction angles at upwards pose. Also there is a peak in humerus rotation over the 50% of the movement because of the singularity of the upwards position of the arm.

Forearm elevation: With humerus flexion and abduction fixed to zero, arm extended (vertically downward) and palm facing the leg, patient elevates only the forearm inside saggital plane until maximum angle is reached. To help this movement, patient pronates allocating palm hand facing to shoulder in the last phase of movement. Elbow flexion, pronation and hand flexion are represented (Figure 13). Rest of measured angles are almost constantly zero figure 12.

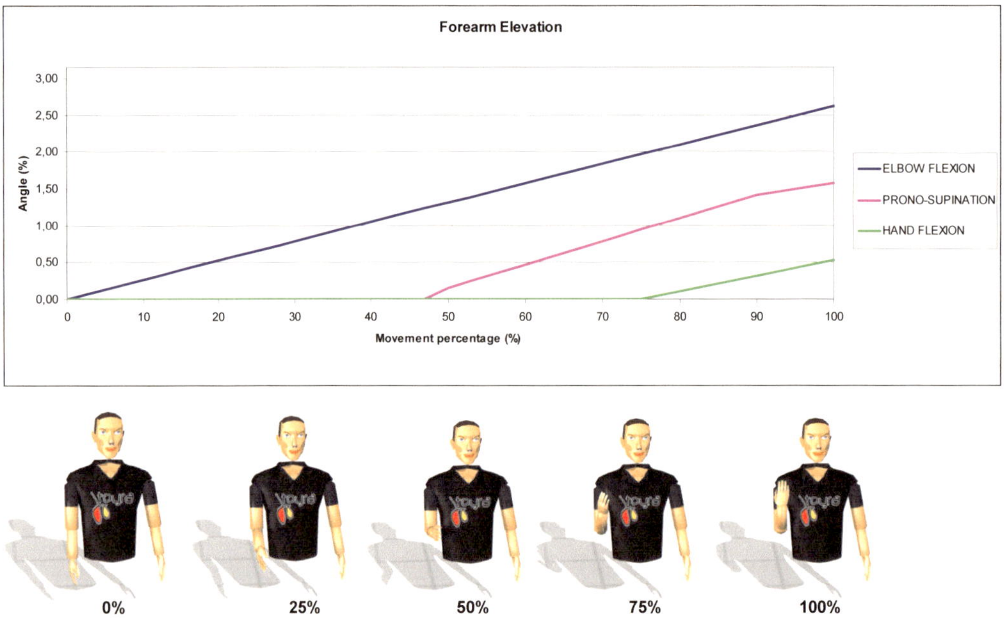

Fig. 13. Forearm elevation

Note that in this exercise elbow flexion raises from 0 to almost PI radians. In the second phase of the movement over transverse plane pronation-supination is performed to facilitate movement towards patient's shoulder. This angle raises from 0 to PI/2 radians. At the end of the movement, also wrist flexion increases a little bit to touch shoulder.

2.4 Estimation of upper-limb biomechanical characteristics based on gyroscopes

Part of the population with SCI presents upper limb involuntary movements, such as tremor, clonus or spasmodic movements (Jankovic and Van der Linden, 1988). There is an absence of studies in the literature centred in the analysis of the involuntary movement behaviour in each articulation of the upper limb. The majority is focused on the measurement of movement at the distal part of the arm. The analysis of involuntary movements at joint level provides information of foremost importance in the design of robotic solutions for rehabilitation, for instance the selection of the appropriate actuator technology to be used by a powered upper limb exoskeleton. In addition, it provides key information to estimate the efforts and to define the exoskeleton structure, (Rocon et al, 2007). This section will introduce an estimation of tremor kinematic parameters by reproducing upper limb kinematics based on a biomechanical model. It will be particularly focused on the estimation of parameters related to tremorous movements but could be extended to other sort of involuntary movements. The method used for the analysis of tremorous movements is based on a combination of solid modelling techniques with anthropometric models of the upper limb, allowing to develop a kinematic and dynamic upper limb model. This model of upper limb musculoskeletal systems allows the estimation of the force contribution of each muscle component during motion, the experimentation of modifications of the musculoskeletal topology as well as the comprehension of complex motion coordination strategies. The input of the model is the angular position, velocity and acceleration of each joint measured by gyroscopes placed at the upper limb of patients suffering from tremor.

The complexity of the musculature together with the difficulty of using non-invasive investigation methods, prevents accurately identifying the function of each muscular component. This work presents the analysis for the development of theoretical kinematic and rigid-body models of the human upper limb, on the basis of former investigations on the upper limb anatomy and biomechanics. A biomechanical model of the upper limb has been built in order to describe its kinematics and dynamic. According to current literature, bones may be regarded as rigid bodies in contrast to soft tissues, with respect to the relevant physiological ranges of motion and force handling. This allows the isolation of the skeletal subsystem from the soft tissues by converting their relations with the bones into external actions. The upper limb kinematics and dynamics may then be analyzed and modelled in considering the skeletal components only, (Maurel, 1999). Neglecting the hand, the human upper limb may be described as composed of five bones, the clavicle, the scapula, the humerus, the ulna and the radius, forming two mechanisms, the shoulder and the elbow. Their association allows a wide range of combined motions, and confers to the human arm the highest mobility in the human body, (Kapandji, 1983). In our study we are only considering the following degrees of freedom: elbow flexion-extension, forearm pronation-supination, wrist abduction-adduction, and wrist flexion-extension, (Rocon et al., 2007).

The forearm movements have been proved to be independent from each other, Youm, et., 1997. Physiologically, no fixed axis or rotation centre can be recognized in a real joint. For most joints, the relative motion between bones is a combination of rolling and gliding with pressure on the contact areas. An accurate joint model should account for all these movements as well as the forces and torques induced on the bones. A 2-D theoretical analysis was lead in this direction by Engin in 1984. The model described the relative motion between two bones, including both geometrical and material nonlinearities as well as the ligament and contact, forces and torques, (Engin, 1984). Another approach towards joint dynamics simulation was presented by Chao et al. The technique, named Rigid Body Spring Model, consisted of modeling the articular surface pressure with distributed compressive springs. When subjected to tensile forces, the compressive springs were removed from the model. An iterative scheme was thus used to solve the system for the equilibrium, whereas the spring redundancy was handled by energy optimization. It was applied to static analysis of the wrist and hand biomechanics, (Chao et al., 1993). In most cases, however, translations appear negligible with respect to rotations, so that the model development and analysis may be simplified using idealized joints. In a 3-D space, an object may be characterized with respect to some reference coordinate system by 6 parameters: 3 related to the position and 3 related to the orientation of the segments. The mobility of a mechanism corresponds to its number of independent kinematic parameters, therefore called degrees of freedom (DOF). Considering these definitions, the skeleton mobility may be completely described by analyzing the joint kinematics. The general procedure is to individually consider the true functional mobility of each joint before considering the interdependencies induced by loops. In most analysis (Kapandji, 1983), the upper limb joints were idealized in the form of 3-DOF Ball & Socket 3-DOF Ball & Socket 2-DOF Hinge or 1-DOF Hinge rotational joints. Regarding dynamics, in most approaches, the upper limb has been assumed to be composed of rigid bodies, including the bones and the soft tissues attached to them, connected by ideal (frictionless) kinematic joints. The rigid bodies have been assumed to possess fixed centres of gravity, and the joints, fixed axes or centres of rotation, (Raikova, 1992).

Our approach has been build taking into account the Leva (de Leva 1996) and Zatsiorsky and Seluyanov tables (Zatsiorsky et al., 1990). These tables are the most widely accepted information within the field of biomechanics in order to perform dynamic analysis. In particular in sports and medical biomechanics. Leva adjustments has been made in order to define accurately the anthropometric measurements required to obtain inertial parameters from Zatsiorsky tables. A solid rigid model of the forearm has been build with the information taken from the above mentioned tables. The model has been parameterized using the Denavit-Hartenber approach. Finally a library has been made to allow a dynamical analysis of the system. This analysis has been done using the recursive algorithm from (Fu et al., 1987).

The model proposed consider the upper limb as a chain composed of three rigid bodies the arm, the forearm and the hand articulated on the rigid basis formed by the trunk and related by ideal rotational joints, (Maurel, 1999). This representation relies on three assumptions: 1) The mechanical behaviour of the upper limb with respect to the trunk is independent of the rest of the human body, 2) Each segment, bones and soft tissues have similar rigid body motions, 3) The deformation of the soft tissues does not significantly affect the mechanical properties of a segment as a whole. Assuming the hand motion has a negligible effect on the large motion dynamics of the upper limb, the hand was considered as a rigid extension of the forearm. Consequently, it has been necessary to determine a rigid body equivalent to the hand and forearm assembly to be substituted in the rigid body dynamic analysis. As a result, four rigid segments have been defined, in order to be able to analyse all the recorded degrees of freedom. Each segment is responsible for a degree of freedom: 1) Elbow flexion-extension, 2) Pronation-supination, 3) Wrist flexion-extension, and 4) Wrist deviation.

Two of these segments were virtual (No mass and no length). Each segment has attached its own Reference System (plus a coordinate frame for the all of them). In the Figure 14 can be seen the coordinate frames the defined and the degree of freedom represented per each system. The Denavit-Hartenberg parameters can be seen in table 1. For rotary elements, the parameter θ determines the position of the joint. That table then indicates the relationship between the parameter and the physiological measured angle represented by β_i for each segment *i*. F_L means forearm length and H_L means hand length.

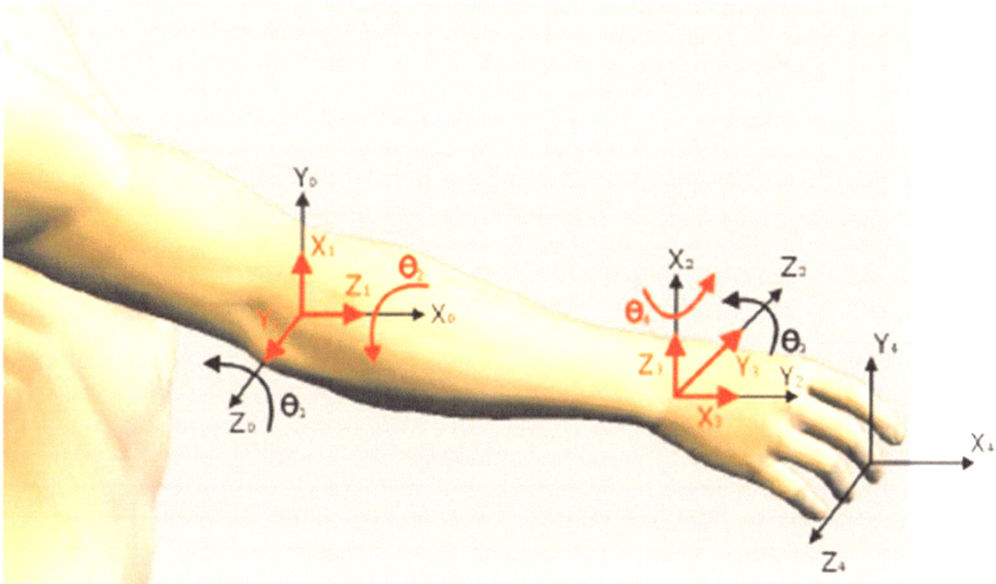

Fig. 14. Solid model representation of the forearm.

Segment	d	a	θ	α
1 - Elbow F/E	0	0	$\beta_1 + \pi/2$	$\pi/2$
2 - Pronation	F_L	0	β_2	$\pi/2$
3 - Wrist F/E	0	0	$\beta_3 + \pi/2$	$\pi/2$
4 - Elbow Dev.	0	H_L	β_4	$\pi/2$

Table 1. DH parameters.

Biomechanical parameters per segment were obtained from previous report (de Leva, 1996). Segment 1 and Segment 3 are virtual; they are only defined to cope with the degrees of freedom of elbow flexion-extension and wrist flexion-extension respectively. However, when these segments are moved, the masses of the "real" segments are moved. All the inertial and mass parameters of a segment are defined below, using the following symbols: B_M, body mass, F_L, forearm length, F_M, forearm mass, H_L, hand length, H_M, hand mass, CoG_M, centre of gravity of each segment (obtained from Leva tables), and M_I inertia matrix. The computational algorithm used is based on the Newton-Euler equations of motion. Thanks to their recursive implementation, these equations of motion are the most efficient set of computational equations for running on a uniprocessor computer, so that implementation in real-time is possible.

$$M_1 = 0$$
$$CoG_1 = [0,0,0]$$
$$MI_1 = \begin{bmatrix} 0 & 0 & 0 \\ 0 & 0 & 0 \\ 0 & 0 & 0 \end{bmatrix}$$
$$M_2 = F_M = 1.6 \cdot \frac{B_M}{100}$$
$$CoG_2 = [0, F_L(0.457 - 1), 0]$$
$$MI_2 = \begin{bmatrix} 0.08 & 0 & 0 \\ 0 & 0.09 & 0 \\ 0 & 0 & 0.15 \end{bmatrix} \cdot F_M \cdot F_L^2$$

$$M_3 = 0$$
$$CoG_3 = [0,0,0]$$
$$MI_3 = \begin{bmatrix} 0 & 0 & 0 \\ 0 & 0 & 0 \\ 0 & 0 & 0 \end{bmatrix}$$
$$M_4 = = M_M = 0.6 \cdot \frac{B_M}{100}$$
$$CoG_4 = [0, H_L(0.79 - 1), 0]$$
$$MI_4 = \begin{bmatrix} 0.55 & 0 & 0 \\ 0 & 0.42 & 0 \\ 0 & 0 & 0.66 \end{bmatrix} \cdot H_M \cdot H_L^2$$

This analysis is intended to estimate the torque and power of the tremorous movement in each joint of the upper limb based on the information provided by the gyroscopes. Gyroscopes provide absolute angular velocity in its active axis, the combination of two independent gyroscopes, placed distal and proximally to the joint of interest, is required. Figure 15 illustrates the placement of the gyroscopes. With the gyroscopes in this position is possible to measure the following movements of the upper limb: Elbow flexo-extension, Forearm prono-supination, Wrist flexo-extension, Wrist deviation. In order to assess tremor biomechanical characteristics we have studied its behaviour in 31 patients suffering from different pathologies of tremor. A set of 6 tasks were select to excite tremor movements during the measurement session.

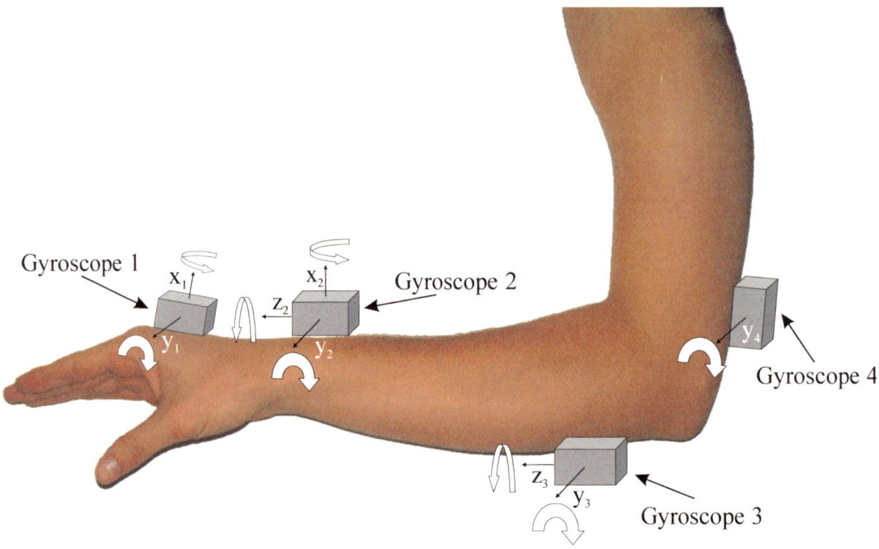

Gyroscope 1: Placed over the third metacarpal
Gyroscope 2: Placed over the edge of the forearm
Gyroscope 3: Placed bellow the olecranon process
Gyroscope 4: Placed over the olecranon process

Fig. 15. Gyroscopes placement.

Active orthoses are intended to counteract tremor by applying controlled forces. Torque is an essential parameter in the choice of the actuator technology that will be used by powered orthoses. Special care should be taken with this parameter since it presents a dynamic behaviour. As can be seen in Figure 16, this parameter presents a dynamic behaviour. The actuator technology that will drive the orthoses must be able to apply the same torque characteristics. Table 2 summarizes the mean value of torque estimated in each joint of the upper limb for the tasks of stretching out the arm and putting finger to nose. These tasks are shown because they are the ones in which maximum values of tremor activity were registered.

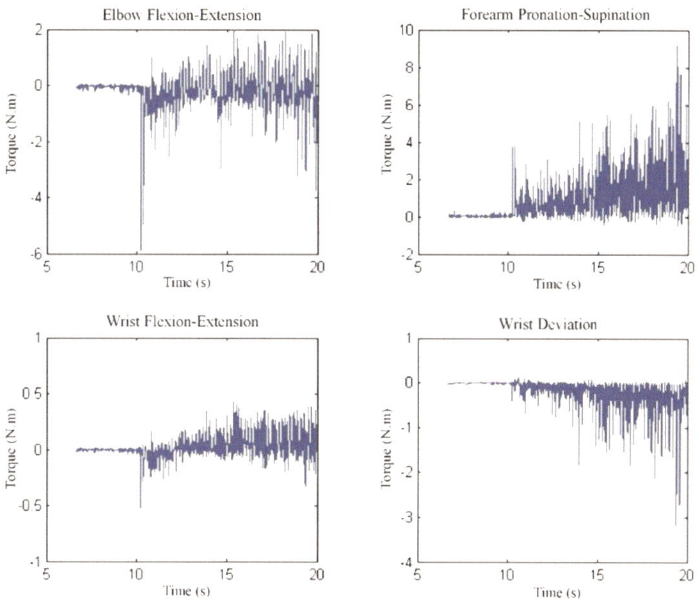

Fig. 16. Arm torques.

Movement	Finger to nose	Outstreched Arm
Elbow Flexo-extension	1.9 *N.m*	1.2 *N.m*
Forearm Prono-supination	3.7 *N.m*	1.9 *N.m*
Wrist Flexo-extension	0.4 *N.m*	0.2 *N.m*
Wrist Deviation	1.1 *N.m*	0.5*N.m*

Table 2. Mean values of the torque estimated in finger to nose and outstretched arm tasks

Movement	Finger to nose	Outstreched Arm
Elbow Flexo-extension	0.2 *W*	0.01 *W*
Forearm Prono-supination	1.8 *W*	0.2 *W*
Wrist Flexo-extension	0.08 *W*	0.03 *W*
Wrist Deviation	0.4 *W*	0.04 *W*

Table 3. RMS values of the power estimated in each joint during execution of finger to nose and outstretched arm tasks

The other important parameter is the power that the device can absorb. The amount of power consumed in relation to tremor is one of the key parameters that need to be taken into account in the design of these devices. The power at the joint plus the performance of the devices will also determine the battery capacity. Tremor is assumed to be a stationary movement and, leaving aside the viscous coefficient of joint braking, there is no effective work done on the joint. That is why the RMS value of the power estimated for the tremorous movement during the putting finger to nose and stretching out arm tasks are presented in Table 3.

The results of this study show the basis of the dynamics of tremorous movement in each joint of the upper limb, information that is required for the design of portable active upper limb exoskeletons. The model presented could be extended to the study of the biomechanical parameters of any other voluntary/involuntary movements associated to SCI patients.

3. Conclusion

Biomechanical analysis systems have turned out to be a powerful tool for a quantitative assessment of movement in all degrees of freedom. Up to now, upper limb biomechanical analysis is not so often presented in the literature and in clinical practice The variety, complexity and range of upper limb movements is a challenge to assessment and interpretation of data and the clinical routines for 3-D analysis in upper limbs are not fully established. There have been presented 4 different clinical applications of developing an upper limb biomechanical model. Clinical daily practice, robotics and virtual reality can be topics to apply upper limb biomechanical models.

4. Acknowledgment

The research for this manuscript has been partially funded by grant from the Spanish Ministry of Science and Innovation CONSOLIDER INGENIO, project HYPER (Hybrid NeuroProsthetic and NeuroRobotic Devices for Functional Compensation and Rehabilitation of Motor Disorders, CSD2009-00067) by grant from Consejería de Sanidad de la Junta de Comunidades de Castilla-La Mancha (Spain), ref: 06006-00 and TOYRA Project (National Hospital for Spinal Cord Injury, FUHNPAIIN; INDRA Sistemas S.A. y Rafael del Pino Foundation).

5. References

Arai, T. & Kragic, D. (1999). Variability of Wind and Wind Power, In: Wind Power, S.M. Muyeen, (Ed.), 289-321, Scyio, ISBN 978-953-7619-81-7, Vukovar, Croatia

Bednarczyk JH, Sanderson DJ. (1994). Kinematics of wheelchair propulsion in adults and children with spinal cord injury. *Archives of Physical Medicine and Rehabilitation* 75: 1327-1334.

Biryukova EV, Roby-Brami A, Frolov AA, Mokhtari M. (2000) Kinematics of human arm reconstructed from spatial tracking system recordings. *Journal of Biomechanics* 33:985-995.

Boninger ML, Cooper RA, Robertson RN, Shimada SD. (1997). Three-dimensional pushrim forces during two speeds of wheelchair propulsion. *American Journal of Physical Medicine and Rehabilitation* 76:420-426.

Boninger ML, Cooper RA, Baldwin MA, Shimada SD, Koontz AL. (1999). Wheelchair pushrim kinetics: body weight and median nerve conduction. *Archives of Physical Medicine and Rehabilitation* 80:910-915.

Brauer RL, Hertig BA. (1981). Torque generation on wheelchair handrims. *American Society Mechanical Engineering* AMD 43:113-116.

Broeks JG, Lankhorst GJ, Rumping K, Prevo AJ (1999). The long-term outcome of arm function after stroke: results of a follow-up study. *Disabilility and Rehabililitation* 21(8):357-364.

Chao E, Lynch J, and Vanderploeg M (1993) Simulation and animation of musculoskeletal joint systems. *Journal of Biomechanical Engineering,* 115: 562 - 568.

Cirstea MC, Levin MF. Compensatory strategies for reaching in stroke (2000). *Brain,* 123 (Pt 5): 940-953.

Clauser CE, McConville JT, Young JW. (1969). Weight, volume and center of mass of segments of the human body. AMRL-TR-69-70. Wright-Patterson Air Force Base, Yellow Springs (OH).

Collinger JL, Boninger ML, Koontz AM, Price R, Sisto SA, Toledrico ML, Cooper RA. (2008). Shoulder biomechanics during the push phase of wheelchair propulsion: a multisite study of persons with paraplegia. *Archives of Physical Medicine and Rehabilitation* 89: 667-676.

Cooper RA. (1995). Biomechanics of mobility and manipulation. En: Cooper RA editor. *Rehabilitation Engineering: applied to mobility and manipulation.* Medical Sciences Series. Bristol: Institute of Physics Publishing. p. 69-144.

Cooper RA, Robertson RN, VanSickle, Boninger ML, Shimada SD. (1996). Projection of the point of force application onto the palmar plane of the hand during wheelchair propulsion. *IEEE Transaction on Neural Systems and Rehabilitation Engineering* 4: 133-142.

Cooper RA, Robertson RN, VanSickle DP, Bonninger ML, Shimada SD. (1997). Methods for determining three-dimensional wheelchair pushrim forces and moments-a technical note. *Journal of Rehabilitation Research and Development* 34 (2):435-446.

Cooper JE, Shweddyk E, Quandbury AO, Miller J, Hildebrand D (1993). Elbow joint restriction: effect on functional upper limb motion during performance of three feeding activities. *Archives of Physical Medicine and Rehabiitation* 74:805-809.

Cooper R, Boninger M, Shimada S, Lawrence B. (1999). Glenohumeral joint kinematics and kinetics for three coordinate system representation during wheelchair propulsion. *American Journal of Physical Medicine and Rehabiitation* 78:435-446.

Curtis KA, Drysdale GA, Lanza RD, Kolber M, Vitolo RS, West R. (1999). Shoulder pain in wheelchair users with tetraplegia and paraplegia. *Archives of Physical Medicine and Rehabilitation* 76:360-367.

Dallmeijer AJ, Kappe YJ, Veeger DH, Janssen TW, van der Woude LH. (1994). Anaerobic power output and propulsion technique in spinal cord injures subjects during wheelchair ergometry. *Journal of Rehabilitation Research and Development* 31: 120-128.

Dallmeijer AJ, van der Woude LHV, Veeger HEJ, Hollander AP. (1998). Effectiviness of force application in manual wheelchair propulsion in persons with spinal cord injuries. *American Journal of Physical Medicine and Rehabilitation* 77:213-221.

De Leva P, Adjustments to Zatsioorsky-Seluyanov' s segment inertia parameters. (1996). *Journal of Biomechanics*. 29(9): 1223 - 1230.

De los Reyes-Guzmán A, Gil-Agudo A, Peñasco-Martín B, Solís-Mozo M, del Ama-Espinosa A, Pérez-Rizo E (2010). Kinematic analysis of the daily activity of drinking from a glass in a population with cervical spinal cord injury. *Journal of NeuroEngineering and Rehabilitation* ,7:41.

Digiovine CP, Cooper RA, Boninger ML. (2001). Dynamic calibration of a wheelchair dynamometer. *Journal of Rehabilitation Research and Development* 38 (1): 41-55.

Dwan LN, McIntosh AS. (2006). Kinematics of the upper limb: A reaching and placing task with resistance in children. *Gait and Posture* 24(S):S235-S238.

Engin A. (1984) On the theoretical modelling of human joints. *Mathematical Modelling in Science and Technology*, J. R. Avula, Ed. Pergamon Press, New York, pp. 560–565.

Finch E (2002) Physical rehabilitation outcome measures: a guide to enhanced clinical decision making. 2nd edition. Hamilton, Ontario, Decker; 2002:ix,292.

Finley M, Rasch E, Keyser R, Rodgers M. (2004). The biomechanics of wheelchair propulsion in individuals with and without upper-limb impairment. *Journal of Rehabilitation Research and Development* 41: 395-402.

Fitoussi F, Diop A, Maurel N, Laassel EM, Pennecot GF (2006). Kinematic analysis of the upper limb: a useful tool in children with cerebral palsy. *Journal of Pediatric Orthopedics* 15(4):247-256.

Fu KS, Gonzalez RC, Lee CSG (1987). *Robotics: Control, Sensing, Vision, and Intelligence*. McGraw-Hill Book Company.

Gellman H, Sie I, Waters RL. (1988). Late complications of the weight-bearing upper-extremity in the paraplegic patient. *Clinical Orthopedic and Related Research* 233: 132-135.

Gil-Agudo A, del Ama- Espinosa A, Pérez-Rizo E, Pérez-Nombela S, Crespo-Ruiz B (2010). Shoulder joint kinetics during wheelchair propulsion on a treadmill at two different speeds in spinal cord injury patients. *Spinal Cord* 48: 290-296.

Gil-Agudo A, Del Ama-Espinosa A, Pérez-Rizo E, Pérez-Nombela S, Rodríguez-Rodríguez LP (2010). Upper limb joint kinetics during manual wheelchair propulsion in patients with different levels of spinal cord injury. *Journal of Biomechanics* 43:2508-2515.

Hanavan EP (1966) A personalized mathematical model of the human body. *Journal of Spacecraft* 3:446-448

Jaennerod M (1984). The timing of natural prehension movements . *Journal of Motor Behaviour* 16:235-254.

Jankovic J, Van der Linden C (1988). Dystonia and tremor induced by peripheral trauma: predisposing factors. *Journal of neurology, neurosurgery, and psychiatry*. 51(12):1512-9.

Kapandji I (1983) The physiology of the joints: Upper limb. Churchill Livingstone, 1983.

Koontz AM, Cooper RA, Boninger ML, Souza AL, Fay BT. (2002). Shoulder kinematics and kinetics during two speeds of wheelchair propulsion. *Journal of Rehabilitation Research and Development* 39:635-650.

Kulig K, Rao SS, Mulroy SJ, Newsam CJ, Gronley JK, Bontrager EL, Perry J. (1998). Shoulder joint kinetics during the push phase of wheelchair propulsion. *Clinical Orthopedics* 354:132-143.

Kulig K, Newsam CJ, Mulroy SJ, Rao S, Gronley JK, Bontrager EL, Perry J. (2001).The effect of level spinal cord injury on shoulder joint kinetics during manual wheelchair propulsion. *Clinical Biomechanics (Bristol, Avon)* 16:744-751.

Laffont I, Briand E, Dizien O, Combeaud M, Bussel B, Revol M, Roby-Brami A (2000). Kinematics of prehension and pointing movements in C6 quadriplegic patients. *Spinal Cord* 38(6):354-362.

Levin MF (1996) Interjoint coordination during pointing movements is disrupted in spastic hemiparesis. *Brain*, 119(1):281-293.

Linden ML, van Valent L, Veeger HE, van der Woude LHV. (1996). The effect of wheelchair handrim tube diameter on propulsion efficiency and force application. *IEEE Transactions on Neural Systems and Rehabilitation Engineering* 4: 123-132.

Magermans DJ, Chadwick EKJ, Veeger HEJ, van der Helm FCT (2005). Requirements for upper extremity motions during activities of daily living. *Clinical Biomechanics (Bristol, Avon)* 20:591-599.

Maurel W (1999) 3D modeling of the human upper limb including the biomechanics of joints, muscles and soft tissues.. Ph.D. dissertation, Ecole Polytechnique Federale de Lausanne.

Maynard FM, Bracken MB, Creasey G (1997). International Standards for Neurological and Functional Classification of Spinal Cord Injury. American Spinal Injury Association. *Spinal Cord* 35:266-274.

McCrea PH, Eng JJ, Hodgson AJ (2002) Biomechanics of reaching: clinical implications for individuals with acquired brain injury. *Disability and Rehabilitation* 24(10):534-541.

Mercer JL, Boninger M, Koontz A, Ren D, Dyson-Hudson T, Cooper R. (2006). Shoulder joint kinetics and patology in manual wheelchair users. *Clinical Biomechanics* 21:781-789.

Michaelsen SM, Luta A, Roby-Brami A, Levin MF (2001). Effect of trunk restraint on the recovery of reaching movements in hemiparetic patients. *Stroke* 32(8):1875-1883.

Mosqueda T, James MA, Petuskey K, Bagley A, Abdala E, Rab G (2004). Kinematic assessment of the upper extremity in brachial plexus birth palsy. *Journal of Pediatric Orthopedics* 24(6):695-699.

Murgia A, Kyberd PJ, Chapell PH, Light CM (2004). Marker placement to describe the wrist movement during activities of daily living in cyclic tasks. Clinical Biomechanics (Bristol Avon), 19(4):248-254.

Murphy MA, Sunnerhagen KS, Johnels B, Willen C. (2006). Three-dimensional kinematic motion analysis of a daily activity drinking from a glass: a pilot study. *Journal of Neuroengineering and Rehabiitation*, 3:18.

Murray IA, Johnson GR (2004). A study of the external forces and moments at the shoulder and elbow while performing every day tasks. *Clinical Biomechanics (Bristol Avon)* 19(6):586-594.

Nakayama H, Jorgensen HS, Raaschou HO, Olsen TS (1994). Compensation in recovery of upper extremity function after stroke: the Copenhagen Stroke Study. *Archives of Physical Medicine and Rehabiitation* 75(8):852-857.

Newsam CJ, Mulroy SJ, Gronley JK, Bonstrager EL, Perry J. (1996). Temporal-spatial characteristics of wheelchair propulsion. Effects of level spinal cord injury, terrain and propulsion rate. *American Journal of Physical Medicine and Rehabilitation* 75: 292-299.

Newsam CJ, Rao SS, Mulroy SJ, Gronley JK, Bontrager EL, Perry J. (1999). Three dimensional upper extremity motion during manual wheelchair propulsion in men with different levels of spinal cord injury. *Gait and Posture* 19:223-232.

Niesing R, Eijskoot F, Kranse R, den Ouden AH, Storm J. (1990). Computer-controlled wheelchair ergometer. *Medicine and Biological Engineering and Computer* 28:329-338.

Parker VM, Wade DT, Langton Hewer R (1986). Loss of an arm function after stroke: measurement, frequency and recovery. *International Rehablitation Medicine* 8(2):69-73.

Petuskey K, Bagley A, Abdala E, James MA,, Rab G (2007). Upper extremity kinematics during functional activities: Three-dimensional studies in a normal pediatric population. *Gait and Posture* 25:573-579.

Praagman M, Stokdijk M, Veeger HEJ. Visser B. (2000). Predicting mechanical load of the glenohumeral joint using net joint moments. *Clinical Biomechanics (Bristol Avon)* 15: 315-321.

Rab G., Petuskey K., Bagley A. (2002). Determination of kinematics of the upper extremity. *Gait and Posture* 15;2:.113-119.

Raikova R (1992) A general approach for modelling and mathematical investigation of the human upper limb. 1992. *Journal of Biomechanics* 25:857 - 867.

Rau G., Disselhorst-Klug., Schmidt R. (2000). Movements biomechanics goes upwards: from the leg to the arm. *Journal of Biomechanics*, 33(10):1207-1216.

Roby-Brami A, Feydy A, Combeaud M, Biryukova EV, Bussel B, Levin MF (2003). Motor compensation and recovery for reaching in stroke patients. *Acta Neurological Scandinavian* 107(5):369-381.

Rocon E, Belda-Lois JM, Ruiz AF (2007). Design and validation of a rehabilitation robotic exoskeleton for tremor assessment and suppression. *IEEE Transactions on Neural Systems and Rehabilitation Engineering* 15(3):367-378.

Rodriguez C., Quintero H., Aschner H. (2005) Movimiento del brazo humano: de los tres planos a las tres dimensiones. Revista de ingeniería de Universidad de los Andes, Bogotá, Colombia, núm 22 (nov-2005), pp. 36-44.

Rodgers MM, Tummarakota S, Lieh J. (1998). Three-Dimensional dynamic analysis of wheelchair propulsion. *Journal of Applied Biomechanics* 14:80-92.

Rodgers MM, Keyser RE, Gardner ER, Rusell PJ, Gorman PH. (2000). Influence of trunk flexion on biomechanics of wheelchair propulsion. *Journal of Rehabilitation Research and Development* 37:283-295.

Rönnqvist L, Rösblad B (2007). Kinematic analysis of unimanual reaching and grasping movements in children with hemiplegic cerebral palsy. *Clinical Biomechanics (Bristol Avon)* 22:165-17.

Safaee-Rad R, Shwedyk E, Quanbury AO, Cooper JE (1990). Normal functional range of motion of upper limb joints during performance of three feeding activities. *Archives of Physical Medicine and Rehabilitation* 71(7): 505-509.

Samuelson K, Larsson H, Tropp H. (1989). Wheelchair ergometer with a device for isokinetic torque measurement. *Scandinavian Journal of Rehabilitation Medicine* 21:205-207.

Sie IH, Waters RL, Adkins RH, Gellman H, (1992). Upper extremity pain in the postrehabilitation spinal cord injury patient. *Archives of Physical Medicine and Rehabilitation* 73: 44-48.

Subbarao J, KlopSiegwart, R. (2001). Indirect Manipulation of a Sphere on a Flat Disk Using Force Information. International Journal of Advanced Robotic Systems, Vol.6, No.4, (December 2009), pp. 12-16, ISSN 1729-8806fstein J, Turpin R. (1995). Prevalence and impact of wrist and shoulder pain in patients with spinal cord injury. *Journal of Spinal Cord Medicine* 18:9-13.

Tupling SJ, Davis GM, Pierrynowski MR, Shephard RJ. (1986). Arm strength and impulse generation: Initiation of wheelchair movement by the physically disabled. *Ergonomics* 29: 303-311.

Van Anden CJ, Wolterbeek N, Doorenbosch AM, Veeger HEJ, Harlaar J (2008). Complete 3D Kinematics of upper extremity functional tasks. *Gait and Posture* 27:120-127.

Van der Helm FCT, Veeger HEJ. (1999). Shoulder modelling in rehabilitation: the power balance during wheelchair propulsion. En: van der Woude LHV, Hopman MTE, van Kemenade C, editors. *Biomedical aspects of manual wheelchair propulsion: state of the art II*. Amsterdam: IOS Press. p. 96-103.

Van der Woude LHV, De Groot G, Hollander AP, van Ingen Schenau GJ, Rozendal RH. (1986). Wheelchair ergonomics and physiology testing of prototypes. *Ergonomics* 29:1561-1573.

Van der Woude LHV, Veeger HEJ, Dallmeijer AJ, Janssen TWJ, Rozendaal LA. (2001). Biomechanics and physiology in active manual wheelchair propulsion. *Medicine Engineering Physics* 23:713-733.

Van Drongelen S, Van der Woude LHV, Janssen TW, Angenot E, Chadwick EK, Veeger DH. (2005). Mechanical load on the upper extremity during wheelchair activities. *Archives of Physical Medicine and Rehabilitation* 86: 1214-1220.

Veeger HEJ, Rozendaal LA, van der Helm FCT.(2002). Load on the shoulder on low intensity wheelchair propulsion. *Clinical Biomechanics (Bristol Avon)* 17:211-218

Villalba M. (2003). Protocolo de análisis de movimiento en los brazos para diagnóstico clínco. Proyecto de grado en Ingeniería Mecánica. Universidad de los Andes. Bogotá. Colombia.

Wyndaele M, Wyndaele JJ (2006) Incidence, prevalence and epidemiology of spinal cord injury: what learns a worldwide literature survey? *Spinal Cord* 44:523-529.

Veeger HEJ, Rozendaal LA, van der Helm FCT.(2002). Load on the shoulder on low intensity wheelchair propulsion. *Clinical Biomechanics (Bristol Avon)* 17:211-218

Wu G, van der Helm F, Veeger H.E.J., Makhsous M, Van Roy P, Anglin C, Nagels J, Karduna A, McQuade K, Wang X, Werner F, Bucholz B (2005). ISB recommendation on definitions of joint coordinate systems of varius joints for the reporting of human joint motion- Part II: shoulder, elbow, wrist and hand. *Journal of Biomechanics* 38:981-992.

Youm Y, Cryer R, Thambyrajah K, Flatt A, Sprague B. (1997) Biomechanical analysis of forearm pronation-supination and elbow flexion-extension. *Journal of Biomechanics* 12:245 - 255.

Zatsiorsky V, Seluyanov V, Chugunova L (1990) Methods of determining mass-inertial characteristics of human body segments. *Contemporary problems of biomechanic.*, G. Cherny and S. Regiror, Eds. CRC Press, 272 - 291.

7

Adaptations of the Motor System in Animal Models of Spinal Cord Injury and Disuse

Pierre A. Guertin
Laval University & Laval University Medical Center
Canada

1. Introduction

More than 1.3 million patients are currently living with a spinal cord injury (SCI) in North America (Reeve Foundation). There is no cure for SCI although recent advances in acute care interventions (*e.g.*, removal of bone fragments, decompression, anti-inflammatory drugs) have increased survival and reduced neurological dysfunctions (Baptiste & Fehlings, 2007). Accordingly with the *American Spinal Injury Association* (ASIA) guideline, tetraplegic (cervical lesions) and paraplegic (thoracic lesions or below) patients are classified either as ASIA-A, ASIA-B, ASIA-C or ASIA-D (see Table 1). Quadriplegia also called tetraplegia is when a person has a SCI within the cervical area which results in paralysis of all four limbs. In addition to the arms and legs being paralyzed, the abdominal and chest muscles will also be affected which result in weakened breathing and the inability to properly cough and clear the chest. Paraplegia is when the level of injury occurs at the thoracic level or lower. Although they typically experience leg movement and abdomen problems, paraplegics can use their arms and hands.

ASIA-A	No voluntary motor control and no sensation below injury level
ASIA-B	No voluntary motor control, some sensations below injury level
ASIA-C	Some motor control (< grade 3) and some sensations below injury level
ASIA-D	Some motor control (> grade 3) and some sensations below injury level
ASIA-E	Normal voluntary motor control and sensation below injury level

Table 1. Classification of SCI severity

Advanced rehabilitation 'activity-based' strategies such as body weight-supported treadmill training or BWSTT (leg movements generated passively by manual assistance from therapists) and functional electrical stimulation (FES)-biking are increasingly used especially with motor-incomplete (ASIA-C and ASIA-D) patients. Indeed, given that spared descending pathways exist and, thus, some voluntary motor control remains in these subclasses of patients, it becomes possible to further increase voluntary ambulation using BWSTT training (Dobkin et al., 2006; Hicks & Ginis, 2008). However, motor system, metabolic outcomes or health benefits associated with these approaches remain unclear (Hicks & Ginis, 2008; Duffell et al., 2009). In turn, chronic SCI patients classified as motor-complete (ASIA-A & ASIA-B) generally experience greater health problems often referred to as 'secondary complications' that are associated with significant changes of the motor, locomotor, skeletal, cardiovascular, circulatory and hematologic problems (Huang & DeVivo, 1990; Bauman, 1999; Riegger et al., 2009; Rouleau et al., 2010,2011; Spungen, 2003). No safe, effective and regulatory agency-approved treatments against these chronic problems exist yet.

In the last few years, great therapeutic hopes for motor-complete SCI patients (ASIA-A and ASIA-B) have emerged from physical activity-based studies performed in adult complete paraplegic cats showing that basic locomotor movements (i.e., hindlimb stepping) can be restored partially with regular treadmill training, weight support, passively generated movement and administration (*i.t.* or *i.p.*) of drugs such as clonidine, an alpha-2 noradrenergic agonist (Barbeau et al., 1993; Chau et al., 1998). Regular assisted training combined with clonidine and a few other monoaminergic drugs have even induced, in some cases, episodes of overground walking with Canadian crutches in previously wheelchair-bound SCI patients (Barbeau et al., 1998). Clear evidence suggests that clonidine can, in fact, facilitate walking through reflex-mediated actions by decreasing spinal reflexes and hence spasticity and clonus (Waindberg et al., 1990; Remy-Neris et al., 1999). Unfortunately, at doses used for locomotor enhancement in some paraplegic patients, clonidine was also found to induce severe side effects even if given *i.t.* (i.e., bradycardia, sedation, hypotension - pers.com. Dr. Hugues Barbeau). It had therefore become imperative to identify other pharmacological strategies and compounds that could safely and more specifically enhance locomotor function recovery or reduce motor system changes and problems in chronic and, if possible, in motor-complete SCI patients (i.e., for whom BWSTT or other comparable approach does not yield beneficial effects). The identification of therapeutic approaches aimed at reducing or preventing motor system alterations in SCI or comparable chronic conditions (e.g., burn patients, AIDS patient with cachexia, etc.) would benefit both patients and health care systems for which associated costs are significant (approximately $100,000 - 400,000 per year/patient, Table 2).

Initial hospitalization	$140,000
1st year paraplegics	$152,000
1st year tetraplegics	$417,000
Averaged life time paraplegics	$428,000
Averaged life time tetraplegics	$1,350,000

Table 2. Costs of SCI in U.S. dollars (source: http://www.sci-info-pages.com/facts.html)

Although, these therapeutic approaches may not be designed to repair or cure SCI, they would nonetheless contribute at preventing (in acutely injured patients), reducing or reversing (in chronic SCI patients) secondary complications associated with motor system changes and significantly reduced physical activity (see also *section 2.6*).

2. Motor system changes associated with spinal cord injury and disuse

The motor system may be divided into several organs and structures. There is the central nervous system (CNS) that comprises the brain and the spinal cord. Its one hundred billion neurons are involved in motor and sensory functions (Kandel et al., 2000). The brain consists of the pyramidal and extrapyramidal system specifically associated with voluntary motor control. These brain structures constitute the main command centres that control voluntary

muscular contraction. Most of their neuronal commands are sent to neurons and motoneurons located in the spinal cord where sensory motor integration and final motor commands sent to muscle are organized for proper induction of coordinated movements.
In contrast, locomotion and other rhythmic and partially involuntary motor behaviours are largely controlled by signals and neuronal commands generated in the brainstem and spinal cord. In fact, complex neuronal circuits located in these non-cortical areas of the CNS are known to be capable of generating motor functions even in absence of descending inputs from cortical areas and other brain regions (Guertin & Steuer, 2009; Guertin, 2010). In fact, locomotion, micturition, ejaculation, scratching, erection, and respiration are amongst the motor behaviours that are mainly controlled by spinal cord and brainstem circuits (see Fig.1).

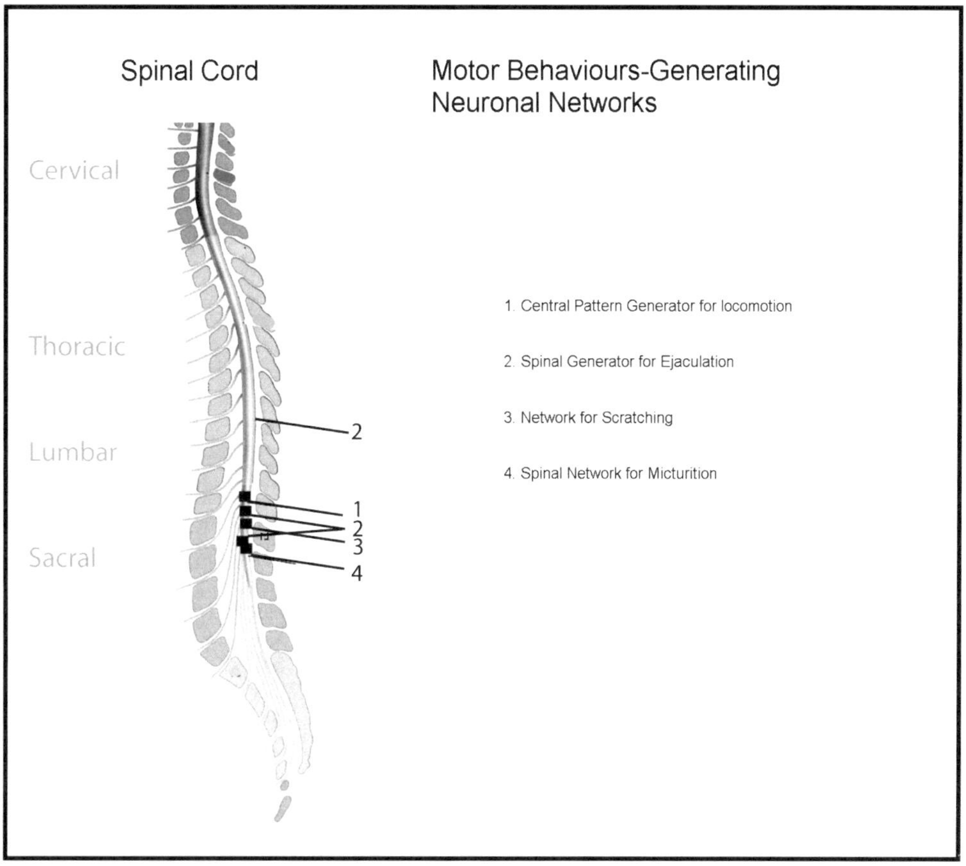

Fig. 1. Neuronal networks in the spinal cord that control, brain-independently, complex motor behaviours. Respiration (not shown here) is also largely controlled by non-cortical structures including the brainstem (e.g., Pre-Bötzinger complex).

Thus, the CNS controls either directly or indirectly the muscular systems. Although some types of muscles such as the cardiac and smooth muscles are considered controlled by the autonomic nervous system and hormones, the striated skeletal muscle system is directly controlled by the CNS. This is the main reason why after SCI, an immediate and irreversible

loss of sensory and voluntary motor control is found. This said, increasing evidence suggests that functions controlled mainly by the spinal cord can nonetheless be elicited despite SCI using specific pharmacological or electrical approaches (see *section 2.6*).
In humans, the striated skeletal muscle system comprises approximately 650 muscles. It is formed by different fiber types and properties including slow-twitch fibers (type I) and relatively fast to very fast-twitch fibers (IIa, IIb and IIx)(Table 3). The main action of skeletal muscles in motor control is to allow movement execution. Almost all skeletal muscles either originate or insert on the skeleton. When a muscle moves a portion of the skeleton, that movement results into flexion, extension, adduction, abduction, etc. (Martini & Nath, 2011).
The human skeleton consists of both fused and individual bones supported by ligaments, tendons, muscles and cartilage. Among several functions, it primarily serves as a scaffold for movements controlled by the CNS and muscles as mentioned earlier. The biggest bone in the body is the femur which is also the main skeletal structure affected after chronic SCI, disuse or immobilization. Finally, energy and other metabolic processes involved in motor control and movements largely depend upon the integrity of the circulatory and hematologic systems - i.e., distribution of erythrocytes and oxygen to muscles.

Type I	Slow twitch, high fatigue resistant, high oxidative, low glycolytic
Type IIa	Moderately fast twitch, fairly high fatigue resistant, high oxidative, high glycolytic
Type IIx	Fast twitch, intermediate fatigue resistant, intermediate oxidative, high glycolytic
Type IIb	Very fast twitch, low fatigue resistant, low oxidative, high glycolytic

Table 3. Muscle fiber types and main properties

All in all, the main components of the motor system described above are changed and altered specifically in patients with complete and motor-complete SCI as well as in patients suffering of chronic disuse and immobilization (burn patients, AIDS patients, some patients with cardiac or pulmonary problems)(Huang & DeVivo, 1990; Bauman, 1999; Riegger et al., 2009; Rouleau et al., 2010,2011; Spungen, 2003; Lainscak et al., 2007).

2.1 Spinal cord-transected murine model of complete paraplegia

In brief, all experimental procedures were conducted in accordance with the Canadian Council on Animal Care guidelines. Mice were generally housed 4-5 animals per cage in a controlled-temperature environment (22 ± 3°C), maintained under a 12h light:dark cycle with free access to water and food. Before surgery, pre-operative care was provided 30 minutes prior to anesthesia. It included subcutaneous injections of 1.0 ml of lactate-Ringer's solution, 0.1 mg/kg of buprenorphine, and 5 mg/kg of Baytril, an antibiotic. Initially, complete anesthesia was conducted using 2.5% isoflurane in a cage of induction. Anesthetized animals were then shaved dorsally (2-cm) from the mid-dorsal area to the neck. Then, each animal was maintained under complete anesthesia using a specially adapted facial mask delivering directly 2.5% isoflurane to the animal. The shaved area was cleaned with 70 % (*v/v*) isopropyl alcohol and, then with 10% (*v/v*) povidone-iodine solution whereas eyes are protected from dryness using ocular lubricant. The first skin incision was made using fine scissors over 2 cm along the midline from the mid-dorsal area to the neck. Fat tissues (interscapularis fat) were cut and removed to expose the high-thoracic segments.

The latissimus dorsi fascia was cut bilaterally to expose the vertebral column between the 4th and 6th thoracic vertebrae. Curved forceps were then used to tightly hold that area of the vertebral column that was cleaned from fascia and muscles to improve the grip. Forceps were also used to gently lift that part of the vertebral column which, once bent upward, eased the transection of the intervertebral ligaments between the 9th and the 10th vertebrae. This last part was critical to offer an open access for insertion of extra fine microscissors between the 9th and 10th thoracic vertebrae for the complete transection of the spinal cord. Then, the inner vertebral walls were explored and entirely, but delicately, scraped three or four times with fine scissors tips in order to sever any small fibres which had not been previously cut. It is important to scrape carefully to avoid severing the intervertebral ligaments located ventrally (i.e., if severed, it may lead to a dislocation of the vertebral column and corresponding bleeding). Throughout the transection procedures, bleeding although minor was controlled by applying pressure with cotton tips. The interscapularis fat was carefully replaced and the opened skin area was closed using 3 or 4 Michel suture clips. Michel suture clips are generally faster to install and are normally associated with less infection problems than typical suture threads. This overall surgical procedure was conducted under aseptic conditions using only perfectly cleaned materials and surgical tools - materials were previously autoclaved and tools were continuously sterilized throughout the procedure using a portable quartz beads-sterilizer).

Once the surgical procedures completed, anesthesia was interrupted and mice were placed in a large cage equipped with a heating pad placed underneath. It is critically important to use only minimal heating intensity (35°C) to avoid rapid dehydration, heat shock and death during the recovery period. Generally, the animals recovered completely within 15 min although we normally left them on the heating pad overnight with free access to food and water. The recovery procedure was found to be critical to ensure a high percentage of survival post-surgery (typically around 95% if everything is performed as described). The next day, the animals were replaced in their initial cage with their initial cage mates in order to reduce potential aggressions and fights.

Fig. 2. Spinal cord histology. Luxol blue and Cresyl violet staining of a longitudinal section of the spinal cord from a non-laminectomized spinal cord-transected mouse one week post-surgery.

Postoperative care, provided a few hours after surgery as well as every day for the next 4 days, included injections of lactate-Ringer's solution (2 x 1 ml/day, s.c.), buprenorphine (2 x

0.1 mg/kg/day, s.c.), and Baytril (5 mg/kg/day). Bladders were also manually emptied twice a day until a spontaneous return of some micturition reflexes. For voiding, the bladder was gently squeezed between the thumb (side of the bladder) and two fingers (e.g., the index and one other finger placed the other side of the bladder). This maneuver requires time and experience. In male mice, it was specifically challenging since, in addition, penises have to be maintained against a paper towel throughout the maneuver to improve successful voiding (i.e., it appeared to contribute, perhaps via capillary action, to urine expulsion outside the urinary tract). The belly and sexual organ were cleaned daily using paper towels and chlorhexidine gluconate solution (0.05 % *v/v*) to prevent urinary infection. Normally, with these procedures, mice that survived the firsts 24 hours, remained relatively healthy for a long period of time (i.e., several months). Finally, Michel suture clips were removed after 10 or 14 days post-surgery. Cages were cleaned regularly (ideally, cages needed to be changed every 3 or 4 days) and mice were cleaned, as described above, on a daily basis to prevent urinary tract infection. All in all, once anesthetized, this surgical procedure took no longer than five minutes whereas another 5-10 minutes was typically required for animals to recover from anesthesia.

This approach led to complete paraplegia (Figs. 2 & 3) - an immediate and irreversible loss of sensory and voluntary motor control below injury level (low-thoracic level). Although, it is possible to maintain these animals relatively healthy for severaonmonths post-spinal transection, a number of neuronal, muscular, skeletal, vascular, and hematologic changes were rapidly displayed. A detailed characterization of these changes is presented in the following subsections.

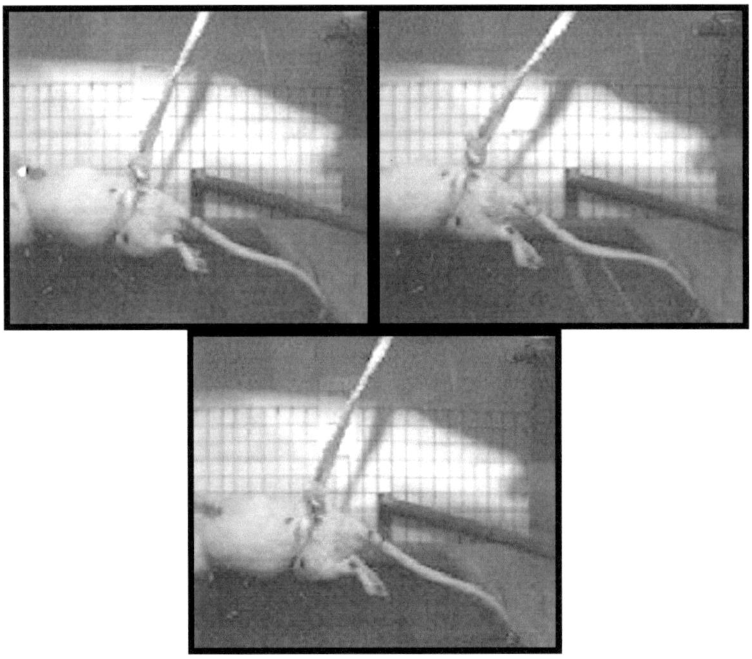

Fig. 3. Video images of a paraplegic mouse placed on a treadmill. A complete loss of hindlimb movement is encountered immediately following the spinal cord transection.

2.2 Disuse-related bone loss, biomechanical property changes and factures

Nearly all SCI individuals experience a drastic loss of bone mineral content (up to 30% at the femoral level) leading to a marked increase of fracture incidence within one year after injury (Ragnarsson & Sell, 1981; Garland et al., 1992; Wilmet et al., 1995; Lazo et al., 2001; Sabo et al., 2001). Although, the basic mechanisms underlying osteoporosis in post-menopausal women have been extensively studied, those involved in chronic immobilization and disuse have received considerably less attention. In animal models of disuse, traditionally in rats, hindlimb immobilization has been found to induce a drastic and sudden loss of femoral bone tissue suggesting that different mechanisms may be involved in disuse vs. estrogen-deficiency/aging-related osteoporosis (Bagi & Miller, 1994). For instance, a 10-30% decrease of cancellous bone has been reported within only a few weeks in the ipsilateral femur of rats that had their hindlimbs immobilized with a cast or an elastic bandage (Ito et al., 1994; Ma et al., 1995; Mosekilde et al., 2000). Comparable changes have been found in other models of disuse such as in tail-suspended rats (Wronski et al., 1989). Some of these disuse-related changes are believed to be mediated by both an increase of osteoclastic bone resorption and a decrease of osteoblastic bone formation (Rantakokko et al., 1999). On the other hand, growing evidence suggests that several factors other than mechanical unloading *per se* can influence the combination of cellular and molecular mechanisms underlying disuse-related bone loss. For instance, in the case of disuse induced by a lesion of the sciatic nerve, the loss of bone tissue in rats is caused partly by a disruption of the neurogenic innervation of the bone marrow (Zeng et al., 1996). Moreover, differential tissue- and biomarker-specific changes have been reported in the tail-suspension vs. sciatic nerve lesion models (Hanson et al., 2005). In the case of microgravity, bone tissue changes have been attributed mainly to a marked decrease of osteblast formation in young adult rats (Matsumoto et al., 1998). Taken together, those data suggest that the combination of various factors specific to each model and condition of disuse may dictate, to some extent, the different sets of molecular mechanisms involved in demineralization and bone loss.

Here, we characterized some of the main structural and functional adaptive changes occurring specifically within a few weeks in adult spinal cord transected mice. In brief, within a few weeks post-transection, paraplegic mice were weighed, sacrificed and the femoral bones dissected and cleaned of soft tissue. The femurs were wrapped in saline-soaked gauze and frozen at -20 degrees C in sealed vials until testing. For histomorphometry, the left femoral bones were fixed with paraformaldehyde, decalcified, paraffin embedded and stained with acid fuchine using the Masson's trichrome procedures. Histomorphometric analyses were performed with a NOVA Prime, Biioquant's image analysis system (R&M Biometric, Nashville, TN) for primary bone morphometric parameters. Three bone slices at the metaphyseal level were analyzed. For densitometry, measurements were made with the rigth femoral bones of sham and paraplegic mice. Bone mineral content (BMC, g) from the femora of each animal was assessed using dual-energy X-ray absoptiometry (DEXA, model Piximus II, Lunar Corporation, Madison WI, for details, see Kolta S, De Vernejoul M.C. et al. 2003). Bone mineral density (BMD, g/cm^2) was calculated as BMC divided by projected bone area. Each femur was scanned separately for whole bone analysis. For biomechanical assessment, on the day of testing, the femur was slowly (4 hours) tawed at room temperature. They were placed horizontally on the three-point bending device (MTS, Eden Prairie, MN). The mechanical resistance to failure was tested using a servo-controlled electromechanical system (Intron, Instron, Canton, MA). The crosshead speed for all tests was 10 mm/sec until the femur fractured. Displacement and load values were acquired at 100 Hz, recorded and stored on PC. Off-line data analyses were performed to calculate maximal strength (N), stiffness (slope of the linear part of the curve to failure, N/cm), and elasticity deformation (N). Bones were kept wet throughout testing and used for histomorphometrical testing (proximal end).

All histomorphometric measurements and analyses were made from the metaphyseal area of the left femora. The cancellous bone volume was found to decrease by 25.2% in paraplegic mice (within 1 month post-transection) compared with control (non-paraplegic). The average trabecular bone thickness was found to decrease by 10.65%. The thickness was initially of 25.55 micron in the control groups and of only 22.83 micron in the paraplegic group. The number of trabecular bone areas decreased rapidly also after injury. In the control group, the average trabecular number was 3.38 nbr/mm2 whereas in the paraplegic group, it decreased to only 2.89 nbr/mm2 representing a 14.50% decrease. On the other hand, the trabecular separation, defined as the space between trabecular bone areas, increased after injury. In fact, on average, the trabecular separation increased by 24.03% within 1 month post-SCI (Picard et al., 2008).

The bone mineral density (BMD) of the left femora measured by dual-energy X-ray absorptiometry (DEXA) significantly changed after injury. The BMD was just below 0.09 g/cm2 in control and of 0.0731 in paraplegic mice. Bone mineral content (BMC) also proportionally decreased after injury (see *sections 2.6* and *2.7* for further details).

The maximum force in N required for the crosshead to fracture the right femora at the mid-diaphyseal level was decreased by 13% on average within a few weeks post-transection (Fig.4D). The stiffness in N/mm was also reduced after injury with average values of 57.23 and 51.08 in control and paraplegic groups, respectively, representing a 10.8% decrease (Fig.4B). The elastic force decreased also by approximately 15% in early spinal transected mice compared with control (Fig.4C).

2.3 Muscular atrophy, muscle fiber-type conversion, and strength loss

It is well-documented in various rat models that the contractile properties of slow twitch muscles change into more fast-like muscles after chronic spinalization (Roy et al., 1991; Talmadge, 2000). Hindlimb extensor muscles such as soleus (SOL) typically exhibit extended atrophy (e.g., up to 50%) and type I to type II muscle fiber conversion following spinalization in rats (Krikorian et al., 1982; Lieber et al., 1986 a,b; Midrio et al., 1988; Talmadge et al., 1995). Contraction and relaxation times as well as maximal tetanic force (Po) and maximal twitch force (Pt) have also been found to be importantly decreased in rat SOL several months after spinalization (Davey et al., 1981; Talmadge et al., 2002).

Evidence from other models of inactivity and immobilization suggests that some of these changes, in fact, are induced very early after inactivity and reduced muscular activity and loading. For example, a 10% loss of body weight (Pierotti et al., 1990) accompanied by a 40-50% decrease of SOL mass, TPT and 1/2 RT (Frenette et al., 2002) and a rapid reduction in slow myofibril proteins (Thomason et al., 1987) have been reported after 1-2 weeks of hindlimb suspension in rats. Comparable results have been found within less than 2 weeks in rats after spinal cord isolation (i.e., de-afferented and spinalized, Grossman et al., 1998) or in microgravity (Fitts et al., 2001). In addition, a 40% reduction of SOL cross sectional area has been found only 10 days post-spinal cord transection in rats (Dupont-Versteegden et al., 1999). The possibility that other early changes may occur after spinal cord transection is largely unexplored.

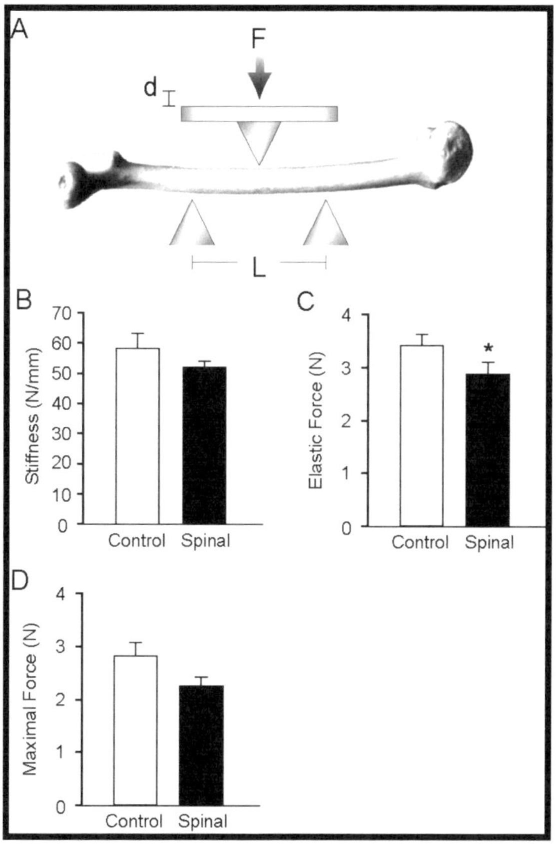

Fig. 4. Bone mechanical properties. Two-point bending test (A) revealed decreased femoral stiffness (B), elasticity (C) and maximal force (D) in untrained spinal transected mice (spinal, black) versus control (intact animals, white)(unpublished data).

Here, we characterized some of the earliest adaptations in gross anatomy and muscle properties at only 7 days following spinal cord transection in adult mice (Landry et al., 2004). In brief, whole body weight was measured daily during the first week post-spinalization. After dissection of SOL for functional tests in vitro (see section below), animals were sacrificed with pentobarbital overdose. Forelimbs and hindlimbs were surgically removed just below the shoulder and the hip joints respectively. Paws as well as all parts of the pectoral and back muscles attached to the forelimbs were removed. Tests included weight measurement of the left forelimb and hindlimb as well as of the right SOL. To further assess muscle atrophy, limbs were weighed in air and in water to measure volume changes. Volume was calculated as follows with a volumic mass of 0.998 for water at room temperature (22°C):

$$\text{Volume} = (\text{weight in air - weight in water}) \text{ x } (\text{volumic mass of water})$$

For measurement of contractile properties, we anesthetized animals with pentobarbital sodium (50 mg/kg). The right SOL was carefully dissected and incubated in fully oxygenated Krebs-Ringer bicarbonate buffer solution maintained at 25°C and supplemented

with glucose (2 mg/ml). *In vitro* measurement of muscle contractile properties was performed as described elsewhere (Côté et al., 1997). In brief, one tendon was attached to a rigid support at the bottom of the bath, and the other end was connected to an isometric force transducer (Grass FT-03) through a stainless steel hook. An initial resting period of 15 min was allowed before testing. Muscles were carefully stretched to their optimal length, defined as the length at which maximal isometric twitch tension is produced. One single twitch contraction was elicited and the following measurements were obtained: maximum twitch tension (Pt), time-to-peak tension (TPT), and one-half relaxation time (1/2 RT). After measurement of twitch parameters, muscles were stimulated for 1 s at frequencies of 10, 20, 35, 50, 80, and 100 Hz to determine maximal tetanic tension (Po, N/cm^2). The value used for muscle density was 1.062 g/cm (Koh & Brooks, 2001) and the ratio of fiber length to muscle length used was 0.71 (Brooks & Faulkner, 1988).
We reported that paraplegic mice at 7 days post-surgery encountered a drastic loss in body weight (Landry et al., 2004). On average, a 24% decrease in weight was found at 7 days post-spinalization. A similar loss was found in another group of paraplegic mice that received instead daily injection of lactate-Ringer's solution (2 ml/day, s.c.) during the first week post-spinalization suggesting that dehydration did not contribute to weight loss.
The specific weight of individual body parts was also examined in paraplegic mice. In intact mice, the average weight of forelimbs and hindlimbs was 436 and 1239 mg respectively. At 7 days post-spinalization, hindlimb weight decreased by 28% compared to intact mice. Interestingly, a 21% reduction in the forelimbs of paraplegic mice was also observed during the same period of time. Relative to body weight, the loss observed in hindlimbs was greater than the one in forelimbs. Similar reductions in volume were found respectively in hindlimbs and forelimbs.
Regarding properties, for soleus mass displayed significantly lower values (-32%) in untrained paraplegic mice at 7 days post-spinalization compared with intact animals. A 33% decrease of Po was measured at 7 days post-spinalization. The absolute tension generated at different frequencies of stimulation showed mainly that SOL force was reduced in paraplegic mice compared to control at stimulation frequencies above 35 Hz. On the other hand, maximal tension was reached at lower stimulation frequencies for paraplegics compared to control.
Our data showed also in soleus a change toward faster-type properties in the first few days post-immobilization (transection).The surprising initial and rapid conversion to slower contractile properties at 7 days post-spinalization is further supported by changes found in contraction and relaxation times (TPT and 1/2 RT respectively). TPT became slower (i.e., increased time of contraction) by 21% at 7 days compared to control. Similar changes were observed with 1/2 RT which became slower (i.e., increased time of relaxation) by 48% at 7 days post-spinalisation.
As mentioned above, it is well-known that there is an important shift in fiber phenotype distribution a few weeks post-SCI even more so in soleus. Generally, slow fibers tend to change for a faster phenotype after 2 weeks post-spinal cord transection. After spinal cord transection, 50-55% of the slow type fibers showed important fiber type conversion, shifting to a hybrid isoform (faster phenotype) whereas fiber type conversion was not observed in another hindlimb muscle, EDL, often classified as a purely fast-twitch muscle (Table 4).

Fiber type %	Non-TX	TX untrained
EDL type II	98.7 ± 0.3	98.7 ± 0.6
EDL hybrid	1.3 ± 0.3	1.3 ± 0.6
SOL type I	54.6 ± 2.6	2.9 ± 1.5
SOL type II	45.4 ± 2.6	46.5 ± 2.5
SOL hybrid	0 ± 0	50.7 ± 3.3

Table 4. Fiber type conversion in normal (non-TX) and untrained paraplegic (TX untrained)(unpublished data).

2.4 Circulatory and hematologic changes associated with increased risks of blood cloth formation and deep vein thrombosis

Among the cardiovascular and pulmonary problems associated with SCI, deep venous thrombosis (DVT) is one of the most serious complications in patients that survive to the accident. Indeed, DVT constitutes the third most common cause of death in SCI patients (Waring & Karunas, 1991; DeVivo, 1999) and, despite prophylaxic methods (e.g. anticoagulant administration), a significant proportion of SCI patients will develop a pulmonary embolism caused by DVT (Deep et al., 2001).

Complete paraplegic and tetraplegic individuals are particularly vulnerable given that spasticity, typically found in incomplete SCI patients, may decrease the risks of DVT formation (Green et al., 2003). Generally, DVT formation is attributed to a combination of factors including also venous stasis, venous injury, and hypercoagulability. In turn, these factors facilitate platelet, LDL-cholesterol, and leukocyte adhesion, procoagulant system activation, and hence, thrombin generation. Although, few animal models of DVT and/or pulmonary embolism exist (Frisbie, 2005), none have been developed to study these complications after SCI which may explain why the specific mechanisms of DVT formation in paralytics remain poorly understood.

Here, we characterized, in spinal cord transected (Tx) mice, some of the physiological changes occurring after SCI that could possibly contribute to DVT formation (Rouleau & Guertin, 2007; Rouleau et al., 2007). Specifically, we characterized also alterations of deep vein diameter in the hindlimbs of Tx mice because venous distensibility and capacity changes may participate to DVT formation (Miranda & Hassouna, 2000). We took advantage of this experimental model to measure with great precision (µm), using *in vivo* fluorescence confocal microscopy, changes in diameter of the femoral and saphenous veins. All tests were performed weekly during one month post-Tx since risks of DVT in patients have been reported to increase by several folds specifically during the first few weeks after SCI (DeVivo et al., 1999).

In brief, we put the tail on a heated cushion to dilate the tail vein 10 min before injection. Then 200 µl of 5 mg/ml fluorescein isothiocyanate-dextran (FD-40) (Sigma, St-Louis, MO) dilute in injectable endotoxin-free dPBS (Sigma), was injected intravenously into the tail vein. Animals were killed by CO_2 asphyxiation around 10 min after injection. The skin was cut to access to the femoral and saphenous veins. Microscope observation and measurement were performed with an Olympus BX61WI confocal system and analysed with Fluoview 300 (Carsen group, Markhan, Canada).

For hematologic data, peripheral blood was collected at various times post-transection by cardiac puncture. Each blood sample was analyzed for platelet quantification with a CELL-DYN 3700® automatic blood cell analyzer (CD3700)(Abbott Laboratories, North Chicago, IL).

We found by measuring deep vein diameter using *in vivo* fluorescent confocal microscopy techniques that the femoral and saphenous veins drastically increased in size after SCI compared with intact mice. This is illustrated in Fig. 5 showing typical examples from a control (left panel) and from a paraplegic mouse at 3 week post-TX (right panel). We can clearly distinguish that the femoral vein drastically increased in size post-transection compared with control. In fact, average values calculated for the femoral vein revealed, for control animals, an average diameter of 319 μm augmented to 458 μm at 3 weeks post-surgery (Fig. 5). Comparable increases of saphenous vein diameter were found after spinal transection (338 μm in control vs 433 in paraplegics)
The hematologic data revealed mild anemia that occurs as early as at 7 days post-transection. Specifically, average counts of erythrocytes (10.11 x 10^{12} /L in control mice) decreased to values ranging from 9.91 to 9.54 x 10^{12} /L in paraplegic mice. Hemoglobin concentrations were decreased from 164.9 ± 2.8 g/L in controls to 153.3 g/L in paraplegic mice. Decreased hematocrit levels were also found in paraplegic mice (range from 0.46 ± 0.01 to 0.44 ± 0.01 L/L) compared with controls (0.48 ± 0.01 L/L, Fig. 1C). In turn, platelet counts remained unchanged after spinal transection with levels of 16.76 ± 0.80 x 10^{11} /L in controls and 17.73 ± 0.75 in paraplegic mice (Rouleau et al., 2007).

2.5 Complex spinal cord network that controls locomotor rhythm generation

The Central Pattern Generator (CPG) for locomotion is a network of neurons located in the lumbar area of the spinal cord that is capable of producing the basic commands for stepping even when isolated from supraspinal and sensory inputs (Grillner & Zangger, 1979, see also Guertin, 2010). Early evidence of a CPG emerged a century ago from the pioneer work of Sherrington (1910) and Brown (1914). In the 70s, low-thoracic spinalized rabbits and cats were used to show that an endogenous release of 5-HT induced by 5-HTP can generate fictive locomotor-like rhythms in the spinal cord (recorded with electroneurograms) of acute spinal cord-transected animals (Viala & Buser, 1971) or increase extensor muscle activity in regularly treadmill-trained and sensory-stimulated spinal animals (Barbeau & Rossignol, 1990, 1991). A clear demonstration of its existence was provided in 1979 by Grillner who could induce, with L-DOPA, locomotor-like neural activity in the motor nerves of completely de-afferented, curarized, and spinal cord-transected cats (Grillner & Zangger, 1979). In rats, the CPG was found, with activity-dependent labeling (e.g., c-fos), to be located mainly in rostral segments of the lumbar spinal cord (Cina & Hochman, 2000). Comparable results were found in mice where CPG activity was found to originate from lumbar segments with critical elements in L1-L2 (Nishimaru et al., 2000).
In the 80s and 90s, *in vitro* isolated spinal cord preparations were extensively used to study the pharmacological control of CPG neurons at the system and cellular levels. Initially discovered in lampreys, bath application of N-methyl-D-asparate (NMDA) was found to induce rhythmic activity (recorded from ventral roots) that shared locomotor characteristics - called 'fictive locomotion'. This provided evidence that even a perfectly isolated CPG can be activated with drugs. Then, neonatal rat and mouse spinal cord isolated preparations were developed and used also to study *in vitro* drug-induced CPG-mediated locomotor-like neurographic activity. These studies have essentially revealed that bath-applied combinations of drugs such as NMDA, 5-HT and DA can best induce robust fictive locomotor-like rhythms in the mammalian isolated spinal cord (Cazalets et al., 1992;

Kjaerulff & Kiehn, 1994). Although, these studies have revealed that several families of drugs need to be combined for enhanced CPG activation, most of the compounds used *in vitro* were synthetic neurotransmitters (e.g. 5-HT and DA) which, unfortunately, do not constitute good candidates for drug treatments because of poor selectivity (e.g. activation of all receptor subtypes) and incapacity to cross the BBB.

In humans, evidence of a CPG was provided after showing that 'automatic' (involuntary) stepping-like movements could be triggered spontaneously under certain conditions or by epidural stimulation at the L2 level in SCI patients confined to a bed (Dimitrijevic et al., 1998). Although a completely isolated CPG can produce locomotor rhythms, sensory inputs (*i.e.* muscle proprioception, vision, etc.) were found to provide useful feedback signals to the CPG that can re-enforce muscle contraction and adapt stepping to external disturbances (Rossignol & Dubuc, 1994). However, none of these studies have identified a full CPG-activating drug that can, upon systemic administration, potently elicit acutely powerful weight-bearing stepping in complete SCI animals with no other stimulation/assistance (e.g., non-therapetically relevant tail pinching or other sensory stimulation).

Changes post-spinal cord transection were also found in sublesionally-located neurons (below injury level). Since most of these changes were found in neurons located in upper lumbar segments of the spinal cord, they were postulated to correspond with changes in CPG neuron candidates. Immediate early genes (IEGs) constitute a large family of genes well-known as early regulators of cell growth, differentiation signals, learning and memory. We reported in low-thoracic spinal cord-transected mice, that IEGs such as *c-fos* and *nor-1* expression respectively increased and decreased within a few days in the segments L1-L2, specifically in the dorsal horn and intermediate zone areas (Landry et al., 2006). Changes in the lumbar spinal cord of rostrally-transected animals were of special interest since some of these segments (e.g., L1-L2 in mice) were shown to contain critical central pattern generator (CPG) elements as mentioned earlier. Given that IEGs are better known for their role in CNS development and plasticity, spontaneous changes of IEG expression (i.e., specifically *c-fos* and *nor-1*) in L1-L2 segments may be considered as among the first sublesional cellular events associated with altered cellular functions and properties post-SCI. This said, some of these changes may be associated also with other phenomena than plasticity or reorganization of spinal motor and locomotor networks. For instance, *c-fos* and nor-1 were used as markers in experimental models of pain and transient global ischemia suggesting a role in several functions (see Landry et al., 2006a).

Other key elements including transmembranal receptors may be considered good candidates for plasticity and reorganization of motor and locomotor networks located sublesionally following a spinal cord-transection (and probably to some extent also after partial injuries). For instance, we found using *in situ* hybridization increased 5-HT_{1A} mRNA levels in L1-L2 segments in 5-HT_7-deficient mice compared with wild-types (Landry et al., 2006b). This was interpreted as evidence suggesting that even greater changes may occur post-trauma in absence of functionally closely-related genes. Results in mice revealed also increased 5-HT_{2A} mRNA levels in lumbar segments (laminae VII, VIII, and IX) several days after a low-thoracic transection (Ung et al., 2009).

All in all, it is unclear how these changes of neuronal properties and gene expression below lesion level may affect functional recovery and, specifically, the development of approach designed to reactivate behaviours-generating neuronal networks (e.g., CPGs for locomotion, micturition, ejaculation, etc.). Nonetheless, it has been postulated by others that such changes may contribute to increase sublesional network excitability and, thus, may facilitate training-induced learning and rehabilitation.

2.6 Advanced locomotor training induced pharmacologically as a treatment against motor system changes in SCI

Given that no cure exists yet to repair the spinal cord, an interesting avenue to prevent or reduce some of the motor system changes described in previous sections of this chapter may be to pharmacologically induce episodes of locomotion. To achieve this, an alternative strategy could be to develop a CPG-activating drug treatment that could temporarily re-activate this sublesional network in tetraplegic and most paraplegic subjects.

Experiments mainly conducted in my laboratory since 2004 have led to a better understanding of pharmacological CPG activation *in vivo*. In brief, we found in completely low-thoracic spinal cord-transected mice that a few subtypes of blood brain barrier (BBB) permeable molecules can elicit partial CPG-activating effects (i.e., locomotor-like movements or LMs that resemble crawling - successive flexions and extensions coordinated in both hindlimbs without weight bearing)(Guertin, 2004a; Landry & Guertin, 2004; Landry et al., 2006; Lapointe et al., 2009). We subsequently found that drug combinations with some of these compounds including dopaminergic and serotonergic compounds (e.g., DA precursors such as L-DOPA combined with a decarboxylase inhibitor such as carbidopa, and a 5-HT1A receptor agonist such as 8-OH-DPAT or buspirone, etc.), could elicit significantly greater CPG-activating effects including large amplitude LMs with some equilibrium, plantar foot placement and weight bearing capabilities (i.e., real stepping rather than crawling, Guertin 2004b; Lapointe & Guertin 2008; Guertin et al., 2010, Guertin et al., 2011)(Fig.6). As mentioned earlier, this idea that drug combinations can produce apparently full CPG-activating effects was also supported by comparable findings in *in vitro* isolated spinal cord preparations (better and more stable fictive locomotor neuronal activities in isolated spinal cords, e.g., Cazalets et al., 1992; Kjaerulff & Kiehn, 1994; Kiehn & Kjaerulff, 1996; Jiang et al., 1999; Whelan et al., 2000).

This identification of a potent CPG-activating tritherapy (Guertin et al., 2010) recently received support from a special NIH program (Rapid Access to Interventional Development program) to conduct some of the preclinical studies (toxicity and safety pharmacology in rats). It has been determined that a tri-therapy composed of L-DOPA, carbidopa and buspirone is safe and ideally suited for further development at the clinical level (i.e., each drug is already FDA approved for diseases other than SCI and no abnormal pharmacology or toxicology data was found) as a first-in-class CPG activating drug treatment candidate. However, although efficacy in early chronic SCI mice has recently been demonstrated (Guertin et al., 2010; Guertin et al. 2011), it remains unclear how repeated administration over several weeks would affect disuse-related motor system changes.

As mentioned earlier, chronic SCI patients (especially motor-complete also called ASIA-A or ASIA-B patients) experience often life-threatening health problems also referred to as 'secondary complications' including motor system changes reported here also in this paraplegic mouse model. Using combination therapy, we obtained preliminary data suggesting that repeatedly-treated paraplegic mice can partially prevent some pathophysiological motor system changes found after SCI (Guertin et al., 2011).

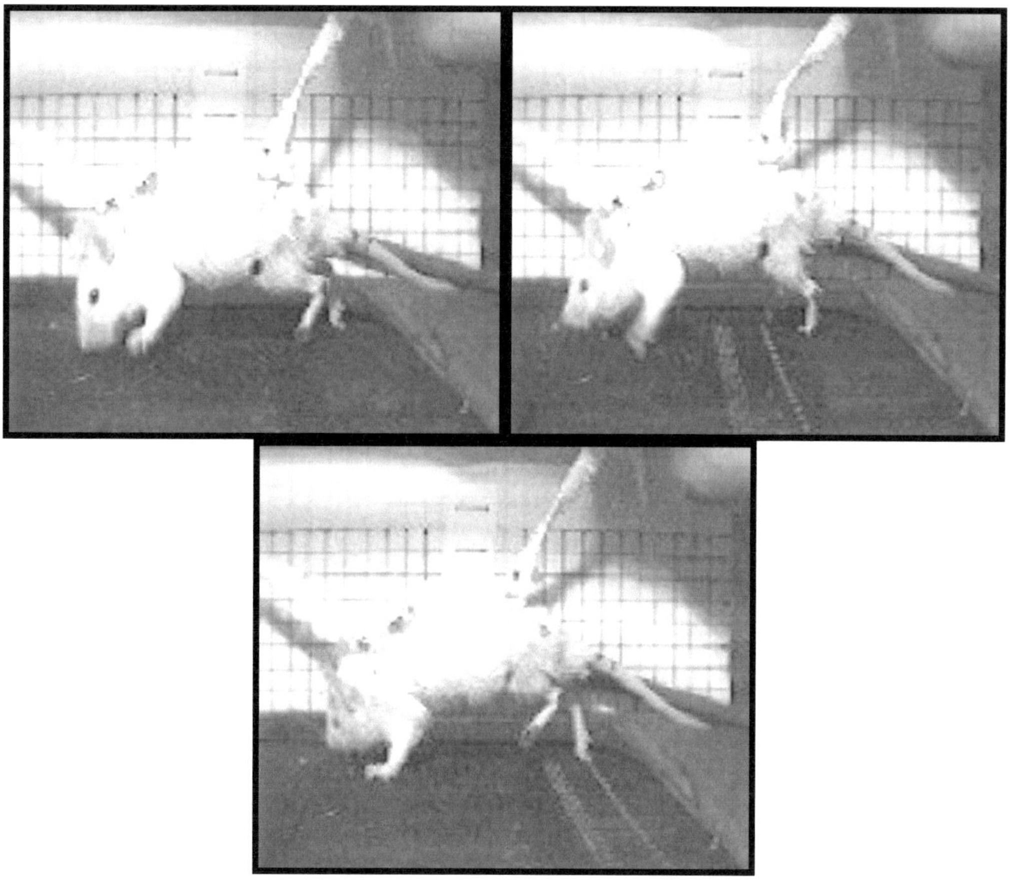

Fig. 5. Video images of a paraplegic mouse placed on a treadmill 15 minutes following administration of a CPG-activation tritherapy. Involuntary movements were generated for approximately 30 to 45 min. Then a complete return to complete paraplegia occurred.

Subcutaneous administration (several times per week) of a first-generation combination treatment was found, upon each injection (within 15 min), to repeatedly induce temporarily (during approx. 30-45 min) episodes of weight bearing stepping in non-assisted paraplegic mice at least during one month.

Regarding body weight values, combination therapy-treated paraplegic animals progressively displayed a moderate increase in weight suggesting that repeated administration of this combination therapy was well-tolerated (i.e., a loss of weight would have suggested toxic effects and additional health problems). No significant difference was found in bone mineral density (BMD) values in femoral bones of tritherapy-treated vs. placebo-treated paraplegic mice. Post-mortem examination of muscle size (whole surface area and fiber cross-sectional area or CSA) measured from cryostat transverse sections prepared from two hindlimb muscles, *soleus* (SOL) and *extensor digitorum longus* (EDL), was performed to assess the effect of combination therapy-induced training on muscular atrophy normally found after SCI. We found values corresponding with larger muscles and muscle fibers in the combination therapy-treated compared with the placebo-treated paraplegic animals. Sol values increased by 24% in combination therapy-treated paraplegic mice (0.61 ± 0.05 mm^2) compared with placebo-treated ones (0.49 ± 0.03 mm^2, fig. 3A). Comparable results were found in EDL (combination therapy-treated 0.91 ± 0.03 mm^2 vs. placebo-treated 0.77 ± 0.06 mm^2)(not shown). At the cellular level, comparisons between combination therapy-treated and placebo-treated animals revealed that type I fiber CSA values non-significantly changed whereas type II fiber and intermediate fiber (type I + II labeled) CSA values significantly increased subsequently both by 8% (Fig. 3C, 3D). An analysis of muscle fiber-type ratios (i.e., proportion among all fibers of type I, type II or type I + II fibers) indicated that no significant changes were found between groups. Subpopulations of red blood cell (RBC) constituents were assessed and compared between groups. Levels of RBC, platelet, hemoglobin and hematocrit were significantly increased by 11%, 19%, 10% and 10%, respectively, in combination therapy-treated vs. placebo-treated paraplegic animals.

All in all, these results revealed that pharmacological activation of the CPG four times per week during 1 month can prevent anemia and prevent partially muscle atrophy. Circulatory systems were not further examined in this study. On the other hand, this study showed that bone loss typically occurring post-transection in this animals can not be prevented in these conditions. Altogether, it is suggested that training conditions or treatments may have to be optimized for further physiological effects on all parts of the motor system.

Along this idea, we recently conducted a study where paraplegic animals received an anabolic agent, namely clenbuterol, in addition to tritherapy-induced locomotor training. We found that tritherapy-treated paraplegic mice with or without clenbuterol treatment displayed significant locomotor function recovery during 2 months upon each administration of the CPG-activating therapy (Fig.7). To further characterize movements induced by the tritherapy-training, angular excursion at the hip, knee and ankle, as well as movement amplitude values were analysed. Typical examples of hindlimb kinematics are shown in figure 7. Hip, knee and ankle angular displacement showed similar patterns in intact, tritherapy-trained alone and tritherapy-trained + clenbuterol paraplegic animals. Untrained paraplegic animals displayed a consistent lack of angular excursion at the hip level although some displacements were found at the knee and ankle levels (hip: 85°, knee: 30-47°, ankle: 28-125°). Hindlimb movement amplitude values measured by calculating toe displacement in X and Y axis (step "length" and "height") revealed that intact mice had greater step length values than both tritherapy-trained paraplegic groups. On the other hand, both groups of tritherapy-trained paraplegic animals showed similar step length values which were significantly greater than those in untrained paraplegic mice. The coefficient of variation (CV) was higher in untrained mice. Intact, tritherapy-trained and tritherapy-trained + clenbuterol paraplegic mice showed similar step height values. However, differences were found in the variability of the step height, as shown by CV, where intact animals displayed less variability than the other groups of tritherapy-trained animals. No Y axis movement amplitude was observed in paraplegic untrained mice since no weight-bearing movement are normally expressed spontaneously. Overall, a significant increase in performances over time was observed in tritherapy-trained groups of paraplegic mice movement kinematic values were comparable with those from intact animals.

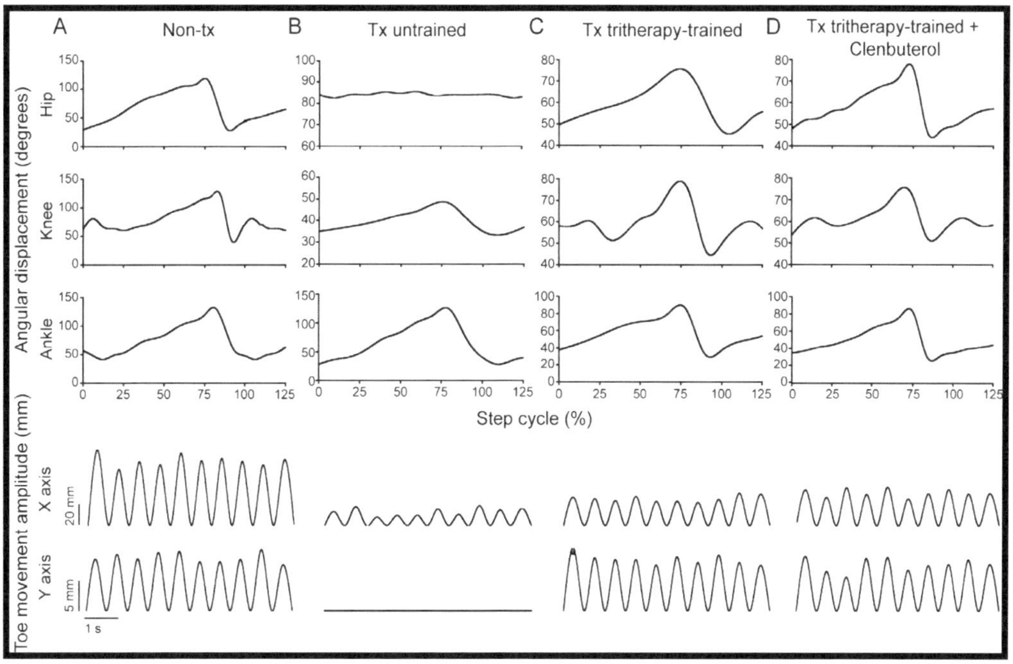

Fig. 6. Kinematic analyses in intact (non-Tx), paraplegic (Tx) untrained, paraplegic tritherapy-trained and tritherapy-trained and treated with clenbuterol. Step parameters from both tritherapy-trained paraplegic mice were similar with those from intact animals suggesting that the tritherapy appropriately restored episodes of locomotor movements.

Femoral BMD and BMC values were measured in order to address whether tritherapy-training alone or combined with clenbuterol can prevent or at least reduce bone loss normally found in untrained paraplegic mice. However, in all groups of paraplegic animals, important losses were found. Untrained paraplegic mice (BMD: 0.0767 ± 0.0010 g/cm^2, BMC: 0.0381 ± 0.0008 g) and tritherapy-trained paraplegic animals (BMD: 0.0766 ± 0.0011 g/cm^2, BMC: 0.0378 ± 0.0009 g) showed comparable values whereas in paraplegic trained + clenbuterol groups, femoral BMD (0.0731 ± 0.0012) and BMC (0.0349 ± 0.0009) further decreased.
Morphometric analyses of soleus and EDL were performed in order to further characterize specific muscular property changes in all groups. Muscle CSA, fiber type-specific CSA and relative distribution values were analysed. For soleus CSA, untrained and tritherapy-trained paraplegic mice had significantly lower muscle CSA values than intact animals and tritherapy-trained + clenbuterol paraplegic groups. However soleus CSA in untrained paraplegic mice was not significantly lower than tritherapy-trained paraplegic animals. For EDL, in contrast with muscle mass changes, CSA values showed statistical differences between groups. Tritherapy-trained + clenbuterol paraplegic mice showed higher EDL CSA values than all the other groups. Untrained and tritherapy-trained paraplegic mice had lower CSA values than intact animals.

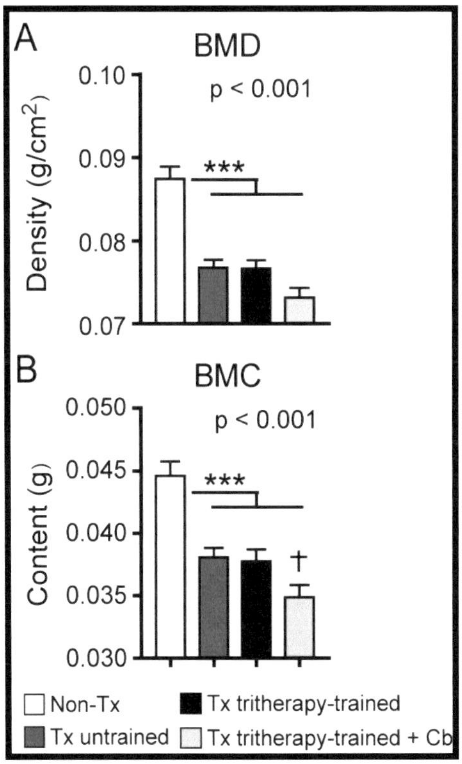

Fig. 7. Femoral BMD and BMC in intact (non-Tx), paraplegic (Tx) untrained, paraplegic tritherapy-trained and tritherapy-trained and treated with clenbuterol. Unfortunately, bone loss was not prevented in both tritherapy-trained paraplegic mice compared with intact animals suggesting that the tritherapy with or without clenbuterol failed to restore bone properties.

Soleus and EDL muscle cross-sectional area				
	Non-Tx	Tx untrained	Tx tritherapy-trained	Tx tritherapy-trained + clen
Soleus	0.85 ± 0.05	0.56 ± 0.05 **††	0.64 ± 0.04 *††	0.93 ± 0.06
EDL	1.10 ± 0.04	0.95 ± 0.04 **††	0.96 ± 0.04 **††	1.25 ± 0.05 **

Table 5. Soleus and EDL cross-sectional area values in intact (non-Tx), paraplegic (Tx) untrained, paraplegic tritherapy-trained and tritherapy-trained and treated with clenbuterol. Although encouraging anti-atrophying effects were found in tritherapy-treated paraplegic mice, only paraplegic animals that received both clenbuterol + tritherapy displayed a complete restoration of muscle size (even a relative hypertrophic effect was induced compared with intact animals).

More differences were found when analysing individually fiber type-specific CSA values. Specifically, for soleus fiber types, all three fiber types from tritherapy-trained + clenbuterol paraplegic animals displayed larger CSA values than all other groups (type I: 1656.7 ± 80.8 μm^2, type II: 987.2 ± 16.7 μm^2, hybrid: 1145.5 ± 18.0 μm^2). Conversely, untrained paraplegic mice displayed the lowest soleus fiber type CSA of all groups (type I: 783.1 ± 15.1 μm^2, type II: 753.2 ± 9.1 μm^2, hybrid: 750.0 ± 8.1 μm^2). In EDL, type II fiber CSA differences between groups were similar to soleus type II (intact: 1063.5 ± 15.9 μm^2, paraplegic untrained: 908.1 ± 11.4 μm^2, paraplegic trained: 963.4 ± 10.9 μm^2, paraplegic trained + clenbuterol: 11.65.2 ± 17.9 μm^2).

3. Conclusion

These findings provided proof-of-concept data strongly supporting the idea that physical activity can prevent or restore motor system adaptations normally expressed after SCI. However, that study was exploratory and thus, it remains unclear the extent to which physical activity elicited with this pharmacological approach can extensively prevent or reverse secondary complications. Although anemia and partial muscle atrophy were prevented in CPG-activating tritherapy-trained paraplegic mice, addition of anabolic aids such as clenbuterol appeared to synergistically affect positively the motor system in paraplegic mice (complete reversal of atrophy, complete lack of anemia, etc.). Effects on other elements of the motor systems such as blood vessels (e.g., deep vein size) or skeleton remain to be explored or improved. From a scientific perspective, it remains also to be determined clearly what role physical inactivity may play on motor system adaptations post-SCI and corresponding health problems in humans. This said, motor system changes post-SCI obtained in this murine model was found to resemble those typically encountered in patients with SCI or disuse. It may therefore be useful to further study basic cellular mechanisms underlying these changes of the musculoskeletal systems in these conditions. It may also serve to accelerate the development of new therapeutic strategies aimed at reducing or preventing completely all musculoskeletal and biomechanical changes in SCI patients or in patients suffering of disuse or immobilization.

4. References

Siegwart, R. (2001). Indirect Manipulation of a Sphere on a Flat Disk Using Force Information. *International Journal of Advanced Robotic Systems,* Vol.6, No.4, (December 2009), pp. 12-16, ISSN 1729-8806

Bagi CM, Miller SC.Comparison of osteopenic changes in cancellous bone induced by ovariectomy and/or immobilization in adult rats.Anat Rec. 1994 Jul;239(3):243-54.PMID:7943756

Baptiste DC, Fehlings MG (2007). Update on the treatment of spinal cord injury. Prog Brain Res, Vol 161, pp.17-33. PMID:17618980

Barbeau H, Rossignol S.The effects of serotonergic drugs on the locomotor pattern and on cutaneous reflexes of the adult chronic spinal cat.Brain Res. 1990 Apr 23;514(1):55-67.PMID:2357531

Barbeau H, Rossignol S.Initiation and modulation of the locomotor pattern in the adult chronic spinal cat by noradrenergic, serotonergic and dopaminergic drugs.Brain Res. 1991 Apr 19;546(2):250-60.PMID:2070262

Barbeau H, Chau C, Rossignol S Noradrenergic agonists and locomotor training affect locomotor recovery after cord transection in adult cats. Brain Res Bull. 1993;30(3-4):387-93.PMID: 8457888

Barbeau H, Norman K, Fung J, Visintin M, Ladouceur M. Does neurorehabilitation play a role in the recovery of walking in neurological populations? Ann N Y Acad Sci. 1998 Nov 16;860:377-92. Review. PMID: 9928326

Bauman WA, Spungen AM, Adkins RH, Kemp BJ.Metabolic and endocrine changes in persons aging with spinal cord injury.Assist Technol. 1999;11(2):88-96. Review.PMID:11010069

Brown TG. On the nature of the fundamental activity of the nervous centres; together with an analysis of the conditioning of rhythmic activity in progression, and a theory of the evolution of function in the nervous system.J Physiol. 1914 Mar 31;48(1):18-46 PMID: 16993247

Cazalets JR, Sqalli-Houssaini Y, Clarac F.Activation of the central pattern generators for locomotion by serotonin and excitatory amino acids in neonatal rat.J Physiol. 1992 Sep;455:187-204.PMID:1362441

Chau C, Barbeau H, Rossignol S.Early locomotor training with clonidine in spinal cats.J Neurophysiol. 1998 Jan;79(1):392-409.PMID:9425208

Cina C, Hochman S.Diffuse distribution of sulforhodamine-labeled neurons during serotonin-evoked locomotion in the neonatal rat thoracolumbar spinal cord.J Comp Neurol. 2000 Aug 7;423(4):590-602.PMID:10880990

Côté CH, Perreault G, Frenette J.Carbohydrate utilization in rat soleus muscle is influenced by carbonic anhydrase III activity.Am J Physiol. 1997 Oct;273(4 Pt 2):R1211-8.PMID:9362282

Davey DF, Dunlop C, Hoh JF, Wong SY.Contractile properties and ultrastructure of extensor digitorum longus and soleus muscles in spinal cord transected rats.Aust J Exp Biol Med Sci. 1981 Aug;59(4):393-404.PMID:7295218

Deep K, Jigajinni MV, McLean AN, Fraser MH.Prophylaxis of thromboembolism in spinal injuries--results of enoxaparin used in 276 patients.Spinal Cord. 2001 Feb;39(2):88-91.PMID:11402364

DeVivo MJ, Jackson AB, Dijkers MP, Becker BE.Current research outcomes from the Model Spinal Cord Injury Care Systems.Arch Phys Med Rehabil. 1999 Nov;80(11):1363-4. No abstract available. PMID:10569428

Dimitrijevic MR, Gerasimenko Y, Pinter MM.Evidence for a spinal central pattern generator in humans.Ann N Y Acad Sci. 1998 Nov 16;860:360-76.PMID:9928325

Dobkin B, Apple D, Barbeau H, Basso M, Behrman A, Deforge D, Ditunno J, Dudley G, Elashoff R, Fugate L, Harkema S, Saulino M, Scott M; Spinal Cord Injury Locomotor Trial Group.Weight-supported treadmill vs over-ground training for walking after acute incomplete SCI.Neurology. 2006 Feb 28;66(4):484-93.PMID:16505299

Duffell LD, de N Donaldson N, Newham DJ. Why is the metabolic efficiency of FES cycling low? IEEE Trans Neural Syst Rehabil Eng. 2009 Jun;17(3):263-9. Epub 2009 Feb 27. Erratum in: IEEE Trans Neural Syst Rehabil Eng. 2009 Dec;17(6):605. PMID:19258202

Dupont-Versteegden EE, Murphy RJ, Houlé JD, Gurley CM, Peterson CA.Mechanisms leading to restoration of muscle size with exercise and transplantation after spinal cord injury.Am J Physiol Cell Physiol. 2000 Dec;279(6):C1677-84.PMID:11078681

Fitts RH, Riley DR, Widrick JJ.Functional and structural adaptations of skeletal muscle to microgravity.J Exp Biol. 2001 Sep;204(Pt 18):3201-8. Review.PMID:11581335

Frenette J, St-Pierre M, Côté CH, Mylona E, Pizza FX.Muscle impairment occurs rapidly and precedes inflammatory cell accumulation after mechanical loading.Am J Physiol Regul Integr Comp Physiol. 2002 Feb;282(2):R351-7.PMID:11792643

Frisbie JH.An animal model for venous thrombosis and spontaneous pulmonary embolism.Spinal Cord. 2005 Nov;43(11):635-9.PMID:15951743

Garland DE, Stewart CA, Adkins RH, Hu SS, Rosen C, Liotta FJ, Weinstein DA.Osteoporosis after spinal cord injury.J Orthop Res. 1992 May;10(3):371-8.PMID:1569500

Green D, Hartwig D, Chen D, Soltysik RC, Yarnold PR.Spinal Cord Injury Risk Assessment for Thromboembolism (SPIRATE Study).Am J Phys Med Rehabil. 2003 Dec;82(12):950-6.PMID:14627932

Grillner S, Zangger P.On the central generation of locomotion in the low spinal cat.Exp Brain Res. 1979 Jan 15;34(2):241-61.PMID:421750

Grossman EJ, Roy RR, Talmadge RJ, Zhong H, Edgerton VR.Effects of inactivity on myosin heavy chain composition and size of rat soleus fibers.Muscle Nerve. 1998 Mar;21(3):375-89.PMID:9486867

Guertin PA.The mammalian central pattern generator for locomotion.Brain Res Rev. 2009 Dec 11;62(1):45-56. Epub 2009 Aug 29. Review.PMID:19720083

Guertin PA, Ung RV, Rouleau P.Oral administration of a tri-therapy for central pattern generator activation in paraplegic mice: proof-of-concept of efficacy.Biotechnol J. 2010 Apr;5(4):421-6.PMID:20349462

Guertin PA, Ung RV, Rouleau P, Steuer I.Effects on locomotion, muscle, bone, and blood induced by a combination therapy eliciting weight-bearing stepping in nonassisted spinal cord-transected mice.Neurorehabil Neural Repair. 2011 Mar;25(3):234-42. Epub 2010 Oct 15.PMID:20952632

Hanson AM, Ferguson VL, Simske SJ, Cannon CM, Stodieck S.Comparison of tail-suspension and sciatic nerve crush on the musculoskeletal system in young-adult mice. Biomed Sci Instrum. 2005;41:92-6.PMID:15850088

Hicks AL, Ginis KA.Treadmill training after spinal cord injury: it's not just about the walking.J Rehabil Res Dev. 2008;45(2):241-8. Review.PMID:18566942

Huang CT, DeVivo MJ, Stover SL.Anemia in acute phase of spinal cord injury.Arch Phys Med Rehabil. 1990 Jan;71(1):3-7. PMID:2297306

Ito T, Ohmori S, Kanda K, Kawano S, Murata Y, Seo H.Changes in serum 1,25-dihydroxyvitamin D3 and mRNAs for osteocalcin and alkaline phosphatase in femur unloaded by tail suspension in rats.Environ Med. 1994;38(2):103-6.PMID:12703522

Kjaerulff O, Barajon I, Kiehn O.Sulphorhodamine-labelled cells in the neonatal rat spinal cord following chemically induced locomotor activity in vitro.J Physiol. 1994 Jul 15;478 (Pt 2):265-73.PMID:7525942

Koh TJ, Brooks SV.Lengthening contractions are not required to induce protection from contraction-induced muscle injury.Am J Physiol Regul Integr Comp Physiol. 2001 Jul;281(1):R155-61.PMID:11404289

Krikorian JG, Guth L, Barrett CP, Donati EJ.Enzyme histochemical changes after transection or hemisection of the spinal cord of the rat.Exp Neurol. 1982 Jun;76(3):623-43. PMID:6211367

Lainscak M, Podbregar M, Anker SD (December 2007). "How does cachexia influence survival in cancer, heart failure and other chronic diseases?". Curr Opin Support Palliat Care 1 (4): 299–305. PMID 18685379

Landry E, Frenette J, Guertin PA.Body weight, limb size, and muscular properties of early paraplegic mice.J Neurotrauma. 2004 Aug;21(8):1008-16.PMID:15319000

Landry ES, Rouillard C, Levesque D, Guertin PA.Profile of immediate early gene expression in the lumbar spinal cord of low-thoracic paraplegic mice.Behav Neurosci. 2006 Dec;120(6):1384-8.PMID:17201484

Landry ES, Lapointe NP, Rouillard C, Levesque D, Hedlund PB, Guertin PA.Contribution of spinal 5-HT1A and 5-HT7 receptors to locomotor-like movement induced by 8-OH-DPAT in spinal cord-transected mice.Eur J Neurosci. 2006 Jul;24(2):535-46. Epub 2006 Jul 12.PMID:16836640

Lazo MG, Shirazi P, Sam M, Giobbie-Hurder A, Blacconiere MJ, Muppidi M.Osteoporosis and risk of fracture in men with spinal cord injury.Spinal Cord. 2001 Apr;39(4):208-14.PMID:11420736

Lieber RL, Johansson CB, Vahlsing HL, Hargens AR, Feringa ER.Long-term effects of spinal cord transection on fast and slow rat skeletal muscle. I. Contractile properties.Exp Neurol. 1986 Mar;91(3):423-34.PMID:3948953

Lieber RL, Fridén JO, Hargens AR, Feringa ER.Long-term effects of spinal cord transection on fast and slow rat skeletal muscle. II. Morphometric properties.Exp Neurol. 1986 Mar;91(3):435-48.PMID:2936616

Ma YF, Jee WS, Ke HZ, Lin BY, Liang XG, Li M, Yamamoto N.Human parathyroid hormone-(1-38) restores cancellous bone to the immobilized, osteopenic proximal tibial metaphysis in rats.J Bone Miner Res. 1995 Mar;10(3):496-505.PMID:7785472

Midrio M, Danieli Betto D, Betto R, Noventa D, Antico F.Cordotomy-denervation interactions on contractile and myofibrillar properties of fast and slow muscles in the rat.Exp Neurol. 1988 Apr;100(1):216-36.PMID:3350090

Mosekilde L, Thomsen JS, Mackey MS, Phipps RJ.Treatment with risedronate or alendronate prevents hind-limb immobilization-induced loss of bone density and strength in adult female rats.Bone. 2000 Nov;27(5):639-45.PMID:11062350

Nishimaru H, Takizawa H, Kudo N.5-Hydroxytryptamine-induced locomotor rhythm in the neonatal mouse spinal cord in vitro.Neurosci Lett. 2000 Feb 25;280(3):187-90.PMID:10675792

Picard S, Lapointe NP, Brown JP, Guertin PA.Histomorphometric and densitometric changes in the femora of spinal cord transected mice.Anat Rec (Hoboken). 2008 Mar;291(3):303-7.PMID:18231968

Rémy-Néris O, Denys P, Daniel O, Barbeau H, Bussel B.Effect of intrathecal clonidine on group I and group II oligosynaptic excitation in paraplegics.Exp Brain Res. 2003 Feb;148(4):509-14. Epub 2002 Nov 22.PMID: 2582835

Ragnarsson KT, Sell GH.Lower extremity fractures after spinal cord injury: a retrospective study.Arch Phys Med Rehabil. 1981 Sep;62(9):418-23.PMID:7283682

Rantakokko J, Uusitalo H, Jämsä T, Tuukkanen J, Aro HT, Vuorio E.Expression profiles of mRNAs for osteoblast and osteoclast proteins as indicators of bone loss in mouse immobilization osteopenia model.J Bone Miner Res. 1999 Nov;14(11):1934-42.PMID:10571694

Reeve Foundation at www.christopherreeve.com.

Riegger T, Conrad S, Liu K, Schluesener HJ, Adibzahdeh M, Schwab JM.Spinal cord injury-induced immune depression syndrome (SCI-IDS).Eur J Neurosci. 2007 Mar; 25(6):1743-7.PMID:17432962

Rossignol S, Dubuc R.Spinal pattern generation.Curr Opin Neurobiol. 1994 Dec;4(6):894-902. Review.PMID:7888774

Rouleau P, Guertin PA.Traumatic and non-traumatic spinal cord-injured patients in Quebec, Canada. Part 2: biochemical profile.Spinal Cord. 2010 Nov;48(11):819-24. Epub 2010 May 11.PMID:20458326

Rouleau P, Guertin PA.Traumatic and nontraumatic spinal-cord-injured patients in Quebec, Canada. Part 3: pharmacological characteristics.Spinal Cord. 2011 Feb;49(2):186-95. Epub 2010 Jun 15.PMID:20548322

Rouleau P, Ung RV, Lapointe NP, Guertin PA.Hormonal and immunological changes in mice after spinal cord injury.J Neurotrauma. 2007 Feb;24(2):367-78.PMID:17376000

Rouleau P, Guertin PA Early changes in deep vein diameter and biochemical markers associated with thrombi formation after spinal cord injury in mice.J Neurotrauma. 2007 Aug;24(8):1406-14. PMID:17711402

Roy RR, Baldwin KM, Edgerton VR.The plasticity of skeletal muscle: effects of neuromuscular activity.Exerc Sport Sci Rev. 1991;19:269-312. Review.PMID:1936088

Sabo D, Blaich S, Wenz W, Hohmann M, Loew M, Gerner HJ.Osteoporosis in patients with paralysis after spinal cord injury. A cross sectional study in 46 male patients with dual-energy X-ray absorptiometry.Arch Orthop Trauma Surg. 2001;121(1-2):75-8.PMID:11195125

Sherrington CS.Flexion-reflex of the limb, crossed extension-reflex, and reflex stepping and standing.J Physiol. 1910 Apr 26;40(1-2):28-121.PMID:1699302

Spungen AM, Adkins RH, Stewart CA, Wang J, Pierson RN Jr, Waters RL, Bauman WA.Factors influencing body composition in persons with spinal cord injury: a cross-sectional study.J Appl Physiol. 2003 Dec;95(6):2398-407. Epub 2003 Aug 8.PMID:12909613

Talmadge RJ, Roy RR, Edgerton VR.Prominence of myosin heavy chain hybrid fibers in soleus muscle of spinal cord-transected rats.J Appl Physiol. 1995 Apr;78(4):1256-65.PMID:7615431

Talmadge RJ, Roy RR, Edgerton VR.Persistence of hybrid fibers in rat soleus after spinal cord transection.Anat Rec. 1999 Jun 1;255(2):188-201.PMID:10359520

Talmadge RJ, Roy RR, Caiozzo VJ, Edgerton VR Mechanical properties of rat soleus after long-term spinal cord transection.J Appl Physiol. 2002 Oct;93(4):1487-97.PMID:12235051

Thomason DB, Herrick RE, Surdyka D, Baldwin KM. Time course of soleus muscle myosin expression during hindlimb suspension and recovery.J Appl Physiol. 1987 Jul;63(1):130-7.PMID:2957349

Ung RV, Landry ES, Rouleau P, Lapointe NP, Rouillard C, Guertin PA.Role of spinal 5-HT2 receptor subtypes in quipazine-induced hindlimb movements after a low-thoracic spinal cord transection.Eur J Neurosci. 2008 Dec;28(11):2231-42. Epub 2008 Nov 3.PMID:19019202

Viala D, Buser P. Methods of obtaining locomotor rhythms in the spinal rabbit by pharmacological treatments (DOPA, 5-HTP, D-amphetamine)].Brain Res. 1971 Dec 10;35(1):151-65.[PMID: 5289621

Wainberg M, Barbeau H, Gauthier S.The effects of cyproheptadine on locomotion and on spasticity in patients with spinal cord injuries.J Neurol Neurosurg Psychiatry. 1990 Sep;53(9):754-63.PMID: 2246657

Waring WP, Karunas RS.Acute spinal cord injuries and the incidence of clinically occurring thromboembolic disease.Paraplegia. 1991 Jan;29(1):8-16.PMID:2023773

Wilmet E, Ismail AA, Heilporn A, Welraeds D, Bergmann P.Longitudinal study of the bone mineral content and of soft tissue composition after spinal cord section.Paraplegia. 1995 Nov;33(11):674-7.PMID:8584304

Wronski TJ, Dann LM, Scott KS, Crooke LR Endocrine and pharmacological suppressors of bone turnover protect against osteopenia in ovariectomized rats.Endocrinology. 1989 Aug;125(2):810-6.PMID : 2502377

Zeng QQ, Jee WS, Bigornia AE, King JG Jr, D'Souza SM, Li XJ, Ma YF, Wechter WJ.Time responses of cancellous and cortical bones to sciatic neurectomy in growing female rats.Bone. 1996 Jul;19(1):13-21.PMID:8830982

8

Biomechanics of the Craniovertebral Junction

Jeffrey G. Clark, Kalil G. Abdullah,
Thomas E. Mroz and Michael P. Steinmetz
Cleveland Clinic
United States of America

1. Introduction

The craniovertebral junction (CVJ) consists of the occiput and the first two cervical vertebrae, and functions as an articulation point capable of complex motions distinct from the remainder of the spinal column. These unique features make the CVJ more mobile than any of the other joints in the cervical spinal column, and important biomechanical properties must be understood in order to properly accommodate instrumentation to stabilize the spine after trauma, neoplasm, or degenerative disease. Each joint (Occiput-C1 and C1-C2) has its own unique biomechanical properties; at the occiput-C1 joint, bony structures are most responsible for stability and motion, while at the C1-C2 joint, ligamentous structures provide greater stability and motion compared to the bony elements.

A fundamental understanding of the biomechanics of the CVJ is important for spinal surgeons, physical therapists, and biomechanical engineers. In this chapter, we will review basic biomechanical and physiological properties of the CVJ, and then discuss common changes in biomechanics that occur via trauma and degenerative disease. This will provide the foundation for a brief discussion on techniques for the fixation of the craniovertebral junction.

2. Anatomy

The biomechanical features of the CVJ arise from the unique characteristics of the structures that comprise this region. It is first important to examine the osteology, joints, ligamentous structures, and blood supply that make up the CVJ.

2.1 Osteology

The osteology of the CVJ consists of three unique bones: the occiput, atlas (C1), and axis (C2). The occiput is the most inferior bone of the skull. The atlas and axis are the first and second cervical vertebrae, respectively.

The occiput is a thin bone that contributes to the calvaria and base of the skull. Its posterior surface is firmly attached to the parietal bones through the lamboid suture. Its lateral surfaces are attached to the temporal bones through the occipitomastoid sutures. Anteriorly, the occiput is attached to the sphenoid bone. On the posterior surface, a large, vertically oriented protuberance projects outwards, which at its highest point is referred to as the inion, which forms the attachment of the ligamentum nuchae. The occiput is especially notable for a large, triangular shaped hole in its inferior surface known as the foramen magnum, through which the brainstem and spinal cord connect at the cervicomedullary junction. A pair of occipital condyles lie anterolateral to the foramen magnum, and constitute the articulation points for the atlas. These articulation points are relatively flat, which limits the axial rotation of the atlanto-occipital joint.

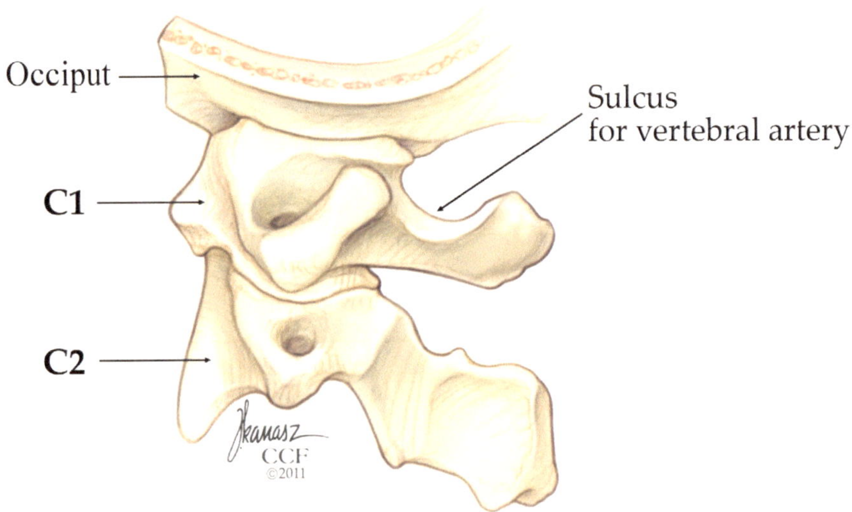

Fig. 1. Sagittal view of the occiput, atlas, and axis.

The atlas is ring-shaped, and contains two upward projecting lateral masses. These lateral masses articulate superiorly with the occipital condyles, forming the atlanto-occipital joint. Inferiorly, they form the atlanto-axial joint by articulating with the superior articular process of the axis. Through these two joints, they form a bridge between occiput and axis. The lateral masses are connected to each other by an anterior and a posterior arch that form a round outline to the spinal canal. The anterior arch is thinner than the posterior arch and is remarkable for a smoothed articulation point that is opposed to the odontoid process of the axis. In a small number of patients, the posterior arch may have a small cleft or rarely, it may have partial or complete aplasia (Gehweiler et al., 1983). The atlas does not have a vertebral body, as the embryological body becomes the odontoid process (dens) of the axis. Consequently, no intervertebral disk exists between the atlas and the axis. Transverse processes protrude horizontally from both sides of the atlas, and they extend more laterally than the transverse processes of the other cervical vertebrae. The foramen transversaria pierce these processes and create a channel through which the vertebral artery flows.
The axis is thicker and narrower than the atlas. On the anterior side, the vertebral body is flanked by two lateral masses. The odontoid process protrudes upwards from the center of the body to articulate with the posterior arch of the atlas, forming the key articulation point for axial rotation of the cervical spine. The lateral masses articulate superiorly with the inferior articular processes of the atlas. The vertebral arch defines the posterior borders of the vertebrae, and encloses a triangular-shaped spinal canal. On the inferior surface of the

vertebral arch, the inferior articular processes of the axis protrude downward and articulate with the superior articular processes of C3. These are located posterior to the superior articular processes of the axis, approximately equidistant from the anterior and posterior portions of the bone. Small transverse processes protrude laterally from between the articular processes and contain transverse foramen. The lamina and spinous process constitute the remainder of the vertebral arch. The spinous process is often, but not always, bifid (Martin et al., 2010).

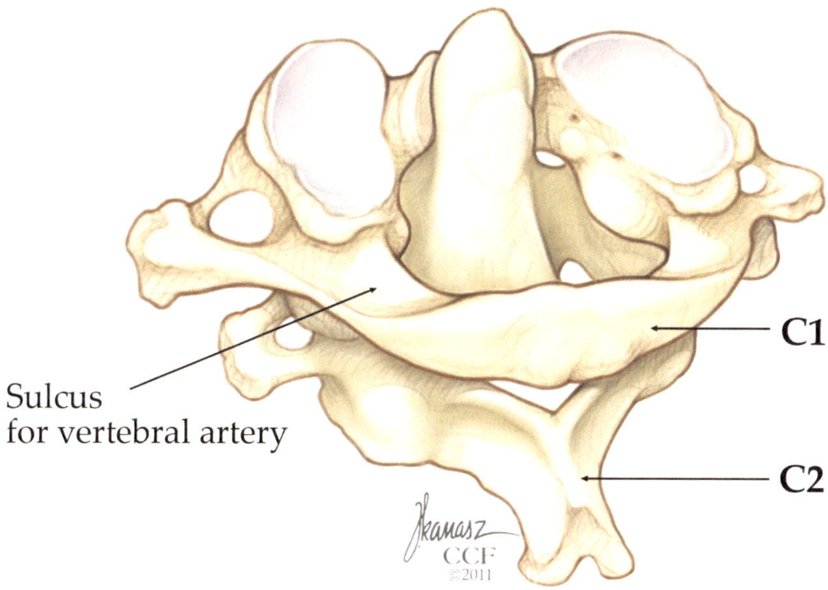

Fig. 2. Articulation between the atlas and the axis.

2.2 Joints

The CVJ consists of two synovial joints: the atlanto-occipital joint and the atlanto-axial joint. Each of these joints has unique anatomical and functional characteristics that contribute to the complex motion of the CVJ.

The atlanto-occipital joint is formed from articulation between the occipital condyles and the superior articular processes of the atlas. The articular processes of this joint are flat, which limits axial rotation and stabilizes flexion and extension. Each articulation forms a synovial joint surrounded by capsular ligaments.

The atlanto-axial joint has two distinct articulation points that act together to enable axial rotation. The first is a set of lateral articulations that are formed between the inferior articular processes of the atlas and the superior articular processes of the axis. The second set of articulations is formed between the odontoid process of the axis and the anterior arch of the atlas. The odontoid process functions as a pivot, and the lateral articulations permit ample rotation. Unlike the relatively flattened articular surfaces of the atlanto-occipital joint, the articular processes of the atlanto-axial joint are biconcave (Swartz et al., 2005). Loose and thin capsular joint ligaments surround the articulations in the CVJ complex, permitting a wide range of motion (Debernardi et al., 2011).

2.3 Ligamentous structures

Eight main ligaments support the CVJ: the tectorial membrane, the alar ligament, the cruciate ligament, the apical ligament, capsular joints, accessory atlantoaxial ligament, and the anterior and posterior atlanto-occipital membranes (Debernardi et al., 2011).

The tectorial membrane is a longitudinal ligament that begins inferiorly as part of the posterior longitudinal ligament of the vertebral column and extends upward to become continuous with the cranial dura mater. It was initially thought that the tectorial membrane functioned to limit extension of the CVJ. However, more recent evidence suggests that the tectorial membrane prevents anterior spinal cord compression by the odontoid process (Tubbs et al., 2007).

The alar ligament is shaped like a flattened V and connects the anterior and superior portion of the odontoid process to the lateral masses of the atlas and to the occiput. (Debernardi et al., 2011). It functions to limit axial rotation of the atlanto-axial joint (Dvorak & Panjabi, 1987).

The cruciate ligament is a thick, cross-shaped ligament with vertical and transverse components. The vertical component travels from the body of the axis to the clivus, while the transverse component (also called the transverse atlantal ligament or transverse ligament) extends from the medial side of the lateral masses of the axis and encloses the articulation formed between the odontoid process and the anterior arch of the atlas. The transverse portion of the cruciate ligament functions as an anatomical seatbelt, pulling the odontoid process tight against its articulation surface on the atlas. The transverse ligament also limits flexion of the CVJ (Debernardi et al., 2011; Panjabi et al., 1991c).

The apical ligament runs between the vertical portion of the cruciate ligament and the anterior atlanto-occipital membrane, connecting the anterior rim of the foramen magnum to the tip of the odontoid process. Some studies suggest that it may be congenitally absent in up to 20% of patients (Tubbs et al., 2000).

The capsular joints enclose the articulations between the occipital condyles and superior articular processes of the atlas, and between the inferior articular processes of the atlas and the superior articular processes of the axis. They also enclose the synovial fluid surrounding the joint and function to limit axial rotation in both joints of the CVJ (Debernardi et al., 2011).

The accessory atlantoaxial ligament connects the body of the axis to the lateral masses of the atlas and then continues cephalad to the occipital bone. In the past, this ligament was thought to be part of the tectorial membrane. However, studies now show that the fibers of these two ligaments are discontinuous (Tubbs et al., 2004). This ligament appears to check the rotation of both CVJ joints. However, its role in preventing hyperrotation is secondary to the function of the alar ligaments (Brolin & Halldin, 2004; Debernardi et al., 2011).

The anterior and posterior atlanto-occipital membranes travel downward to connect the anterior and posterior rims of the foramen magnum to the anterior and posterior arches of the atlas. These ligaments, however, do not appear to be an important contributor to biomechanical stability of the CVJ (Debernardi et al., 2011).

2.4 Blood supply

Blood is principally supplied to the CVJ through branches from the vertebral arteries. The vertebral arteries arise from the subclavian arteries and travel superiorly through the transverse foramen of the cervical spinal column. Upon leaving the transverse foramen of

C2, the vertebral artery is only minimally protected by dorsal bony structures as compared to when the artery runs through the subaxial spine. It also travels laterally to tunnel through the more lateral transverse foramen of the atlas. Upon leaving the atlas, the vertebral artery turns medially and pierces through the posterior ligaments and dura before ascending through the foramen magnum. As these arteries approach the alar ligament, they anastomose with the apical arcade that surrounds the odontoid process. Because the odontoid process is attached to the body of the axis by a cartilaginous plate, no vascular communication occurs between these portions of the axis (Menezes & Traynelis, 2008).

3. Normal biomechanics

The CVJ plays an important role in the overall motion of the cervical spine, accounting for 25% of the flexion and extension and up to 50% of the axial rotation of the neck (Menezes & Traynelis, 2008). Although the CVJ consists of two distinct joints (atlanto-occipital and atlanto-axial), it still functions as a single mobile unit, with the atlas acting like a washer between the cervical spine and the occiput. Each of these joints, however, has unique kinematic properties that contribute to the complex motion of the CVJ.

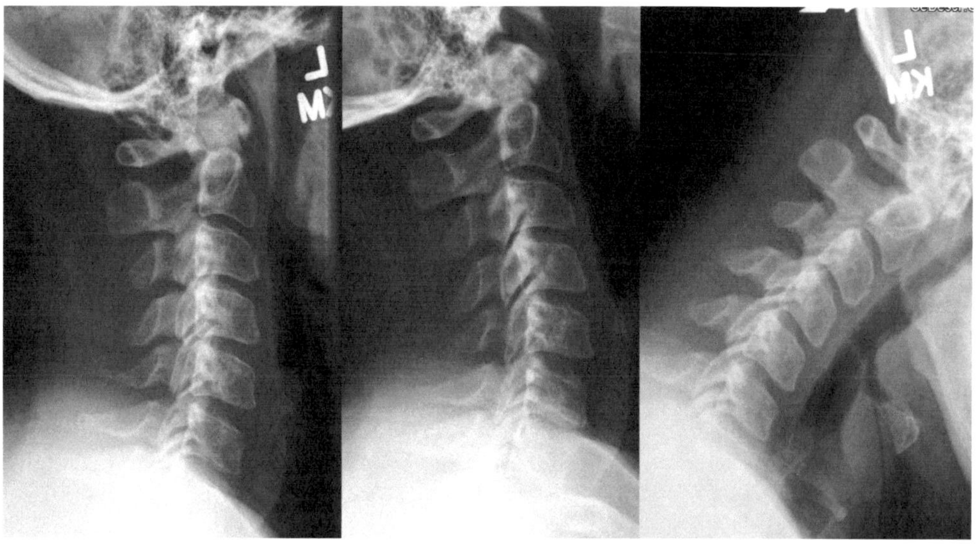

Fig. 3. Plain films of the cervical spine in neutral, extension, and flexion positions.

3.1 Kinematics of the cervical spine

The kinematics of the cervical spine are well established. In one classic study, the range of motion of 150 asymptomatic adults of both genders was determined using a three-dimensional motion measuring device. Each subject was seated in a chair that immobilized the subcervical spine and then subjected to five passive motions: flexion/extension, lateral bending, axial rotation, axial rotation out of maximum flexion, and axial rotation out of maximum extension (table 1). On average, women had a greater range of motion than men. Overall, range of motion decreased with age. Evaluation of these motions is an important component in the examination of patients with suspected cervical injury (Dvorak et al., 1992).

Age	Flexion and Extension		Lateral Bending		Axial Rotation		Rotation from Flexion		Rotation from Extension	
	M	F	M	F	M	F	M	F	M	F
20-29	152.7	149.3	101.1	100.0	183.8	182.4	75.5	72.6	161.8	171.5
30-39	141.1	155.9	94.7	106.3	175.1	186.0	66.0	74.6	158.4	165.8
40-49	131.1	139.8	83.7	88.2	157.4	168.2	71.5	85.2	146.2	153.9
50-59	136.3	126.9	88.3	76.1	166.2	151.9	77.7	85.6	145.8	132.4
> 60	116.3	133.2	74.2	79.6	145.6	154.2	79.4	81.3	130.9	154.5

Table 1. Kinematic measurements of the cervical spine by gender and age (Reproduced from Dvorak et al., 1992).

3.2 Biomechanics of the atlanto-occipital joint

Although the atlanto-occiptal joint contributes to flexion, extension, lateral bending, and rotation, cadaveric studies indicate that its principle motion is flexion and extension. This motion is primarily restricted by bony elements (Wolfla, 2006). Approximately 24.5 degrees of motion is possible in flexion and extension, with the majority of motion in the direction of extension (Panjabi et al., 1988). Flexion is ultimately restricted by contact between the odontoid process and the occiput, while extension may be limited by the tectorial membrane. However, some evidence suggests that the tectorial membrane is not involved in limiting extension, but that it may act to reduce spinal cord compression by the odontoid process (Tubbs et al., 2007). Rotation and lateral bending are both restricted by bony articulation points, tight alar ligaments, and the capsular ligaments, causing them to account for 2.5-7.2 and 3.5-5.5 degrees of motion in a single direction, respectively (Debernardi et al., 2011; Goel et al., 1988; Panjabi et al., 1988). In the horizontal plane, the instantaneous axis of rotation for the atlanto-axial joint is located in the anteromedial foramen magnum (Iai et al., 1993).

3.3 Biomechanics of the atlanto-axial joint

The atlanto-axial joint also contributes to flexion, extension, lateral bending, and rotation. However, its primary function has been demonstrated to be rotation. These motions are primarily restricted by ligamentous elements (Wolfla, 2006). In a cadaver, axial rotation in one direction can account for 23.3-38.9 degrees (Goel et al., 1988; Panjabi et al., 1988). Using radiographic studies of live patients, one group confirmed a 38 degree motion, accounting for 77% of the 49 degrees of axial rotation of the cervical spine. Rotation in C3-C7 accounted for an additional 15 degrees, while a 4 degree negative rotation in the atlanto-occipital joint accounted for the remainder of the motion. In other words, rotation of the atlanto-axial joint is accompanied by a smaller rotation of the atlanto-occipital joint in the opposite direction. The odontoid process acts as a pivot point for rotation, with the instantaneous axis of rotation located at the center of this process (Iai et al., 1993). The contralateral alar ligament is pulled tight during rotation, limiting motion. Thus the right alar ligament limits rotation to the left, and the left alar ligament limits rotation to the right (Dvorak & Panjabi, 1987). Capsular joint ligaments also play an important role in limiting atlanto-axial rotation (Debernardi et al., 2011). The accessory atlantoaxial ligament also functions to check rotation. However, its contributions are of questionable significance in the presence of functional alar ligaments (Brolin & Halldin, 2004).

Flexion and extension of the atlanto-axial joint account for a total of 10.1-22.4 degrees of motion, with both directions accounting for about the same range of mobility (Goel et al., 1988; Panjabi et al., 1988). The transverse portion of the cruciate ligament holds the dens tight against the anterior arch of the atlas and limits flexion of the C1-C2 joint. Extension is limited by the bony articulation points, and possibly by the tectorial membrane. An in vivo radiographic study demonstrated that the instantaneous axis for flexion and extension of the atlanto-axial joint is on the posterior surface of the odontoid process, approximately halfway between the base and the tip (Dvorak et al., 1991).
Lateral bending accounts for 6.7-11 degrees of motion in one direction (Iai et al., 1993; Panjabi et al., 1988). As in the atlanto-occipital joint, the alar ligaments, bony articulation points, and capsular ligaments are responsible for maintaining lateral rigidity (Dvorak et al., 1988).

4. Pathological destabilization

The biomechanical properties of the CVJ can be disrupted by trauma, degenerative disease, neoplasm, infection, iatrogenic injury, and congenital defects. In this chapter, we focus on disruptions due to trauma, rheumatoid arthritis, and Down syndrome. .

4.1 Traumatic alterations in biomechanics

Trauma to the cervical spine typically occurs through high energy events such as falls, sports injuries, motor vehicle crashes, and diving accidents. CVJ instability should be suspected if there is weakness in the arms, dislocation, subluxation, or any of the radiographic findings listed in table 2 (White & Panjabi, 1990). Destabilization can occur due to fractures of any of the bones and some of the supporting ligaments of the CVJ.

>8°	Axial rotation C0-C1 to one side
>1 mm	C0-C1 translation (sagittal plane)
>7 mm	Overhang C1-C2 (total right and left)
>45°	Axial rotation C1-C2 to one side
>4 mm	C1-C2 translation (sagittal plane)
<13 mm	Posterior body C2-posterior ring of C1
	Avulsed transverse ligament

Table 2. Criteria for CVJ instability (Reproduced from White & Panjabi, 1990)

Although many occipital condyle fractures are asymptomatic, some have the potential to cause major CVJ destabilization. These fractures are classified as type I, type II, and type III fractures. Type I fractures occur from comminution of the occipital condyle without significant bone fragment displacement into the foramen magnum. Excessive axial loading is believed to be the biomechanical cause of these injuries. In rare cases the alar ligament may also be damaged to produce instability. However, a competent contralateral alar ligament and tectorial membrane are generally more than sufficient to maintain stability. Type II fractures occur when a linear fracture crosses over from the base of the skull with extension to the occipital condyle. These fractures remain attached to the base of the skull and are typically stable. Type III fractures occur from condylar avulsion due to excess force form lateral bending or axial rotation (Karam & Traynelis,

2010). The alar ligaments are often compromised in type III fracture, causing them to generally be considered unstable, and the condylar fragments can be displaced into the crowded foramen magnum, which can cause neurovascular injury (Anderson & Montesano, 1988). Damage to the occipital condyle has been modelled in cadaveric studies with progressive, unilateral condylectomies. Hypermobility was noted in all of the motions of the atlanto-occipital joint (flexion, extension, axial rotation, and lateral bending) with a fifty percent resection of the condyle. In the atlanto-axial joint, hypermobility was achieved with 25% resection for flexion and extension, 75% resection for axial rotation, and 100% resection for lateral bending. Taken together, these results indicate that condylar injuries have great potential to disrupt the stability of the atlanto-occipital joint (Vishteh et al., 1999).

Fractures of the atlas most commonly occur in the anterior or posterior arches. The Jefferson fracture, first characterized by Geoffrey Jefferson in 1919, is a lesion of both arches that has unique biomechanical significance (Jefferson, 1919). A classical Jefferson fracture is characterized by two fractures in each of the vertebral arches, resulting in four distinct bone fragments. However, significant variability exists, resulting in fractures with two to five fragments. This fracture can occur as the result of hyperextension of the neck causing a blow to the back of the head which transmits significant force to the CVJ. Alternatively, strong axial forces from an extraphysiological load—such as would occur in a dive into shallow water—cause axial loading on the skull which translates force to the cervical spine through the occipital condyles. This downward load causes the lateral masses of the atlas to spread apart, introducing strain and potential fracture into the thin anterior and posterior arches (Bozkus et al., 2001). In a cadaveric study of atlantal fractures, high-speed axial force produced fragmentation in the classical pattern described by Jefferson. These cervical segments also had significant destabilization, resulting in range of motion increases of 40% in flexion and extension, and 20% in lateral bending (Panjabi et al., 1991b). The axial loading that causes Jefferson fractures is also implicated in the genesis of transverse ligament damage, and the identification of a coexisting ligament injury is of utmost clinical importance. These two pathologies often coexist, causing significantly increased cervical destabilization. The biomechanical changes associated with transverse ligament damage are explained below.

The axis is susceptible to three categories of fractures: fractures of the odontoid process, fractures of the pars interarticularis, and fractures of the axis body. Fractures of the odontoid process and pars interarticularis are the most common, and have the largest effects on CVJ instability.

Fractures of the odontoid process are the most common traumatic lesion of the axis. These are categorized by the location of the fracture, and occur near the tip of the odontoid process (type I), at the junction between the body and the odontoid process (type II), or within the body of the axis (type III). Of these, type II fractures are the most common and the most unstable. One finite element model of type II odontoid fractures suggests that a combination of lateral force and axial rotation are responsible for this fracture. Lateral force causes displacement of the first two vertebrae and places the inferior articular process of the atlas on the odontoid process. Axial rotation in turn puts tension on the alar ligament, placing torque on the dens. These two forces together contribute to fracture and potential displacement of bone into the spinal canal (Puttlitz et al., 2000).

Damage to the pars interarticularis of the axis is referred to as Hangman's fracture or traumatic spondylolisthesis of the axis. The name Hangman's fracture has its origins due tothe similarities these axial fractures have to lesions reported in judicial hangings (Rayes et al., 2011). Although once widely believed to contribute to death in many hangings, a study of cervical vertebrae from 34 judicial hanging victims revealed only 6 axial fractures, of which only 3 were Hangman's fractures (James & Nasmyth-Jones, 1992). However, the biomechanical mechanism of injury is clear. In a judicial hanging, the submental knot pulls upward on the jaw, jerking the head backwards in relation to the neck. The more extensible atlanto-occipital joint is not affected by this movement and the hanging body causes distraction and extension of the subaxial spine. This causes the atlanto-axial joint to undergo abrupt hyperextension, causing compression and fracture in the pars interarticularis. Today, hangman's fracture is most commonly seen in head-on collisions between automobiles. When a car crashes, the head continues forward relative to the restrained body. This motion, however, cannot explain the hangman's fracture. When modelled in primates, this form of trauma resulted in antlanto-occipital dislocation, but never axial fracture. The more likely explanation for the hangman's fracture is rapid backwards deceleration of the head from contact with the steering wheel or dashboard. This results in compressive hyperextension that affects only the craniovertebral junction, causing the axis to fracture (Penning, 1995).

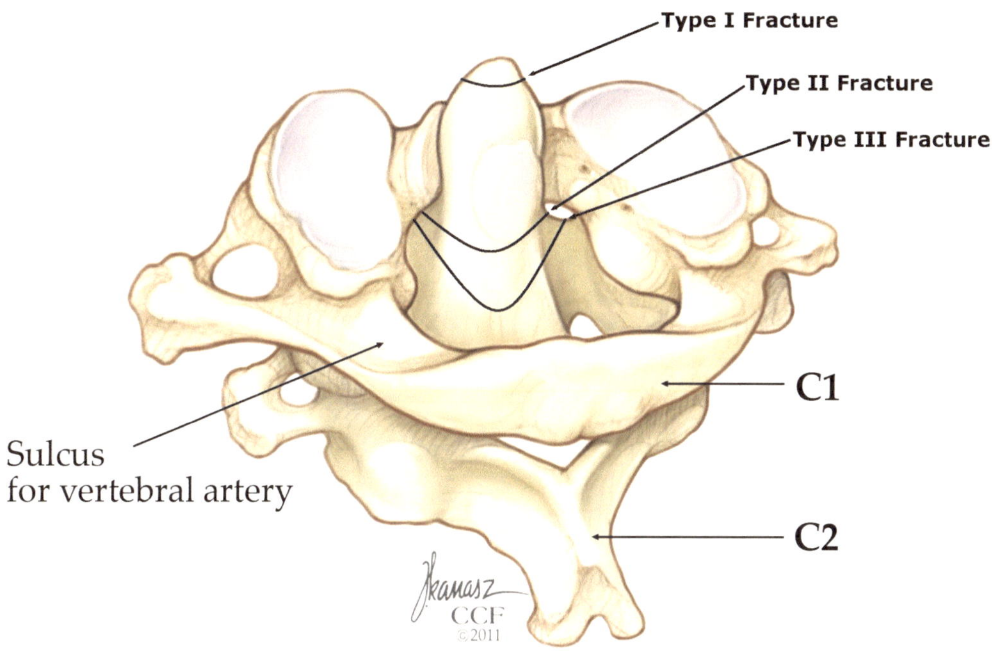

Fig. 4. Fractures of the odontoid process.

Of all axial lesions, the biomechanics of surgically-induced transoral odontoidectomy may be the best understood. This procedure is normally used to treat cervicomedullary compression. In a study of cadaveric human spines, transoral odontoidectomy was found to significantly increase translational motion from less than one millimeter in all directions to 10.2, 6.7, and 2.0 millimeters in the anterior-posterior, lateral, and superior-inferior directions, respectively. Surprisingly, axial rotation had no quantitative change. However, lateral bending, flexion, and extension increased by 95%, 71%, and 104%, respectively. Each of these changes was principally due to expansion of the neutral zone (Dickman et al., 1995).

Damage to the transverse ligament can occur in isolation, but it usually accompanies damage to other regions of the CVJ, especially fractures of the atlas. Likewise, associated damage to the alar and apical ligaments is also common. The transverse ligament is susceptible to midsubstance tearing, or it can be disrupted by avulsion from the lateral mass of the atlas. In one study, axial loading was shown to cause damage to the transverse ligament, both with and without fractures of the atlas (Panjabi et al., 1991b). Other reports suggest that neck flexion can also cause transverse ligament disruption (Jackson et al., 2002). This explains why head-on collisions are more likely to result in transverse ligament injury than rear-end crashes (Debernardi et al., 2011). Experimental damage to the transverse ligament produces biomechanical instability that is similar to iatrogenic odontoidectomy, resulting in substantially increased translational motion, lateral bending, flexion, and extension (Saldinger et al., 1990).

The alar ligament is most susceptible to injury in rear-end collisions. In this situation, a sudden, unexpected collision of a slightly rotated head induces maximal rotation and whiplash flexion. Since the limitation of axial rotation is the most important function of the alar ligament, this pathological motion produces overstretch and potential rupture (Saldinger, 1990). In cadaveric models, unilateral transection of the alar ligament produced a small increase in axial rotation in the atlanto-axial joint. However, bilateral transection was linked to significant increases in axial rotation, flexion, extension, and lateral bending (Panjabi et al., 1991a).

4.2 Biomechanical implications of rheumatoid arthritis and down syndrome

In the absence of trauma or surgery, the craniovertebral junction tends to remain stable over time. Some congenital conditions can cause CVJ instability and some degenerative conditions, such as osteoporosis, do make the CVJ much more susceptible to fracture with age. Two of the most significant disorders that contribute to CVJ instability are rheumatoid arthritis and Downs syndrome.

Severe rheumatoid arthritis can cause erosion of the bony components of the CVJ. In particular, these degenerative changes can affect the insertions of the transverse ligament into the atlas, causing ligamentous laxity and atlanto-axial instability in 20-86% of patients with rheumatoid arthritis (Krauss et al., 2010). These osteoarthropathies may contribute further instability as they progress to include disruption of the alar ligament, the occipital condyles and the odontoid process. This condition, known as basilar impression, is hallmarked by translation of the odontoid process in the cranial direction and subluxation or dislocation of the atlanto-occipital joint (Martin et al., 2010). Additionally, an odontoid pannus often develops, which has the potential to compress the spinal cord (Krauss et al., 2010). A recent study using computed tomography (CT) of patients with rheumatoid arthritis in the cervical spine reported instability in sagittal translation in a large percentage of patients. In this study, 8 of 24 patients had occipital condyle deformity, while 15 of 24 had lesions in one or more lateral masses of the axis. Damage to the condyles caused the atlanto-occipital joint to undergo translation in the posterior direction during flexion. In contrast, deformity in the lateral masses caused the atlanto-axial joint caused translation in the anterior and inferior directions during flexion. These movements contribute to pathological instability that should be considered when working with rheumatoid arthritis patients (Takatori et al., 2010).

Down syndrome is a relatively common genetic disease which is associated with craniocervical instability. Although the majority of these cases are asymptomatic, radiographic screening is still recommended before competition in athletic events like the Special Olympics. Instability can be due to abnormalities in either the atlanto-occipital or atlanto-axial junction (Hankinson & Anderson, 2010). Two main hypotheses have been proposed to explain the instability of the atlanto-axial joint. First, the occipital condyles and the superior articular processes of the atlas remain flatter than in children without Down syndrome. CT data clearly suggests that the flattened surfaces of these condyles become more rounded as children age. In principle, this abnormal bone formation fails to restrict the lateral and anterior motions of the atlanto-axial joint, resulting in instability (Browd et al., 2006, 2008). The second theory suggests that ligamentous laxity is the principle cause of instability in these patients. However, it is currently unknown which of these two theories explains the majority of the effect. Instability of the atlanto-axial joint is generally due to a loose articulation between the odontoid process and the anterior arch of the atlas. This results in marked instability in rotation, flexion, and extension. The cause of this instability is probably due to a combination of factors. These may include disconnection of the odontoid process from the body of the axis (os odontoideum) and ligamentous laxity due to collagen defects and chronic inflammation. Proper management of these instabilities is essential before these patients compete in contact sports or organized, strenuous events (Hankinson & Anderson, 2010).

5. General biomechanical principles of fixation

The complex anatomy of the CVJ introduces significant challenges to appropriate fixation. Fortunately, many of the fractures of the cervical spine can be treated nonsurgically with orthosis alone. However, multiple fractures, fracture displacement, instability and neurological compression are all factors that can require surgical intervention. Although a thorough treatment of CVJ fixation is beyond the scope of this chapter, it is important that certain principles of fixation be understood when considering proper surgical fixation of the CVJ.

Fixation to the occiput is best accomplished through the use of screws and rods/plates. In pull-out experiments, bicortical screws resisted 50% more force than unicortical screws or wires. The most stable location for screw placements was within the midline keel of the occiput (Haher et al., 1999). The thickness of the occipital protuberance decreases significantly in the lateral and caudal bone. Therefore, screws placed at or just lateral to the keel have the most pullout resistance. In one cadaveric study, constructs utilizing screws placed in the lateral occiput were found to better resist lateral bending, while screws placed more medially were better for resisting axial rotation. These considerations make the evaluation of individual patient characteristics vital in the selection of fixation technique (Anderson et al., 2006; Steinmetz et al., 2010).

The atlas can be a challenging site for fixation, especially when it is disrupted by CVJ pathology. Although the lateral masses can accept sublaminar wiring, lateral mass screws withstand greater pullout forces. Bicortical placement should also be utilized, as it also appears to enhance pullout resistance (Steinmetz et al., 2010). However, caution should be used when using bicortical screws, as the internal carotid artery can be at risk for puncture in a subset of patients (Currier et al., 2008). Another successful approach has been to place screws that penetrate both the posterior arch and the lateral mass (Tan et al., 2003).

Fixation to the axis can be accomplished through sublaminar wiring, or through screws placed in the pedicle or lamina. Alternatively, screws may be placed transarticularly, allowing them to span both the atlas and the axis (Steinmetz et al., 2010).

Once a plan has been made to place screws, wires, rods or plates, constructs and longitudinal members must be developed to stabilize the CVJ. Since the atlanto-axial joint is responsible for the axial rotation, stabilization of pathological rotation can be accomplished by fixation of the atlas to the axis. This is best accomplished through transarticular screws (Oda et al., 1999). A screw that goes through the lateral mass of the atlas and then through the axis can also be effective, although this method has been shown to provide significantly less stiffness (Finn et al., 2008). Although the principle motion of the atlanto-occipital joint is flexion and extension, stabilization of this motion cannot be adequately prevented with fixation of the occiput to the atlas. However, fixation of the occiput to the axis can produce optimal stabilization of aberrant flexion and extension (Hurlbert et al., 1999; Steinmetz et al., 2010).

6. Conclusions

The craniovertebral junction is an intricate structure with unique anatomy and complex biomechanical characteristics. These characteristics allow for significant flexion, extension, and axial rotation with remarkable stability under normal circumstances. However, trauma, degenerative disease, and some congenital disorders can cause instability in this region. A thorough understanding of the biomechanics of the CVJ is necessary to design strategies to stabilize the pathologies of the upper cervical spine.

7. References

Anderson, P., & Montesano, P. (1988). Morphology and Treatment of Occipital Condyle Fractures. *Spine*, Vol.13, No.7, (July 1988), pp. 731-736, ISSN 1528-1159

Anderson, P., Oza, A., Puschak, T., & Sasso, R. (2006). Biomechanics of Occipitocervical Fixation. *Spine*, Vol.31, No.7, (April 2006), pp. 755-761, ISSN 1528-1159

Bozkus, H., Karakas, A., Hancı, M., Uzan, M., Bozdag, E., & Sarıoglu, A., (2001). Finite Element Model of the Jefferson Fracture: Comparison with a Cadaver Model. *European Spine Journal*, Vol.10, No.3, (June 2001), pp. 257-263, ISSN 0940-6719

Brolin, K., & Halldin, P. (2004). Development of a Finite Element Model of the Upper Cervical Spine and a Parameter Study of Ligament Characteristics. *Spine*, Vol.29, No.4, (February 2004), pp. 376-385, ISSN 1528-1159

Browd, S., Healy, L., Dobie, G., Johnson, J., Jones, G., Rodriguez, L., & Brockmeyer, D. (2006). Morphometric and qualitative analysis of congenital occipitocervical instability in children: implications for patients with Down syndrome. *Journal of Neurosurgery: Pediatrics*, Vol.105, No.1, (July 2006), pp. 50-54, ISSN 1933-0715

Browd, S., McIntyre, J., & Brockmeyer, D. (2008). Failed age-dependent maturation of the occipital condyle in patients with congenital occipitoatlantal instability and Down syndrome: a preliminary analysis. *Journal of Neurosurgery: Pediatrics*, Vol.2, No.5, (November 2008), pp. 359-364, ISSN 1933-0715

Currier, B., Maus, T., Larson, D., & Yaszemski, M. (2008). Relationship of the internal carotid artery to the anterior aspect of the C1 vertebra: implications for C1-C2 transarticular and C1 lateral mass fixation. *Spine*, Vol.33, No.6, (March 2008), pp. 635-639, ISSN 1528-1159

Debernardi, A., D'Aliberti, G., Talamonti, G., Villa, F., Piparo, M., & Collice, M. (2011). The Craniovertebral Junction Area and the Role of the Ligaments and Membranes. *Neurosurgery*, Vol.68, No.2, (February 2011), pp. 291-301, ISSN 0148-396X

Dickman, C., Crawford, N., Brantley, A., & Sonntag, V. (1995). Biomechanical effects of transoral odontoidectomy. *Neurosurgery*, Vol.36, No.6, (June 1995), pp. 1146-1152, ISSN 0148-396X

Dvorak, J., & Panjabi, M. (1987). Functional anatomy of the alar ligaments. *Spine*, Vo.12, No.2, (March 1987), pp. 183-189, ISSN 1528-1159

Dvorak, J., Schneider, E., Saldinger, P., & Rahn, B. (1988). Biomechanics of the craniocervical region: The alar and transverse ligaments. *Journal of Orthopaedic Research*, Vol.6, No.3, (May 1988), pp. 452-461 ISSN 0736-0266

Dvorak, J., Panjabi, M., Novotny, J., & Antinnes, J. (1991). In vivo flexion/extension of the normal cervical spine. *Journal of Orthopaedic Research*, Vol.9, No.6, (November 1991), pp. 828-834, ISSN 0736-0266

Dvorak, J., Antinnes, J., Panjabi, M., Loustalot, D., & Bonomo, M. (1992). Age and gender related normal motion of the cervical spine. *Spine*, Vol.17, No.10 Supplement, (October 1992), pp. S393-S398, ISSN 1528-1159

Finn, M., Fassett, D., Mccall, T., Clark, R., Dailey, A., & Brodke, D. (2008). The cervical end of an occipitocervical fusion: a biomechanical evaluation of 3 constructs. *Journal of Neurosurgery: Spine*, Vol.9, No.3, (September 2008), pp. 296-300, ISSN 1547-5654Gehweiler, J., Daffner, R., & Roberts, L. (1983). Malformations of the atlas vertebra simulating the Jefferson fracture. *American Journal of Roentgenology*, Vol.140, No.6, (June 1983), pp. 1083-1086, ISSN 1546-3141

Goel, V., Clark, C., Gallaes, K., & Liu, Y. (1988). Moment-Rotation relationships of the ligamentous occipito-atlanto-axial complex. *Journal of Biomechanics*, Vol.21, No.8, (August 1990), pp. 673-680, ISSN 0021-9290

Haher, T., Yeung, A., Caruso, S., Merola, A., Shin, T., Zipnick, R., Gorup, J., et al. (1999). Occipital Screw Pullout Strength: A Biomechanical Investigation of Occipital Morphology. *Spine*, Vol.24, No.1, (January 1999), pp. 5-9, ISSN 1528-1159

Hankinson, T., & Anderson, R. (2010). Craniovertebral junction abnormalities in Down syndrome. *Neurosurgery*, Vol.66, No.3 Supplement, (March 2010), pp. 32-38, ISSN 0148-396X

Hurlbert, R., Crawford, N., Choi, W., & Dickman, C. (1999). A biomechanical evaluation of occipitocervical instrumentation: screw compared with wire fixation. *Journal of Neurosurgery: Spine*, Vol.90, No.1 Supplement, (January 1999), pp. 84-90. ISSN 1547-5654

Iai, H., Moriya, H., Goto, S., Takahashi, K., & Tamaki, T. (1993). Three-dimensional motion analysis of the upper cervical spine during axial rotation. *Spine*, Vol.18, No.16, (December 1993), pp. 2388-2392 ISSN 1528-1159

Jackson, R., Banit, D., Rhyne, A., & Darden, B. (2002). Upper cervical spine injuries. *Journal of the American Academy of Orthopedic Surgeons*, Vol.10, No.4, (July-August 2002), pp. 271-280 ISSN 1067-151X

James, R., & Nasmyth-Jones, R. (1992). The occurrence of cervical fractures in victims of judicial hanging. *Forensic Science International*, Vol.54, No.1, (April 1992), pp. 81-91, ISSN 0379-0738

Jefferson, G. (1919). Fracture of the atlas vertebra. Report of four cases, and a review of those previously recorded. *British Journal of Surgery*, Vol.7, No27, (1919), pp. 407-422, ISSN 1365-2168

Karam, Y., & Traynelis, VC. (2010). Occipital condyle fractures. *Neurosurgery*, Vol.66, No.3 Supplement, (March 2010), pp. A56-A59, ISSN 0148-396X

Krauss, W., Bledsoe, J., Clarke, M., Nottmeier, E., & Pichelmann, M. (2010). Rheumatoid Arthritis of the Craniovertebral Junction. *Neurosurgery*, Vol.66, No.3 Supplement, (March 2010), pp. A83-A95, ISSN 0148-396X

Martin, M., Bruner, H., & Maiman, D. (2010). Anatomic and Biomechanical Considerations of the Craniovertebral Junction. *Neurosurgery*, Vol.66, No.3 Supplement, (March 2010), pp. A2-A6, ISSN 0148-396X

Menezes, A., & Traynelis, V. (2008). Anatomy and biomechanics of normal craniovertebral junction (a) and biomechanics of stabilization (b). *Child's Nervous System*, Vol.24, No.10, (October 2008), pp. 1091-1100, ISSN 1433-0350

Oda, I., Abumi, K., Sell, L., Haggerty, C., Cunningham, B., & McAfee, P. (1999). Biomechanical Evaluation of Five Different Occipito-Atlanto-Axial Fixation Techniques. *Spine*, Vol.24, No.22, (November 1999), pp. 2377-2382, ISSN 1528-1159

Panjabi, M., Dvorak J., Duranceau, J, Yamamoto, I., Gerber, M., Rauschning, W., & Bueff H. (1988). Three-Dimensional Movements of the Upper Cervical Spine. *Spine*, Vol.13, No.7, (July 1988), pp. 726-730, ISSN 1528-1159

Panjabi, M, Dvorak, J, Crisco, J., Oda, T, Wang, P., & Grob, D. (1991). Effects of alar ligament transection on upper cervical spine rotation. *Journal of Orthopaedic Research*, Vol.9, No.4, (July 1991), pp. 584-593, ISSN 0736-0266

Panjabi, M, Oda, T, Crisco, J, Oxland, T., Katz, L., & Nolte, L. (1991). Experimental Study of Atlas Injuries I: Biomechanical Analysis of Their Mechanisms and Fracture Patterns. *Spine,* Vol.16, No.10 Supplement, (October 1991), pp. S460-S465, ISSN 1528-1159

Panjabi, M., Oxland, T., & Parks, E. (1991). Quantitative anatomy of cervical spine ligaments. Part I. Upper cervical spine. *Journal of Spinal Disorders,* Vol.4, No.3, (September 1991), pp. 270-276, ISSN 0895-0385

Penning, L. (1995). Kinematics of cervical spine injury. A functional radiological hypothesis. *European Spine Journal,* Vol.4, No.2, (April 1995), pp. 126-132, ISSN 1432-0932

Puttlitz, C., Goel, V., Clark, C., & Traynelis, V. (2000). Pathomechanics of Failures of the Odontoid. *Spine,* Vol.25, No.22, (November 2000), pp. 2868-2876, ISSN 1528-1159

Rayes, M., Mittal, M., Rengachary, S., & Mittal, S. (2011). Hangman's fracture: a historical and biomechanical perspective. *Journal of Neurosurgery: Spine,* Vol.14, No.2, (February 2011), pp. 198-208, ISSN 1547-5654

Saldinger, P., Dvorak, J., Rahn, B., & Perren, S., (1990). Histology of the Alar and Transverse Ligaments. *Spine,* Vol.15, No.4, (April 1990), pp. 257-261, ISSN 1528-1159

Steinmetz, M. P., Mroz, T. E., & Benzel, E. (2010). Craniovertebral Junction: Biomechanical Considerations. *Neurosurgery,* Vol.66, No.3 Supplement, (March 2010), pp. A7-A12, ISSN 0148-396X

Swartz, E., Floyd, R., & Cendoma, M. (2005). Cervical spine functional anatomy and the biomechanics of injury due to compressive loading. *Journal of Athletic Training,* Vol.40, No.3, (July-September 2005), pp. 155-161, ISSN 1062-6050

Takatori, R., Tokunaga, D., Hase, H., Mikami, Y., Ikeda, T., Harada, T., Imai, K. (2010). Three-dimensional morphology and kinematics of the craniovertebral junction in rheumatoid arthritis. *Spine,* Vol.35, No.23, (November 2010), pp. E1278-1284, ISSN 1528-1159

Tan, M., Wang, H., Wang, Y., Zhang, G., Yi, P., Li, Z., Wei, H. (2003). Morphometric evaluation of screw fixation in atlas via posterior arch and lateral mass. *Spine,* Vol.28, No.9, (May 2003), pp. 888-895, ISSN 1528-1159

Tubbs, R., Grabb, P., Spooner, A., Wilson, W., & Oakes, W. (2000). The apical ligament: anatomy and functional significance. *Journal of Neurosurgery: Spine,* Vol.92, No.2 Supplement, (April 2000), pp. 197-200, ISSN 1547-5654

Tubbs, R., Salter, E., & Oakes, W. (2004). The Accessory Atlantoaxial Ligament. *Neurosurgery,* Vol.55, No.2, (August 2004), pp. 400-404, ISSN 0148-396X

Tubbs, R., Kelly, D., Humphrey, E., Chua, G., Shoja, M., Salter, E., Acakpo-Satchivi, L. (2007). The tectorial membrane: Anatomical, biomechanical, and histological analysis. *Clinical Anatomy,* Vol.20, No.4, (May 2007), pp. 382-386, ISSN 1098-2353

Vishteh, A., Crawford, N., Melton, M., Spetzler, R., Sonntag, V., & Dickman, CA. (1999). Stability of the craniovertebral junction after unilateral occipital condyle resection: a biomechanical study. *Journal of Neurosurgery: Spine,* Vol.90, No.1 Supplement, (January 1999), pp. 91-98, ISSN 1547-5654

White, A., & Panjabi, M. (1990). *Clinical Biomechanics of the Spine* (Second Edition), J.B. Lippincott Company, 0-397-50720-8, Philadelphia, Pennsylvania

Wolfla, C. (2006). Anatomical, biomechanical, and practical considerations in posterior occipitocervical instrumentation. *The Spine Journal*, Vol.6, No.1 Supplement, (November-December 2006), pp. S225-S232, ISSN 1529-9430

9

A Pure Moment Based Tester for Spinal Biomechanics

Ti-Sheng Chang[1], Jia-Hao Chang[2] and Ching-Wei Cheng[3]
[1]*Department of Neurosurgery, Taichung Armed Force General Hospital*
[2]*Department of Physical Education, National Taiwan Normal University*
[3]*Department of Bio-industrial Mechatronics Engineering, National Chung Hsing University, Taiwan*

1. Introduction

1.1 History of spine biomechanics

Spine biomechanics is the physical science that forms a substantial portion of the foundation of modern spine surgery. Plato's conceptualization of mathematics as the life force of science created the birth and growth of the science of mechanics and spine biomechanics. Aristotle was the first to discuss human kinesiology and spine biomechanics under pure logical analysis. Leonardo da Vinci was the first to accurately describe the human adult S-shape spinal posture with its curvature, articulations and vertebrae. Borelli provided many calculations regarding spine biomechanics [1]. Bone trabecular architecture to its mechanical and load-bearing attributed to the Wolff's law [2]. It contributed to the development of spine biomechanics as a discipline.

1.2 Classification of spinal testers

The lumbar spine incorporates a complex combination of accompanying rotations or translation with each primary movement. In vitro testing have insufficiently replicated in life conditions are in the limitation of the number of degree of freedom available to move the specimen during testing. The kinematic patterns of the lumbar spine are dynamic condition under physiological loading. The ideal testing facilities are capable of adequately modeling the complex, dynamic, six degree of freedom nature of the lumbar spine.

A number of devices designed to spinal biomechanics have been described in the literature. The first measurement of lumbar spine movements was performed by Weber on three cadavers in 1827 [3]. They investigated the reduction in length of an individual muscle during contraction and devoted much study to the role of bones as mechanical levels. This degree of freedom is a translation. Adams [4] described a jig that was capable of converting translational motion into forward flexion. This testing facility could create two degrees of freedom, allowing translation in the sagittal direction and rotation about frontal direction. This facility could not be used to test a motion segment in other modes of movement as it is not able to incorporate accompanying rotation. Goertzen et al. [5] used servo motor with planetary gearbox were connected to an articulating arm, which applied the moment to the cranial end of the specimen. Lysack et al. [6] involved the use of a linear actuator with cable system and roller bearings to produce moments. Their apparatus allowed continuous cycling loading. They could supply continuous loading, however, the direction of movement was limited. In the meantime, they needed to change the position of the specimen under different loading (such as flexion-extension-flexion). More complicated apparatus have been constructed to allow for loading to be controlled in more than one plane of rotation. Goel et al. [7] used deadweights and cables acting about pulleys to produce force couples. Yamamoto et al. [8] defined the implementation of pneumatic actuators. They used paired vacuum-operated low friction glass cylinders to produce pure moment condition. Wilke et al. [9] suspended the stepper motors and a pneumatic system over the specimen and used a gimbal joint and XYZ slide to allow the motors to follow the motion and orientation of the upper fixtures. These testing facilities are force controlled rather than displacement controlled and cannot reproduce the kinematic patterns of the lumbar spine. This force application is also under quasi-static conditions, rather dynamic conditions. Quasi-static conditions are a poor representation of dynamic loading [10]. Hence, these methods are incapable of reproducing physiological loading of the specimen. Stokes et al. [11] used a series of six linear actuators to enable the six degrees of freedom to be independently controlled. Six linear encoders were utilized to measure and control the displacement of the testing machine. This facility was displacement-control mode, they usually needs complex mathematical calculation before data analysis.

A robot [12] is capable of motion in six degree of freedom (DOF) and is able to dynamically test a specimen throughout its entire range of motion. When coupled with an appropriate force transducer, a robot material testing facility is able to provide kinetic information for the simulated condition in life spinal motion. This is an ideal facility for spine biomechanical study. However, the price of this facility was relative high. Not every institute has the resource to use it. Under this thinking process, a pure moment based spinal tester with the backbone of robot and relative cheap price to perform spinal biomechanical study should be developed.

2. Biomechanical parameters

2.1 Clinical associated biomechanical parameters

Several parameters may be obtained through biomechanical tests of flexibility to quantify mechanical properties [13]. Such parameters include range of motion (ROM), neutral zone (NZ) and elastic zone (EZ). NZ is the displacement at the zero-load point measure from the neutral position [13-14]. EZ is the displacement from the zero-load point to the maximum load point. ROM is the displacement from the neutral position to the maximum load point, that is, the sum of NZ and EZ. In biomechanical study, the ROM represents the stability of the specimen before and after additional procedures (including destructive and stabilizing procedures). The NZ indicates the laxity around the neutral position of a motion segment and residual deformation after removing a defined pure moment load from a motion segment. Mimura et al. [15] revealed that, in flexion-extension and lateral bending, ROM decreases and NZ increases during disc degeneration. In the early stage of disc degeneration, ROM increases while in the late stage of disc degeneration, ROM decreases. If only ROM is used as the measurement parameter, misinterpretations are likely. Previous in vitro studies indicated that NZ typically increases after experimentally induced injuries [16-17], and that it decreases with the addition of muscle forces and spinal instrumentation [18].

2.2 Flexibility and stiffness

Flexibility is ratio of strain to stress that is the ability of the structure to deform under the application of a load. Stiffness is the opposite. It is ratio of stress to strain in a loaded material that is the stress divided by the relative amount of change in the structure's shape. Panjabi [19] outlined the biomechanical testing of a spinal segment as including both stiffness and flexibility methods. In stiffness method (displacement-control), the free end of specimen was displaced, and the resulting forces and moments in the specimen were measured. The application of a given displacement at the superior-most vertebral body imposed complex loads of varying magnitudes along the spinal segment because of coupling behavior of the spine. This method provided kinetic information for the simulated condition in life spinal motion. Although the magnitude of the complex load could be quantified with a six-axis load cell, it was not practical to measure those all along the spinal segment. It usually needs complex mathematical calculation. In the flexibility method (load-control), a load was applied to the free vertebra of the specimen and the resulting displacements of the vertebra were measured. This method allowed complete freedom of movements of all the vertebra of the spine, thereby allowing natural behavior of the spinal column to take place. The in vitro biomechanical study could be standardized under this way [20].

2.3 Pure moment

The most common method used currently is flexibility protocol. Panjabi [19] emphasized that non-constraining pure moment load is warranted. Pure moment means that pure bending moments or the pure shear moments depend on the direction of action. There is no force during measurement. Pure bending moments include flexion, extension, left and right lateral bending direction. Pure shear moments include right and left axial rotation direction. The spinal anatomy is not a uniform structure. The loads at a cross section are proportional to the bending moment (force × level arm) at the cross section. An anterior directed horizontal force or eccentric compression load cannot produce uniform bending moment through the whole length of the specimen. The purpose of pure moment loading is to supply the same magnitude at each cross section throughout the whole length of the construct [19]. Non-constraining construct means that one side is fixed to the apparatus and the other end is free to move, allowing the natural spinal movements. The use of non-constraining pure moments ensures that the load experienced by a specimen remains constant along its length independent of its geometry, motion or, stiffness. This means that, throughout the loading cycle, the loading conditions at any two cross-sections in the spinal column are identical. The major advantage of pure moment loading is that it allows for the comparison of the biomechanical properties of different spinal constructs.

3. Self-design pure moment based spinal tester

3.1 Equipment and hardware

This pure moment based spinal tester contained power supply unit, measurement unit, associated hardware and control unit. Power supply unit included 4 servo motors and planetary reduction gearbox. Measurement unit included load cell and multi-axis force/torque sensor controller. The control unit included computer and 2 RS-232 PCI Cards. These set up allows for communications with both tester and load cell through single purpose written program on one PC. The picture of this tester was shown in Figure 1.

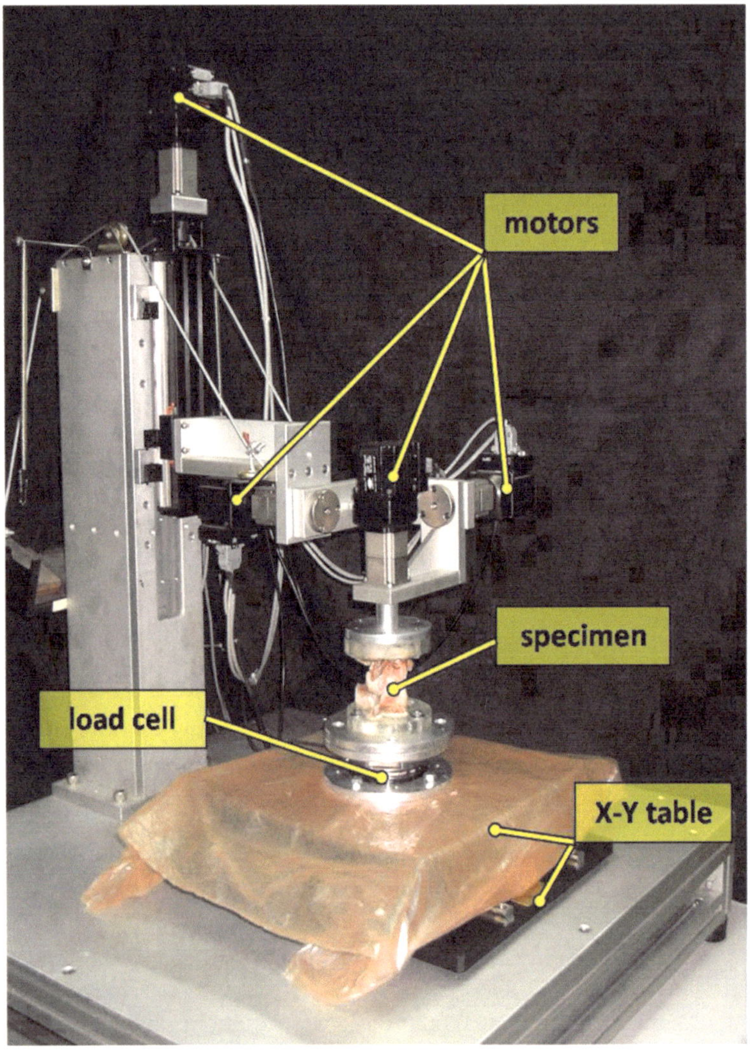

Fig. 1. The testing machine and mounting system with a specimen during performance of a flexibility test. Various component of this tester is illustrated. Reprinted from Journal of Medical and Biological Engineering, vol 29, No 1, Chang, T.S. et. al, a new multi-direction tester for evaluation of the spinal biomechanics, p 7-13, 2009, with kind permission from Taiwanese Society of Biomedical Engineering [21].

3.2 Machine composition

The mechanism is based on a modular aluminum extrusions 800 mm wide* 800 mm deep *1120 mm height. This material was selected for good corrosion resistant qualities when exposed to a moist, salt environment, such as spinal specimen. The drive apparatus included 4 servo motors combined with a planetary reduction gearbox. The Motors 1, 2, and 3 were used to provide the right-left axial rotation, flexion-extension and right-left lateral bending respectively. Motor 4 was provided a consistent force along the Z-axis during specimen testing. [21]

3.3 Coordinated system

The coordinate system was the junction of the posterior one-third and anterior two-third of the intervertebral disc. The +z-axis was described upward from the origin, the +y-axis pointed to the left, and the +x-axis pointed forward. The +Fx/-Fx, +Fy/ -Fy and +Fz/-Fz represented anterior/posterior, left/right and decompression/compression axial force, and +Mx/-Mx, +My/-My and +Mz/-Mz represented right/left bending, flexion/extension and right/left rotation moment, respectively.

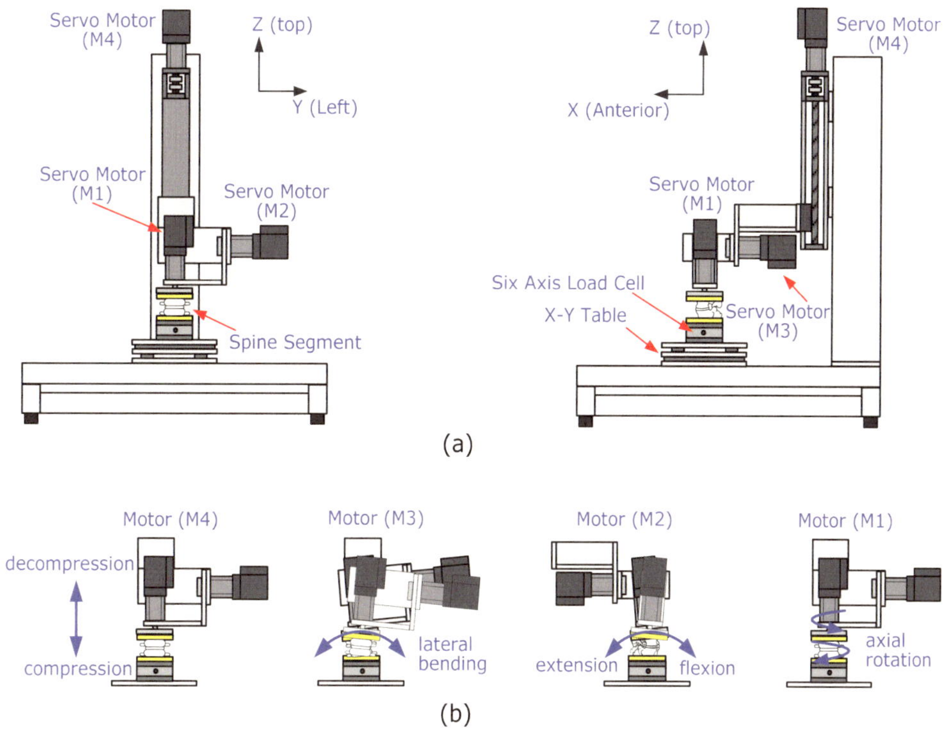

Fig. 2. The Multi-degree spine tester (a) full view (b) close-up of the apparatus set for each motion . Reprinted from Journal of Medical and Biological Engineering, vol 29, No 1, Chang, T.S. et. al, a new multi-direction tester for evaluation of the spinal biomechanics, p 7-13, 2009, with kind permission from Taiwanese Society of Biomedical Engineering [21].

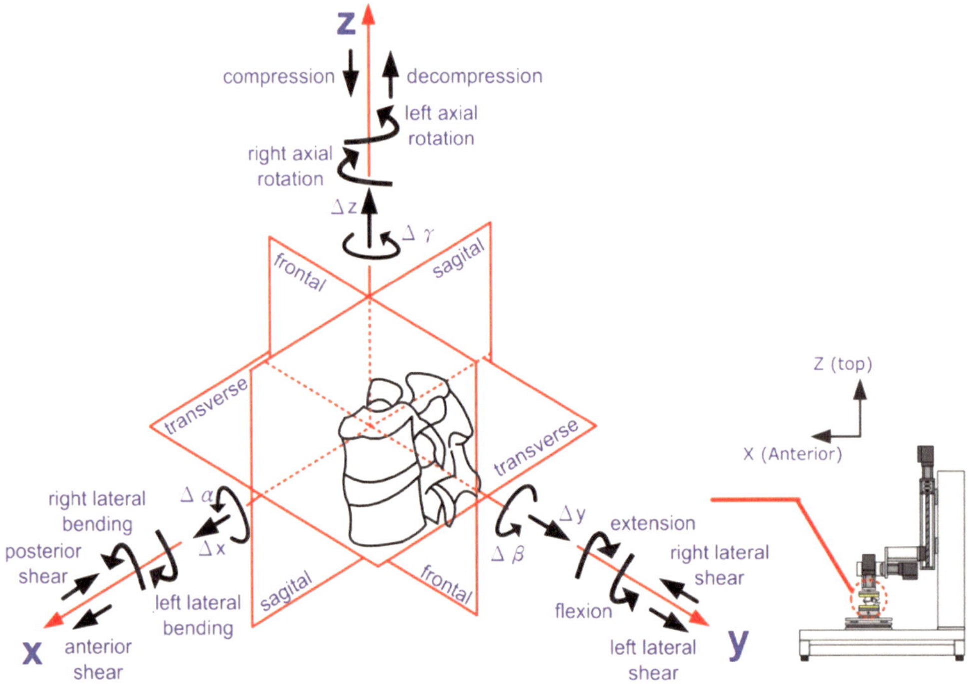

Fig. 3. Coordinated system used for tester . Reprinted from Journal of Medical and Biological Engineering, vol 29, No 1, Chang, T.S. et. al, a new multi-direction tester for evaluation of the spinal biomechanics, p 7-13, 2009, with kind permission from Taiwanese Society of Biomedical Engineering [21]

A multi-segment spine specimen can be mounted in the apparatus using two stainless steel pots and dental plaster. This allows for easy extraction of the specimen after mechanical testing. The bottom pot rigidly fixes the caudal end of the spinal segment to the base of the frame through a six axis load cell while the top pot holds the cephalad end of the spine. Below the load cell, an X -Y table with double rail track and slide was used to prevent shear force. The inertia is drastically reduced while the movement of the X-Y table. Unconstraint, pure bending moment was achieved during test.

3.4 Software

Software had to be written to send desired positional information to the tester and receive actual position and force information from the tester and load cell.

3.4.1 Control and data collected

The main control unit included preload, load cycle setting and the data of force, moment and motor position data was shown on the scene of computer. A software package running in Borland C^{++} Builder provided an interface allowing the user to define desired motions, and to collect load and displacement data. The signal from the load cell was conditioned and connected to the computer to provide a feedback signal for load control testing. The interface between each motor was independent, and each motor could be adjusted as if necessary. The direction of the specimen was maintained at a constant speed until the feedback signal of the load cell was observed. Motor and load cell data were recorded in the computer. The computer enabled various control and measuring devices to communicate with each other across different interface. Regulation, control, and measurements were automatically performed by the computer. The flowchart of spinal tester connected was illustrated on figure 4.

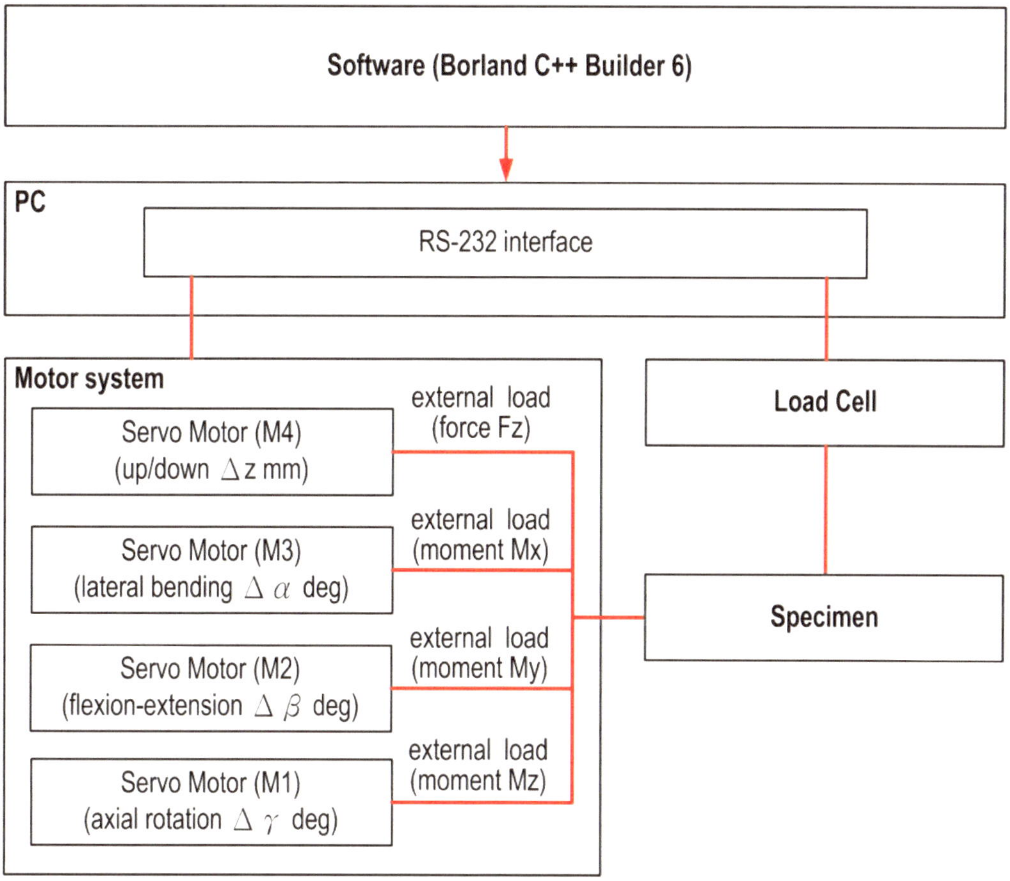

Fig. 4. Spine tester connections . Reprinted from Journal of Medical and Biological Engineering, vol 29, No 1, Chang, T.S. et. al, a new multi-direction tester for evaluation of the spinal biomechanics, p 7-13, 2009, with kind permission from Taiwanese Society of Biomedical Engineering [21].

The raw load cell data and the corresponding raw position data were processed using self-written software to yield, in six DOF. To account for the effect of off-axis loads, the raw load cell data, which were transmitted at the caudal end of the specimen, were transformed into the local body coordination system. Relative angles were calculated at Cardan angles with sequence X (bending), Y (flexion-extension), Z (rotation). Noise was reduced by passing the data through a digital second-order Butterworth low-pass filter with a cutoff frequency of 5 Hz. Using commercial software (Matlab, The Method Works, US), these transformed load and displacement data were processed to yield flexibility curves (angle versus moment) for the flexion-extension, lateral bending and rotation tests.

3.5 Verification of spine tester

To verify this spine tester, a circular cylinder was used. The cylinder was formed from polyurethane (PU diameter 25 mm, length 90 mm), which is a homogenous polymer. Table 1 shows the physical properties of PU. The PU could be mounted on the apparatus using two aluminum pots and polyester resin plaster. Two stainless steel screws inserted above and below the pots rigidly secured the PU to the tester. The test protocol was to apply pure bending moments to the PU to a maximum of 2 Nm in right-left lateral bending (M3), flexion-extension (M2) and right-left axial rotation (M1) in sequence. Rotation velocity was 1°/sec. A real-time graphical display of servo motor angle and applied moment was available during the test. The direction was reversed when the moment reached ±2 Nm. After cycling the PU five times, mean values and standard deviations were calculated. No compressive preloads were applied. Torque was measured ten times at intervals of 0.4 Nm.

Physical property	Value
Hardness (kg/mm^2)	8
Specific gravity (g/cm^3)	0.904
Heat distortion temperature (kg/cm^2)	90
Hydraulic strength (kg-cm/cm)	1.6
Elastic modulus of bending (kg/cm^2)	18500
Elastic modulus of shear (kg/cm^2)	46500
Poisson's ratio	0.23~0.38

Table 1. Physical property of polyurethane (PU).

The calculated value was from equation (A) and (B) [22].
Which

$$T = GI_p \frac{d\phi}{dx} \quad (A)$$

Where
T = torque.
$d\phi/dx$ = twist rate.
Ip = polar moment of inertia
G = shear modulus of elasticity

$$M = -EI\frac{\theta}{L} \quad (B)$$

Where
M = bending moment
E = elastic bending modulus
I = inertia
L = length
θ = angle of bending

The error rates for flexion-extension, lateral bending and axial rotation were about 2.16 %, 2.66% and 1.36%, respectively. The PU examination results revealed larger errors in flexion-extension and in lateral bending than in rotation (2.16%, 2.66% and 1.36%, respectively). This may have been due to the X-Y table. The error even reach around 5% at the beginning of flexion-extension (5.15% and 4.22% at -0.4 and +0.4 Nm). More loading was needed to start the X-Y table. Fortunately, the error rate decreased progressively as load approached maximum. In most biomechanical studies, data are recorded from the end loading. This condition did not substantially affect the final results, and it could be eliminated entirely if a servo motor is used to drive the X-Y table [21].

4. Application of this tester

4.1 Spinal unit function evaluating the changes in ROM and NZ after discectomy and implantation by sheep spine

One motion segment of L4/5 from one sheep lumbar spine was used for testing of this tester. The specimen was tested intact to serve as its own control. The various surgical procedures (figure 5) including laminectomy, discectomy and transpedicular screw fixation were performed. Laminectomy was performed with Kerrison rongeur, after resection of the spinous process and the interspinous and supraspinous ligaments. The lamina was removed out to the most medial portion of the articular facet. Care was taken to preserve the pars interarticularis. The cranial limit of the resection was the corresponding pedicle. The ligamentum flavum was removed, also. The posterior longitudinal ligament and the annulus were incised using No. 15 blade. Discectomy was practiced at the L4/5 intervertebral space. It was accomplished through an incision of square shape in the annulus fibrosis just anterior to the plane of the pedicle, and approximately 70% of the disc material was removed with disc forcep and curret. Transpedicular screw fixation was practiced within the L4 and L5 pedicle, and an ISOLA system was connected.

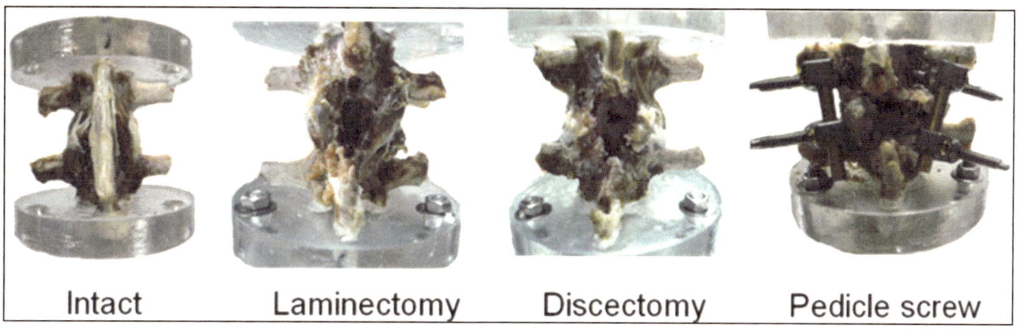

Fig. 5. Various surgical procedures was illustrated.

Biomechanical testing of sheep lumbar spine was performed using a non-destructive, flexibility method of testing under non-constraining pure moment loads. Pure bending moments were applied to the specimen to a maximum of 2 Nm in right-left lateral bending (M3), flexion-extension (M2) and right-left axial rotation (M1) in sequence after different surgical procedure. The velocity of rotation is 1 degree per second. The load cell provided a feedback signal to the computer through RS-232 interface with 40 Hz sampling rate. A real time graphical display of servo motor angle and applied moment was available during the test. The direction was reversed when the moment reached ±2 Nm. The specimen were cycled for a total of five cycles- the first four cycles were considered preconditioning and the fifth cycle was used for analysis. No compressive preloads were applied, and approximately five minutes were allowed between tests for viscoelastic recovery.

ROM, NZ and NZ/ROM of flexion-extension and lateral bending increased after laminectomy and discectomy, while the ROM, NZ and NZ/ROM of flexion-extension and lateral bending decreased after fixation. However, the ROM, NZ and NZ/ROM of rotation still increase after decompressive procedure and fixation. ROM of flexion-extension (Figure 6), lateral bending and rotation of the specimen after different surgical procedures was demonstrated. The NZ increased after decompressive procedure and recovered after fixation procedure.

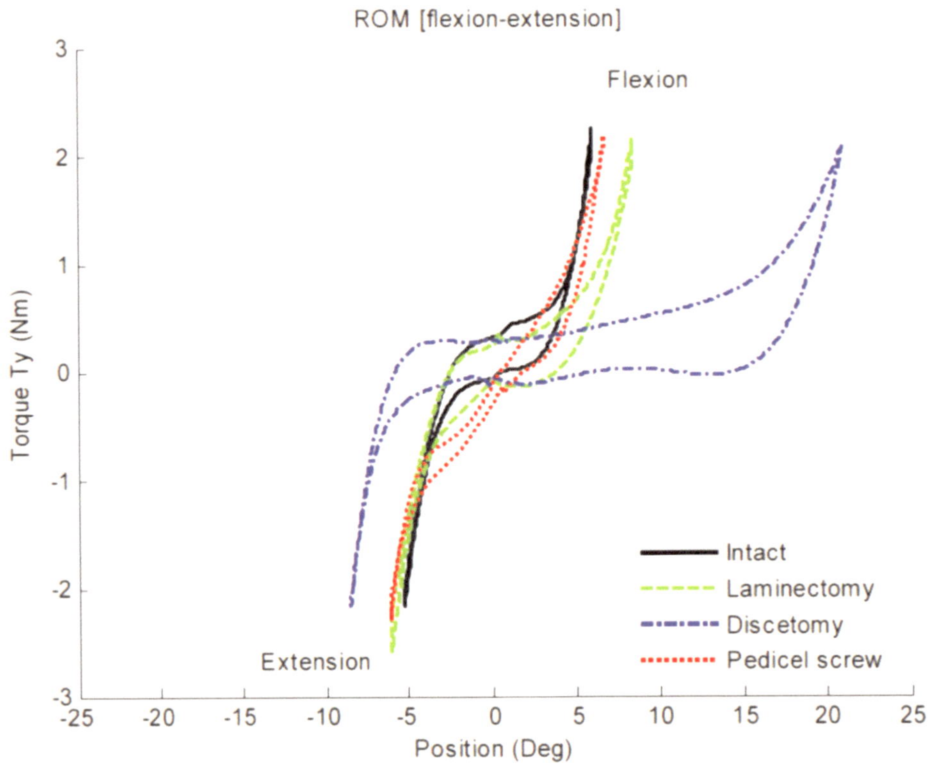

Fig. 6. Demonstration of the ROM of flexion-extension of the specimen after different surgical procedures . Reprinted from Journal of Medical and Biological Engineering, vol 29, No 1, Chang, T.S. et. al, a new multi-direction tester for evaluation of the spinal biomechanics, p 7-13, 2009, with kind permission from Taiwanese Society of Biomedical Engineering [21].

4.2 Compare the biomechanical stability between unilateral and bilateral cage-instrumented for lumbar spine

In this study the specimens were divided into two equal group unilateral PLIF (Posterior Lumbar Interbody Fusion) group and bilateral PLIF group. All biomechanical testing was performed with use of a spinal tester. Nondestructive, unconstrained loading parameters applied to the upper end vertebrae included the following: lateral bending (± 2 Nm, 100 axial preload), flexion-extension (± 2Nm, 100 axial preload), axial rotation (± 2Nm, 100 axial preload). The spinal tester analyzed biomechanical parameters include ROM and NZ.

Twelve motion segments of L4/5 from twelve sheep lumbar spines were studied for this in-vitro investigation. At the time of salvage, the animals were 12-18 months old and weighted 60 kg (53 to 65 kg). Following preparation, the specimens were stored frozen at -20°C then thawed at room temperature for 24 hours prior to testing. Care was taken to completely preserve the bony and ligamentous structures of the locomotor segment of each specimen, and only muscular and fatty tissue was removed. The cranial and caudal vertebrae of each functional spinal unit was anchored with stainless-steel screws and embedded with custom-designed metal fixtures using polyester resin. The intervening segments were left unconstrained.

The specimens were divided into two equal groups (figure 7). Group 1 included specimens that were tested intact. The following surgical procedures were then performed:

1. left hemilaminectomy,
2. left medial facectomy,
3. left discectomy,
4. left cage insertion (one, 8*8*12 mm),
5. left transpedicular screw fixation (two screws-4.75*25 cm and one rod- ISOLA system)

The group 2 specimens underwent the same sequence of procedures as the Group 1 except the bilateral sides, which included:

1. total laminectomy,
2. bilateral medial facetectomy,
3. bilateral discectomy,
4. two cage insertion (8*8*12 mm)
5. bilateral transpedicle screws fixation (four screws-4.75*25 cm and two rods- ISOLA system)

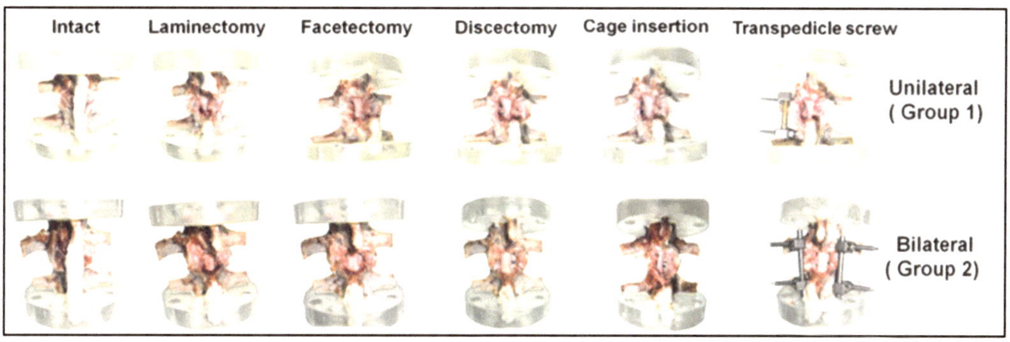

Fig. 7. Various surgical procedures between unilateral and bilateral groups were illustrated.

The lower vertebrae were centered over the load cell and maintained in neutral position by using the set coordinate system described previously [21]. After being mounted on the spine tester, each specimen was tested for right-left lateral bending, flexion-extension and right-left axial rotation at a constant speed of 1°/sec in sequence before and after different surgical procedures. A compressive preload of 100 N was applied. The direction was reversed until the moment detected by the load cell reached ±2 Nm. The load cell provided a feedback signal to the computer through RS-232 interface with 40 Hz sampling rate. The load and displacement data were collected and recorded during testing. A real-time graphical display of servo motor angle and applied moment was available during the test.

The bilateral group's ROM of flexion-extension was increased significantly after facetectomy (1.7±0.7, $p<0.05$) procedure in comparison with the unilateral group (0.5±0.6). The bilateral group's ROM of lateral bending was increased significantly after discectomy (3.7±1.0,

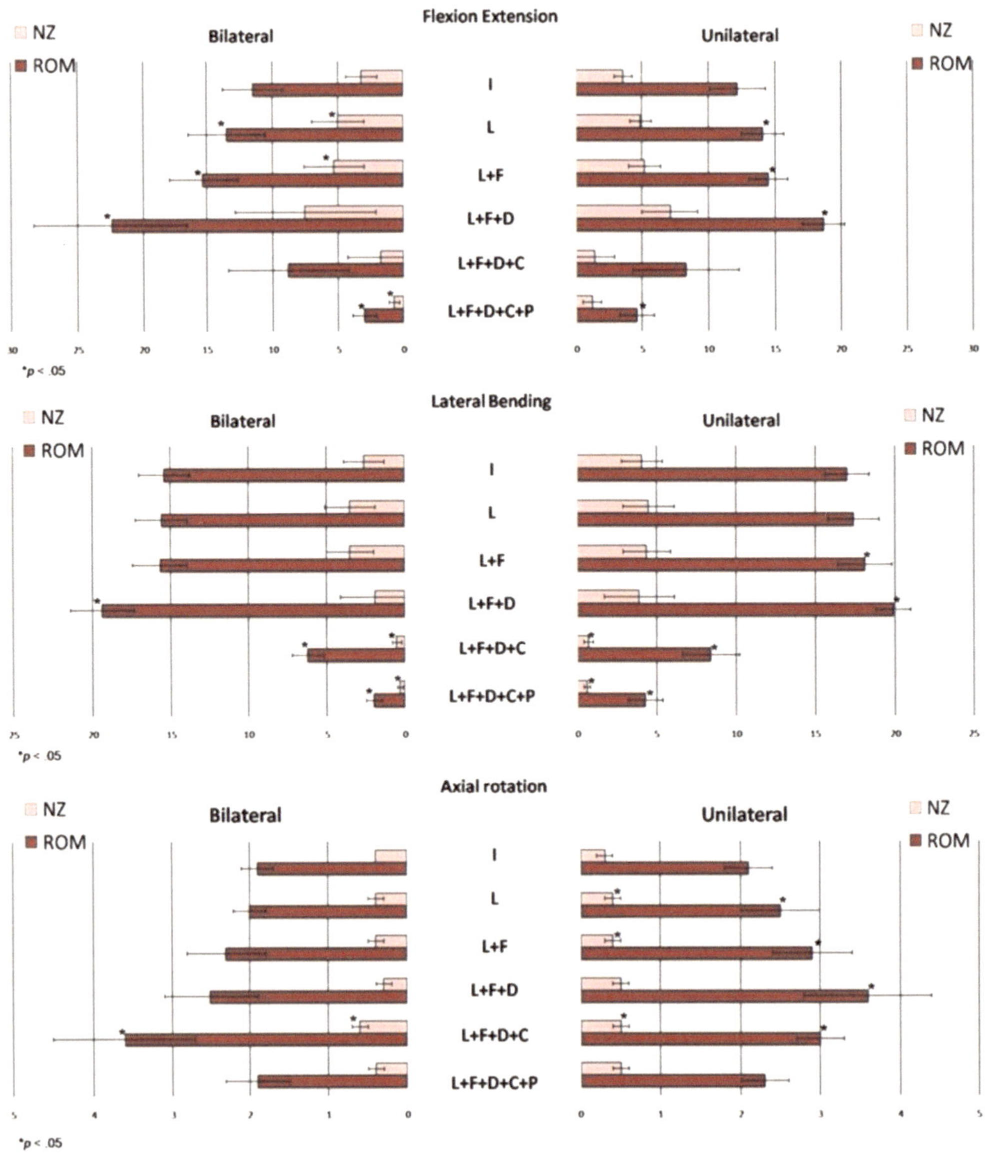

Fig. 8. Effects of destructive and stabilizing procedures on the ROM and NZ of unilateral and bilateral group. (L: Laminectomy, F: Facetectomy, D: Discetomy, C: Interbody Cage, P: Pedicle screw)

$p<0.05$) procedure in comparison with the unilateral group (1.8±1.6). The bilateral group's ROM of axial rotation was increased significantly after cage insertion (1.1±0.9, $p<0.05$) procedure in comparison with the unilateral group (-0.6±0.6). The bilateral group's ROM of axial rotation was decreased significantly after discectomy (0.2±0.3 vs 0.7±0.4, $p<0.05$) and transpedicle screw insertion (-1.7±0.8 vs -0.7±0.4, $p<0.05$) procedure in comparison with the unilateral group. The bilateral group's NZ of axial rotation was increased significantly after cage insertion (0.3±0.1, $p<0.05$) procedure in comparison with the unilateral group (0.0± 0.2).The bilateral group's NZ of axial rotation was decreased significantly after laminectomy (0.0±0.1 vs 0.1±0.0, $p<0.05$) and discectomy (-0.1±0.1 vs 0.1±0.1, $p<0.05$) procedure in comparison with the unilateral group (figure 8). Based on the results of this study, both ROM and NZ, unilateral cage-instrumented PLIF and bilateral cage-instrumented PLIF, transpedicle screw insertion procedure did not revealed a significant difference between flexion-extension, lateral bending and axial rotation direction except the ROM in the axial rotation.

5. Conclusion

This pure moment based spinal tester is capable of motion in six degree of freedom and is able to dynamically test a specimen throughout its entire range of motion. It can provide kinetic information for the simulated condition in life spinal motion. This is an ideal facility for spine biomechanical study. It has minimal weight moving over the specimen, thus minimizing friction and inertial effects. This allows the plotting of complete moment-displacement curves from which the characteristic flexibility parameters of interest can be calculated for each spine specimen in real time. The ability of calculated ROM and NZ is of particular importance given the clinical instability of a spinal segment. This multi-directional spinal tester is an effective and practical machine in the biomechanical study of spine.

6. Reference

[1] S. Naderi, N. Andalkar, and E, Benzel, "History of spine biomechanics: Part I- the pre-Greco-Roman, Greco-Roman, and Medieval roots of spine biomechanics", Neurosurgery 60: 382-391, 2007.
[2] S. Naderi, N. Andalkar, and E. Benzel, "History of spine biomechanics: Part II- from the renaissance to the 20th century", Neurosurgery 60: 392-404, 2007.
[3] E.H. Weber, "Anatomical and physiological tests on some systems of human spine mechanism", Arch. anat .physiol 1: 240-271, 1827.
[4] M.A. Adams, "Spine update mechanical testing of the spine- an appraisal of methodology, results, and conclusions" Spine 20: 2151-2156, 1995.
[5] D.J. Goertzen, C. Lane, and T. R. Oxland, "Neutral zone and range of motion in the spine are greater with stepwise loading than with a continuous loading protocol. An in vitro porcine investigation" Journal of Biomechanics 37: 127-261, 2004.
[6] J.T. Lysack, J.P. Dickey, G.A. Dumas and D. Yen, "A continuous pure moment loading apparatus for biomechanical testing of multi-segment spine specimens", J. Biomech 33: 765-770, 2000.

[7] V.K. Goel, S. Goyal, and C. Clark, "Kinematics of the whole lumbar spine: effect of discectomy", Spine 10: 543-554, 1985.

[8] Yamatoma, M.M. Panjabi, T. Criso and T.R. Oxland, "Three-dimensional movements of the whole lumbar spine and lumbosacral joints", Spine 14:1256-1260, 1989.

[9] H.J. Wilke, L . Claes, H. Schmitt and S. Wolf, "A universal spine tester for in vitro experiments with muscle force stimulation", Eur. Spine. J 3:91-97, 1994.

[10] V, Yingling, J. Callaghan, and S. McGill, "Dynamic loading affects the mechanical properties and failure site of porcine spines" Clinical Biomechanics 12: 301-305, 1997.

[11] I.A. Strokes, M. Gardner-Morse, D. Churchill, and J.P. Laible, "Measurement of a spinal motion segment stiffness matrix", J. Biomech 35: 517-521, 2002.

[12] R.E. Thompson, T.M. Barker and M.J. Pearcy, "Defining the neutral zone of sheep intervertebral joints during dynamic motions: an in vitro study" clinical Biomechanics 18: 89-98, 2003.

[13] M.M. Panjabi, "The stabilizing system of the spine. Part II. Neutral zone and instability hypothesis", J. Spinal Disord 5: 390-397, 1992.

[14] M.M. Panjabi, "The stabilizing system of the spine. Part I. Function, dysfunction, adaptation, and enhancement",J. Spinal Dis,5: 383-389, 1992.

[15] M. Mimura, M.M. Panjabi, T.R. Oxland, T.J. Criso, I.I. Yamamoto, and A .Vasavada, "Disc degeneration affects the multidirectional flexibility of the lumbar spine", Spine 19: 1371-1380, 1994.

[16] M.M. Panjabi, M. Kifune, W. Liu, M. Arand, A. Vasavada, and T.R. Oxland, "Graded thoracolumbar spine injuries: development of multidirectional instability", Eur Spine J 7: 332-339, 1998.

[17] T.R. Oxland, and M.M. Panjabi, "The onset and progression of spinal injury: a determination of neutral zone sensitivity", J. Biomech 25: 1165-1172, 1992.

[18] H.J. Wilke, S. Wolf, L.E. Claes, M. Arand, and A. Wiesue, "Stability increase of the lumbar spine with different muscle groups. A biomechanical in vitro study", Spine 20: 192-198, 1995.

[19] M.M. Panjabi, "Biomechanical evaluation of spine fixation devices: I A conceptual framework", Spine 13:1129-1134, 1988.

[20] V.K. Goel, D.G Wilder, M.H. Pope and W.E. Edwards, "Biomechanical testing of the spine: Load-controlled versus displacement-controlled analysis", Spine 20:2354-2357, 1995.

[21] T.S. Chang, C.W. Cheng, C.S. Wang, H.Y. Chen, and J.H. Chang, "A New Multi-direction Tester for Evaluation of the Spinal Biomechanics", Journal of Medical and Biological Engineering 29(1): 7-13, 2009.

[22] R.R. Craig, "Mechanics of Materials", First ed, Toronto: John Wiley & Sons Inc, pp 175-179, 1996.

[23] T.S. Chang, J.H. Chang, C.S. Wang, H.Y. Chen, and C.W. Cheng, "Evaluation of unilateral cage-instrumented fixation for lumbar spine", Journal of Orthopaedic Surgery and Research 5:86

Part 3

Musculoskeletal Biomechanics

10

Analysis of the Dynamic Sagittal Balance of the Lumbo-Pelvi-Femoral Complex

Legaye Jean
University of Louvain, Mont-Godinne
Belgium

1. Introduction

The acquisition of bipedalism has enabled the human species an intellectual, technological and social development. However, the transition to the standing position was possible only through morphological adaptations, particularly in the lower limbs, the pelvis and the spine. The pelvis has changed from an elongated shape (called "in tension", typical of quadrupeds), to a more squat morphology (called "in pressure", characteristic of bipedalism). The pelvis was indeed a key holder of these transformations as a pivot basis submitted to the loads of gravity from the trunk and to the reaction forces from the ground, transmitted by the femoral heads. Parallel to the adaptation of the pelvis, the appearance of the spinal curvatures has allowed establishing a balance defined as stable and economic in terms of stress on the musculo-ligamentous structures and of muscle contractions necessary for its maintenance. However, maintaining this balance when standing was precarious: all the stresses of gravity were to be maintained within this entire vertical body and inside a narrow sustentation polygon. (Figure 1).

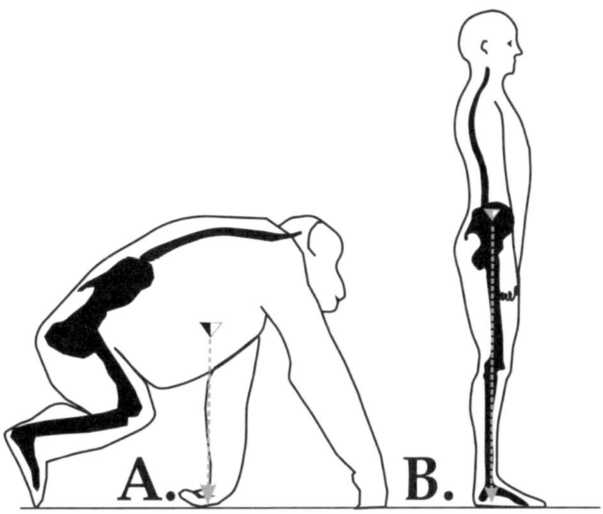

Fig. 1. Differences in lombo-pelvi-femoral morphology, gravity line and sagittal balance between a quadruped chimpanzee (A.) and a standing human (B.).

Dynamic management of the position of gravity was therefore essential. For the standing human, any unbalancing disruption has negative effects inducing pain and anatomical deterioration. An effective analysis of the sagittal balance in standing position was so primordial for biomechanical and medical purposes. This procedure was reported here. It involves both a morphological evaluation of the lumbo-pelvi-femoral complex by the analysis of the relations between pelvic anatomy and spinal curvatures, and a mechanical assessment of the strengths of gravity on each of the vertebral and pelvic anatomical structures. The integration of such data allowed a personalized analytical and functional assessment of the sagittal balance in vivo for a standing individual.

2. Morphological analysis of the lumbo-pelvi-femoral complex

2.1 Prior descriptions

Many sagittal morphotypes have been described by anthropologists. Stagnara has proposed a classification based on the intensity and the topography of the spinal curvatures. So, he defined the morphotypes as "normal", “kyphosis”, “lordosis”, “kypho-lordosis”, in “total lordosis or kyphosis”, “inverted back”, “flat back" according to the angular and millimetric values of the respective curves. Subsequently, authors have reported the influence of the lordosis on the sagittal rotation of the pelvis, expressed by the tilt of the sacral plate. Several spinal parameters were proposed. The “lumbar lordosis” was defined as the angle between the upper plate of the first sacral vertebra S1 (or the sacral plate) and the upper plate of L1, “lordosis” was differently described according to the authors: the bottom limit was either the sacral plate or the lower plate of L5, the top limit either the most backward tilted plate or other specified vertebrae. The normality was assessed by comparing the observed value to a range of normal mean values. Using the mean values of these parameters, however, remained inadequate for an individual assessment of spinal curvatures because of the great range of variations for physiological values (Table 1 for lordosis and kyphosis), greater than simply due to differences in the measurement techniques.

	“Lordosis” (°)			“Kyphosis” (°)		
	Min.	**Max.**	**range**	**Min.**	**Max.**	**range**
Duval-Beaupère (1998)	46	87	41	33	71	38
Guigui (2003)	37	89	52	7	65	58
Vaz (2002)	26	76	50	25	72	47
Gelb (1995)	38	84	46	9	66	57
Jackson (2000)	35	90	55	22	75	52

Table 1. Ranges of variation of normal values of “Lordosis” and “Kyphosis” reported by several authors.

2.2 Descriptive morphological parameters

2.2.1 The “Pelvic radius” and the “Lumbo-pelvic lordosis”

Jackson emphasized sagittal descriptive parameters of the pelvis and spine. (Jackson, 2000) (Figure 2) They aimed to compare an individual with ranges of values proposed as the normality.

2.2.1.1 The anatomical parameter

The "Pelvic Lordosis" or "Pelvic Radius" (PR-S1): the angle between the upper plate of S1 and the line connecting the posterior point of the sacral plate to the bi-coxo-femoral axis.

2.2.1.2 The positional parameters

The "Sacral Inclination" (SI): the angle between the vertical and the posterior edge of S1
The "Pelvic Angle" (PA): the angle between the vertical and the line connecting the posterior point of the sacral plate to the bi-coxo-femoral axis.
The "Lumbo-Pelvic Lordosis": the angle between the upward extension of the line defining PR-S1 and the upper plate of T12.

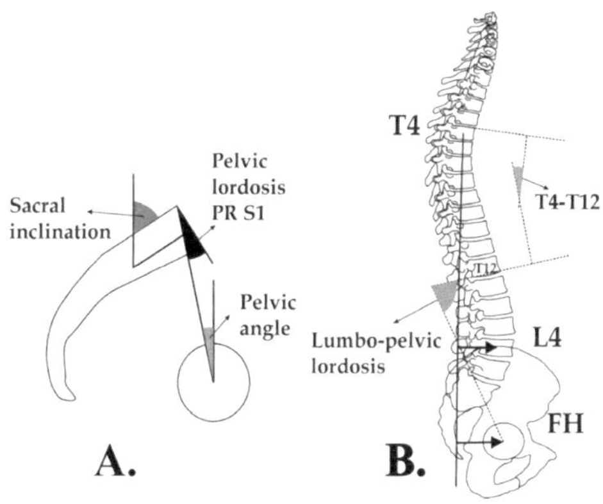

Fig. 2. The angular anatomical and positional parameters described by Jackson (2000).

2.2.1.3 Method of evaluation

3 criteria were defined as the normality:

- The center of the femoral heads and the center of the body of L4 are positioned in front of the vertical downwards of the center of the body of T4 (Figure 2 B)
- "Pelvic Angle" between 0 and 35 °
- "Lumbo-Pelvic Lordosis" between 60 and 120

Moreover, the quotient of the angles "Thoracic Kyphosis" (T4-T12) / "Lumbo-Pelvic Lordosis" had to be between 0.15 and 0.75 (Figure 2 B)

2.2.2 The sagittal "Overhangs"

2.2.2.1 The Overhang of C7

Many authors considered the plumb-line from C7 on the underlying structures as an evidence of the overall sagittal balance of the lumbo-pelvi-femoral complex. Jackson assessed that C7 has to be projected at the upper posterior angle of S1, with a margin of 60 mm in front and behind. (Jackson, 2000) The more important was the global lordosis or the segmental lordosis L4L5 and L5S1, the greater was C7 projected behind. C7 was also observed to project optimally 35 mm behind the femoral heads (25 mm forwards to 85 mm backwards) in normal subjects. The overhang of C7 on the sacral plate was observed significantly correlated with the lumbar lordosis (r=0.36), but not the overhang of C7 on the femoral heads. It was considered specific to characterize the sagittal balance of the individual.

The overhangs of C7 on the body of T12 were analyzed by Vedantam: the more C7 was behind the sacrum, the more the apex of the thoracic curve was located upwards and the more T12 and the lumbar apex were forwards. (Vedantam, 1998) Unfortunately, the radiological definition of the body of C7 was often imprecise and makes this reference unusable. The two plates of C7 were reported visible only in 50 to 63% of the cases, due to the superposition of the shadow of the shoulders. On 150 radiographs of adolescents, Vedantam reported that 41% of the cases were rejected because of this lack of precision. The definition of T1 was even worse. (Vedantam, 1998) These two markers were so difficult to use in clinical practice. Moreover, nor the pelvis sagittal morphology or the femoral heads were taken into account by these techniques. They were unable to detect a pelvic well or mal rotation. They appraised only the global balance, but not an eventual reciprocal pelvic or spinal adaptation to a local disturbance.

2.2.2.2 The Overhang of the ear canals

Gangnet reported a normal projection of the ear's canals 28 mm posterior to the femoral heads. (Gangnet, 2003) Nevertheless, this overhang was greatly affected by the position of the heads or an eventual disturbance of the cervical lordosis.

2.2.2.3 The Overhang of T4

For normal subjects, the vertical down from the center of T4 was observed behind the center of L4 and the femoral heads. (Jackson, 2000) (Figure 2B)

2.3 The analytical parameters of the sagittal balance

Using the parameters described above and comparing the observed values to normal standards provided purely descriptive analysis of sagittal balance. Dubousset proposed in 1984 to consider the pelvis as the foundation of the spine: a mobile base interposed between the spine and the lower limbs. (Dubousset, 1984) In 1998, Duval-Beaupère defined an essential anatomical sagittal pelvic parameter, the "Pelvic Incidence", and pelvic and spinal positional parameters (i.e. varying with the position of the subject). The evaluation of the harmony of their values allowed an analytical study of the individual sagittal balance of the lumbo-pelvi-femoral complex. (Duval-Beaupère, 1998)

The position of the arms was reported greatly influential on the sagittal shape of the spine. (Vedantan, 2000) The arms lying on a support were considered as reproducible and minimally influencing the position of the spine.

The angular parameters were expressed in degrees, the dimensional parameters in millimeters. A positive value was posterior, a negative anterior.

2.3.1 Positional pelvic parameters (Figure 3A)

- "Sacral Slope" (SS): angle between the upper plate of S1 (or sacral plate) and a horizontal line. A vertical sacrum was described by a low value of SS, a horizontal sacrum by a high value. The reported values (expressing a forward tilt of the sacral plate) were negative (-40.6 ° ± 8.5 from 25 to 59);
- "Pelvic Tilting" (PT): angle between the vertical and the line joining the middle of the sacral plate to the bi-coxo-femoral axis (11.4 ° ± 5.9 from -0.1 to 29.2);
- "Overhang of S1" (OVH S1): distance between the bi-coxo-femoral axis and the vertical projection of the middle of the sacral plate (21mm ± 10.8 from 43.5 to -1.5);

- "Pelvic Thickness" (PT): distance between the middle of the sacral plate and the bi-coxo-femoral axis (95mm ± 9 from 83 to 112).

2.3.2 Spinal positional parameters (Figure 3B)

- "Lordosis" (L): angle between the sacral plate and the more backward tilted plate of another lumbar or thoracic vertebra (63.5 ° ± 10.9 from 45 to 87);
- "Kyphosis" (K): angle between the more backward tilted plate used for "LA" measurement and the more forward tilted upper vertebral plate (49.3 ° ± 9.2 from 33 to 71).

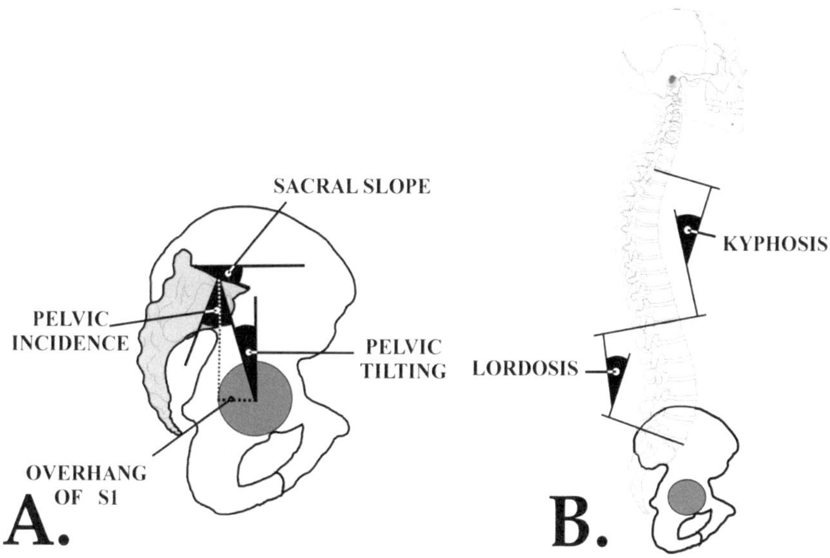

Fig. 3. The sagittal pelvic and spinal parameters

2.3.3 The anatomical parameter "pelvic incidence" (Figure 3A)

"Pelvic Incidence" (PI): angle between the line perpendicular to the sacral plate at its midpoint and the line connecting this point to the bi-coxo-femoral axis. This angle was anatomical (i.e. independent of the position of the pelvis) and specific for each individual. It reflected the mutual relations between the ilium and the sacrum through the sacroiliac joints, whose mobility was considered negligible, but in which were concentrated the forces of the weight of the trunk and these provided by the femoral heads from the ground. The mean value of PI was 53 ° ± 9 (min 33.7, max 77.5) for Duval-Beaupère, corroborated by numerous publications. (Boulay, 2006; Duval-Beaupère, 1998; Guigui, 2003; Marty, 2002; Vaz, 2002; Vialle, 2005a) A geometric relationship demonstrated that the anatomical parameter "Pelvic Incidence" was equal to the sum of the positional parameters "Sacral Slope" and "Pelvic Tilting" (PI = SS + PT).

2.3.4 Correlations between pelvic and spinal parameters (Figure 4)

A sequence of significant correlations between parameters was reported by Duval-Beaupère, confirmed by other authors (Boulay, 2006; Duval-Beaupère, 1998; Marty, 2002; Guigui, 2003; Vaz, 2002).

The first fundamental correlation linked the anatomical parameter "Pelvic Incidence" and the positional parameter "Sacral Slope" (r = 0.86). The second highly significant correlation was between the "Sacral Slope" and the "Lordosis" (r = 0.84). The relation between "Lordosis" and "Kyphosis" was poorly significant (r=0.36).

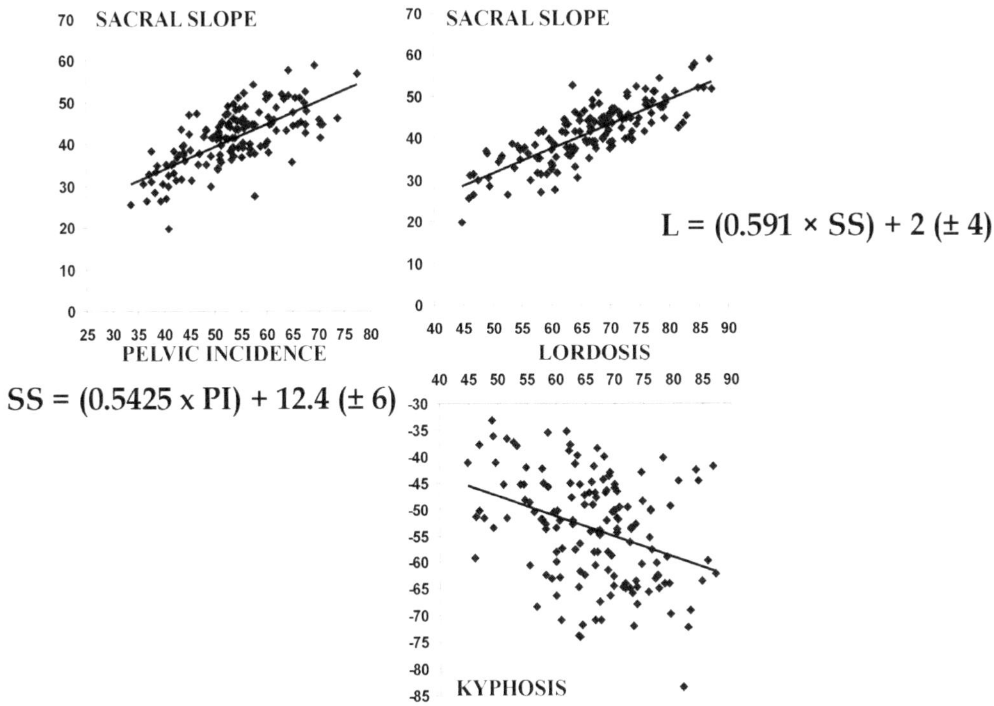

Fig. 4. Significant correlations between parameters and their predictive equations

These correlations allowed establishing the essential role of the pelvic morphology in the regulation of the sagittal spinal curves: high value of "Pelvic Incidence" was associated to high "Sacral Slope" value and an important "Lordosis" (Figure 5 A), low "Pelvic Incidence" value was associated with low "Sacral Slope" value and a more flat "Lordosis". (Figure 5 B)

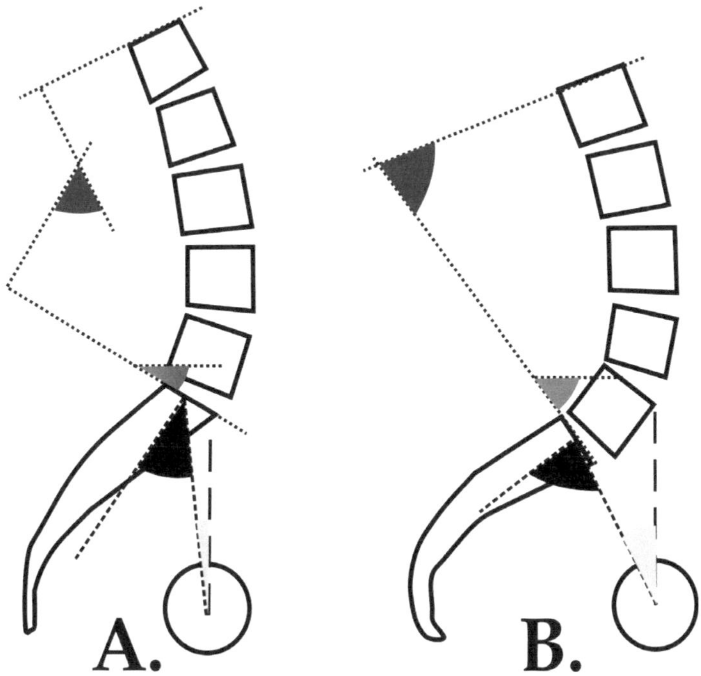

Fig. 5. Low (A.) and great (B.) value of "Pelvic Incidence" and sagittal lumbar shape.

The normality of a sagittal shape was attested by the harmony of these relationships, and not by comparing observed and average values. Using these equations, it became possible to assess the "Sacral Slope" adapted to the individual value of "Pelvic Incidence". The difference between the observed and this optimal value was named "ΔPS". Similarly, the value of "Lordosis" adapted to the observed "Sacral Slope" was determinable (the difference between observed and calculated value was named "Δlord") and even the optimal value of "Lordosis" according to the "Sacral Slope" adapted by the "Pelvic Incidence" (the difference with the observed value was named "Δlord optimal"). This analytic evaluation allowed detecting a global or a local disturbance (pelvic, lumbar, kyphotic ...). A pelvic tilt was considered significant if "ΔPS" exceeded 12 °, lordosis was unsuited to the observed sacral slope if "Δlord" was more than 8 ° or unsuited to the pelvic incidence if "Δlord optimal" was more than 8 °.

2.3.5 Individual pelvic sagittal shapes

Individual anatomical variations of the pelvis were related to the value of "Pelvic Incidence". Greater was the value of the "Pelvic Incidence" more was the sacral plate forwards tilted and the sacrum curved, greater were the values of "Pelvic Tilting" and "Overhang of S1" relatively to the femoral heads and lower the value of "Pelvic Thickness". (Figure 6)

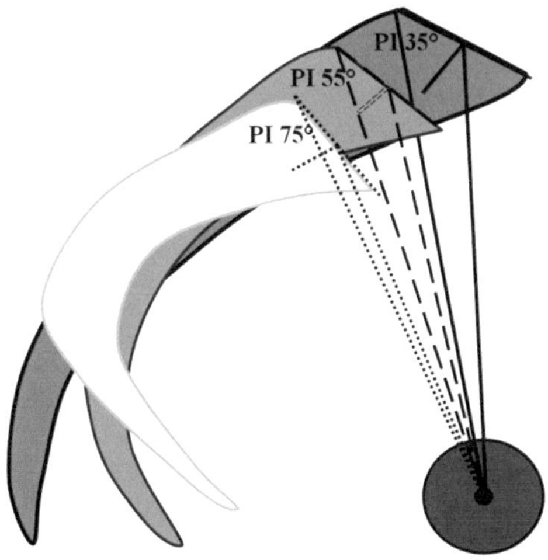

Fig. 6. Individual shapes of the sacrum and of the pelvis according the value of "Pelvic Incidence".

It was interesting to differentiate the application of this concept to an individual and to the population. At the population scale (normality of the harmony between the parameters), the value of "Pelvic Tilting" increases with the value of the "Sacral Slope", but inversely at the individual scale, the value of "Pelvic Tilting" decreases with the value of the "Sacral Slope" by pelvic retroversion (in case of disturbance). This apparent paradox highlighted the necessity of an individualized analysis of the harmony between parameters rather than a comparison with standard values.

2.3.6 Reported values, correlations and gender differences

After the first description of these sagittal parameters (Duval-Beaupère, 1998), several studies reported similar observations, both for the values and for the significant chain of correlations. This confirms the validity and reproducibility of these parameters and the usefulness of the method. (Tables 2 and 3)

	Duval-Beaupère (1998)		Guigui (2003)		Vaz (2002)	
Parameters	**Mean**	**sd**	**Mean**	**sd**	**Mean**	**sd**
Pelvic Incidence (°)	52	*11*	55	*11*	52	*12*
Sacral Slope (°)	41	*9*	42	*9*	39	*9*
Pelvic Tilting (°)	11	*6*	13	*6*	12	*6*
Lordosis (°)	64	*11*	61	*13*	47	*11*
Kyphosis (°)	49	*9*	41	*9*	47	*9*
Coefficients "r"						
"PI"/"SS"	0.84		0.81		0.86	
"SS"/"L"	0.86		0.86		0.75	
"L"/"K"	0.34		0.31		0.36	

Table 2. Reported angular values expressed of the parameters and Spearman's coefficients "r" for the significant relation between parameters.

	Duval-Beaupère (1998)			Guigui (2003)		
	Women	Men	Sign.	Women	Men	Sign.
Pelvic Incidence (°)	49	58	**	57	54	*
Sacral Slope (°)	39	45	**	44	41	**
Lordosis (°)	57	65	**	63	59	***
Kyphosis (°)	45	46	ns	39	42	ns

Table 3. Values of the parameters: differences according to gender (* $p<0.05$ ** $p<0.01$ *** $p< 0.001$)

2.3.7 Relationships between the descriptive and analytic methods

The most important factor missing on the descriptive method (Jackson, 2000) was the low correlation between the anatomical parameter (PR-S1) and the positional parameters, whereas these correlations were strong for the analytic parameters of Duval-Beaupère (1998). (Table 4) The parameter "PR-S1", although significantly correlated with the "Pelvic Incidence" ($r = 0.998$, $p<0.001$), was less related with lordosis ($r = 0.66$, $p<0.01$). This was because, unlike the "Pelvic Incidence", it involved in its measure the slightly trapezoidal shape of S1 (Marty, 2002). In addition, the "Lumbo-Pelvic Lordosis" incorporates both anatomical and positional components. The descriptive method, however, was complex because it required a lot of measures. It was also imprecise as a consequence of the numerous physiological values and the large areas of overlap with the pathological situations.

	Gelb (1995)	Vedantam (1998)	Jackson (2000)		Duval (1998)	Guigui (2003)	Vaz (2002)
SI/ lordosis	0.47	0.68	0.56	**SS/ lordosis**	0.86	0.85	0.75
PRS1/ lumbo-pelvic lordosis			ns	**PI/ lordosis**	0.60		

Table 4. Reported Spearman's coefficients (r) between parameters

2.3.8 Analytic evaluation of a clinical imbalance

Three types of disturbances may arise, leading to a displacement of the trunk forwards and inducing an sagittal unbalance with excessive stresses of the anatomical structures and necessitating muscle contractions, possibly painful:

- Type A: lack of "Lordosis" with a "Sacral Slope" value too low for the value of PI; (Figure 6A) It was the most frequently observed disturbance in clinical practice for low back pain. The loss of "Lordosis" was the consequence of lumbar disorders, mostly at the lower levels (disc diseases with local inter vertebral reduction of the lordosis, fractures ...), the result of fusion in inadequate lordosis or the result of muscular atrophy (often with obesity, sometimes by muscular or neurological disorders s as Parkinson's disease). The pelvic reaction to this loss of lordosis was a backward rotation (retroversion) achievable by extension of the hips, and then by flexion of the knees (and flexion of he ankles).

- Type B: excessive "Sacral Slope" value reflecting a forward pelvic rotation (anteversion), by stiff flexion of the hips, sufficiently or not compensated by an accentuation of the "Lordosis". (Figure 6 B) This situation occurred mostly in cases of hip (and knee) osteoarthritis. Only the treatment of the origin was useful (as by hip arthroplasty).
- Type C: "Lordosis" insufficient to compensate an excessive kyphosis, with backwards pelvic rotation (low value of SS), and finally flexion of the hips and the knees. (Figure 6 C) This situation occurred mostly with aging, by disc thoracic narrowing or osteoporotic factures, after traumatic fractures or in majors Scheuerman's diseases cases.

Each of these 3 situations tends to induce an anterior translation of the gravity loads, unfavorable for the evolution of the subject.

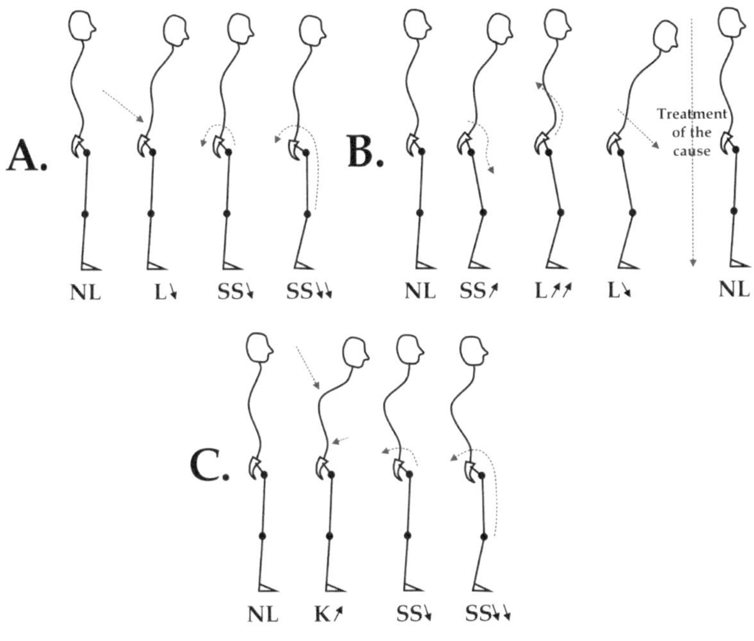

Fig. 6. Types of sagittal disturbances and their evolution

The value of "Pelvic Incidence" determines the stability of a balanced attitude, the ability of a subject to react to a disturbance and also the individual risks of a loss of "Lordosis". A subject with a low "Pelvic Incidence" value has a lower capacity to adapt to a disturbance because of low potential of "Lordosis", contrary to those with a great value of "Pelvic Incidence" with a great reserve of compensation. Conversely, the risk of insufficient "Lordosis" will be greater for the subjects with high "Pelvic Incidence" value, necessitating a high "Lordosis" value to be adapted. In case of lumbar fusion, the risk of insufficient "Lordosis" will be greater than in subjects with small "Pelvic Incidence" value, necessitating less "Lordosis" to compensate. Similarly, interventions not allowing an increase of lordosis (as inter-somatic cages, disc prosthesis, inter spinous blocks) should be avoided for cases with high "Pelvic Incidence" value, easily resulting in a disturbed sagittal balance by loss of "Lordosis" (and a late compensation on the overlying levels, difficult to treat).

The analytic evaluation is so individual. It must be integrated into the evolution of the subject. In further paragraph 4, this analytic method will also be functional because it allows integrating the biomechanical loads of gravity on the spine and pelvis.

3. The sagittal balance in spinal diseases

3.1 The spondylolisthesis

3.1.1 Isthmic spondylolisthesis

Significantly higher values of "Pelvic Incidence" and "Sacral Slope" were reported by several authors. (Hanson, 2002; Huang, 2003; Labelle, 2004, 2005; Vialle, 2005b, 2007a, 2007b) The sacral plate was described more tilted, inducing a marked lordosis and a slip of L5 on S1. This generated a forward shift of the center of gravity of the trunk. The correction was attempted by flattening of the kyphosis (the decrease in the sagittal slope of T9 expressed the anterior displacement of the trunk). (Figure 7) Additionally, the increased lordosis L4L5 L5S1 was considered damaging the isthmus. The importance of the value of pelvic incidence may be considered a prognostic factor for the progression of the listhesis. (Hanson, 2002; Huang, 2003; Labelle, 2004; Vialle, 2005b, 2007a, 2007b)
The adult form of the sacrum was also described more curved in kyphosis, particularly between S1 and S2, and nearly similar to the sacrum of children before the acquisition of standing position with a lower angle between the frontal edge of S1 and the sacral plate. (Marty, 2002)

3.1.2 Degenerative spondylolisthesis

In degenerative spondylolisthesis, the sagittal balance was described differently: the angle of kyphosis was not influenced, but the lordosis was significantly flattened with pelvic retroversion (lower value of the "Sacral Slope"). (Morel, 2005) In this way, the slope of T9 was in the range of normal values. (Figure 7) The "Pelvic Incidence" was reported greater than for younger subjects. An accentuation of this age-related value can be attributed to torsion stresses on the sacroiliac joints during life.

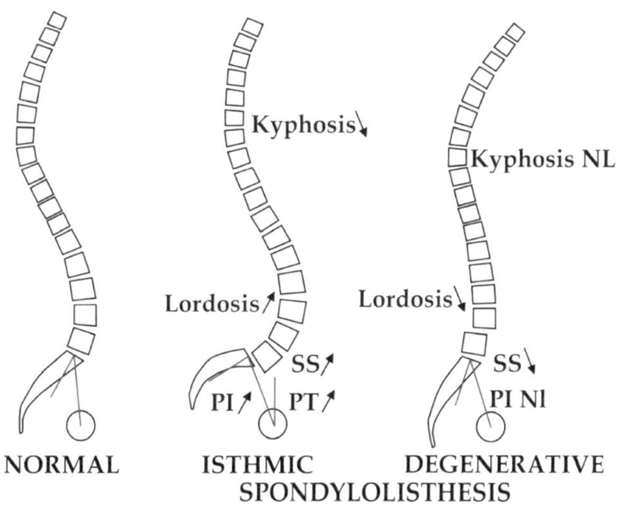

Fig. 7. Sagittal shape in normal case and in isthmic and degenerative spondylolisthesis

3.2 Lombo-arthritis – Low back pain

The pelvic incidence values were identical to the normal adult population. In most cases, the essential of the disturbance was a loss of lumbar lordosis (by disc degeneration, by pelvic retroversion reacting to obesity ...) sometimes associated with stiffness in flexion of the hip. It induced an anterior displacement of the trunk often progressive because of the muscular weaknesses frequently occurring in aging individuals. This more anterior application of gravity on the pelvis tends to tilt the sacrum forwards, but the ground reaction forces transmitted through the femoral heads tend to tilt the iliac bones backwards. (Figure 8) This induced a twisting phenomenon into the sacroiliac joints, which was source of back and leg pain (the "Pyriform Syndrome"), and eventually of an increasing of the value of "Pelvic Incidence". The loss of lordosis (occurring mainly in the lower levels) was then compensated by a pelvic retroversion and a hyperextension in the higher lumbar levels.

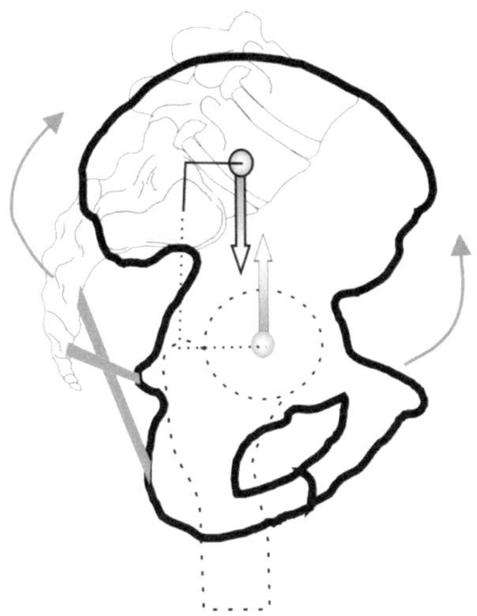

Fig. 8. Torsion stresses on the sacro-iliac joint induced by the inverse move of the ilium and sacrum in case of forwards displacement of the loads of the trunk

3.3 Herniated discs

A lower pelvic incidence (47.3°) was observed only in patients under 40 year old with a herniated lumbar disc. (Guigui, 2003) A pelvic retroversion was frequently observed, independently of the age.

3.4 Implications on the result of surgical lumbar fusion

Respect of the harmony of the parameters was crucial in such surgical procedures. A significant pelvic retroversion was reported in patients remaining painful after lumbar fusion comparing to painless cases. (Gottfried, 2009; Kawakmi, 2002; Lazennec, 2000) Similarly, Kumar reported degenerative changes in the adjacent levels 5 years after surgery only in 8% of the well balanced cases but in 50% of the unbalanced cases. (Kumar, 2000) The twisting phenomenon into the sacroiliac joints occurred when lumbar lordosis was inadequate, especially if L5-S1 was included in the fusion. In addition, the critical effect of the upper lordosis with compensation by retro- (or ante-) listhesis of the overlying disc in a hypo-lordotic fusion was to fear. (Figure 9)

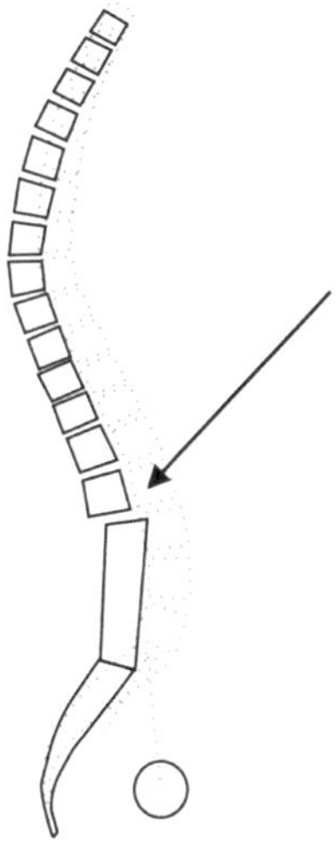

Fig. 9. Retro listhesis of the upper lordosis in compensation of a fusion insufficiently curved

Any imbalance, no matter the indication (degenerative disease or deformity such as scoliosis) was detrimental to clinical outcome in the short and long term. The origin was vertebro-discal stresses, painful muscle cramps and twisting in the sacroiliac joints.

3.5 Deformations on osteoporosis

The negative factor was the progressive thoracic kyphosis by disc narrowing for which lumbar and pelvic compensation became progressively inadequate. (Figure 10) The same principle applied in the event of osteoporotic spinal fractures, in kyphosis or badly reduced. The forward displacement of the trunk, especially if lumbar compensation was reduced, had to be avoided. The hyper kyphosis produced by osteoporotic fractures induced a forward tilting of the trunk that compensated as much as possible an accentuation of the lumbar lordosis, in the limits of possible as far as age and lumbar discs go. A pelvic retroversion occurred to help compensate this evolutionary hyper-kyphosis in intensity and topographic extension, and finally a flexion of the hips and of the knees.

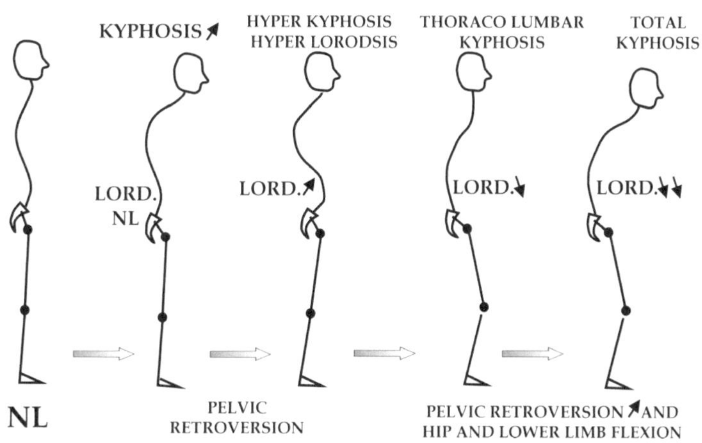

Fig. 10. Sagittal evolution with aging for kyphotic osteoporosis

3.6 The aging

Aging was observed to be accompanied with an accentuation of the thoracic kyphosis: 30 ° for 30-39 y.o., 40 ° for 50-59 y.o., 50 ° increasing from 60 to 80 y.o.. (Korovessis, 1998) In parallel, the lumbar lordosis disappeared gradually: 68 ° for 40 - 49 y.o., 62 ° for 50 - 69 y.o., less than 60 ° after 70 y.o. . (Gelb, 1995) This induced a progressive displacement forwards of the trunk, resulting in the projection of C7 more anterior to the sacral promontory: 4.3 cm behind for 40 - 49 y.o., 3.7 for 50 - 59 y.o., 2.4 for 60 - 69 y.o., only 1.9 cm after 70 y.o. . (Gelb, 1995; Jackson, 1994) A significant correlation between PI and age (r = 0.14) was reported (Guigui, 2003). These alterations of the curves imposed an evaluative and functional analysis considering the impact on the stresses of gravity.

3.7 Hyper-kyphosis related to age

The loss of lordosis by aging induced in the early evolution a decrease of kyphosis with a pelvic retroversion. The displacement forwards of gravity of the trunk relatively to the thoracic and especially the lumbar vertebrae accentuates the curving stresses on the thoracic spine that will finally decompensate, resulting in accentuation of the kyphosis which is related to age (loss of disc height, osteoporotic fractures). T9, and the loads of gravity on the thoracic and lumbar structures, were too much forward, requesting the disco-ligamentar structures and inducing more rebalance muscle contractures, themselves becoming painful.

3.8 Sheuerman's disease

This disease was local to the thoraco-lumbar vertebrae. The "Pelvic Incidence" was so similar to the normal population, as well as "Pelvic Tilting" and "Sacral Slope" although "Lordosis" was increased in compensation.

3.9 Influence of the sport activities

The pelvic incidence was observed significantly higher (p <0.0001) among soccer players (55.7 °) than in non-athletic subjects (50.3 °). (Wodecki, 2002)

4. Functional analysis by assessment of the gravity loads on the lumbo-pelvi-femoral complex: The mechanical model

The analytic concept of the harmony of the pelvi-spinal balance expressed a balance "economical" in terms of loads on the disco-ligamentar structures and muscular efforts required for its maintenance. This concept was developed by Duval (1987) in conjunction with an innovative individual determination of the gravity loads on the spine in station and in vivo: the "barycentremetry". In this way, the sagittal analysis has become "functional".

4.1 Measurement of the gravity loads

4.1.1 The mathematical models

Mathematical models were performed to evaluate the mechanical stress applied to the spine. The first were based on analysis of the axial compression of the spine in a standing position from the lever arms of action of muscles and other structures. The initial assessment was from the body cross sections, (Shultz, 1981) then the finite element models reproducing these forces were developed. Used for research or hardware design, they were totally useless in clinical practice.

4.1.2 The platform of force

Therefore many authors have used the platforms of force in conjunction with radiographs to assess the gravity loads on the spine and pelvis. The position of gravity was assimilated to be vertical from the application point of the whole body weight on the ground. (Gangnet, 2003; During, 1985) However, these techniques remained imprecise because they failed to access to the position in height of gravity and especially were inaccurate because they integrated the whole body (including the legs underlying to the pelvis) in establishing the position of the gravity loads applied to the segmental spinal and pelvic structures. If it was a good approximation in normal standing position, it was inaccurate in case of spinal or pelvic disturbance because the gravity of the whole body was no more assimilative to segmental gravity (of the trunk, of bodily segments supported by each vertebra...). (Figure 11)

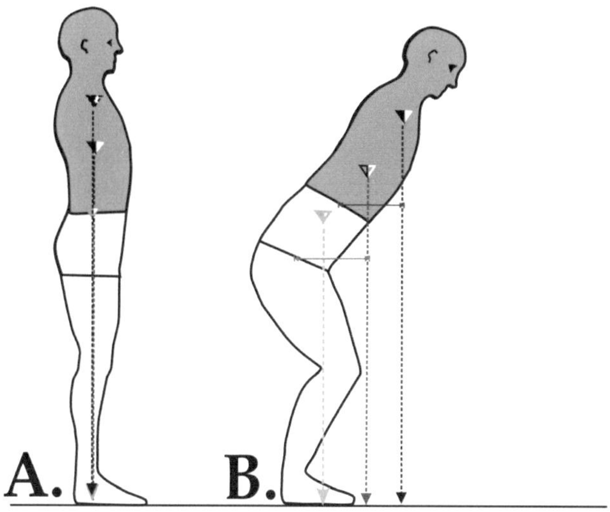

Fig. 11. Segmental lever arms and centers of gravity in normal (A) and unbalanced (B) standing position

4.1.2.1 Barycentremetry

A prototype gamma-ray scanner (whose absorption was proportional to the crossed mass) has provided access in patients in vivo to the position of gravity of 1 centimeter thick body slices. (Duval, 1987) This scanner was coupled to a system of three-dimensional reconstruction of the spine and pelvis from bi-planar X-rays. After matching the two reference systems, a process of integration provided the lever arms and the loads of gravity on all discs and vertebral levels as well as on the pelvis and on the femoral heads in a standing position: "the barycentremetry". (Figure 12)

In this way, it was found that the application points of gravity were projected within a cylinder of 1 centimeter diameter, located forwards at the thoracic levels, backwards at the lumbar levels (26 mm behind the middle the upper plate of L3) and crossed the upper plate of the sacrum behind its middle, and backwards to the femoral heads (36 mm). The centre of gravity of the body segment supported by the femoral heads was more often in front of T9 (0 to 14 mm when the thoracic kyphosis was less than 35 °, 20 to 32 mm if it was higher). (Duval 1992 & 2008)

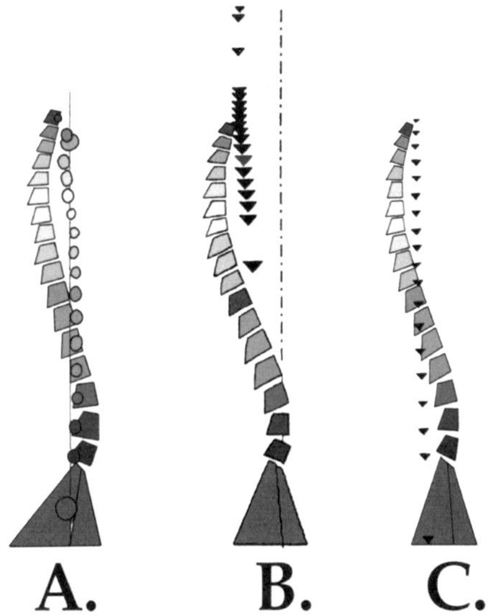

Fig. 12. Barycentremetry by gamma ray scanner providing the elementary center of gravity of body slices centered on vertebrae and pelvis (A), the location in upright position of the centers of gravity supported by each vertebrae and pelvis (B), the projected lever arm of gravity applied on each level of the spinal and pelvic structures (C).

	Mean (in mm)	sd	min	max
L3	25	25	-18	96
S1	18	27	-31	111
Femoral heads	36	21	9	52

Table 5. Values of the lever arms of the gravity on L3, S1 and the femoral heads axis.

4.1.2.2 Barycentremetry confronted to the force platforms

Using force platforms for standing normal subject, the position of the center of gravity of the whole body (including the legs) was observed projected 28 mm (SD 14) behind the femoral heads by Gangnet (2003), 12 mm (SD 12) behind the sacral promontory by During (1985). These data were similar to the barycetremetric observations, testifying the liability of both techniques in such normally balanced position. Nevertheless, only the barycentremetry allowed to determine real segmental centers of gravity for each pelvic and vertebral levels, and to take into account the individual variation of each segments relatively to the others in case of misbalanced position. (Duval, 1992 & 2008)

4.1.2.3 Biomechanical implications of the position of gravity

The loads of gravity backwards to the lumbar levels were balanced by the abdominal muscle chains, saving the back muscles at rest. At the thoracic levels, the forward position was compensated by the posterior spinal muscles and the stiffness of the rib cage. This optimal balance was defined as economical, in accordance to the analytic definition of the harmonious relations of spinal and pelvic parameters. (Figure 13)

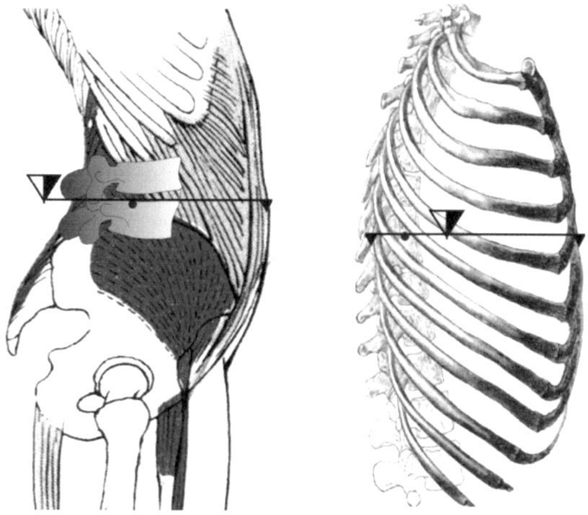

Fig. 13. Optimal balance between gravity and the abdominal muscles at lumbar levels, the rib cage and spinal muscles at the thoracic levels.

It has been found by simultaneous muscle activity detection through direct electromyography recordings and by the gamma ray scanner, that only the respect for the harmonious personal relationships between the parameters allowed a "muscle silent" balance: it is both economical and stable. In cases of pelvic retroversion or anteversion, or inadequate lumbar curve, the lever arm of gravity became relatively forwards to lumbar or femoral structures, thereby inducing excessive mechanical stresses and muscle counterbalancing contractures accentuating the excessive loads on the anatomical structures: the balance was no more economical and instable. (Figure 14)

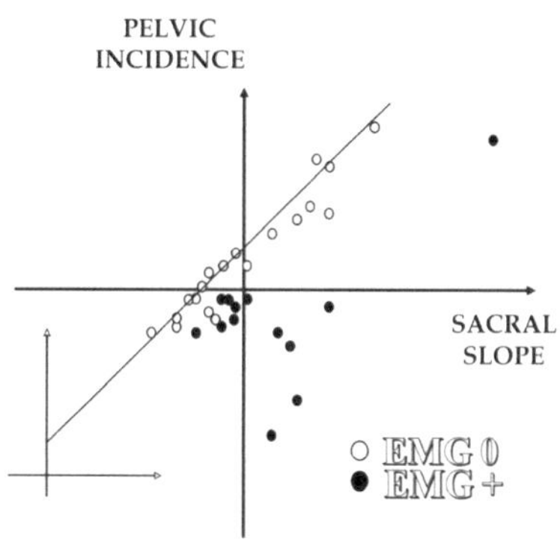

Fig. 14. Correlation between muscular contractions of the posterior muscles of the lumbar spine and the respect of the harmonious relations between the analytic parameters

4.1.2.4 Validation of the mechanical model

The data obtained by barycentremetry were similar to the data obtained by force platform for a normal standing balance. To complete the validation of the method, the values obtained by using the lever arms of the forces defined by barycentremetry were compared with data reported from the biomechanical model of Shultz-Andersson and with experimental data of the loads on the disc L3-L4 measured directly in vivo by Nachemson. (Nachemson, 1981; Shultz-Andersson, 1982)

	Standing	Sitting
Nachemson (1981)	330 N	420 N
Schultz (1982)	440 N	380 N
Duval (27 y.o., 69 kg)	362 N	396 N

Table 6. Comparison of the values of loading forces on the disc L3-L4 determined by barycentremetry and the data published by Schultz and Nachemson.

4.1.2.5 The "barycentremetry" as mechanical model of the sagittal balance

The sagittal balance of the spine was economical in terms of levers arms of the loads of gravity at each levels of the lumbo-pelvi-femoral unit, well-balanced by minimal muscular activity exerting a low flexing force in a long lever arm (the abdominal muscles, the posterior spinal muscles being inactive) or strengths in the bone or ligament structures (the rib cage). It was possible if:

- For each lumbar level, the supported center of mass was projected behind the center of rotation (which was at the posterior third within the disc)
- The center of gravity of the body segment supported by the femoral heads was projected behind the femoral heads. It was assimilated to a point located forwards of T9.

An application of gravity too far anterior will induce compressive forces and shear stresses on the vertebral structures, the discs and the ligaments, and induce rebalancing muscle contractions, which can become painful and further accentuate the excess loads on inter-vertebral structures. A twisting effect was also induced in the sacroiliac joints, the source of postural back and lower limb pain.

In reaction to a position of gravity much too anterior, the pelvic retroversion with flattening of the lordosis will bring back gravity behind the femoral heads, but the loads will be more anterior at the lumbar level because of backwards movement of the lumbar vertebrae relatively to the gravity line. Thereafter, the flexion of the hips and lower limbs will accentuate this situation less and less economical. The stresses of the posterior spinal muscles will become more important and deleterious and a source of pain throughout the spine and pelvis. (Figure 15)

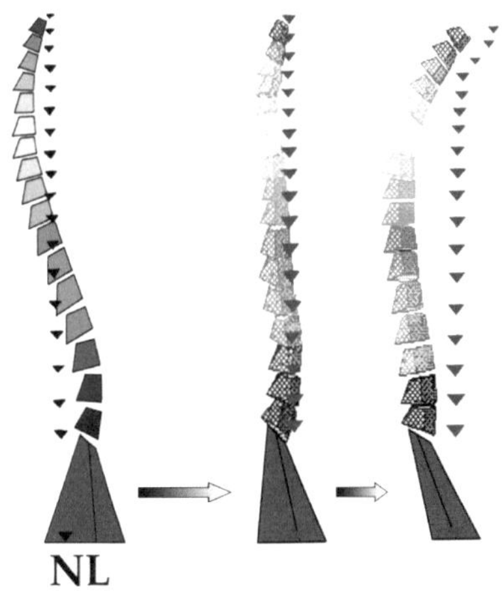

Fig. 15. Lever arms of gravity in normal and progressive anterior sagittal disturbance

4.2 Approximation of the mechanical model using the data of the barycentremetry

The barycentremetry was a laboratory technique substantiating the observations of harmonious relations between the parameters for a sagittal balance economically stable in terms of mechanical stresses. Nevertheless, such a functional evaluation of the sagittal balance appeared of first interest. Therefore, a method usable in daily medical clinical practice was elaborated, easily applicable for an individual sagittal analysis.

4.2.1 The simili-barycentremetry

For a series of 42 asymptomatic subjects and 39 scoliotic cases, the data of gravity obtained by barycentremetry and radiographic were available in concordance. From these radiographic data, several additional parameters have been defined. Since it was possible to produce an equation providing the lever arm of gravity supported at the levels L3, S1 and the femoral heads: the "simili-barycentremetry".

The evaluation was based on the fact that the center of gravity of the trunk supported by the femoral head was at the level of T9 in height. The used data were the relative overhangs of the vertebrae, the number of vertebrae included in the curvatures, anthropometric data, slopes of L3, T9, T1. (Figure 16)

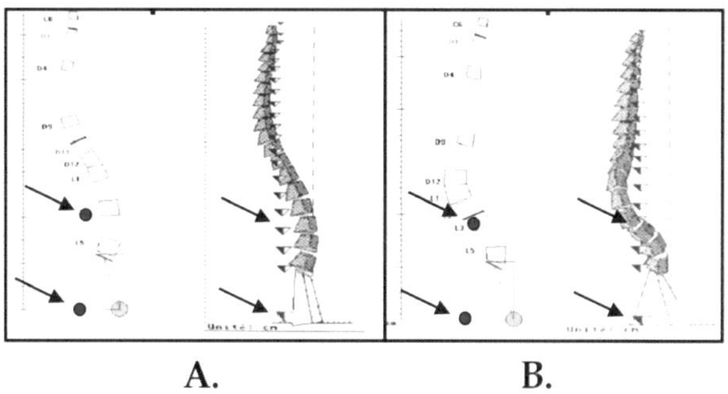

Fig. 16. Simili-barycentremetry compared to Barycentremetry for 2 cases visualizing the similarity of the location of the gravity loads at L3 and the femoral heads levels.

In order to validate the method, the results of this equation were compared with the data of the barycentremetry for the same patients on the same radiographs. (Figure 17)

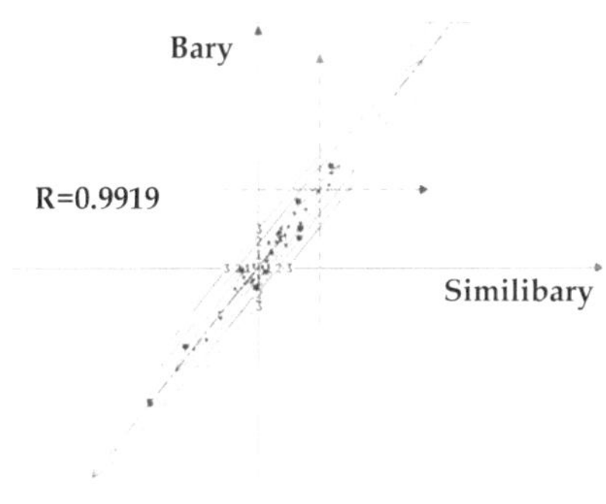

Fig. 17. Correlation of the data of the gravity loads at the level L3 by barycentremetry and using the predictive equation of simili-barycentremetry for 42 normal subjects.

Various media for three-dimensional reconstruction of the spine have integrated this simili-barycentremetry in an automated manner. Biomod 3S® (AXS Ingenery, Bordeaux-Mérignac, France) used semi-automated method for 3D reconstruction of the spine and integrated automatically the measurement of the parameters and the data of simili-barycentremetry numerically and visually. (Figure 18)

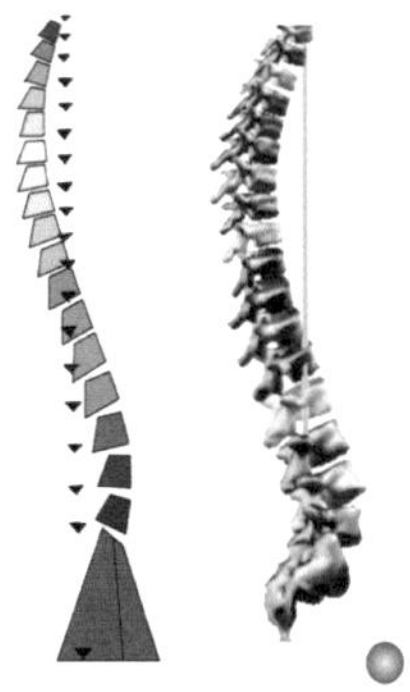

Fig. 18. Barycentremetry and simili-barycentremetry by Biomod 3S®

4.2.2 The parameters

The automated simili-barycentremetry might not be available for everyone. However, the use of individual parameters allowed an approximated functional analysis of sagittal balance finer than the analytical analysis initially described (2.3.8.) (Figure 19)

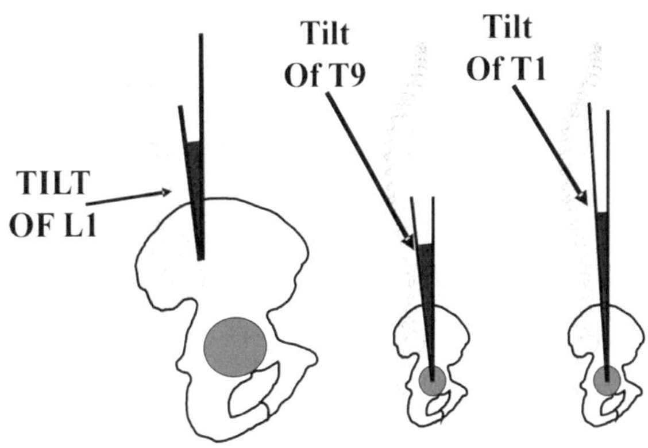

Fig. 19. The tilt parameters used for the simili-barycentremetry

4.2.2.1 The tilt of T9

The position of the center of gravity of the trunk supported by the femoral head was observed in height at T9 level (rarely T8 or T10), in front of the vertebral body from 0 to 14 mm if the kyphosis angle was less than 35 °, 20 to 32 mm if the kyphosis exceeded 35 °. Its projection was 36 mm (sd 21mm) behind the femoral heads. T9 was considered reflecting the position of center of gravity of the trunk. This position was assimilated to the tilt of T9 (angle between the vertical and the line between the hip-axis and the centre of the body of T9 (10.5° backwards, sd 3). This tilt has been observed correlated significantly (r = 0.62) with the projection of the center of gravity of the trunk on the femoral heads.

4.2.2.2 The tilt of L1

This angle was defined as the angle between the vertical and the line between the center of L1 and the lower plate of L5. It expressed the slope of the lumbar spine, independently of the pelvis orientation. Its value for asymptomatic subjects was -8 degrees (i.e. forwards), sd 5. It reflected the result at the lumbar level of the global balance, of an eventual correction of an upper disturbance in kyphosis by both the pelvis and the lumbar curve.

4.2.2.3 The tilt of T1

This angle was defined as the angle between the vertical and the line between the center of T1 and the lower plate of L5. It expressed the global tilt of the whole spine, but excluding the analysis of the pelvis rotation. This global slope value was reported to be of 3 degrees (sd 3).
It suffered of the same inconvenient as the overhang of C7.
Significant correlation between the tilt parameters were observed, testifying once more the harmony in the lumbo-pelvi-femoral complex in standing position. (Table 7)

Correlation	r=
Tilt T9 - Kyphosis	0.4214
Tilt L1 - Tilt T9	0.5935
Pelvic Incidence - Tilt L1	-0.1707

Table 7. Significant correlations between the "tilt parameters"

4.2.2.4 The role of the "Overhang of S1" and the "Pelvic thickness"

This "Overhang of S1" on the femoral heads was correlated with the "Pelvic Incidence" by the intermediary of the "Pelvic Tilting" (OVH S1/ PT r = 0.80, PT/ PI r = 0.54). Therefore, the overhang was the greater in case of major value of "Pelvic Incidence", the greater were the gravity loads of the trunk projected behind the femoral heads. Also the "Pelvic Thickness" (inversely related to Pelvic Incidence r=0.334) was observed to affect the lever arm of action of the lumbo-pelvic muscles. As well, the lever arms of action of the gluteus maximus was important in case of high value of PI, PT, OVH S1 and low value of Pelvic Thickness. Contrarily, in case of low value of pelvic incidence, the gravity was projected less backwards to the femoral heads (and so the risk of disruption of the balance was greater), the values of PT and OVH S1 were lower, but the pelvic thickness was greater (the static and dynamical structures are so more vertical and such less efficient) and the lever arm of the gluteus maximus was shorter.(Figure 20) It these cases, the risk of torsion strength in the sacro-iliac joints would be greater.

5. Conclusion

In his search for the economy, the organism creates and manages moderate curves closer to the line of gravity. The lever arm of gravity remains as small as possible.
The use of the described parameters allows a functional personalized analysis of the sagittal balance of an individual.
But some questions remain:

- what is the acceptable lordosis deficit, related to the ideal value for the spine that will be able to support the age-related changes without decompensate and induce pain? We can just affirm that the lordosis (and the pelvic and spinal parameters) must be as close as possible to the ideal values

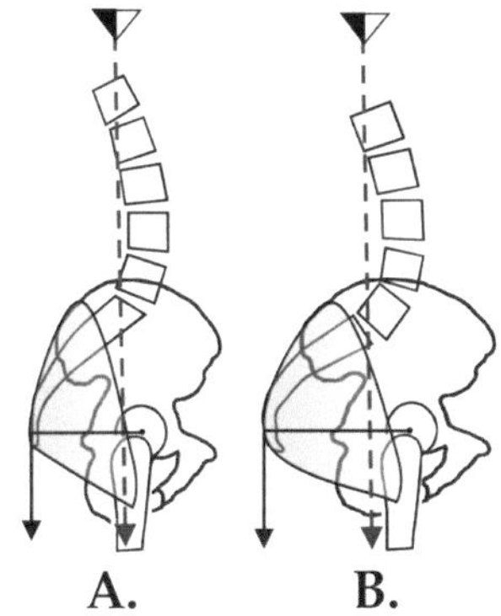

Fig. 20. Relation between Pelvic incidence (A low value, B high value) and the lever arm of gravity on the femoral heads and the lever arm of action of the gluteus maximus.

- what are the real and practical ways to restore a sufficient lordosis, either surgically or functionally? Probably, the use of a navigation device of the lumbar curve during surgery has a place for the surgical regulating. The real question is concerning a truly lordosing surgery (a vertebral osteotomy). But in this case, the correction must be complete and does not tolerate a residual deficit.
- what is the optimal ratio of benefit- risk in such serious and potentially iatrogenic procedures? Also the restoration of an adequate value according to the harmony between the parameters must be made. The global balance of the individual must be taken into account, including the cervical spine, the hips and the lower limbs including the knees and the ankles.

It can be concluded and counseled to fuse only when necessary, and in any case never lose any lordosis (by installation of the hips in extension and not in flexion, not fusing longer than indispensable, avoiding the often kyphosing surgical procedures (as inter-spinous blocks or other devices). The balancing factors take precedence over segmental lesions. Surgical procedures as inter-body fusion or disc prosthesis should not be performed in case of pre-operative loss of lordosis, because results will be unsatisfactory and involve adjacent complications. (Figure 21)

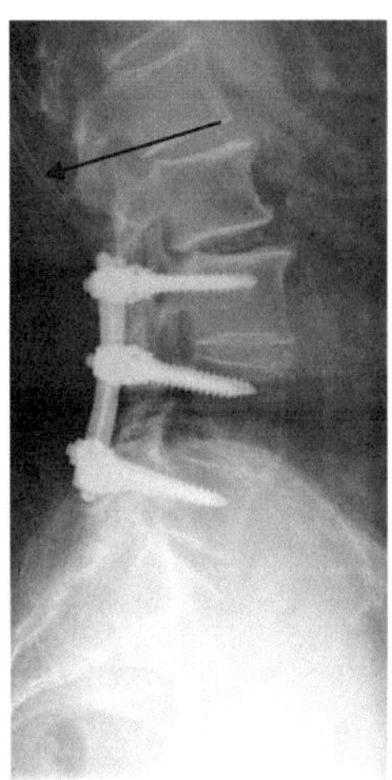

Fig. 21. Retro-listhesis in compensation to a loss of lordosis induced by the device

6. Prospects

The data reported allowed now to access an individualized functional analysis of the sagittal total balance of the lumbo-spino-pelvic complex in standing position.
However, this analysis is static and not integrated into the movement and the daily activity of the subject. The immobile bipedal station is exceptional. The acquisition of dynamic data incorporating the described parameters could assess the loads supported by the spino-pelvic structures during daily activities.
Nevertheless, actual technical devices for measuring parameters require irradiation which could become significant if the acquisitions had to be repeated, especially dynamically. For this reason, optical acquisition techniques have been developed. Currently static and repeated over time, they allowed an analytical study of the sagittal balance of a subject, its evolution and individual strategies of adaptation, after an initial radiograph using the parameters described. (Figure 22A) The simulation of the position of bony structures within the skin envelope was actually elaborated and validated. (Figure 22 B)

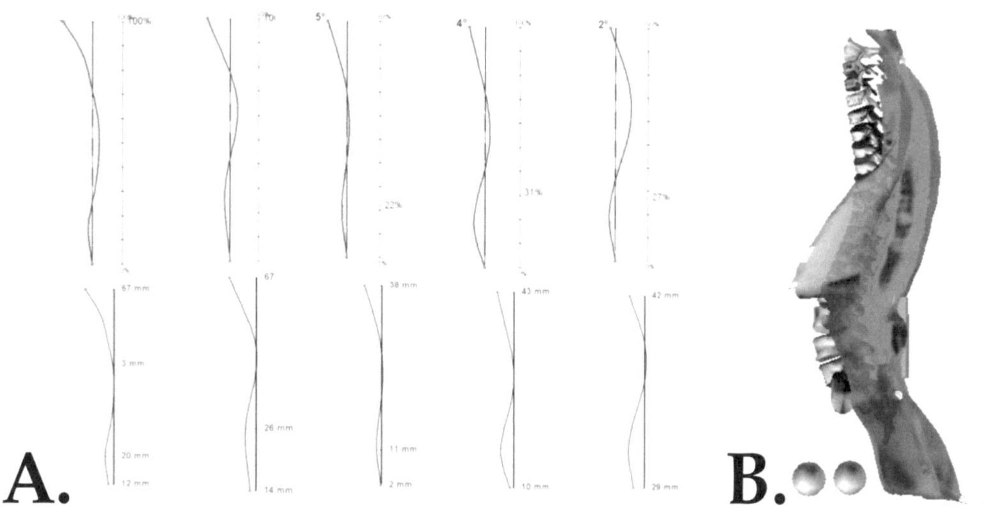

Fig. 22. Sagittal evolution of the shapes of a case during 2 years by optical assessment (A) and bony structures related to the back skin surface (B) (Biomod L® and Biomod 3S®)

Dynamic acquisitions of skin surfaces by these methods allow now an optical motion analysis, the detection of abnormal movements or segmental stiffness. The acquisition of three-dimensional envelope allows an assessment of the mass of body segments and thus the position of the centers of gravity into the body. Combined with an X-ray, real or extrapolated, this promising technology will allow a functional evaluation of all individual lumbo pelvic-femoral balance in the real life in movement.

7. References

Boulay, C. et al. (2006). Sagittal alignment of spine and pelvis regulated by pelvic incidence: standard values and prediction of lordosis. *Eur Spine J*, Vol. 15, pp. 415–422

Dubousset, J. (1984). The pelvis « intercalary bone ». *Monograph of the GES*, Paris, p. 15-22

During, J. et al. (1985). Toward standards for posture. Postural characteristics of the lower back system in normal and pathologic conditions. *Spine*, Vol. 10, Issue 1, pp. 83-7

Duval-Beaupère, G. & Robain, G. (1987). Visualization on full spine radiographs of the anatomical connections of the centres of the segmental body mass supported by each vertebra and measured in vivo. *Int Orthop*, Vol 11, Issue 3, pp. 261-9

Duval-Beaupère, G.; Schmidt, C. & Cosson, P. (1992). A Barycentremetric study of the sagittal shape of spine and pelvis: the conditions required for an economic standing position. *Ann Biomed Eng*, Vol. 20, Issue 4, pp. 451-62

Duval-Beaupère, G. et al. (1998). Pelvic incidence: a fundamental parameter for three-dimensional regulation of spinal sagittal curves. *Eur Spine J*, Vol. 7, pp. 99-103

Duval-Beaupère, G. (2008). Gravitational forces and sagittal shape of the spine. Clinical estimation of their relations. *Int Orthop*, Vol. 32, Issue 6, pp. 809-16

Gangnet, N. et al. (2003). Variability of the spine and pelvis location with respect to the gravity line: a three-dimensional stereoradiographic study using a force platform. *Surg Radiol Anat*, Vol. 25, pp. 424-33

Gelb, D.E. (1995). An analysis of sagittal alignment in 100 asymptomatic middle or aged volunteers. *Spine*, vol. 20, pp. 1351-8.

Gottfried, O.N. et al. (2009). Spinopelvic parameters in postfusion flatback deformity patients. *Spine J*, Vol. 9, Issue 8, pp. 639-47

Guigui, P. et al. (2003). Physiological value of pelvic and spinal parameters of sagital balance: analysis of 250 Healthy volunteers. *Rev Chir Orthop Reparatrice Appar Mot*, vol. 89, Issue 6, pp. 496-506

Hanson, D.S. et al. (2002) Correlation of pelvic incidence with low- and high-grade isthmic spondylolisthesis. *Spine*, Vol. 27, Issue 18, pp. 2026-9

Huang, R.P.; Bohlman, H.H. & Thompson, GH. (2003). Predictive value of pelvic incidence in progression of spondylolisthesis. *Spine*, Vol. 28, pp. 2381-2385

Jackson, R.P. & McManus, A.C. (1994). Radiographic analysis plane alignment and balance in standing volunteers and patients with low back an matched for age, sex and size. *Spine*, Vol. 19., Issue 14, pp. 1611-8

Jackson, R.P. & Hales, C. (2000). Congruent spinopelvic alignment on standing lateral radiographs of adult volunteers. *Spine*, Vol. 25, pp. 2808-2815

Kawakami, M. et al. (2002). Lumbar sagittal balance influences the clinical outcome after decompression and posterolateral spinal fusion for degenerative lumbar spondylolisthesis. *Spine*, Vol. 27, Issue 1, pp. 59-64

Korovessis, P.G.; Stamatakis, M.V.& Baikousis, A.G. (1998). Reciprocal angulation of vertebral bodies in the sagittal plane in an asymptomatic Greek population. *Spine*, Vol. 23, Issue 6, pp. 700-5

Kumar, M.N.; Baklanov, A. & Chopin, D. (2001). Correlation between sagittal plane changes and adjacent segment degeneration following lumbar spine fusion. *Eur Spine J*, Vol. 10, Issue 4, pp. 314-9

Labelle, H. et al. (2004). Spondylolisthesis, pelvic incidence, and spinopelvic balance: A correlation study. *Spine*, Vol. 29, Issue18, pp. 2049-2054

Labelle, H. et al. (2005). The importance of spino-pelvic balance in L5-s1 developmental spondylolisthesis: a review of pertinent radiologic measurements. Spine, Vol. 30, Issue 6, pp. S27-34

Lazennec, JY. Et al. (2000). Sagittal alignment in lumbosacral fusion: relations between radiological parameters and pain. *Eur Spine J*, Vol. 9, Issue 1, pp.47-55

Marty, C. et al. (2002). The sagittal anatomy of the sacrum among young adults, infants and spondylolisthesis patients. *Eur Spine J*, Vol. 11, pp. 119-25

Morel, E. et al. (2005). Sagittal balance of the spine and degenerative spondylolisthesis. *Rev Chir Orthop Reparatrice Appar Mot*, Vol. 91, Issue 7, pp. 615-26

Nachemson, A.L. (1981). Disc pressure measurements. *Spine*, Vol. 6, Issue 1, pp. 93-7

Schultz, A. & Andersson, G. (1981). Analysis of loads on the lumbar spine. Spine, Vol.6, Issue 1, pp. 76–82

Schultz, A.; Andersson, G. et al. (1982). Loads on the lumbar spine. Validation of a biomechanical analysis by measurements of intradiscal pressures and myoelectric signals. *J Bone Joint Surg Am*, Vol. 64, Issue 5, pp. 713-20

Vaz, G. et al. (2002). Sagittal morphology and equilibrium of pelvis and spine. *Eur Spine J*, Vol. 11, pp. 80–87

Vedantam, R. et al. (1998). Comparison of standing sagittal spinal alignment in asymptomatic adolescents and adults. *Spine*, vol. 23, pp. 211-5

Vedantam, R. et al. (2000). The effect of the variation in arm position on sagittal spnal alignment. *Spine*, Vol. 25, Issue 17, pp. 2204-9

Vialle, R. et al. (2005). Radiographic Analysis of the Sagittal Alignment and Balance of the Spine in Asymptomatic Subjects. *J Bone Joint Surg (Am)*, Vol. 87, Issue 2, pp. 260-267

Vialle, R. et al. (2005). Radiological assessment of lumbosacral dystrophic changes in high-grade spondylolisthesis. *Skeletal Radiol*, Vol. 34, Issue 9, pp. 528-35

Vialle, R. et al. (2007) Sacral and lumbar-pelvic morphology in high-grade spondylolisthesis. *Orthopedics*, Vol. 30, Issue 8, pp. 642-9

Vialle, R. et al. (2007). Is there a sagittal imbalance of the spine in isthmic spondylolisthesis? A correlation study. Eur Spine J, Vol. 16, Issue 10, pp. 1641-9

Wodecki,P. et al. (2002). Sagittal alignment of the spine: comparison between soccer players and subjects without sports activities. *Rev Chir Orthop Reparatrice Appar Mot*, Vol. 88, Issue 4, pp. 328-36

Part 4

Human and Animal Biomechanics

11

Potentialities and Criticalities of Plantar Pressure Measurements in the Study of Foot Biomechanics: Devices, Methodologies and Applications

Claudia Giacomozzi
Istituto Superiore di Sanità (Italian National Institute of Health)
Italy

1. Introduction

Literally speaking, Biomechanics is the discipline that applies the principles and laws of Mechanics to biological systems. As for the human body and, more specifically, the human foot, biomechanics focuses on the understanding of those laws of the Physics by which the human being moves within the Earth gravitational environment by adopting a bipedal posture and using a complex interfacing structure such as the foot-and-ankle system. Keeping the focus on the most common human displacement activity, i.e., gait, we may state that the main target of a functional gait is to push the body centre of gravity forward. To do that, gait has to deal with a set of forces the body exchanges with the environment - especially with the ground - and with a set of movements which represent both causes and effects of force transmission. A thorough description of the foot biomechanics should then mainly rely on the observation of both kinematic and kinetic variables, namely, i) forces and moments of force external to the body; ii) forces and moments of force internally generated by the musculo-skeletal system; and iii) movements and timing of the movements in terms of linear and angular displacements, linear and angular velocities, linear and angular accelerations of the whole body or of specific body segments. On the other hand, the effects of loading under the sole of the foot in terms of plantar pressure have been reported since the late 1800's; and since the first attempts to measure it, its use has been ever increasing worldwide. In fact, plantar pressure assessment alone is not enough to thoroughly investigate biomechanics - in terms of neither kinematics nor kinetics - being pressure related to the only component of the force vector which is normal to the examined surface. Plantar pressure, however, has great potentialities in the field of Research but even more in Clinics and Podiatry. When compared with other assessment devices typically used in gait analysis, pressure measurement systems are easier to implement and use, less time-consuming and cumbersome to the patient, less expensive than complex gait analysis equipment; measurements are more easily acquired, processed and interpreted, and - last but not least - they are meaningful and effective in the assessment or in the monitoring of any foot or ankle treatment. In the last ten years, a significant increase has been observed in peer-reviewed publications dealing with studies focussed on plantar pressure measurements. However, despite the great interest of the scientific world in this potentially valuable assessment tool, little evidence has been gathered so far of the effectiveness, appropriateness and generalisability of the plantar pressure measurement methodology. This fact is attributable to several reasons, the most important one being the lack of standardisation. In the following paragraphs, a brief literature overview will be given to better introduce the role pressure measurements have in the scientific and clinical context, but also to better explain how and to what extent the lack of standardisation of instrumentation and procedures has frustrated all researchers' and clinicians' efforts at giving this methodology the role it deserves in the investigation, understanding and management of foot biomechanics.

2. Literature overview

The main source this brief literature overview relies on is the PubMed Web Resource, the specific tool to search in databases of peer-reviewed scientific literature in the biomedical field. PubMed is freely accessible on the web (http://www.ncbi.nlm.nih.gov/pubmed/), and its more than 20 million citations for biomedical literature come from MEDLINE – the biomedical database of the U.S. NLM -, life science journals, and online books. This precious free resource has been developed and is maintained by the National Center for Biotechnology Information (NCBI), at the U.S. National Library of Medicine (NLM), located at the National Institutes of Health (NIH).

Search combination	Search date	Total number of publications	Publications in the last ten years	Year of the first publication
„foot" & „biomechanics"	Jan 17th, 2011	3975	2132 (54%)	1950
„foot" & „biomechanics" & „pressure"	Jan 17th, 2011	767	470 (61%)	1966
„foot" & „pressure"	Jan 17th, 2011	5605	2807 (50%)	1918
„foot pressure"	Jan 17th, 2011	473	275 (58%)	1980
„foot biomechanics"	Jan 17th, 2011	58	40 (69%)	1973
„plantar pressure" or „plantar loading" or „foot pressure" or „foot loading"	Jan 17th, 2011	1124	748 (66%)	1976

Table 1. Publications cited in PubMed resulting from different combinations of search terms that regard foot biomechanics and plantar pressure.

The Author has used a few research combinations just to understand whether and how human plantar pressure measurements are used and associated with the concepts of foot biomechanics and gait. Table 1 briefly indicates the most interesting combinations of search terms, and the main results obtained for each of them up to January 2011 in terms of: i) the overall number of papers found that contain the search terms in all PubMed fields of research; ii) the subset of papers published in the last ten years; iii) the year of the first publication.

Table 1 clearly shows that, generally speaking, foot biomechanics is quite a recent field of scientific investigation which is rapidly gaining interest worlwide. All search combinations proved in fact that at least 50% of the literature is concentrated in the last ten years. With special attention to pressure, it is worth noticing that 20% of all the publications containing "foot" & "biomechanics" also contain "pressure"; the percentage rises to 22% when referred to the last ten years, showing a more frequent association of the concept of "pressure" with the concept of "biomechanics". As for the great number of publications found for the "foot" & "pressure"combination, it should be noted that some of them do not deal with foot pressure proper, being sometimes focussed on clinical applications and/or on patients with concurrent blood pressure pathologies. Thus, the literature overview was finally focussed on the search combination reported in the last row of Table 1, i.e., „plantar pressure" or „plantar loading" or „foot pressure" or „foot loading", which turned out to be wide enough and appropriate. From now on, the paper will only deal with this combination of literature research.

As shown in Table 1, the first peer-reviewed publication is quite recent (Gordon, 1976). Actually, the very first paper resulting from the PubMed research is dated 1953 (Cram, 1953), but it is a misprint since the true title is "A sign of sciatic nerve root pressure" rather than "A sign of sciatic nerve foot pressure" as stored in the database, and it has nothing to do with plantar pressure measurement. In about 35 years, 1124 publications have been produced in all, 66% of which in the last ten years. The brief literature overview that follows is based on only 119 publications dated 2010, so as to give an idea of the most recent issues taken into account in this field. Here is a summary of a few interesting observations:

- 86 out of the 119 papers (72% of the total amount) indeed deal with plantar pressure measurements; they have been listed in the Reference section from (Morrison et al, 2010) to (Tessutti et al, 2010).
- Of the 86 publications, 75 (87%) deal with clinical or research applications, while the remaining 11 (13%) address methodological issues. On one hand, this shows the great potential of plantar pressure measurements in the Clinics or in the field of Applied Research; on the other hand, however, the presence of more than 10% of methodological papers may be read as a sign of a moderate but increasing interest towards methodological and standardisation issues. For a more detailed description of Clinical, Sport or Research applications, Table 2 classifies the 86 papers according to the main pathology or issue treated. It is worth highlighting that some pathologies are almost always investigated with the support of plantar pressure measurements – i.e., foot, ankle and hip pathologies, foot surgery, orthosis design and assessment, musculo-skeletal performance -, some do not require pressure measurement investigation as is the case with Parkinson's disease, a few others are partly investigated by involving pressure measurements and partly only relying on different investigation methods – i.e. balance control, diabetes, gait biomechanics, foot injuries -. As for Diabetes, it should be observed that in the last years most scientific studies on Diabetes and foot biomechanics did rely almost exclusively on plantar pressure measurements, both barefoot and inside prescribed footwear and orthoses. The main reason for this is probably the interest of researchers on the most evident effect of biomechanical alterations, i.e. abnormal peak pressures so often associated with the ulceration process. Only recently has the need been felt for a more complete investigation of biomechanical alterations Diabetes induces in all the structures involved in gait i.e. joints, muscles, tendons, soft tissues, skin, bone, cartilage, peripheral vascular system, motor and sensory nervous system.

- Back to Table 2, it is also extremely important to underline that all 2010 methodological studies are related to pressure measurements.
- With respect to the specific field of application, the 86 papers can be grouped as follows: 69 papers strictly related to the clinical context; 1 to the military environment; 8 to sports; 8 to technology.
- Only 45 out of the 86 publications do report absolute pressure values. This concept is critical indeed, and will be further discussed later on; however, it is worth anticipating that reporting absolute pressure values obtained within a certain study may help understand the appropriateness of the whole methodological setup designed and used in the study, and surely helps researchers to better judge the comparability of his/her own results with those reported in the study.
- As for the technology used in the 86 publications, an increasing interest in wearable devices has been observed with respect to previous years. In detail: in 46 studies a pressure platform was used, i.e. a rigid sensor matrix made integral with the floor; 32 used an in-shoe wearable pressure system; 2 used a custom-made platform purposely designed for pressure and shear measurements; 1 used a footprinting mat; 5 used discrete pressure sensors.
- Still on technology, in a commercial versus prototype pressure devices context, it can be observed that about 60% of the 86 studies used commercial pressure measurement devices. The involved Companies/Products ordered according to a decreasing number of citations are: Novel; Tekscan; Rsscan; Biofoot/IBV(®) in-shoe system; Zebris; Medilogic; Harris footprinting mat; Vista Medical. Only 5 studies described and used prototypes among which a quite new in-shoe prototype of a textile device (Shu L et al, 2010) is worth citing. In the remaining cases, the device was not clearly described, which, together with the lack of absolute pressure values, might represent an obstacle for correct data interpretation and comparison.
- As for the pressure-related parameters used, the situation is quite confusing. Just a few comments to give the reader a rough idea of the need for standardisation, and to well justify the current difficulty in performing proper comparisons among studies:
  - Some "conventional" parameters are frequently cited and used in the papers, e.g., peak pressure, mean pressure, pressure-time integral, peak force, force-time integral, center of pressure, stance period, and symmetry indices, but almost none of the studies describe the way each parameter has been obtained; thus, while some of them are undoubtedly always obtained in the same manner, for others critical differences in the computation algorithm surely lead to different results. Mean pressure is a clear example: its value changes dramatically according to whether it is based on the whole stance period or only on the period of each sensor activation.
  - Meaningful regional masks are used in several papers but they are hardly defined, and even rarer is the detailed description of the algorithm used to select the foot sub-areas.
  - There is an increasing interest towards pressure-derived quantities and novel numerical analysis: while acknowledging the great potential of such computational approach, the risk to obtain poorly comparable results is in this case even greater than when traditional parameters are used, unless comparison is assured and proved with respect to the source datasets. Besides this aspect, derived quantities should be even better described than traditional ones because sometimes their

clinical association, relevance and meaning are not straightforward for an effective worldwide use.

- The final observation is rather a criticism to the superficial attitude and the lack of attention shown by the main actors of a publication, i.e. authors, reviewers, editors, and even readers: peer-reviewed 2010 publications, similarly to the publications of previous years, sometimes present data that may not be, in any way, related to a properly conducted study. Five examples of dubious measurements are briefly reported below. papers are not clearly cited in order to be respectful with colleagues who did not pay the proper attention while preparing, reviewing or simply reading them. Example 1: according to a study, electronic footprints do not match ink footprints: it is reasonable to hypothesize that the statement came out from comparison with a platform which was not well calibrated or not sensible enough, or even with a very low spatial resolution, but none of these aspects was taken into account in the paper. Example 2: a platform made of resistive sensors is used for static tests lasting more than 30s. Since resistive sensors suffer from hysteresis and creep, their use under static conditions is usually not recommended, unless a preliminary assessment proved that the device can be reliably used for a long loading time. Again, the issue is not discussed in the paper. Example 3: a paper dealing with obese patients (BMI > 35kg/m^2) reported dynamic peak pressures not greater than 250kPa. These values are suspiciously low: for comparison, consider that a paper published in 2001 (Hills AP et al, 2001) reported more than 500kPa of averaged peak pressure values for both men and women. Example 4: a paper reports peak pressures under the forefoot not greater than 35kPa, which is almost impossible: even if the authors meant mean rather than peak pressure - mean being obviously much lower than peak pressure - the result would have been obtained from a person with a body mass of about 35kg standing on a support surface of 100cm^2, thus greater than the EU size 38 or US size 7. Example 5: a paper deals with pressure measurements obtained with a pressure platform while wearing shoes: this means that the measurements are inconsistent for they refer to the interface between the platform and the sole of the shoe.

Main Pathology/Issue	Number of papers dealing with pressure measurements (% of 86)	Publications dealing with pressure measurements	Number of papers in 2010 -not all dealing with pressure measurements (% of 119)
Ankle pathology	2 (2.3%)	Morrison et al, 2010 Rouhani et al, 2010 a	2 (1.7%)
Anthropology	1 (1.2%)	Hirasaki et al, 2010	3 (2.5%)
Balance control	2 (2.3%)	Hirata et al, 2010 Vuillerme & Boisgontier, 2010	10 (8.4%)
Children	4 (4.6%)	Pau et al, 2010 Bosch et al, 2010 Bosch & Rosenbaum, 2010 Pauk et al, 2010	5 (4.2%)

Main Pathology/Issue	Number of papers dealing with pressure measurements (% of 86)	Publications dealing with pressure measurements	Number of papers in 2010 -not all dealing with pressure measurements (% of 119)
Diabetes	8 (9.3%)	do Carmo Dos Reis et al, 2010 Zequera & Solomonidis, 2010 Cisneros Lde et al, 2010 Hastings et al, 2010 See et al, 2010 Z. Pataky et al, 2010 Chen et al, 2010 Rao et al, 2010	14 (11.8%)
Elderly	1 (1.2%)	Battaglia et al, 2010	1 (0.8%)
Falls	2 (2.3%)	Abu-Faraj et al, 2010 Mickle et al, 2010	2 (1.7%)
Foot injuries	4 (4.6%)	Goffar et al, 2010 Hirschmüller et al, 2010 Schepers et al, 2010 Hetsroni et al, 2010	7 (5.9%)
Foot pathology, anatomy and function	15 (17.4%)	Navarro et al, 2010 Yalçin et al, 2010 Kaipel et al, 2010 Lee et al, 2010 Hyslop et al, 2010 Ribeiro et al, 2010 Mackey et al, 2010 Yavuz et al, 2010 Martínez-Nova et al, 2010 Gu et al, 2010 Barberà i Guillem et al, 2010 Yavuz & Davis, 2010 Nordsiden et al, 2010 Putti et al, 2010 b Menz et al, 2010	17 (14.3%)
Foot surgery	7 (8.1%)	Schuh et al, 2010 a Bayomy et al, 2010 Wagenmann et al, 2010 Yoon et al, 2010 Ellis et al, 2010 Jeans & Karol, 2010 Najafi et al, 2010	7 (5.9%)

Table 2. Part A. 2010 Publications dealing with plantar pressure measurement, classified according to the main pathology or the main issues investigated.

Main Pathology/Issue	Number of papers dealing with pressure measurements (% of 86)	Publications dealing with pressure measurements	Number of papers in 2010 -not all dealing with pressure measurements (% of 119)
Footwear and/or insoles	6 (7.0%)	Hong et al, 2010 Deleu et al, 2010 Stöggl et al, 2010 Schuh et al, 2010 b Tong & Ng, 2010 Queen et al, 2010	7 (5.9%)
Gait strategy/biomechanics	6 (7.0%)	Putti et al, 2010 b Teyhen et al, 2010 C.M. Senanayake & S.M. Senanayake, 2010 a C.M. Senanayake & S.M. Senanayake, 2010 b Rouhani et al, 2010 b M. D'Amico et al, 2010	8 (6.7%)
Knee pathology	4 (4.6%)	Bek et al, 2010 Wang et al, 2010 Lidtke et al, 2010 Aliberti et al, 2010	4 (3.4%)
Lower limb amputees	2 (2.3%)	Kendell et al, 2010 Tura et al, 2010	2 (1.7%)
Lower limb injuries	1 (1.2%)	Kelly et al, 2010	1 (0.8%)
Muscolo-skeletal performance	5 (5.8%)	Braz & Carvalho, 2010 Girard et al, 2010 Stolwijk et al, 2010 No authors, 2010 Tessutti et al, 2010	5 (4.2%)
Postmenopausal women	4 (4.6%)	Monteiro et al, 2010 a Monteiro et al, 2010 b Faria et al, 2010 Monteiro et al, 2010 c	4 (3.4%)
Pregnancy	1 (1.2%)	Karadag-Saygi et al, 2010	1 (0.8%)
NONE (research; methodology;..)	11 (12.8%)	Giacomozzi, 2010 a Natali et al, 2010 Oliveira & Tavares, 2010 Giacomozzi, 2010 b Zammit et al, 2010 Miller, 2010 Ramanathan et al, 2010 Giacomozzi, 2010 c Shu et al, 2010 Chevalier et al, 2010 Keijsers et al, 2010	11 (9.2%)
Total	86 (100%)		119* (100%)

* the list of 2010 papers also included papers – not related to pressure measurements - dealing with: gait rehabilitation (1); ground interfaces (1); obesity (2); Parkinson's disease (4).

Table 2. Part B. 2010 Publications dealing with plantar pressure measurement, classified according to the main pathology or the main issues investigated.

3. Pressure measurement devices (PMDs): Technical and performance issues

In 2010 great attention was paid to the technical aspects of plantar pressure measurement. Awareness is growing in the scientific environment about the key point: in order to render pressure measurements appropriate, comparable, meaningful and effective, the process towards standardisation has to start with the assessment of the technical performance of the pressure measurement devices (PMDs) through which pressure is quantified. Some proposals have been published and disseminated so far through publications (Giacomozzi C, 2010 a; Giacomozzi C, 2010 b; Giacomozzi C, 2010 c), meetings, on-line forums[1], and an ongoing attempt within the Pedobarographic Group of the International Foot and Ankle Biomechanics Community (i-FAB-PG) for a Consensus Document on the topic. The following paragraphs aim at giving the reader a brief description of the currently available pressure sensor technology, the technical features which mainly interfere with overall PMD performance, some suggestions for implementing an adequate PMD technical assessment.

3.1 Basic concepts on PMD sensor technology

Generally speaking, the measurement of pressure can be obtained with a transducer that quantifies the effect of a force acting perpendicularly to a certain surface. This definition must be clearly kept in mind when investigating foot biomechanics with a PMD because, independently of sensor technology, a pressure sensor alone cannot measure the effect of forces which are not oriented perpendicularly to its surface. Even more important is the concept that, if the sensor surface is not parallel to the ground - as it may happen with in-shoe systems or when the floor is not rigorously horizontal -, the measured quantity is not only, or not completely, related to the vertical component of the Ground Reaction Force (GRF).

Along the years valuable reviews have been delivered on the available sensor technology, novel prototypes, their main features and quality of performance. The first interesting and thorough review was written by Lord in 1981 (Lord M, 1981). Another very good technical review was disseminated by Cobb and Claremont in 1995 (Cobb J, Claremont DJ, 1995): interestingly enough, it also addressed transducers applied to the measurement of shear forces. Albeit highly desirable, none of them have been successfully integrated into commercial pressure measurement systems yet. A further very useful review on the issue of plantar assessment was published in 2000 (Orlin MN, McPoil TG, 2000): it contains not only a thorough review of the available pressure measuring techniques, but also a stimulating discussion on most used parameters and potential clinical applications.

Right now -at the beginning of 2011- commercial PMDs and most prototypes are still focussed on pure pressure measurements, and are essentially based on optical devices, pneumatic discrete sensors, discrete -or matrices of- resistive sensors, and discrete -or matrices of- capacitive sensors. Worthy of note is a novel textile sensor prototype. Low-cost, semiquantitative pressure measurement solutions are not taken into account here, while they are discussed in (Orlin MN, McPoil TG, 2000). Each of the above sensing solutions will

[1]A) The Italian National Institute of Health (ISS) hosts an on-line moodle-based Forum dedicated to PMDs at http://vcms.iss.it/moodle19/. Registration is free. Contact c_giacomozzi@yahoo.com for assistance. B) The international community of Foot and Ankle Biomechanics (i-FAB) hosts an on-line moodle-based Forum of the i-FAB Pedobarographic Group at http://moodle.i-fab.org//. Free registration is suggested. Contact c_giacomozzi@yahoo.com for assistance.

be briefly described here below, but a first important aspect -which is common to all PMDs with the only exception of optical technology- is **sensor size**. In fact, the smaller the sensor, the higher its sensitivity and its potential to accurately detect localized peak pressures - otherwise underestimated because averaged over the entire surface of a wider sensor. Conversely, the electrical noise of extremely small sensors may increase owing to the necessary greater amplification of the signal, and may thus interfere with sensor accuracy and repeatability. Besides this, the simultaneous electrical management of a very high number of sensors on the same sensor matrix at a high scanning rate might become a critical issue to cope with. For a proper detection of localized peak pressures under the human foot, a linear size of 2-3mm might be reasonable for a sensor, basing this estimation on location and dimension of the metatarsal heads and on the expected local pressure curve.

Brief description of current sensor technologies.

Optical devices

Obviously, they are only aimed at measuring pressures through platforms fixed to the measurement environment, thus this kind of technology is not usable for in-shoe assessment. A good example of an optical pedobarograph - namely the Sheffield pedobarograph - was first described in 1982 (Duckworth T et al, 1982). Basically, the pedobarograph is made of an illuminated glass plate covered with a plastic sheet. When the sheet is pressed on the glass, light scatters and generates a foot image which is captured by a camera at the bottom of the device, and then digitized. Pressure variations are thus measured by quantifying the variations of voltage level in the camera output, which are associated with the variations of intensity of the captured image. It is worth noting here that spatial resolution -further discussed in the following paragraphs as a critical PMD technical feature- is in this case extremely high. The relevance of the use of the optical device in Clinics was reported soon after (Duckworth T et al, 1985), and is still reported in the lastest papers (Ramanathan AK et al, 2009).

Pneumatic discrete sensors

A hydrocell-based technology is used within the commercial in-shoe Parotec System. Unlike the optical technology, this one is only used for in-shoe pressure measurements under specific local foot areas. Basically, each sensor is made of a small volume of an incompressible fluid contained in a small polyurethane pack, integral with a microsensor placed just beneath it, and isolated by a thin dielectric foil. An interesting technical paper which analyses some aspects of the performance of the Parotec system was published in 2000 (Chesnin KJ et al, 2000). The paper reports the following relevant technical features: 24 sensors on each insole; pressure range up to 625kPa; pressure resolution 2.5kPa; good accuracy (2%FS); high precision (0.4%FS); negligible hysteresis and drift; very low temperature drift, humidity drift and non-linearity; insole height 3mm; sampling rate 100Hz.

Textile sensor

An interesting novel prototype of a fabric pressure sensor is described in Shu's 2010 paper (Shu L et al, 2010). In brief, each pressure sensor is obtained by fixing a conductive sensing fabric onto a conductive yarn and on a top-bottom conversion layer made of different silicon rubbers. The paper illustrates the main technical features of a prototype insole containing 6 sensors, suggesting it for sports and fitness assessment, i.e.: sampling rate 100Hz; pressure range 0-1000kPa; pressure resolution 1kPa; life-time > 100000 cycles; negligible temperature and humidity effects; low cost. The height of the insole is not reported in the paper, which might be a relevant issue to be taken into account.

Resistive sensors

One of the two most widely used sensor technologies (the other being the capacitive technology briefly discussed soon after), which may be arranged under the form of arrays of discrete sensors, platforms, or in-shoe systems. Available commercial systems are delivered worldwide by the following Companies: Diagnostic Support (platforms), Imago (platforms), Loran (platforms and in-shoe systems), Medilogic (platforms), Rsscan (platforms), Tekscan (platforms and in-shoe systems), Vista Medical (platforms). There are other brands on the market, but the products are usually made by one of the above Companies. A common functioning principle of the different resistive sensors is that they rely on an electrical current flow whose intensity depends on the pressure exerted on the sensor surface. When the effective contact area of the sensor increases due to pressure, electrical conductivity increases as well, in a roughly linear fashion, within a certain range of pressure. In some cases the change of conductivity is due to a volume effect rather than a contact surface effect, and an elastic deformation takes place in the conductive material. In general, manufacturers have to deal with low-impedance sensors - hence the good performance with respect to noise immunity –, but with some drawbacks such as hysteresis, fast ageing, instability. A special type of resistive devices is also on the market, i.e. long platforms which only act as resistive "contacts" and which are addressed to the measurement of spatial and temporal parameters of gait. Even though some of them - as for example the GaitRite (www.gaitrite.com) - deliver some "pressure" levels rather than only an on-off answer, it is extremely important to keep in mind that they only represent a qualitative output, in no way appropriate for quantitative pressure analysis.

Capacitive sensors

Their functioning principle is the variation of capacitance induced by a variation of pressure exerted on the sensor surface. The different commercial products use two types of capacitive sensors:

i. Platforms and in-shoe systems by Novel, and platforms by Zebris use elastomer-based capacitive sensors, thus exploiting the variation of thickness of an elastic dielectric material: the higher the pressure, the smaller the thickness and the higher the capacitance, according to a linear law. In general, manufacturers have to deal with greater difficulties than with resistive sensors to obtain fast measurements, and cope with high impedance, which may entail noise or interference. On the other hand, this kind of sensors show higher stability, lower hysteresis, higher resistance to the deteriorating effects of ageing.
ii. Platforms by AMCube and Loran use air-based capacitive sensors also known as "touch mode" sensors: air separates the upper part of the capacitor from the lower part, which is covered by a thin dielectric sheet. The whole system is more rigid than with elastomer-based sensors, and usually the range of linear answer is smaller.
iii. Capacitive technology is also used in the Biofoot in-shoe system by the Institute of Biomechanics of Valencia, Spain (IBV). The system was first described in 2008 (Martínez-Nova A et al, 2008). Its main technical features are: thickness insole 0.7mm; 64 capacitive sensors for each insole; lifetime 3000 steps; pressure range 0-1220kPa; calibration range 0-500kPa; pressure resolution 0.1kPa, measurement uncertainty 10% of calibration range; in-factory calibration; suggested re-calibration after two years. Unfortunately, no further details are available as for the sensor technology they use.

3.2 Basic concepts on PMD technical assessment

Technical assessment of PMD performance is desired, and worldwide claimed to verify appropriateness, reliability and comparability of pressure measurements. It becomes mandatory when such measurements are used for clinical purposes, since in this case the PMD is addressed as a medical device with measuring function, and must comply with specific market regulations. On the other hand, when used in a research or sports context, or if it is a prototype, the device may or may not be considered a medical device - the classification depending on the specific intended use -, but it must always remain safe for users (i.e. minimisation of electrical and mechanical risks, toxicity,...).

PMD performance should be fully characterised in-factory before the device is delivered, or in the research lab in case of prototypes. Owing to ageing effects, however, it is not sufficient to guarantee its appropriate use over time. Thus, the periodic, simplified checking of some technical features should also be implemented on-site, so as to early detect any deterioration of the device entailing the worsening of its measuring performance.

Pressure output of PMDs may significantly differ due to the above-discussed variability in pressure sensor technology, but also due to several equally important factors like the number and arrangement of sensors, the material used to cover, sustain and seal the sensors, the hardware and software used to supply or calibrate the sensors and to acquire data. Thus, PMDs technical performance should be assessed accounting for their final arrangement. In case of in-shoe systems, assessment is even more complex since the devices should also be tested under flexed but repeatable conditions, and with respect to surfaces with adequate elasticity so as to reproduce as much as possible their most frequent working conditions.

With respect to pressure platforms, they may essentially differ for size; thickness; material the mechanical frame is made from; individual sensor technology and performance; individual sensor size; spatial resolution; pressure resolution and range; sampling rate; hardware and software supply and data acquisition equipment. Almost the same holds for in-shoe systems, but for size which is almost always fixed, and for the material of mechanical frame - actually the cover material - which should have specific elastic characteristics and should be appropriate for sealing procedures.

A suitable testing equipment should perform equally well with different sensor technologies and different arrangements. Basically, it should be able to apply a well-controlled and uniform load/pressure over defined PMD areas for a given time period and, in case of dynamic loading, at a controlled and proper rate. Its precision and accuracy should be higher than those expected for the PMD.

The assessment should mainly investigate PMD response in terms of: pressure variability over the whole active area and for the whole pressure range; pressure accuracy; hysteresis; creep and answer stability over short as well as long periods - the latter being mandatory if the device is going to be used for posturographic purposes -; accuracy and repeatability of center of pressure (COP) estimation.

Testing procedures should be properly designed to assess PMDs intended for use in specific scenarios like running, jumping, sprinting, jogging.

More technical details can be found in two 2010 publications (Giacomozzi, 2010 a; Giacomozzi, 2010 b) and on the above on-line forums[2] . Briefly, recommended features of testing equipment for pressure platforms to be used for gait analysis in Clinics (i.e. Medical

---

[2] http://vcms.iss.it/moodle19/; http://moodle.i-fab.org// (see note 1 for explanations)

PMDs) are, at minimum: pressure resolution below 10kPa; force resolution below 1N; spatial positioning re-positioning error lower than 2mm, and sinusoidal loading-unloading cycles applied with a frequency in the range 0.5-1.0Hz.
An example of in-factory testing equipment is widely described together with some suggested testing protocols in (Giacomozzi C, 2010 c): essentially it consists in a wide press machine for delivering pressure steps over the entire PMD surface, and a sensorized, ad hoc testing device which applies controlled static or varying pressure - through pneumatic valves and proper circuitry - as well as force over small active areas.
An example of testing equipment thought for on-site periodic checking is instead described and discussed in (Giacomozzi C, 2010 b). Basically, is consists in a light graduated round table placed on three small pylons, to be used with some weights and a positioning mask. When properly used, the testing device may help to periodically check the accuracy of COP estimation as well as local load and mean pressure under the pylons.
Specific for optical pedobarographs, instead, a very interesting testing equipment and methodology has been described in a 1997 paper with applications to the Sheffield optical pedobarograph (Franks CI, 1997).

4. Pressure measurement protocols and parameters

A wide variety of measurement protocols are currently implemented in the field of plantar pressure assessment, obviously according to the scenario and target of each investigation, e.g., the diagnosis of a pathologic condition, the outcome of a treatment, a patient's monitoring, a footwear/orthosis design and testing, the assessment of a sports performance, a specific study of applied biomechanical research, the identification of reference normative data, and so on. Similarly, there are plenty of pressure-related parameters which are currently considered relevant, some of them directly measured by means of PMDs, some other successively derived or estimated, and, again, the selection of parameters does depend on the final goal of each study. However, there is the need for the identification of some standardisation guidelines -at least to define a few basic parameters and measurement protocols to be taken as reference quantities and reference procedures so as to guarantee the comparability among studies. Moreover, if innovative parameters or measuring conditions were to be compared with some reference parameters and protocols, a better and more correct comprehension would be guaranteed, of new approaches to plantar pressure investigation. The following paragraphs briefly discuss relevant points for both issues.

4.1 Parameters: Traditional and novel ones

With respect to the entire plantar surface of the foot and to the way it is loaded during walking or standing, the following parameters are mostly used and known by the majority of researchers, clinicians and operators in the field:
Peak pressure: For each sensor, it is the highest pressure value experienced during the measurement. It is usually expressed in kPa, even though it is sometimes reported as PSI, N/cm^2, bar. Software applications associated to PMDs usually deliver a peak pressure map which contains the maximum pressure value reached by each sensor: this represents a spatial rather than a temporal map, since there is no association with the time frame each peak pressure occurres at. There is no confusion or misunderstanding on this parameter, the only doubt is associated with those devices which only deliver relative data rather than absolute values of pressure.

Mean pressure: For each sensor, it is the pressure value averaged over the measurement period. Measurement units are the same as for peak pressure. Two approaches may be followed to compute this parameter: averaging pressure over the entire measurement time period or only over the time period the specific sensor had been loaded, which may be much shorter than the entire duration of the test . Thus, in order to avoid interpretation mistakes, the computation algorithm should be clearly stated. Mean pressure output is usually delivered in the form of spatial maps.

Peak pressure curve (usually known as PPC): For the entire measurement surface, it represents the time process of the instantaneous maximum pressure value along the entire measurement period. In an x-y Cartesian graph, the horizontal axis x represents the time process expressed in absolute values (usually s or ms) or as percentage of the whole stance phase, while the y axis represents the instantaneous peak pressure expressed in absolute pressure units (kPa is recommended). Unlike the peak pressure map, this plot contains temporal information while it does not associate such information to the different areas of the plantar surface which instantaneously registers the highest pressure. PPC curve smoothing depends on PMD sampling rate and on eventual smoothing algorithms.

Force curve: Similarly to PPC, it represents the time evolution of the instantaneous value of the vertical component of the GRF. Absolute force values are expressed in N; for inter-subject comparisons, force is normalised to each subject's body weight, and thus expressed as %N or %b.w. This parameter is especially relevant for assessment issues, since the curve can be directly compared with the corresponding curve obtained with a standard force platform.

Pressure-time integral or impulse (usually indicated as PTI): It represents the area under PPC. If peak pressure is expressed in kPa, PTI should be expressed as kPa*s. Great differences might be found in the final PTI value due to the specific computation algorithm and to the PMD sampling rate, which must therefore be clearly stated. Just to explain the concept, if PTI is calculated as the sum of the products of instantaneous pressure by sampling interval, the final value will be much more accurate when using higher sampling rates.

Force-time integral or impulse (usually indicated as FTI): Similarly to PTI, this parameter is obtained by calculating the area under the force curve and is usually expressed as N*s or %N*s. As for PTI, computation procedures should be clearly stated.

Contact area: It is the instantaneous value of loaded PMD area. It is usually expressed in cm^2, and a curve similar to PPC is usually plotted to show contact area evolution along the measurement period. Differences in the estimated area are mainly due to PMD spatial resolution, sensor size and pressure threshold. Thus, proper information should be delivered together with this parameter.

COP trajectory: Represented by a two-dimensional array formed by the instantaneous COP coordinates, it is usually expressed in cm or PMD pixel units, for the whole measurement period. Again, differences may be found due to PMD spatial resolution, which must be clearly stated. A clear statement of the reference coordinate system used must be given too. In case of posturographic analyses, when parameters like COP sway or area or frequency content are of great interest, PMD sampling rate and frequency response may significantly affect the final COP values.

Besides the above parameters, other interesting indicators are used in specific pressure-related studies, as is for specific pressure gradients (Mueller MJ et al, 2008) or indicators related to COP velocity or acceleration (Wang Y, Watanabe K, 2008). Novel computational approaches have been tried, validated and used in recent publications dealing with neural networks (Betker AL et al, 2005), fuzzy logics (Senanayake CM, Senanayake SM, 2010 a), cluster analysis (Giacomozzi C., Martelli F, 2006), finite element models (Shiang TY, 1997; Petre M et al, 2008; Gu YD et al, 2010; Chen WM et al, 2010), image processing techniques (Pataky TC et al, 2009; Oliveira FP, Tavares JM, 2010) and so on. Usually, the inputs of such models are represented by the above traditional parameters, their reliability strongly relying on the quality and reliability of raw data. For all these interesting new approaches, proper background knowledge and details should be delivered to readers and potential users so that they may deeply understand the meaning, clinical relevance and applicability, limitations, potential, and proper field of application of each new pressure-related parameter.

Proposals for innovative parameters: pressure-integral map, actual mean pressure map, loading time map.

Pressure-integral map: the computation of PTI as the area under PPC is a useful parameter, but it is not able to discriminate those areas of the plantar surface which undergo higher, prolonged and more dangerous loading, i.e., it does not contain spatial information. Moreover, it is associated with an ideal sensor which is loaded with the instantaneous maximum pressure for the entire measurement period: being this almost impossible in dynamic measurement, the final PTI value almost always represents an overestimation even with respect to the most "stressed" region of the foot (conversely, PTI values represent a good estimation of the true local impulse in the case of a regional analysis, as will be described in the following paragraph). The proposed Pressure-integral maps should rather request the calculation of the 'local' PTI for each activated sensor. As for peak pressure maps, pressure-integral maps would contain temporal besides spatial loading information and might indeed have a high clinical relevance.

Actual mean pressure map: while most of the current PMD softwares deliver mean pressure maps which result from averaging pressure values over the whole measurement period, the actual mean pressure map should contain values averaged only over the time frame of each sensor activation. This may render the map more helpful in detecting those areas loaded for a limited amount of time, but with a potentially dangerous mean load.

Loading time map: this is again an attempt to add temporal to spatial information on load distribution. In this case, a previous agreement is needed on the definition of a certain number and duration of contact phases. As a suggestion, the conventional contact phases might be used, i.e. initial contact and loading response (initial 16% of stance), midstance (successive 32% of stance), propulsion (successive 33% of stance) and push-off (remaining 19% of stance) (Vaughan CL et al, 1999). If different colours are associated with the different phases, and with the persistence of loading across several phases, a specific colour - and a specific numeric value - may be associated to each activated sensor on a spatial-temporal map.

4.2 Regional parameters: potentialities of different methodological approaches

Regional analysis of plantar pressure maps and parameters is commonly used, and most of the more recent publications do implement procedures and algorithms to identify specific regions of the plantar surface of the foot. Great potential should be recognised to regional analysis, since it allows to focus on specific areas of interest and to better quantify local alterations of biomechanical parameters. This is particularly important when the effectiveness of a surgical or orthotic treatment has to be exactly quantified. However, what has been discussed in the previous paragraphs with respect to PMD variability of response, lack of standardisation and risk for misleading or missing comparisons, is here amplified, and even greater attention must be paid when designing, implementing and reporting plantar pressure investigations. The increased difficulties, in fact, are essentially due to the variability of the criteria for defining plantar regions, and to the percentual increased weight of computational errors related to smaller areas of interest. While the latter can only be minimised by better characterising PMD technical performance as already pointed out in previous paragraphs, it is interesting here to focus on the criticalities of the regionalisation procedures. Basically, two main approaches are currently followed to identify foot regions: one exploits the geometry of the footprint and the background knowledge of the anatomical structure of the foot; the other uses the information coming straight from the anatomy of the analysed foot.

Geometry-based approach: each and every selection method based on the acquired footprint does start from the longitudinal bisection of the footprint, which is usually computed from: i) the bisecting line of the foot; ii) the line going from the center of the heel to the second toe; iii) the midline of the rectangular box which contains the footprint. As a second step, the transversal selection of the main foot regions with respect to the longitudinal axis of the footprint is usually done by using lines which are perpendicular to it, and roughly located in correspondence with anatomical structures such as the Lisfranc or the Chopart line or the projection of the ankle joint axis, or structures that represent specific percentages of the footprint length. As a successive step in the regionalisation process, toes and individual metatarsal areas are identified on the basis of least square error algorithms, anatomically related assumptions, or other specific criteria. While, as already said, almost all 2010 published studies rely on regional analysis, none of them describe the way regions have been obtained. Sometimes, algorithms are known within a certain community, i.e. groups of researchers who are using the same commercial product. In any case, no procedure for footprint regionalisation has been "standardised" so far. Therefore, in order to avoid misleading conclusions it is mandatory that selection criteria are clearly described in the papers. With discrete sensors the regionalisation phase can be simplified, since they are indeed positioned under well-defined anatomical locations, thus variability in the final outcome of regional analysis will be mainly related to variability in sensor positioning.

Anatomy-based approach: this quite complex approach calls for the simultaneous use of a PMD and a kinematics measurement system to acquire instantaneous positions of foot anatomical landmarks, which are then projected onto the footprint and used for the anatomically-based region selection. This approach greatly improves the reliability of regional analysis in case footprints are not complete or strongly altered by the pathology. Dedicated algorithms must be designed and implemented to properly use the kinematic foot model, superimpose all the involved reference systems, and project the anatomical landmarks. Up to now, the anatomical masking approach has been applied to a prototype pressure platform and dedicated integration software by the Italian National Institute of Health together with a five-segment foot model by Istituti Ortopedici Rizzoli (Giacomozzi C et al, 2000; Stebbins JA et al, 2005), and to Novel platforms and dedicated integration software together with the Oxford Foot Model (Giacomozzi C et al, 2010). A further methodological study based on a Tekscan platform (Miller AL, 2010) only dealt with reference system integration issues.

4.3 Thoughts on protocols

Human walking and standing show intrinsic variability due to the high number of variables which play a role in the gait biomechanical model. In particular, the instantaneous pressure distribution obtained while interacting with the ground suffers from even greater variability due to fast local adjustments of the whole system while bearing and transferring load. The best approach to assess foot biomechanics through reliable and reproducible pressure measurements should therefore be based on the characterisation and control, as complete as possible, of measurement conditions. Here below a limited – certainly not exhaustive - list of concepts and suggestions is given, which should be taken into account to render investigations reliable and reproducible. Most concepts are equally applicable to both platforms and in-shoe systems when performing dynamic gait analysis; system-specific issues, and issues only related to posturographic analysis are identified separately.

- **Measurement environment:** environment conditions should always be controlled and described in order to render measurements reproducible. Any change introduced in a "standard" measurement environment should be well characterised and described: it may have relevant impact on pressure measurements. Barefoot gait analysis focussed on level walking is usually performed in a laboratory environment with good control of light, noise, temperature and humidity; the platform is inserted flush in a comfortable walking pattern, parallel and integral to the ground (patients should not be aware of the exact position of the platform); the walkway is large and long enough to guarantee the performance of a certain number of "at-regimen" steps. Walkways usually consist of quite rigid surfaces; wherever soft carpets are used, even though they do not cover the platform, it must be clearly stated in the study. It may happen that thin portable pressure platforms are placed over soft carpets rather than directly on the floor: this unstable installation should always be avoided and, in any case, it surely entails some alteration in platform performance. When in-shoe systems are used, the measurement scenario may be more varied, and must definitely be described as for: i) the environment itself (a laboratory context, a room or a place into a clinic, outdoors, ...); ii) the walkway (a level hard/soft surface, a slope, stairs, a treadmill, ...).
- **Number and kind of steps:** owing to gait variability, pressure parameters cannot be calculated over one step only; a certain number of steps are thus necessary to perform stable and reliable averages. A study published in 1996 showed that data averaged over 12 steps have quite an adequate standard deviation, which improved only slightly by increasing the number of steps (Macellari V, Giacomozzi C, 1996); however, this number of steps might be indeed too high to be obtained in a clinical context, especially with compromised patients. Five or six is the usual number of steps to obtain mean values of pressure quantities acquired through a platform; more steps are used in case of in-shoe systems, since they are acquired quite easily and the acquisition process is less time consuming. As for which step is to be included in the analysis, standardised approaches with pressure platforms commonly take into account the first, the second, or the third step: the three approaches may be valid, the choice mainly depending on the measurement environment and the main target of the investigation. With in-shoe systems, it is quite common to discard the initial and last steps and to average data over a fixed number of central steps (usually 5-10 steps for each foot).
- **Assessment tasks:** according to the target of the investigation, patients or volunteers are asked to perform specific locomotor tasks (posturographic tasks are briefly discussed as the last point of this list). With the only reference to platform-based gait

analysis during walking, some "requirements" of the measurement protocol are already worldwide agreed upon, i.e.: patients have to be tested barefoot, with arms moving freely along the body; they should become acquainted with the task before acquiring data; artefacts due to sudden noise, light or movements of people should be avoided; patients should look straight ahead, walk naturally and avoid looking at their feet; overtly altered trials must be discarded. As for walking speed, two main approaches are followed: i) the patient has to keep a fixed progression speed- usually with the help of a metronome -; ii) the patient walks at a self-selected speed. Changes in the measurement protocol should be clearly described, as is for example for purposely faster or slower walk, walk on treadmill, dual tasks such as cognitive, acoustic or visual tasks requested during walking. When an in-shoe system is used, changes from the above protocol are frequent: variation in progression speed, true and proper modification of the gait path - i.e. non straight paths, slopes, stairs, treadmill, etc.

- **Specific in-shoe system assessment requirements:** one of the most challenging targets of PMD measurement standardisation is the identification of a reference measurement protocol to be used with in-shoe systems. As a point of fact, these systems are only used in conjunction with an interface between the foot and the floor - i.e. the footwear - which not only modifies and interferes with pressure measurement from a technical point of view, but significantly alters gait as well. For both reasons it is not possible to use barefoot measurement as a reference: rather, it would be useful to standardise the footwear to be used for reference measurements. This is usually done in individual studies, i.e., each research group identifies and uses the measurement conditions and the footwear which are considered the most suitable in terms of feasibility, reproducibility, patient's wearing and equipment burden, allowed gait pattern. Most common in-shoe reference measurements are performed while wearing special socks (with no shoes on), sandals, or a well defined type of sports shoes.
- **Posturographic assessment:** standard measurement protocols do exist even though they are usually implemented with force, rather than pressure, platforms. These protocols account for several aspects, i.e., foot position, patient's position and behaviour, platform position and environment, task duration, etc. (Kapteyn TS et al, 1983). Any deviation from the standardised measurement conditions should thus be clearly described and motivated.

4.4 The role of pressure data processing

This issue is of special relevance in the field of plantar pressure measurements, being the third critical factor, together with PMD technical performance and measurement protocols, to be taken into account in the standardisation process. Several controversies are currently open in the scientific world as for the proper way to process pressure raw data. At the same time, the lack of relevant processing details in some PMD commercial softwares and in the scientific literature renders any description of the state of the art quite complex. The issue will be widely discussed in the i-FAB-PG in the next future, and the eventual agreement on standardised proposals will be shared with the scientific community. As for the discussion on the topic in the present document, the author is here only contributing with two very general, but basic, suggestions. The first is the strong recommendation to clearly describe each and every step of the data processing that takes from pressure raw data to derived parameters: this description is mandatory to render researchers aware of whether, and to what extent, some datasets may be compared with those extracted from their own studies.

The second is a suggestion to a proper selection and use of statistical analysis: in fact, most investigations strongly rely on parametric statistics, i.e., data are usually reported and analysed in terms of mean values and standard deviations. It is not infrequent, however, that the number of samples used and/or of experiments conducted in the study is too small to guarantee the normal distribution of the measured quantities, as is mandatory for a correct use of parametric statistics. In some cases non-parametric statistics are more suitable to describe and interpret datasets, and to infer on the relevance of differences among populations or treatments.

5. Conclusions

Plantar pressure measurements do have a great potential to support the study of foot biomechanics both in a research context and in the clinic. The literature overview reported hereby, even though it only focusses on the 2010 peer-reviewed publications indexed in PubMed, clearly shows that PMD measurements are increasingly used - alone or in conjunction with other kinetic/kinematic parameters - to deeply investigate clinical outcomes of surgical interventions, rehabilitation treatments, preventive actions, disease evolution, as well as to implement new biomechanical models or validate novel methodological approaches. Even though PMDs have been used for several years now, criticalities are still present, which still prevent the complete exploitation of all their potentialities. In the sequence from the design and construction of a PMD to its use on the field, such criticalities may be identified as: i) lack of standardisation of the procedures to assess and compare PMDs technical performance; ii) lack of comparability of measurement protocols; iii) lack of standardisation of the definition and use of data processing procedures. The scientific community is currently demonstrating increasing interest in the above issues. With respect to the first one, attempts towards consensus agreement have already been started in 2010 and are currently implemented within international scientific communities; basic concepts and preliminary recommendations have been described and discussed in the present document. As for the second issue, a short overview of the main measurement parameters and protocols has been reported, along with some suggestions to parameters which might be relevant and meaningful especially in the clinic. The last issue is still at a preliminary discussion phase, and only two basic suggestions have been briefly given in the document, which mainly point to the importance of a clear description of processing procedures and to the proper identification of statistical analysis tools.

Fast advances in technology as well as in computational mechanics are already showing new promising scenarios for the investigation of foot biomechanics, where pressure measurements might become more reliable and suitable (as might be the case with more flexible, wearable textile sensors), and successfully integrated with local friction and shear measurements -at the foot-floor or the foot-insole interface-, reliable low-cost kinematics systems, and 3D dynamic FE models.

6. Acknowledgment

The Author gratefully acknowledges Ms. Monica Brocco for the English editing of the manuscript.

7. References

Abu-Faraj, Z.O., Akar, H.A., Assaf, E.H., Al-Qadiri, M.N. & Youssef, E.G. (2010). Evaluation of fall and fall recovery in a simulated seismic environment: A pilot study. *Conf Proc IEEE Eng Med Biol Soc.* 1:3954-7.

Aliberti, S., Costa, M.S., Passaro, A.C., Arnone, A.C. & Sacco, I.C. (2010). Medial contact and smaller plantar loads characterize individuals with Patellofemoral Pain Syndrome during stair descent. *Phys Ther Sport.* 11(1):30-4.

Barberà i Guillem, R., Gómez Sendra, F., Bermejo Bosch, I. & Garcés Pérez, L. (2010). Reducing the pressure on heel and foot-sole areas by means of Allevyn Gentle, Gentle Border and Gentle Border Heel dressings. *Rev Enferm.* 33(3):51-6.

Battaglia, G., Bellafiore, M., Bianco, A., Paoli, A. & Palma, A. (2010). Effects of a dynamic balance training protocol on podalic support in older women. Pilot Study. *Aging Clin Exp Res.* 22(5-6):406-11.

Bayomy, A.F., Aubin, P.M., Sangeorzan, B.J. & Ledoux, W.R. (2010). Arthrodesis of the first metatarsophalangeal joint: a robotic cadaver study of the dorsiflexion angle. *J Bone Joint Surg Am.* 92(8):1754-64.

Bek, N., Kinikli, G.I., Callaghan, M.J. & Atay, O.A. (2010). Foot biomechanics and initial effects of infrapatellar strap on gait parameters in patients with unilateral patellofemoral pain syndrome. *Foot (Edinb).* Dec 9. [Epub ahead of print]

Betker, A.L., Moussavi, Z.M. & Szturm, T. (2005). On modeling center of foot pressure distortion through a medium. IEEE Trans Biomed Eng. 52(3):345-52.

Bosch, K., Rosenbaum, D. (2010). Gait symmetry improves in childhood--a 4-year follow-up of foot loading data. *Gait Posture.* 32(4):464-8.

Bosch, K., Gerss, J. & Rosenbaum, D. (2010). Development of healthy children's feet--nine-year results of a longitudinal investigation of plantar loading patterns. *Gait Posture.* 32(4):564-71.

Braz, R.G., Carvalho, G.A. (2010). Relationship between quadriceps angle (Q) and plantar pressure distribution in football players. *Rev Bras Fisioter.* 14(4):296-302.

Chen, W.M., Lee, T., Lee, P.V., Lee, J.W. & Lee, S.J. (2010). Effects of internal stress concentrations in plantar soft-tissue-A preliminary three-dimensional finite element analysis. *Med Eng Phys.* 32(4):324-31.

Chesnin, K.J., Selby-Silverstein, L. & Besser, M.P., (2000). Comparison of an in-shoe pressure measurement device to a force plate: concurrent validity of center of pressure measurements. Gait and Posture 12: 128–133.

Chevalier, T.L., Hodgins, H. & Chockalingam, N. (2010). Plantar pressure measurements using an in-shoe system and a pressure platform: a comparison. *Gait Posture.* 31(3):397-9.

Cisneros, Lde. L., Fonseca, T.H. & Abreu, V.C. (2010). Inter- and intra-examiner reliability of footprint pattern analysis obtained from diabetics using the Harris mat. *Rev Bras Fisioter.* 14(3):200-5.

Cobb, J., Claremont, D.J. (1995). Transducers for foot pressure measurement: survey of recent developments. Med Biol Eng Comput. 33(4):525-32.

Cram, R.H. (1953). A sign of sciatic nerve foot pressure J Bone Joint Surg Br. 35-B(2):192-5.

D'Amico, M., D'Amico, G., Paniccia, M., Roncoletta, P. & Vallasciani, M. (2010). An integrated procedure for spine and full skeleton multi-sensor biomechanical analysis & averaging in posture gait and cyclic movement tasks. *Stud Health Technol Inform.* 158:118-26.

Deleu, P.A., Leemrijse, T., Vandeleene, B., Maldague, P. & Devos Bevernage, B. (2010). Plantar pressure relief using a forefoot offloading shoe. *Foot Ankle Surg.* 16(4):178-82.

do Carmo Dos Reis, M., Soares, F.A., da Rocha, A.F., Carvalho, J.L. & Rodrigues, S.S. (2010). Insole with pressure control and tissue neoformation induction systems for diabetic foot. *Conf Proc IEEE Eng Med Biol Soc.* 1:5748-51.

Duckworth, T., Betts, R.P., Franks, C.I. & Burke, J. (1982). The measurement of pressures under the foot. Foot Ankle 3(3): 130-41.

Duckworth, T., Boulton, A.J.M., Betts, R.P., Franks, C.I. & Ward, J.D. (1985). Plantar pressure measurements and the prevention of ulceration in the Diabetic foot. The Journal of Bone and Joint Surgery 67-B (1): 79-85.

Ellis, S.J., Yu, J.C., Johnson, A.H., Elliott, A., O'Malley, M. & Deland, J. (2010). Plantar pressures in patients with and without lateral foot pain after lateral column lengthening. *J Bone Joint Surg Am.* 92(1):81-91.

Faria, A., Gabriel, R., Abrantes, J., Brás, R. & Moreira, H. (2010). The relationship of body mass index, age and triceps-surae musculotendinous stiffness with the foot arch structure of postmenopausal women. *Clin Biomech (Bristol, Avon).* 25(6):588-93.

Franks, C.I. (1997). Calibration of optical foot pressure systems. Med. & Biol. Eng. & Comput. 35: 69-72.

Giacomozzi, C. (2010). Performance of plantar pressure measurement devices (PMDs): update on consensus activities. *Ann Ist Super Sanita.* 46(4):343-5. a

Giacomozzi, C. (2010). Hardware performance assessment recommendations and tools for baropodometric sensor systems. *Ann Ist Super Sanita.* 46(2):158-67. b

Giacomozzi, C. (2010). Appropriateness of plantar pressure measurement devices: a comparative technical assessment. *Gait Posture.* 32(1):141-4. c

Giacomozzi, C., Martelli, F. (2006). Peak Pressure Curve: an effective parameter for early detection of foot functional impairments in diabetic patients. Gait & Posture 23:464-470.

Giacomozzi, C., Macellari, V., Leardini, A. & Benedetti, M.G. (2000). Integrated pressure-force-kinematics measuring system for the characterisation of plantar foot loading during locomotion. Med Biol Eng Comput. 38(2):156-63.

Giacomozzi, C., Stebbins, J. & Kalpen, A. (2010). Footprint masks: reproducibility of the Oxford anatomically-based selection by means of novel geometrical masks. Procs of Scientific Meeting ESM2010, Providence, RI, USA, August 14-17 2010.

Girard, O., Eicher, F., Micallef, J.P. & Millet, G. (2010). Plantar pressures in the tennis serve. *J Sports Sci.* 28(8):873-80.

Goffar, S.L., Naylor, J., Reber, R.J., Rodriguez, B.M., Christiansen, B.C., Walker, M.J., Miller, R.B. & Teyhen, D.S. (2010). Dynamic plantar pressure changes during loaded gait. *US Army Med Dep J.* Jul-Sep:77.

Gordon, V. (1976) Treatment of the patient with calcaneal and plantar pressure ulcers of neurogenic etiology. J Am Osteopath Assoc. 75(5):525-6.

Gu, Y., Li, J., Ren, X., Lake, M.J. & Zeng, Y. (2010). Heel skin stiffness effect on the hind foot biomechanics during heel strike. *Skin Res Technol.* 16(3):291-6.

Hastings, M.K., Gelber, J.R., Isaac, E.J., Bohnert, K.L., Strube, M.J. & Sinacore, D.R. (2010). Foot progression angle and medial loading in individuals with diabetes mellitus, peripheral neuropathy, and a foot ulcer. *Gait Posture.* 32(2):237-41.

Hetsroni, I., Nyska, M., Ben-Sira, D., Mann, G., Segal, O., Maoz, G. & Ayalon, M. (2010). Analysis of foot structure in athletes sustaining proximal fifth metatarsal stress fracture. *Foot Ankle Int.* 31(3):203-11.

Hills, A.P., Hennig, E.M., McDonald, M. & Bar-Or, O. (2001). Plantar pressure differences between obese and non-obese adults: a biomechanical analysis. International Journal of Obesity 25, 1674–1679

Hirasaki, E., Higurashi, Y. & Kumakura, H. (2010). Brief communication: Dynamic plantar pressure distribution during locomotion in Japanese macaques (Macaca fuscata). *Am J Phys Anthropol.* 142(1):149-56.

Hirata, R.P., Arendt-Nielsen, L. & Graven-Nielsen, T. (2010). Experimental calf muscle pain attenuates the postural stability during quiet stance and perturbation. *Clin Biomech (Bristol, Avon).* 25(9):931-7.

Hirschmüller, A., Konstantinidis, L., Baur, H., Müller, S., Mehlhorn, A., Kontermann, J., Grosse, U., Südkamp, N.P. & Helwig, P. (2010). Do changes in dynamic plantar pressure distribution, strength capacity and postural control after intra-articular calcaneal fracture correlate with clinical and radiological outcome? *Injury.* Nov 12. [Epub ahead of print]

Hong, Y., Wang, L., Li, J.X. & Zhou, J.H. (2010). Changes in running mechanics using conventional shoelace versus elastic shoe cover. *J Sports Sci.* Dec 20:1-7. [Epub ahead of print]

Hyslop, E., Woodburn, J., McInnes, I.B., Semple, R., Newcombe, L., Hendry, G., Rafferty, D., De Mits, S. & Turner, D.E. (2010). A reliability study of biomechanical foot function in psoriatic arthritis based on a novel multi-segmented foot model. *Gait Posture.* 32(4):619-26.

Jeans, K.A., Karol & L.A. (2010). Plantar pressures following Ponseti and French physiotherapy methods for clubfoot. *J Pediatr Orthop.* 30(1):82-9.

Kaipel, M., Krapf, D. & Wyss, C. (2010). Metatarsal Length does not Correlate with Maximal Peak Pressure and Maximal Force. *Clin Orthop Relat Res.* Oct 13. [Epub ahead of print]

Kapteyn, T.S., Bles, W., Njiokiktjien, C.J., Kodde, L., Massen, C.H. & Mol, J.M.F. (1983). Standardization in Platform Stabilometry being a Part of Posturography. Agressologie 24, 7: 321-326.

Karadag-Saygi, E., Unlu-Ozkan, F. & Basgul, A. (2010). Plantar pressure and foot pain in the last trimester of pregnancy. *Foot Ankle Int.* 31(2):153-7.

Keijsers, N.L., Stolwijk, N.M. & Pataky, T.C. (2010). Linear dependence of peak, mean, and pressure-time integral values in plantar pressure images. *Gait Posture.* 31(1):140-2.

Kendell, C., Lemaire, E.D., Dudek, N.L. & Kofman, J. (2010). Indicators of dynamic stability in transtibial prosthesis users. *Gait Posture.* 31(3):375-9.

Kelly, L.A., Racinais, S., Tanner, C.M., Grantham, J. & Chalabi, H. (2010). Augmented low dye taping changes muscle activation patterns and plantar pressure during treadmill running. *J Orthop Sports Phys Ther.* 40(10):648-55.

Lee, K.M., Chung, C.Y., Park, M.S., Lee, S.H., Cho, J.H. & Choi, I.H. (2010). Reliability and validity of radiographic measurements in hindfoot varus and valgus. *J Bone Joint Surg Am.* 92(13):2319-27.

Lidtke, R.H., Muehleman, C., Kwasny, M. & Block, J.A. (2010). Foot center of pressure and medial knee osteoarthritis. *J Am Podiatr Med Assoc.* 100(3):178-84.

Lord, M. 1981. Foot pressure measurement: a review of methodology. J Biomed Eng 3 91-9.

Macellari, V., Giacomozzi, C. (1996). Multistep pressure platform as a standalone system for gait assessment. Med & Biol. Eng. & Comput., 34 (4), pp. 299-304.

Mackey, R.B., Thomson, A.B., Kwon, O., Mueller, M.J. & Johnson, J.E. (2010). The modified oblique keller capsular interpositional arthroplasty for hallux rigidus. *J Bone Joint Surg Am.* 92(10):1938-46.

Martínez-Nova, A., Sánchez-Rodríguez, R., Pérez-Soriano, P., Llana-Belloch, S., Leal-Muro, A. & Pedrera-Zamorano, J.D. (2010). Plantar pressures determinants in mild Hallux Valgus. *Gait Posture.* 32(3):425-7.

Martínez-Nova, A., Sánchez-Rodríguez, R., Leal-Muro, A., Sánchez-Barrado, E. & Pedrera-Zamorano, J.D. (2008). Percutaneous distal soft tissue release-akin procedure, clinical and podobarometric assessment with the BioFoot in-shoe system: a preliminary report. Foot Ankle Spec. 1(4):222-30.

Menz, H.B., Munteanu, S.E., Zammit, G.V. & Landorf, K.B. (2010). Foot structure and function in older people with radiographic osteoarthritis of the medial midfoot. *Osteoarthritis Cartilage.* 18(3):317-22.

Mickle, K.J., Munro, B.J., Lord, S.R., Menz, H.B. & Steele, J.R. (2010). Foot pain, plantar pressures, and falls in older people: a prospective study. *J Am Geriatr Soc.* 58(10):1936-40.

Miller, A.L. (2010). A new method for synchronization of motion capture and plantar pressure data. *Gait Posture.* 32(2):279-81.

Monteiro, M.A., Gabriel, R.C., Sousa, M.F., Castro, M.N. & Moreira, M.H. (2010). Temporal parameters of the foot roll-over during walking: influence of obesity and sarcopenic obesity on postmenopausal women. *Maturitas.* 67(2):178-85. a

Monteiro, M.A., Gabriel, R.E., Neves e Castro, M., Sousa, M.F., Abrantes, J.M. & Moreira, M.H. (2010). Exercise effects in plantar pressure of postmenopausal women. *Menopause.* 17(5):1017-25. b

Monteiro, M., Gabriel, R., Aranha, J., Neves e Castro, M., Sousa, M. & Moreira, M. (2010). Influence of obesity and sarcopenic obesity on plantar pressure of postmenopausal women. *Clin Biomech (Bristol, Avon).* 25(5):461-7. c

Morrison, K.E., Hudson, D.J., Davis, I.S., Richards, J.G., Royer, T.D., Dierks, T.A. & Kaminski, T.W. (2010). Plantar pressure during running in subjects with chronic ankle instability. *Foot Ankle Int.* 31(11):994-1000.

Mueller, M.J., Zou, D., Bohnert, K.L., Tuttle, L.J. & Sinacore, D.R. (2008). Plantar stresses on the neuropathic foot during barefoot walking. Phys Ther. 88(11):1375-84.

Najafi, B., Crews, R.T., Armstrong, D.G., Rogers, L.C., Aminian, K. & Wrobel, J. (2010). Can we predict outcome of surgical reconstruction of Charcot neuroarthropathy by dynamic plantar pressure assessment?--A proof of concept study. *Gait Posture.* 31(1):87-92.

Natali, A.N., Forestiero, A., Carniel, E.L., Pavan, P.G. & Dal Zovo, C. (2010). Investigation of foot plantar pressure: experimental and numerical analysis. *Med Biol Eng Comput.* 48(12):1167-74.

Navarro, L.A., Garcia, D.O., Villavicencio, E.A., Torres, M.A., Nakamura, O.K., Huamani, R. & Yabar, L.F. (2010). Opto-electronic system for detection of flat foot by using estimation techniques: Study and approach of design. *Conf Proc IEEE Eng Med Biol Soc.* 1:5768-71.

(No authors listed) (2010). Monitoring of Posture Allocations and Activities by a Shoe-Based Wearable Sensor. *IEEE Trans Biomed Eng.* Apr 15. [Epub ahead of print]

Nordsiden, L., Van Lunen, B.L., Walker, M.L., Cortes, N., Pasquale, M. & Onate, J.A. (2010). The effect of 3 foot pads on plantar pressure of pes planus foot type. *J Sport Rehabil.* 19(1):71-85.

Oliveira, F.P., Tavares, J.M. (2010). Novel framework for registration of pedobarographic image data. *Med Biol Eng Comput.* Nov 3. [Epub ahead of print]

Orlin, M.N., McPoil, T.G. (2000). Plantar pressure assessment. Phys Ther. 80:399–409.

Pataky, T.C., Keijsers, N.L., Goulermas, J.Y. & Crompton, R.H. (2009). Nonlinear spatial warping for between-subjects pedobarographic image registration. Gait Posture. 29(3):477-82.

Pataky, Z., de León Rodriguez, D., Allet, L., Golay, A., Assal, M., Assal, J.P. & Hauert, C.A. (2010). Biofeedback for foot offloading in diabetic patients with peripheral neuropathy. *Diabet Med.* 27(1):61-4.

Pau, M., Corona, F., Leban, B. & Pau, M. (2010). Effects of backpack carriage on foot-ground relationship in children during upright stance. *Gait Posture.* Nov 25. [Epub ahead of print]

Pauk, J., Daunoraviciene, K., Ihnatouski, M., Griskevicius, J. & Raso, J.V. (2010). Analysis of the plantar pressure distribution in children with foot deformities. *Acta Bioeng Biomech.* 12(1):29-34.

Petre, M., Erdemir, A. & Cavanagh, P.R. (2008). An MRI-compatible foot-loading device for assessment of internal tissue deformation. J Biomech. 41(2):470-4.

Putti, A.B., Arnold, G.P. & Abboud, R.J. (2010). Differences in foot pressures between Caucasians and Indians. *Foot Ankle Surg.* 16(4):195-8. a

Putti, A.B., Arnold, G.P. & Abboud, R.J. (2010). Foot pressure differences in men and women. *Foot Ankle Surg.* 16(1):21-4. b

Queen, R.M., Abbey, A.N., Wiegerinck, J.I., Yoder, J.C. & Nunley, J.A. (2010). Effect of shoe type on plantar pressure: a gender comparison. *Gait Posture.* 31(1):18-22.

Ramanathan, A.K., Herd, F., Macnicol, M. & Abboud, R.J. (2009). A new scoring system for the evaluation of clubfoot: the IMAR-Clubfoot scale. Foot (Edinb). 19(3):156-60.

Ramanathan, A.K., Kiran, P., Arnold, G.P., Wang, W. & Abboud, R.J. (2010). Repeatability of the Pedar-X in-shoe pressure measuring system. *Foot Ankle Surg.* 16(2):70-3.

Rao, S., Saltzman, C.L. & Yack, H.J. (2010). Relationships between segmental foot mobility and plantar loading in individuals with and without diabetes and neuropathy. *Gait Posture.* 31(2):251-5.

Ribeiro, A.P., Trombini-Souza, F., Tessutti, V.D., Lima, F.R., João, S.M. & Sacco, I.C. (2010). The effects of plantar fasciitis and pain on plantar pressure distribution of recreational runners. *Clin Biomech (Bristol, Avon).* Sep 13. [Epub ahead of print]

Rouhani, H., Crevoisier, X., Favre, J. & Aminian, K. (2010). Outcome evaluation of ankle osteoarthritis treatments: Plantar pressure analysis during relatively long-distance walking. *Clin Biomech (Bristol, Avon).* Dec 16. [Epub ahead of print] a

Rouhani, H., Favre, J., Crevoisier, X. & Aminian, K. (2010). Ambulatory assessment of 3D ground reaction force using plantar pressure distribution. *Gait Posture.* 32(3):311-6. b

Schepers, T., Kieboom, B., van Diggele, P., Patka, P. & Van Lieshout, E.M. (2010). Pedobarographic analysis and quality of life after Lisfranc fracture dislocation. *Foot Ankle Int.* 31(10):857-64.

Schuh, R., Adams, S., Hofstaetter, S.G., Krismer, M. & Trnka, H.J. (2010). Plantar loading after Chevron osteotomy combined with postoperative physical therapy. *Foot Ankle Int.* 31(11):980-6. a

See, C.K., Acharya, U.R., Zhu, K., Lim, T.C., Yu, W.W., Subramaniam, T. & Law, C. (2010). Automated identification of diabetes type-2 subjects with and without neuropathy using eigenvalues. *Proc Inst Mech Eng H.* 224(1):43-52.

Senanayake, C.M., Senanayake, S.M. (2010). A computational method for reliable gait event detection and abnormality detection for feedback in rehabilitation. *Comput Methods Biomech Biomed Engin.* Sep 30:1. [Epub ahead of print] a

Senanayake, C.M., Senanayake, S.M. (2010). Computational intelligent gait-phase detection system to identify pathological gait. *IEEE Trans Inf Technol Biomed.* 14(5):1173-9. b

Schuh, R., Trnka, H.J., Sabo, A., Reichel, M. & Kristen, K.H. (2010). Biomechanics of postoperative shoes: plantar pressure distribution, wearing characteristics and design criteria: a preliminary study. *Arch Orthop Trauma Surg.* Jun 12. [Epub ahead of print] b

Shiang, T.Y. (1997). The nonlinear finite element analysis and plantar pressure measurement for various shoe soles in heel region. Proc Natl Sci Counc Repub China B. 21(4):168-74.

Shu, L., Hua, T., Wang, Y., Qiao Li, Q., Feng, D.D. & Tao, X. (2010). In-shoe plantar pressure measurement and analysis system based on fabric pressure sensing array. *IEEE Trans Inf Technol Biomed.* 14(3):767-75.

Stebbins, J.A., Harrington, M.E., Giacomozzi, C., Thompson, N., Zavatsky, A. & Theologis, T.N. (2005). Assessment of sub-division of plantar pressure measurement in children. Gait Posture 22(4):372-6.

Stöggl, T., Haudum, A., Birklbauer, J., Murrer, M. & Müller, E. (2010). Short and long term adaptation of variability during walking using unstable (Mbt) shoes. *Clin Biomech (Bristol, Avon).* 25(8):816-22.

Stolwijk, N.M., Duysens, J., Louwerens, J.W. & Keijsers, N.L. (2010). Plantar pressure changes after long-distance walking. *Med Sci Sports Exerc.* 42(12):2264-72.

Tessutti, V., Trombini-Souza, F., Ribeiro, A.P., Nunes, A.L. & Sacco, I.C. (2010). In-shoe plantar pressure distribution during running on natural grass and asphalt in recreational runners. *J Sci Med Sport.* 13(1):151-5.

Teyhen, D.S., Stoltenberg, B.E., Eckard, T.G., Doyle, P.M., Boland, D.M., Feldtmann, J.J., McPoil, T.G., Christie Iii, D.S., Molloy, J.M. & Goffar, S.L. (2010). Static Foot Pressure Associated With Dynamic Plantar Pressure Parameters. *J Orthop Sports Phys Ther.* Oct 22. [Epub ahead of print]

Tong, J.W., Ng, E.Y. (2010). Preliminary investigation on the reduction of plantar loading pressure with different insole materials (SRP--Slow Recovery Poron, P--Poron, PPF--Poron +Plastazote, firm and PPS--Poron+Plastazote, soft). *Foot (Edinb).* 20(1):1-6.

Tura, A., Raggi, M., Rocchi, L., Cutti, A.G. & Chiari, L. (2010). Gait symmetry and regularity in transfemoral amputees assessed by trunk accelerations. *J Neuroeng Rehabil.* 19;7:4.

Vaughan, C.L., Davis, C.L. & O'Connor, J.C.(1999). Dynamics of human gait, 2nd Edition. Kiboho Publishers, Cape Town, South Africa. ISBN: 0-620-23558-6.

Vuillerme, N., Boisgontier, M. (2010). Changes in the relative contribution of each leg to the control of quiet two-legged stance following unilateral plantar-flexor muscles fatigue. *Eur J Appl Physiol.* 110(1):207-13.

Wagenmann, B., Schuh, R. & Trnka, H.J. (2010). Functional Outcome of Cheilectomy for the Treatment of Hallux Rigidus. *Z Orthop Unfall.* Mar 8. [Epub ahead of print]

Wang, C.H., Li, F., Zhang, R. & Shi, Y.Z. (2010). Application study of gait analysis on different syndrome types based on musculature zones of the knee osteoarthritis *Zhongguo Zhen Jiu.* 30(3):183-7.

Wang, Y., Watanabe, K. (2008) The relationship between obstacle height and center of pressure velocity during obstacle crossing. Gait Posture 27(1):172-5.

Yalçin, N., Esen, E., Kanatli, U. & Yetkin, H. (2010). Evaluation of the medial longitudinal arch: a comparison between the dynamic plantar pressure measurement system and radiographic analysis. *Acta Orthop Traumatol Turc.* 44(3):241-5.

Yavuz, M., Davis, B.L. (2010). Plantar shear stress distribution in athletic individuals with frictional foot blisters. *J Am Podiatr Med Assoc.* 100(2):116-20.

Yavuz, M., Husni, E., Botek, G. & Davis, B.L. (2010). Plantar shear stress distribution in patients with rheumatoid arthritis: relevance to foot pain. *J Am Podiatr Med Assoc.* 100(4):265-9.

Yoon, H.K., Park, K.B., Roh, J.Y., Park, H.W., Chi, H.J. & Kim, H.W. (2010). Extraarticular subtalar arthrodesis for pes planovalgus: an interim result of 50 feet in patients with spastic diplegia. *Clin Orthop Surg.* 2(1):13-21.

Zammit, G.V., Menz, H.B. & Munteanu, S.E. (2010). Reliability of the TekScan MatScan(R) system for the measurement of plantar forces and pressures during barefoot level walking in healthy adults. *J Foot Ankle Res.* 3:11.

Zequera, M.L., Solomonidis, S. (2010). Performance of insole in reducing plantar pressure on diabetic Patients in the early stages of the disease. *Conf Proc IEEE Eng Med Biol Soc.* 1:2982-5.

12

Mammalian Oral Rhythms and Motor Control

Geoffrey Gerstner, Shashi Madhavan and Elizabeth Crane
University of Michigan
U.S.A.

1. Introduction

Mastication is a derived mammalian trait, characterized by rhythmic jaw movements associated with intra-oral food handling, reduction and bolus formation. Hiiemae defined it as "a key feature of mammalian feeding that involves the coordination of complex movements and precise dental occlusion during a distinct power stroke of the chewing cycle (Hiiemae, 2000). Lund and Kolta refer to mastication as the time "during which the food is mechanically broken down and mixed with saliva to create a slurry of small particles or bolus that can be easily swallowed" (Lund & Kolta, 2006).

There is a debate as to whether to define mastication in general or precise terms. The debate focuses on whether to include in its definition the requirements of precise post-canine occlusion, unilateral food bolus placement, and transverse motion of the mandible during the power stroke. Given that feeding in most mammalian and non-mammalian species has yet to be studied and characterized, we opt to use fewer qualifiers and to rely on a more general definition of mastication or chewing in this chapter.

The variety of masticatory kinematics and dentoskeletal morphologies (Ungar, 2010) across mammals is almost as striking as plumage variation is among birds. The increased efficiency afforded by masticatory forms and functions may have been necessary to keep pace with another mammalian synapomorphy, the increased energy demands of endothermy. Alternatively, given that erupted enamel cannot be replaced, and that healthy teeth are requisite for longevity and fecundity, efficiency may be required to maximize the life of teeth.

Whatever the case, mastication is only one of several distinct oral motor behaviors, which also include (a) suckling, a mammalian-specific trait involved in milk ingestion, (b) lapping or sucking which are used to ingest liquids, fruit juices or insects, (c) rumination or chewing of cud, (d) gnawing of bones or tough food items, (e) tongue rasping used by cats as a food softening behavior, (f) incising, chopping or cutting food, (g) tooth sharpening or thegosis, (h) speech, whistling and communication, (i) facial expressions such as smiling or gritting teeth aggressively, (j) protective behaviors such as sneezing, coughing, gagging or vomiting, (k) tool use such as blowing on, holding or catching objects, (l) respiratory behaviors such as breathing and panting (m) sensory pleasures such as tasting or kissing.

2. Significance of masticatory biomechanics

Although motor behaviors "above the neck" are underrepresented in biomechanics studies, the oral apparatus affords several important and compelling features and advantages for such studies, which we discuss in this section.

2.1 Jaw tracking

The dentition is a sturdy set of anchors for kinematic tracking purposes. Teeth are anchored by the periodontal ligament to the mandibular bone, which prevents significant tooth movement in healthy mouths. Orthodontic brackets or custom clutches with small footprints are often attached to teeth for holding jaw tracking markers (Flavel et al., 2002; Gerstner & Fehrman, 1999; Gerstner & Kinra, 1999; Gerstner et al., 1999; Gerstner & Parekh, 1997; Hiiemae et al., 1996; Plesh et al., 1993; Wintergerst et al., 2004). More invasive tracking methods such as anchored bone markers or cineradiography are easily used in non-human mammals (Byrd, 1981; Gerstner & Goldberg, 1991; Hylander et al., 1987; Kobayashi et al., 2002a; Schwartz et al., 1989; Yamada et al., 1988). The development of X-ray reconstruction of moving morphology (XROMM) has been used to study oral movements and promises to revolutionize comparative biomechanical studies of oral function (Brainerd et al., 2010).
It is also possible to track certain jaw movement features with marker-less methods (Gerstner & Goldberg, 1994; Ross et al., 2009). This is possible, because most species remain relatively motionless while masticating. Hence, special equipment is often unnecessary.

2.2 Unique motor control characteristics

Because they involve the movement of a single bone, i.e., the mandible, masticatory movements can be relatively simple to track. Yet, mastication has some complex aspects that can provide significant insights into biomechanical issues. For instance, the mandible crosses the midline and articulates with the temporomandibular joints (TMJ), each of which possesses six degrees of freedom in humans and many other species. The jaw is driven by at least 18 muscle groups, and the masticatory movements, which these muscles generate, are usually asymmetrical. Hence, activity in masticatory muscle pairs is asynchronous, but carefully controlled so that mandibular positions and movements are precise and accurate to sub-millimeter levels especially near tooth-to-tooth contact.

2.3 Unique muscle characteristics

The masticatory muscles contain a number of unique features and properties that need to be further explored to understand their functional significance (for review, see Korfage et al., 2005a, 2005b). These include the presence of Type IIX, α-cardiac and neonatal myosin heavy chains in fairly high levels in all adult human masticatory muscles. Furthermore, > 40% of jaw-closer muscle fibers are hybrids, consisting of two or more myosin heavy chain types. Also, whereas in the limbs and trunks, type IIA fibers have larger diameters than type I fibers, the opposite is true in masticatory muscles. Type I fibers are about the same diameter in jaw muscles as they are in limb and trunk muscles; however, the masticatory type IIA fibers are three times smaller in diameter than they are in limb and trunk muscles. The reasons for these unique features remain unclear; however, candidate hypotheses include: (1) the need for fine jaw motor control, (2) energetic demands of jaw function and posture maintenance, (3) the heavy daily use of the jaw, and/or (4) unique adaptive requirements.

2.4 Unique proprioception

Masticatory proprioception has several unique features. For instance, although jaw closer muscles are populated by muscle spindles, jaw opener and tongue muscles have few to no muscle spindles. Tendon organs are absent in jaw closer muscles, but occur in jaw openers albeit at relatively low densities. Mechanoreceptors in the periodontal ligaments, the connective tissue that holds the teeth in their sockets, likely play important proprioceptive roles, essentially replacing the tendon organs in this function.

Also, the mesencephalic nucleus (MeV) is essentially a dorsal root ganglion residing in the brain stem. It contains the cell bodies of primary afferents involved with proprioception of the face and jaw and of mechanoreceptors from the teeth. Interestingly, the MeV is found in all vertebrates with jaws, whereas it does not exist or exists in very rudimentary form in vertebrates without jaws. This suggests that its unique design is somehow tied to jaw function requisites. Cells within the nucleus are electrically coupled, with chemical synapses being absent from the nucleus. Spindle afferents, whose cell bodies are in MeV, are unipolar and form a monosynaptic jaw closing reflex with jaw closer motoneurons.

Skin and hair receptors especially around the corners of the mouth play a role in proprioception; however, they are mostly rapidly-adapting and appear to require tactile stimulation. Proprioception also plays unique and important feedback and feed-forward roles in masticatory control as will be discussed below.

2.5 Central pattern generation and timing

Mastication is controlled by brainstem central pattern generator circuitry (Section 4). The circuitry develops from rhombomeres distinct from respiration, and it has some unique features in the adult. Interestingly, the rhythm generator is anatomically distinct from circuitry that orchestrates muscle activity patterns. Why the rhythm and muscle activity pattern generators are separate is unknown, but probably neurobiologically significant. We believe it may be related to the fact that chewing cycle rhythmicity is relatively invariant. This invariance is curious, given that rhythmic behaviors such as locomotion, heart rate and respiration can vary considerably with changes in functional demands.

2.6 Comparative studies

Although mastication is a mammalian derivation, other non-mammalian species chew rhythmically including teleost fishes (Gintof et al., 2010), some larval amphibians (Larson & Reilly, 2003), and many invertebrates (Marder et al., 2005). Although larval amphibians manifest rhythmic feeding, the adult forms manifest mainly non-rhythmic forms of feeding (Deban et al., 2001). The diversity of chewing patterns among all animals is striking; however, this chapter will focus on mammalian chewing or mastication.

It is generally believed that the masticatory motor program is conserved across mammals (Langenbach & Van Eijden, 2001) and other vertebrate classes as well (Gintof et al., 2010). Although little comparative work at the neurobiological level has been done, it is likely that the fundamental brain stem circuitry that produces mastication is found in many if not most mammals and other vertebrate classes. For the comparative biomechanists, this provides a potentially rich source of questions to address including: (1) does the nervous system constrain evolutionary pathways involving the masticatory apparatus, (2) how are dentoskeletal form and masticatory function interrelated, and (3) how does the centrally generated rhythm differ among species.

2.7 Biomechanics

Oral and mandibular biomechanics are complex due to numerous features including the six degrees of freedom of movement in both TMJs, the 3-dimensional shapes of the mandible the TMJs and the occluding dental surfaces, the material properties of the periodontal ligaments, the complexity of the force-producing muscles including their mechanical redundancy and pennation, and the largely unknown forces generated by muscles of the cheeks, tongue and lips that are in play during rest and function.

Because of these complexities, experimental and modeling studies have made slow inroads to understanding oral biomechanics. Recent finite element modeling (Korioth & Versluis, 1997; Strait at al., 2007), dynamic modeling (Peck & Hannam, 2007), experimental work (Herring et al., 2001) and combinations of experimental and modeling techniques (Gallo, 2005; Peck & Hannam, 2007) have begun to show promise. One of the greatest challenges is to achieve reasonable agreement between experiments and models (Daegling & Hylander, 2000). Biomechanical data and issues with respect to the oromandibular complex are discussed in detail elsewhere (Daegling & Hylander, 2000; Douglas, 1996, Gallo, 2005; van Eijden, 2000). Examples of some of the challenges and issues will be presented, below.

It is tempting to think of the mandible as a Class III lever, with the TMJs serving as fulcra. However, this is an oversimplification, and there is a long-standing alternate argument that the mandible serves as a link with the dentition bearing the load rather than the TMJs (Douglas, 1996). A recent model of the TMJs using MRI and 3-D kinematic data suggests that the joints are loaded during mastication, with the balancing condyle loaded more than the working condyle (Gallo, 2005). The model has not yet captured all functional movements, however, and so it remains possible if not likely that the mandible can act as link, Class III lever or even Class II lever under appropriate conditions (Douglas, 1996). Importantly, biomechanical parameters of interest, e.g., stress, strain, shear, tension, compression, torsion, bending in mandibular corpus, condyles and alveolar bone can be very sensitive to experimental designs or model assumptions.

Of interest to us is whether the time during which opposing teeth are either in contact or are forcibly working on food stuffs, i.e., the occlusal phase of chewing, is related to the rate of tooth wear over the lifetime of an individual. Hence, the forces achieved during mastication are critical parameters to know. These forces have been reported as being 3 - 18 N (reviewed in Douglas, 1996). These are considerably less than the maximum voluntary forces that can be produced in humans, which average about 350 N, with males being able to produce higher (> 400 N) forces on average than women (~ 260 N). Human bite forces are considerably less than those reported in other mammals. Moreover, the maximum voluntary bite forces, above, are higher when the posterior molars and premolars on both left and right sides of the arch are simultaneously maximally intercuspated, as during clenching; maximum voluntary forces drop sharply when the teeth are in eccentric positions, e.g., when anterior teeth are edge-to-edge, where fewer teeth remain in contact.

More investigations are needed to determine how tooth position and bone morphology may be influenced by functional and resting forces, as the above-reported forces are within the range of forces used by orthodontists to move teeth and to alter bone growth patterns.

One of the most promising biomechanical models of the oral complex has been developed in conjunction with the Artisynth project at the University of British Columbia (Peck & Hannam, 2007). This "whole-jaw" modeling project uses morphological and muscle attachment data obtained from imaging real subjects and functional models of muscle physiology, the latter of which can vary in complexity from Huxley-type to Hill-type models. Recently, flexible finite-element model methods have been incorporated to study tissue distortion in the TMJs and tongue associated with function. Jaw movements have been integrated with laryngeal models to explore swallowing and even speech. The ultimate promise is to create subject-specific models and to understand joint loading, movement constraints and neuromotor activation strategies associated with real function. The project is of interest to the issues presented in this chapter, because it is likely that inertial and neuromotor properties of the tongue and hyoid complex may impact chewing rate and rhythmicity. Therefore, a more complete understanding of chewing motor control will require insights from biomechanical models such as those available through Artisynth.

2.8 Clinical significance

There are numerous clinical issues of the orofacial complex, which require biomechanical insights. These include congenital dentoskeletal and neuromuscular anomalies, such as cleft lip and palate, as well as abnormal jaw growth and tooth eruption patterns. Other often serious neuromotor conditions include oral dyskinesias, akinesias, bradykinesias, dystonias, and neurological problems such as aphasias, tics, swallowing disorders and speech disorders. Several common chronic pain conditions occur including temporomandibular disorders (TMD), which are second in prevalence to lower back pain only, and TMD co-morbidities ranging from tinnitus to fibromyalgia. There are issues of physical rehabilitation for denture wearers and cancer survivors who have lost oral structures. Numerous age-related changes in muscle tone, muscle fiber type, oral coordination and eating habits also occur. Several sleep disorders involve the oral apparatus including nocturnal bruxism, sleep-related eating disorder, nocturnal eating syndrome, somniloquy, and obstructive sleep apnea. Many psychosocial disorders involve the orofacial region including facial expressive disorders and eating disorders among others.

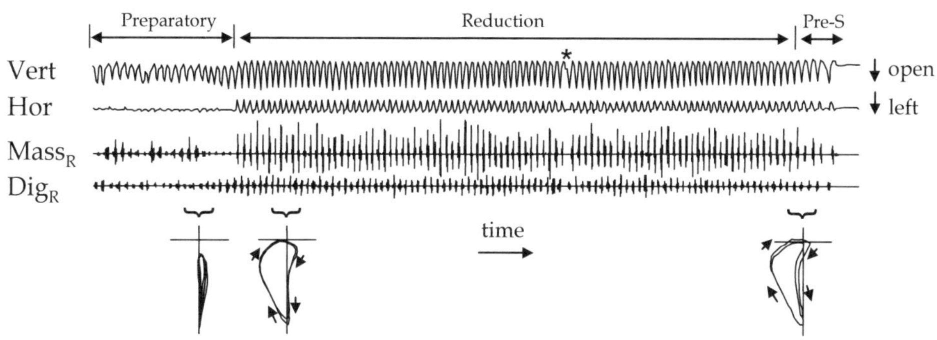

Fig. 1. A chewing sequence. Top: Sequence divided into preparatory, reduction and pre-swallow (Pre-S) series. Traces top to bottom: vertical (Vert) and horizontal (Hor) jaw movement components, right masseter (Mass$_R$), right digastric (Dig$_R$). Asterisk (Vert trace) identifies an O_2 phase. Bottom: Frontal plane projections of jaw movements from each series. Arrows depict jaw movement directions. Crosses on each of the three projections identify the animal's midline (vertical line), and jaw position at maximum closure (horizontal line). Modified and redrawn from Yamada & Yamamura, 1996.

3. Nomenclature: Chewing sequences, series, cycles and phases

Chewing typically occurs in **sequences** beginning with food ingestion and ending with swallowing of the bolus (Fig. 1). A typical chewing sequence is made up of rhythmical chewing **cycles**, which involve successive jaw openings and closings (Fig. 2). Each cycle is then made up of a jaw opening component and a jaw closing component. Many investigators further divide chewing cycles into four **phases** (Fig. 2), viz., slow opening (SO), fast opening (FO), fast closing (FC) and slow closing (SC). We should add that, although these phase names have become fairly commonly used, they may be somewhat misleading. For instance, in some cases, investigators have demonstrated that SO velocities can be faster than velocities occurring during FO (Lund & Enomoto, 1988).

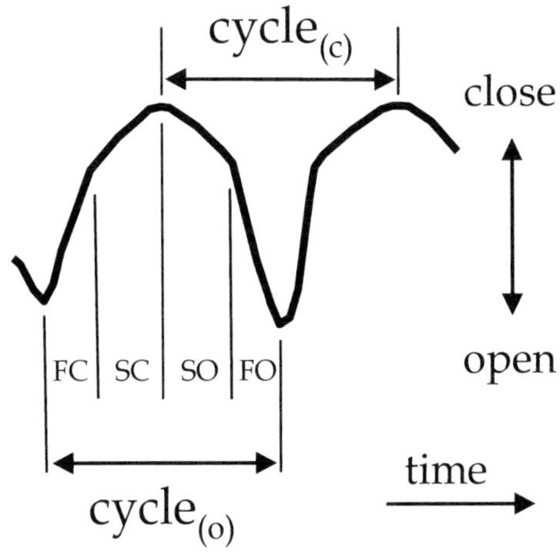

Fig. 2. Masticatory cycles and phases, defined by the vertical jaw movement component using the anterior midpoint of the jaw as a referent (see also Fig. 1). Cycles can be defined from successive maximum jaw closures (cycle$(_c)$) or maximum gapes (cycle$(_o)$). The phases, fast close (FC), slow close (SC), slow open (SO) and fast open (FO) are also shown.

Chewing cycles that introduce food into the mouth are the **preparatory series** (Fig. 1). These cycles are also called Stage I chewing (Masuda et al., 1997; Morimoto et al., 1985), the food preparatory period (Narita et al., 2002; Ootaki et al., 2004; Yamamura et al., 2002), or Type I chews (Schwartz et al., 1989). Those involved with working the food into a bolus are the **reduction series,** Stage IIa chewing (Masuda et al., 1997; Morimoto et al., 1985), rhythmic chewing period (Narita et al., 2002; Ootaki et al., 2004; Yamamura et al., 2002), or Type II chews (Schwartz et al., 1989). Those involved with preparing the food for swallowing by introducing the food into the pharynx are the **preswallow series**, Stage IIb chews (Masuda et al., 1997; Morimoto et al., 1985), the preswallow period (Narita et al., 2002; Ootaki et al., 2004; Yamamura et al., 2002), or Type III chews (Schwartz et al., 1989).

3.1 Type I chews

During a sequence, the food is manipulated initially in the incisor, canine and pre-molar region with a series of rhythmic jaw movements that have been called the preparatory series (Fig. 1). These Type I jaw movement cycles bring the food into the mouth and allow it to undergo initial handling by the anterior teeth as it is moved backwards towards the molars to begin the reduction of the food into a bolus. The preparatory series typically do not involve tooth contact or strong jaw closer muscle activity. They may often have high jaw opener muscle activity. They also tend to be relatively short-duration cycles, i.e., the cycles occur at a relatively fast frequency.

3.2 Type II chews

The rhythmic jaw movements that reduce the food to a bolus are termed the reduction series (Fig. 1). The cycles that constitute this series are the prototypical chewing cycles and involve tooth intercuspation and strong jaw closer muscle activity. Each of these chewing cycles typically consists of FC and SC phases. Whether the opening consists of a single phase, or has two (SO and FO) or even three phases (the third one involves a short pause in jaw movements, see asterisk in Fig. 1) varies, both within chewing sequences and probably across species. The SC phase is the power stroke during which jaw closing muscle force increases to handle the food resistance. Feedback from proprioceptors is used to recruit muscle at a rate that is directly proportional to the resistance offered by the food; the tougher the food, the faster the muscle recruitment rate. This results in each chewing cycle being relatively similar in duration, despite variation in load and concomitant variation in muscle force. This phenomenon is a main part of the discussion in Section 5.

3.3 Type III chews

As the food is reduced and mixed with saliva to form a bolus, tongue movements prepare the food for swallowing by moving the bolus towards the pharynx. The chewing cycles that occur at this time in the sequence are called the pre-swallowing series (Fig. 1) and tend to be the longest duration chewing cycles.

Some chewing cycles may involve a brief pause occurring during opening. When this happens, three opening phases occur, viz., O_1, O_2 and O_3. O_1 and O_3 are similar to SO and FO, respectively, with O_2 being the brief pause (Fig. 1, asterisk). Alternatively, the O_1 and O_2 phases may be lumped together into the SO phase (Lund & Enomoto, 1988). The O_2 phase is associated with a significant increase in cycle duration.

3.4 Caveats

Chewing sequences, cycles and phases can vary considerably, especially under free-roaming conditions, when reduction, ingestion and swallowing can occur at varying time points in a sequence. Under laboratory conditions when a single bite of food is given, the chewing series often proceeds in the order described, above.

Also, it is likely that future investigations will identify species-specific differences in food processing that will be characterized in chewing sequences. One of the future challenges will be to identify what commonalities exist in chewing sequences across species and within species under free-roaming conditions.

We are presently refining methods for use in comparative masticatory studies (see chapter entitled Functional data analysis for biomechanics, in Biomechanics / theory). One of the main goals of this work will be to use these advanced statistical methods to identify functionally and kinematically distinct chewing cycles, to determine why these distinctions exist from biomechanical, developmental, evolutionary and functional perspectives, and ultimately to use the categories to help refine neurophysiologic work so that it becomes possible to address issues regarding how the nervous system switches between chewing cycle forms.

3.5 Summary

A chewing sequence involves ingesting a food morsel and reducing the particle sizes while mixing them with saliva to create a bolus with properties that allow it to be swallowed (Fig. 1).

The chewing sequence consists of rhythmically-occurring chewing cycles (Fig. 2). Over the course of a chewing sequence, the functional nature of chewing shifts from ingestion and initial food handling in the front or anterior part of the mouth (preparatory series) to grinding and reducing the food in the molar region (reduction series) to introducing the food into the pharynx in preparation for swallowing (pre-swallow series). Chewing cycles tend to have the shortest durations during the preparatory series and the longest durations during the pre-swallow series as detailed in (Schwartz et al., 1989).

4. The neuromotor basis of mastication

This section provides a very brief overview of the central and peripheral neural mechanisms involved in the control of oral rhythmic behaviors.

4.1 Central pattern generators (CPG) and central timing networks (CTN)

As is the case for locomotion and respiration, rhythmic oral behaviors including mastication, suckling and licking are controlled by CPG circuits. Unique features to be emphasized below include: (1) anatomical distinctions between CTN also called central rhythm generators (CRG) and the circuits that coordinate output to lower motoneurons, (2) relative invariance in the rhythmicities produced, (3) relatively high variation in the duration of the phases that make up the fundamental cycles.

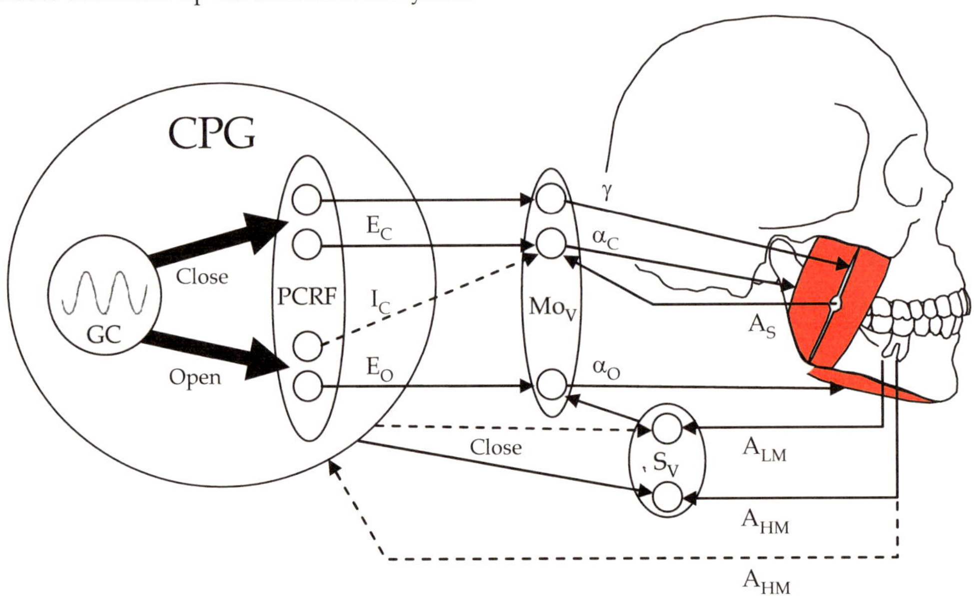

Fig. 3. Simplified diagram of neural components of mastication. Gray ovoids are brain stem nuclei. Solid arrows are excitatory and dotted arrows inhibitory pathways. Abbreviations: Central pattern generator (CPG), nucleus gigantocellularis (GC), parvocellular reticular formation (PCRF), trigeminal motor nucleus (Mo_V), trigeminal sensory nuclei (S_V); afferents: spindle afferents (A_S), low (A_{LM}) and high (A_{HM}) threshold mechanoreceptors; premotoneurons: excitatory to jaw closers (E_C) and to jaw openers (E_O), inhibitory to jaw closers (I_C); lower motoneurons: gammas (γ), alphas to closer (α_C) and opener (α_O) muscles.

4.1.1 Mastication

Fig. 3 shows a diagram of a popular model of CPG circuitry involved in the production of mastication (Nakamura, 1985; Nakamura & Katakura, 1995), reviewed also in (Lund & Enomoto, 1988). The model is based on sophisticated and elegant *in vivo* labeling and electrophysiological work done mainly in the guinea pig and domestic cat. Mastication appears to be largely under the control of CPG circuits located in the pontine and medullary brain stem. Input from higher cortical sites descends through a corticobulbar tract that is a part of the pyramidal system and synapses in the nucleus paragigantocellularis (PGC, not shown in Fig. 3; however, see Fig. 4). The PGC appears to act as a relay between corticobulbar and CPG circuits, because an experimental stimulus frequency applied to the pyramidal tract is recorded in the PGC without modification. However, in the nucleus gigantocellularis (GC), an experimental stimulus applied to the pyramidal tract is packaged into bursts that recur at the rate at which the animal chews. This region within the GC has been termed the central timing network (CTN) or central rhythm generator (CRG).

Output from the GC goes to premotoneurons in the parvocellular reticular formation (PCRF, Fig. 3). These premotoneurons organize output to lower motoneurons, which are located in the trigeminal motor nucleus (Mo_V, Fig. 3). Three main premotoneuron populations have been identified. This includes two excitatory populations, one that synapses on jaw opening lower motoneurons (E_O) and one that synapses on jaw closing motoneurons (E_C). A third population is inhibitory to the jaw closing lower motoneurons (I_C). The E_O and I_C populations burst in synchrony and are involved in jaw opening. The I_C population is believed to suppress the spindle-mediated jaw closing reflex during jaw opening, so that opening is unencumbered by this monosynaptic stretch reflex. The E_C premotoneuron pool bursts out of phase with the other two populations and is involved with jaw closing.

It is likely that there are premotoneurons regulating gamma (γ) motoneuronal activity in spindles; this pathway is depicted as an unlabeled pathway from the PCRF to the γ motoneuron pool in Fig. 3. Both dynamic and static γ motoneurons have been identified (reviewed in Lund, 1991); the dynamic γ motoneurons are tonically active during mastication, whereas the static γ motoneurons are active during jaw closing only. It is likely that α–γ co-activation plays an important role in maintaining a relatively constant chewing cycle frequency in the face of varying loads associated with the ever changing physical properties of ingestants (Ross et al., 2007b).

4.1.2 Licking and suckling

Although most work has focused on the masticatory CPG, there is also interest in the neural correlates of other rhythmic oral behaviors such as spontaneous licking and suckling. Based on evidence from acute animal studies, investigators have suggested that licking and chewing (and other oral rhythmic behaviors) share a common CTN (Carvalho & Gerstner, 2004; Gerstner & Goldberg, 1991; Goldberg & Chandler, 1990). Evidence exists that the licking CTN is located at the same site as the masticatory CTN (Brozek et al., 1996). The concept of a shared CTN probably does not conflict with the more recent model presented by Lund and Kolta describing how CPG circuitry could be modified to produce distinct chewing forms (Lund & Kolta, 2006); at issue is whether the modifiable masticatory CPG output of the Lund-Kolta model in fact produces the licking "form".

There is also debate among scientists about the relationship between suckling and mastication. Iriki, et al. (Iriki et al., 1988) have demonstrated that suckling and mastication are represented at anatomically distinct cortical sites (Fig. 4). In the guinea pig, suckling can only be evoked by stimulation to cortical sites anterior to those that stimulate mastication in adult animals. Stimulating the cortical suckling area (CSA) in adults induces no rhythmic movements. However, in pre-weaned neonates, stimulating the CSA sites produces rhythmic movements that resemble suckling. Stimulating cortical masticatory areas (CMA) in neonates produces no rhythmic jaw movements; however, in the same animals upon weaning, stimulation of these CMA sites produces rhythmic chewing-like movements.

Although suckling and chewing are distinct at the cortical level, the brain stem sites involving the two appear to overlap (Fig. 4, bottom). Future work is required to determine if suckling and chewing share brain stem circuitry.

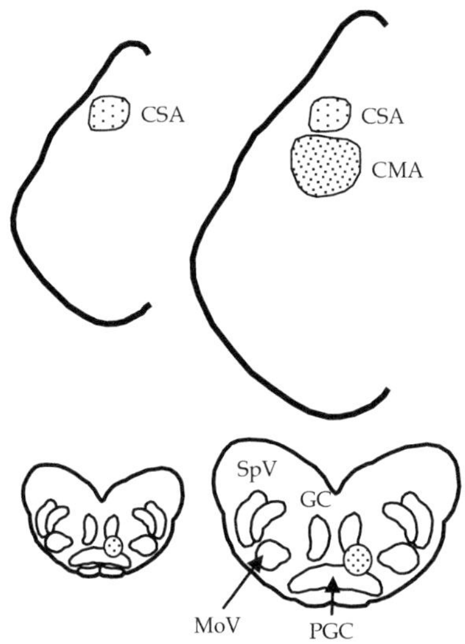

Fig. 4. Top. Left cortical hemispheres of neonate (left) and adult (right) guinea pigs. Bottom. Brain stem sections of neonate (left) and adult (right) guinea pigs. Abbreviations: CSA, cortical suckling area; CMA, cortical masticatory area; SpV, spinal trigeminal system (nucleus is medial, tract is lateral); MoV, trigeminal motor nucleus; GC, nucleus gigantocellularis; PGC, nucleus paragigantocellularis. Modified from Iriki et al., 1988.

4.1.3 Tooth eruption and the transition from suckling to chewing

The above findings (Iriki et al., 1988) are interesting, given that guinea pigs used in the experiments, are born with erupted teeth, which show wear from intra-uterine grinding. However, neonatal guinea pigs do not feed or chew until weaning, indicating that tooth eruption is not sufficient to produce chewing. Rather, events surrounding weaning are apparently required to make the transition from suckling to chewing. What the events are that induce the transition are presently unknown. In any case, discoveries in this area will contribute importantly towards understanding the development of motor systems.

A developmental study of dogs demonstrated that the normal weaning period was prolonged when either the tooth buds were enucleated or the trigeminal afferents to the teeth were blocked (Iinuma et al., 1994). In the case of the afferent block, the puppies ultimately made a transition from suckling to rhythmic chewing. However, in the enucleated group, rhythmicity never developed. The puppies in the enucleated group ate food by "biting" rather than by chewing. In a third experimental group, puppies' teeth were removed after they had erupted and after the puppies had learned to chew rhythmically; this group maintained a rhythmic chewing pattern after the removal of the teeth.

These findings suggest that the teeth and associated afferents are important for developing a normal chewing rhythm, even if chewing starts considerably after tooth eruption. Carefully designed future experiments may be able to uncover a critical developmental window when the brainstem CTN circuits are most responsive and adaptive to such peripheral feedback or cues. This could also be useful for insights into allometric scaling (see Section 5).

4.2 Afferent systems

There are also several afferent systems that regulate and are, in turn, regulated by the CPG circuitry. Among these are muscle spindles found mainly in the jaw closer muscles, tendon organs found in small numbers in jaw opener and tongue muscles, joint receptors (e.g., Ruffini and Pacinian receptors, ligamentous organs and free-nerve endings), high- and low-threshold mechanoreceptors in the oral mucosa, tongue and periodontal ligaments around tooth roots, skin and hair receptors, temperature receptors and nociceptors. For simplicity, Fig. 3 only shows spindle afferents in the masseter, a jaw closer (A_S), and high (A_{HM}) and low (A_{LM}) threshold mechanoreceptors from the periodontal ligament of a lower molar. The spindle and mechanoreceptor afferents are believed to play important roles in minimizing tooth breakage and wear during mastication among other functions (Ross et al., 2009).

Feedback from afferents is carefully modulated by CPG circuitry throughout the masticatory cycle (for review, see Lund, 1991). During jaw opening, the monosynaptic spindle-mediated jaw closing reflex (A_S to α_C, Fig. 3) must be inhibited, and this duty is performed by the inhibitory premotoneuron pool (I_C, Fig. 3). Likewise, during closing the CPG modulates feedback from afferent mechanoreceptors (A_{LM} and A_{HM}, Fig. 3). These afferents mediate a multisynaptic jaw opening reflex, which plays a protective role so that teeth and mucosa are not damaged during jaw closing. Generally, feedback from the A_{LM} is inhibited by the CPG, probably so that low loads do not result in jaw opening during food reduction, whereas feedback from the A_{HM} is enhanced by the CPG, probably so that the opening reflex responds efficiently when potential damage is most likely to occur.

Fig. 3 also shows that feedback from the A_{HM} probably directly inhibits CPG activity so that chewing is halted when potential damage has occurred (Fig. 3, bottom). Similar inhibitory feedback to CPG circuitry probably involves other mechanoreceptors, nociceptors and joint receptors. Activation of these inhibitory feedback arms is responsible for the familiar responses that occur when the tongue or cheeks are accidentally bitten or when something too hard for chewing is bitten.

4.3 Model limitations

The above description is a considerable simplification. Moreover, most of the known details of brainstem control of mastication stem from work involving guinea pigs, cats, rabbits, rats and mice. Hence, knowledge of masticatory neuromotor control is based on a few, mainly inbred laboratory animal models. Virtually nothing is known about the control of mastication in humans or the other 5400+ mammalian species.

There is a broadly-held assumption that masticatory neural circuitry is conserved among mammals. On the other hand, the variation in mammalian dentoskeletal and masticatory muscle forms is striking. It seems likely, therefore, that masticatory neural circuitry would show equally variant characteristics across species. More comparative work is required before the assumption of conserved masticatory neural circuitry can be substantiated.

5. Problems and issues

This section introduces issues involving chewing rate, F_C, or its inverse chewing cycle duration, T_C. We discuss first the surprising relationships between T_C, which is relatively invariant, and the durations of chewing cycle phases, which are relatively variant. Functional and developmental issues with respect to these relationships will be discussed. Next, we tackle issues and experiments relating the scaling of T_C across species and finish by introducing experiments that beg for better biomechanical models of chewing rhythmicity.

5.1 Chewing cycle invariance and phase variance

Ross, et al. (Ross et al., 2010; Ross et al., 2007b) have described chewing variability via the coefficient of variation, CV,

$$CV = SD / Y \tag{1}$$

where SD is the standard deviation of a sample and Y is the mean. CV standardizes variation for comparison purposes. It has been used as an uncorrected statistic (equation 1) (Ross et al., 2010; Ross et al., 2007b) or corrected (Gintof et al., 2010),

$$CV = (1 + 1/4n) * SD / Y \tag{2}$$

where n is the sample size used in the calculation (see Sokal & Braumann, 1980).

Of interest are two important facts. First, the CV for cycle duration, T_C, is surprisingly low in mammals (21%) compared with lizards (32%) (Ross et al., 2007b). Second, the CVs of the phases, which constitute a cycle (cf. Fig. 2) are relatively high, ranging on average from 38% for FC to 73% for FO. In fact, FO and FC phases are significantly more variant in mammals than they are in lizards, and SC variability is similar in mammals and lizards (Ross et al., 2007b). These findings suggest that time-sharing must occur among cycle phases so that T_C remains relatively constant in mammals.

Investigators have extensively studied the correlations between chewing cycle durations and phase durations and the correlations among phase durations. Below, we review work in this area, which reveals as yet resolved complexities. Further work in this area will provide important insights into neural control mechanisms.

5.1.1 Phase modulation and chewing series (preparatory, reduction, pre-swallow)

Work with cats (Hiiemae, 1976; Thexton et al., 1980) and rabbits (Morimoto et al., 1985) suggested that the durations of opening phases (particularly SO, Fig. 2) were correlated with T_C. By contrast, the durations of the closing phases did not correlate with T_C.

However, further work in rabbits demonstrated that correlations between phase durations and T_C depended on cycle type, viz., Type I (preparatory series), II (reduction series), and III (pre-swallow series) (Schwartz et al., 1989). These investigators found positive correlations between opening phases and T_C during Type I and III chews, but not during Type II chews. Likewise, FC and T_C were positively correlated during Type I and III chews, but not during Type II chews. Also SC and T_C were positively correlated during Type II chews, but negatively correlated during Type III chews. It was concluded that three major changes occurred in the chewing motor program during a chewing sequence (Schwartz et al., 1989).

Although these results suggest that kinematic and functional distinctions are important considerations in understanding phase modulation, there are several other important factors that have profound effects on phase modulation as well (see below).

5.1.2 Phase modulation and food properties

It has been shown in rabbits that food properties can influence the relationship between phase durations and T_C. During Type II (reduction series) chews, the opening and FC phases were positively correlated with T_C when the animals chewed bread, whereas these correlations were not present when the animals chewed rice or rabbit chow (Yamada & Yamamura, 1996). By contrast, SC was positively correlated with T_C when the animals chewed rice; however, this correlation was absent when the animals were chewing on bread or rabbit chow (Yamada & Yamamura, 1996).

5.1.3 Phase modulation in driven chewing

A few studies have been done to determine how individual phases are modulated during driven mastication in humans. This typically involves chewing to the beat of a metronome, starting at speeds similar to that of "natural" chewing and increasing the frequency to several times that of natural chewing. Morimoto, et al. (Morimoto et al., 1984) determined that, although the duration of all phases was reduced as driven chewing speed was increased, it was mainly the durations of the opening phase and the occlusal phase (the occlusal phase being the time when the teeth on both arches are crushing the food) that were most significantly correlated with the reduction in T_C. The duration of closing was not as shortened as were the durations of the opening and occlusal phases during the experimental reduction in T_C via increased metronome speeds. The authors suggested that their results for the opening phase corroborated the findings for the cat (Thexton et al., 1980), which findings we presented in Section 5.1.1; however, because the cat lacks an occlusal phase, the cat would not be expected to have an occlusal phase to modulate.

On the other hand, in a similar experiment performed by Plesh, et al. (Plesh et al., 1987), all phases showed similar reductions in duration as the driven speed of mastication was increased. These investigators concluded that all phases were variant.

We believe it is important to recognize that the metronome-driven chewing studied by these investigators is probably controlled or strongly modulated by the cortex (and possibly by cerebellar circuits). It is highly likely that the cortex plays little role in ongoing mastication of the sort being studied in animal models. Hence, what these human experiments demonstrate is that, even with the cortex heavily involved in the production of mastication, there can be complex phase modulation relationships.

5.1.4 Phase modulation individuality

Many if not all of the studies, above, report considerable variation in mean phase and T_C durations at the individual level. We have recently completed a study of data used in a previous publication (Gerstner & Parekh, 1997), in which 22 healthy adult subjects chewed an 8-10 mm diameter gum base pellet first on the right side and then on the left. Twenty-second samples of right-sided and 20-s samples of left-sided chewing were digitized, and then filtered and processed using the functional data analysis methods we present in our chapter on Functional Data Analysis for Biomechanics.

The results revealed individual differences in phase-T_C correlations. Specifically, of the 44 trials (22 subjects x left- and right-sided chewing trials), 18 had positive correlations between SO and T_C, 15 had positive correlations between FO and T_C, one had a negative correlation between FO and T_C, 7 had positive correlations between FC and T_C, and 14 had positive correlations between SC and T_C. Interestingly, in no case were the same correlations found for the left and right-sided chewing trials for a given subject. These findings suggest two things: (1) that left and right-sided chewing within individuals is unique in terms of phase modulation and (2) that phase modulation is unique among individuals. It is important to recognize that all subjects were chewing gum with the same material properties and probably performing mainly Type II (reduction series) chewing cycles.

This suggests several possibilities to us. First, these findings may be unique to humans. Humans have a dense corticobulbar tract relative to other species. If this tract played a role in modulating chewing phases in our human subjects, it may impart individual-specific characteristics in the form of unique phase modulation patterns.

Alternatively, phase modulation patterns may be species-specific and vary across species. Any species-specificity tendencies that may exist may be further amplified by the heavy inbreeding that occurs among laboratory animals, the various results from which were presented, above. We believe it will be important in future work to determine (a) whether the correlations observed within individuals are stable through time, (b) whether there is evidence of heritability in the patterns, and (c) whether the patterns are species-specific.

Perhaps the most intriguing issues are, why does phase modulation vary within chewing sequences, between foods and between individual humans? And what can comparative studies and carefully-designed experiments tell us about the function, stability and behavior of rhythmic motor programs?

5.2 Why and how is chewing rate allometrically-scaled across mammals?

Chewing cycle duration, T_C, scales with body mass across mammalian species (Druzinsky, 1993; Gerstner & Gerstein, 2008; Ross et al., 2009). The scaling takes the mathematical form:

$$y = aM^b \tag{3}$$

or its logarithmic transformation:

$$\log(y) = b*\log(M) + \log(a) \tag{4}$$

Where y is, for instance, T_C or its inverse F_C, and M is usually a size variable, e.g., body mass, M_B, jaw mass, M_J, or jaw length, L_J. The logarithmic transformation linearizes the relationship between y and M, so that log(a) is the y-intercept and b is the slope. Among mammals, the scaling exponent, b, ranges from 0.14 - 0.20, when $y = T_C$ and $M = M_B$ (Druzinsky, 1993; Gerstner & Gerstein, 2008). Among primates, the scaling exponent ranges from 0.514 - 0.583, when $y = T_C$ and $M = L_J$ (Ross et al., 2009).

The slope or scaling exponent is important for several reasons. For one, it describes the relationship between size and the dependent variable, y, over as many as 10 orders of magnitude in M (e.g., Turvey et al., 1988). Furthermore, in comparative studies, the exponent suggests the existence of laws governing biomechanical, morphological, physiological or behavioral variation within taxa. Also, allometric scaling probably represents the manifestation of general organizing principles. Therefore, the promise is that an understanding of allometric scaling may lead to a better understanding of many biological relationships, including those governing many motor control problems.

F_C ranges from < 1 Hz for large species such as elephants and giraffes to > 7 Hz for small species such as mice. Although the scaling of chewing rate with size makes intuitive sense, there are no unequivocal reasons why or how the scaling comes to be. This opens up several interesting questions, which will form much of the remaining discussion in this chapter.

Biologists believe that the masticatory CPG, including the rhythm-generating CTN discussed previously (Fig. 3), is highly conserved among mammals. If one takes this literally, then all mammalian species should possess a CTN that produces a similar masticatory rhythmicity, i.e., the mean and variance in F_C should be nearly the same within individuals of a species, between individuals of a species, and between species.

Secondly, studies to be discussed, below, have demonstrated that the masticatory rhythm adjusts to load variation, probably via feedback from proprioception during chewing. If we take these results at face value, then all mammals should chew at about the same rate because the masticatory system is designed to hold chewing rate constant despite variation in load, including presumably load variation due to jaw mass.

Obviously, what we are omitting from this literal interpretation is whether size-dependent variation in such things as CTN circuitry, peripheral nerves, muscle contractile properties, the size of orofacial structures, tooth biting surface area, metabolic and vascular properties, etc., can influence the fundamental rhythm generated by the CTN. However, in order to shed light on our issue of interest, we are focusing on the observations and claims reported in the literature that: (1) chewing rate is centrally generated by the CTN, (2) the frequency generated by the CTN is relatively invariant, (3) the CTN is a conserved phenotype across mammals, and (4) proprioception serves to hold frequency relatively constant against variation in load. Given these observations and claims, it is unclear how neurobiological factors are being adjusted so that the size-dependent scaling among mammals occurs. In other words, that chewing rate scales with size indicates that there are details with respect to the timing of chewing and chewing rhythmicity, which need to be elucidated.

5.2.1 Acute oral rhythmicity experiments

An obvious missing 'detail' of the model presented in Section 4 is the possibility that cellular or molecular mechanisms exist that adjust chewing rhythmicity to match load variation due to, say, jaw mass independent of load variation due to food properties. Numerous experiments seem to refute this possibility, however.

Using an anesthetized guinea pig model, which can be made to produce rhythmic chewing upon stimulation to a specific region of the cortex known as the cortical masticatory area (CMA, Fig. 4), Chandler and Goldberg were able to demonstrate that affixing 20- and 50-g weights to the lower jaw did not significantly change the rate of oral rhythmicities, although it did increase both the amplitude and duration of masseter (jaw closer) EMG activity (Chandler et al., 1985). The authors believed this was most likely due to an increase in the excitability of jaw closer motoneurons produced by activation of muscle spindles within the jaw closer muscles.

Similarly, Ross' group recently demonstrated that bite force was modulated during SC, primarily by varying the rate at which force was generated in the jaw closers of macaques (Ross et al., 2007a). In other words, as the resistance in food properties increased, not only did the number of recruited muscle fibers increase, but the rate at which muscle fibers were recruited increased as well, so that the increased load did not significantly impact the

duration of jaw closure. The group hypothesized that the reported low variance in chewing cycle durations might be attributable at least in part to rate modulation of bite force during SC (Ross et al., 2010).
These acute experiments demonstrate that, in the short term, the masticatory neuromotor system seems designed to hold chewing rate constant.

5.2.2 Chronic oral rhythmicity experiments

The above experiments demonstrate that chewing rate adjusts to acute load variations. But what about chronic load variations? Is it possible that chronic-tonic changes in load could lead to rhythm adjustments? That is, might the rhythm adapt to load due to jaw mass by slowing or speeding up accordingly, whereas it would adapt to load due to food stuffs by varying jaw closer muscle recruitment levels?
In order to test this, we placed submandibular gold implants in test rats, which doubled the weight of the jaws, and acrylic implants in control rats, which increased the weight of the jaws by only 10%. We then monitored licking rates for 3 months (Carvalho & Gerstner, 2004). (Licking rates are also relatively invariant. Also, as we presented, above, licking and chewing are believed to share the same CTN.) The licking rates remained not significantly different between test and control animals. Interestingly, each animal maintained an individual-specific licking rate such that individuals could be identified at the study's end by reference to their baseline licking rates.
This study showed that chronically loading the jaws for 3 months did not lead to changes in licking rates. However, this experiment was done in grown rats. Perhaps there is a critical window in development when CTN circuitry is particularly plastic and adaptable to jaw mass or load properties. Two such studies, one using a mutant mouse strain and one using dog breeds of various sizes, have been done that shed light on this issue.
Work has been done with the osteopetrotic mouse (op/op), a genetic mutant that results in unerupted teeth and the lack of an important proprioceptive feedback from mechanoreceptors around the dental roots (Kobayashi et al., 2002b). The question was, do these animals chew similarly to normal mice? Although some aspects of feeding were different between the mutant and normal mice, one surprising feature was that the mean ± SD duration of T_C for the mutant mice was similar to that of normal mice (205.6 ms ± 20.5 vs. 205.5 ms ± 34.0, respectively). The authors concluded that these results suggested that the CPG may be genetically pre- programmed, needing no feedback from peripheral receptors to develop.
We evaluated 31 dog breeds in conjunction with 31 size-matched non-domestic mammalian species as a control group with body masses ranging from about 2 kg - 50 kg in both groups. For the dog breeds, T_C did not scale to M_B ($r = 0.299$, $P > 0.1$) nor to L_J ($r = 0.33$, $P > 0.05$); however, T_C did scale to M_B among the mammalian species ($r = 0.63$, $P < 0.001$). We interpreted the results for the dogs to mean that the CTN rhythmicity does not necessarily adjust, even in developmental time scales to the size of the adult animal. The fact that we did see T_C - M_B scaling in the size-matched non-domestic mammals suggested to us that we should have seen scaling in the dogs if scaling necessarily occurred.

5.2.3 Hypothesis 1: Scaling is a result of natural selection

The dog-study results suggested to us that allometric T_C - M_B scaling may be due to natural selection, based on the following arguments. First, the non-domestic mammals manifested

T_C - M_B scaling, indicating that non-domestic species possess chewing rates that scale to M_B. Moreover, all members of a given non-domestic species manifested similar T_C durations and M_B. These results would most likely occur via one of two means: (1) if M_B and T_C were genetically inherited, or (2) if T_C came to scale with M_B as a result of neural feedback in developmental time scales.

If the results had occurred via the first means, i.e., that M_B and T_C were genetically inherited, then M_B and T_C could either be regulated by independent genes, or they could be regulated by the same genes, and thus represent a pleiotropy.

If both M_B and T_C were regulated by independent genes, then the observed T_C - M_B scaling would suggest that the scaling was a result of selection. Alternatively, if T_C - M_B scaling were a pleiotropy, then the scaling should have been observed in the dog breeds. This is because, as breeders select for specific M_B, T_C would have been modified as well. This was not the case, suggesting that M_B and T_C are genetically independent.

It is also important to note that we specifically evaluated L_J in the dogs. Breeders have selected for variation in head size independently of M_B in many breeds. Hence, it is revealing that the dog breeds manifested a lack of either T_C - M_B scaling or of T_C – L_J scaling, because this argues against both the pleiotropy hypothesis and the neural control hypotheses. Based on these results, it would appear that chewing rate may be genetically inherited, and that the scaling occurs as a result of natural selection mechanisms.

5.2.4 Hypothesis 2: Chewing rate is fixed during a critical developmental window

The "selection" hypothesis, above, is primarily based on work with adult animals. It is important to stress that the developmental studies of dogs and guinea pigs presented in Section 4.1.3 suggest an alternative hypothesis, which considers infant size.

The infants of most dog breeds are similarly sized for several weeks before weaning (Hawthorne et al., 2004). If canid T_C were adjusted to scale with L_J or M_B during an early developmental window prior to weaning, then T_C - M_B scaling would not be observed among adult dogs representing breeds differing significantly in adult M_B.

By contrast, there is a correlation between adult M_B and infant M_B among many mammals (Calder, 1996). As for the dogs, if T_C were adjusted to L_J or M_B during an early developmental window prior to weaning in the mammals we studied, then T_C - M_B scaling would be observed among the adult mammals as a result of the correlation between adult and infant M_B.

Given that the erupting teeth appear to play a role in the development of rhythmicity (Section 4.1.3), it seems plausible that the duration of the adult T_C could be determined during a critical developmental window. We would hypothesize that during this window, the nascent CTN circuitry could have its rhythmic output adapted to load due to jaw size, tongue size, oral cavity size, size of a mouthful of ingestant, etc. via peripheral feedback. After this critical window closes, the CTN would only be able to adjust to load variations by modulating muscle recruitment to hold the rhythm constant. The rhythm frequency carried into adulthood would then reflect the time at which the CTN circuitry reached a critical maturation point and/or the time at which the sensory systems modulating muscle recruitment matured.

To begin evaluating the potential role of development, we have undertaken studies of humans between the ages of 4 – 6 yrs (n=20), 11 – 13 yrs (n=20) and 18 - 21 yrs (n=20), sampling mean chewing rates by videotaping gum chewing for 2 minutes and calculating L_J

using lateral cephalograms, a radiograph of the head in the sagittal plane used by orthodontists to perform morphometric analyses of jaw sizes. Our preliminary results suggest that T_C continues to slow down during childhood and adolescence. Hence, a critical developmental window does not appear to occur in human chewing rhythmicity.

However, as introduced earlier in the chapter, humans are characterized by a large corticobulbar fiber tract, which is not present in most other mammalian species. It is possible that this tract provides a means, relatively unique to humans, for continuous adaptation of the oral rhythm. Intriguingly in this regard, the changes in chewing rhythm appear to correlate better with biological age than with L_J among our subjects. This may suggest that CTN maturation is delayed among humans but not indefinitely so.

Why would adjustments leading to T_C - LJ or T_C - M_B scaling during development be critical? Mammals as endotherms require significant energy for sustenance, and maternal milk production in conjunction with infant suckling are two inextricably linked mammalian characteristics necessary for mammalian infant survival. Efficient ingestion of milk is, therefore, critical to individual survival. It has been suggested that the invariant rhythmicity of chewing, with the rhythmicity matched to the natural resonance frequency of the jaw, are necessary for efficient energy acquisition and food processing (see Ross et al., 2010 for a review). Although this suggestion has been made for chewing in adult animals (Ross et al., 2010), it is arguable that an efficient suckling rhythm is even more critical for infant survival.

To evaluate the efficiencies associated with masticatory rhythmicity, we have begun studies of the metabolic costs of chewing at various rates. These have proven somewhat challenging, as the increase in metabolic rate associated with chewing is very small compared to resting metabolic rate. This, however, may be rather telling; if metabolic costs associated with chewing are easily lost in the fluctuations of resting metabolic rate, how metabolically costly can chewing be? If we confirm that chewing at different rates does not result in significant metabolic changes, it will be important to turn our attention to metabolic issues associated with suckling in infancy. If metabolic issues are more significant in infant suckling than in adult chewing, this would provide some important clues as to why the rhythmicity would be determined in infancy and not in adulthood.

5.2.5 Other chewing rhythm observations

Numerous biomechanical models have been presented in the literature to predict the relationship between L_J and T_C (Druzinsky, 1993; McMahon, 1975, 1984; Ross et al., 2009; Turvey et al., 1988). These models predict that L_J is directly proportional to T_C and, therefore, inversely proportional to F_C. In other words, as the length of the jaw lever arm (L_J) increases, F_C should decrease and T_C should increase.

As the food shifts from the front of the mouth during preparatory series chews to the back of the mouth during pre-swallow series chews, L_J, defined by where the food is with respect to the jaw joint fulcrum, gets progressively shorter (Fig. 5). Therefore, if chewing could be approximated by any of the lever-arm models, one would expect that the preparatory series chews would have relatively long durations and pre-swallow series chews would have relatively short durations. However, this is the opposite of what is seen, as the shortest-duration chews occur at the beginning of chewing sequences and the longest-duration at the end of chewing sequences (Fig. 1). This observation indicates that, within individuals, T_C does not appear responsive to feedback regarding the functional L_J; rather, T_C is being determined by the cycle type. Therefore, whatever is responsible for modulating cycle type is key in this regard.

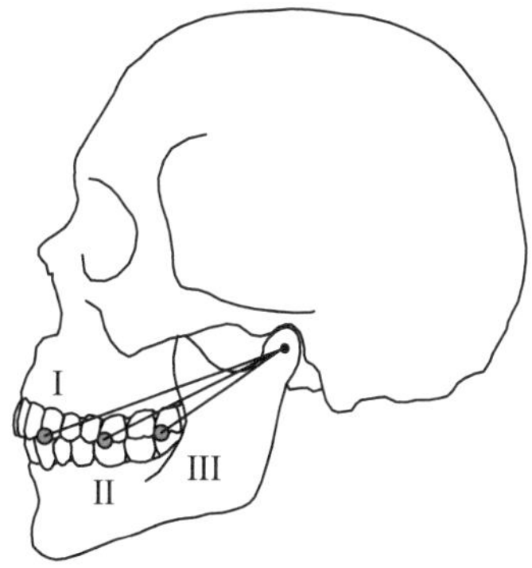

Fig. 5. Jaw lever lengths for preparatory (I), reduction (II) and pre-swallow (III) series cycles.

In humans, males have larger jaws (longer L_J) than females. Therefore, the lever-arm models would predict that males should chew more slowly than females. However, adult human males chew more rapidly than age-matched young adult females (F_C = 1.4 Hz ± 0.3 for 45 males versus 1.2 Hz ± 0.3 for 44 females; our unpublished observations).

Males tend to have more masticatory muscle mass, and male masticatory muscle tends to have more fast fatigable fibers than does female masticatory muscle. Thus, an important set of studies should be performed to identify the relationship between gender, chewing rate and muscle fiber characteristics. Additionally, if results of other studies determine that the rhythmicity is determined during infancy (Section 5.2.4), it would be critical to identify relationships between gender and suckling with respect to gender-specific chewing rates.

These observations suggest some of the intellectual challenges to understanding masticatory control. One important challenge is to develop appropriate biomechanical models of mastication and/or suckling. Another challenge will be to understand the role and function of chewing cycle phases, especially with respect to why phases are added or deleted from ongoing chewing sequences. Finally, it will be critical to identify why and how chewing cycle rhythmicity is so tightly controlled.

6. Conclusion

Rhythmic oral behaviors are under-represented in biomechanics studies; however, the neural mechanisms that produce them, coupled with the biomechanical issues of moving the jaw, tongue and teeth during behaviors such as mastication, licking and suckling present challenges to traditional biomechanical modeling and thinking. Oral rhythmicities are generated by a central timing network, CTN, and associated proprioception, which together produce a relatively invariant rhythmicity. Load variability results in modulation of the rate of muscle recruitment, which results in a chewing rhythm with low variability. Most of the variability in the chewing rhythm is linked to shifts between chewing cycle types. Numerous studies and observations indicate that traditional pendulum and mass-spring biomechanical models are inadequate. The rhythm may be set early in infancy during suckling or it may be genetically pre-programmed and matched to jaw size via natural selection to produce efficient chewing. The problems with understanding the jaw system may expose limitations in other biomechanical models and provide new challenges to more traditional biomechanics studies and paradigms. Future studies will require approaches as diverse as neuroscience, evolutionary, developmental, and comparative biology in order to address biomechanical problems effectively. Because the oral system is a feature shared among humans, mammals and most vertebrates, these studies promise broad impacts and insights to biomechanical issues.

7. References

Brainerd, E. L.; Baier, D. B.; Gatesy, S. M.; Hedrick, T. L.; Metzger, K. A.; Gilbert, S. L. & Crisco, J. J. (2010). X-Ray Reconstruction of Moving Morphology (XROMM): Precision, Accuracy and Applications in Comparative Biomechanics Research. *Journal of Experimental Zoology,* Vol. 313A, pp. 262-279, ISSN 1932-5223

Brozek, G.; Zhuravin, I. A.; Megirian, D. & Bures, J. (1996). Localization of the Central Rhythm Generator Involved in Spontaneous Consummatory Licking in Rats: Functional Ablation and Electrical Brain Stimulation Studies. *Proceedings of the National Academy of Sciences USA,* Vol. 93, No. 8, pp. 3325-3329, ISSN 0027-8424

Byrd, K. (1981). Mandibular Movement and Muscle Activity During Mastication in the Guinea Pig (Cavia Porcellus). *Journal of Morphology,* Vol. 170, pp. 147-169, ISSN 0022-2887

Calder III, W. A. (1996). *Size, Function, and Life History.* Dover Publications, ISBN 0-486-69191-8, Mineola

Carvalho, T. & Gerstner, G. E. (2004). Licking Rate Adaptations to Increased Mandibular Weight in the Adult Rat. *Physiology and Behavior,* Vol. 82, No. 2-3, pp. 331-337, ISSN 0031-9384

Chandler, S. H.; Goldberg, L. J. & Lambert, R. W. (1985). The Effects of Orofacial Sensory Input on Spontaneously Occurring and Apomorphine-Induced Rhythmical Jaw Movements in the Anesthetized Guinea Pig. *Neuroscience Letters,* Vol. 53, pp. 45-49, ISSN 1872-7972

Daegling, D. J. & Hylander, W. L. (2000). Experimental Observation, Theoretical Models, and Biomechanical Inference in the Study of Mandibular Form. *American Journal of Physical Anthropology,* Vol. 112, pp. 541-551, ISSN 0002-9483

Deban, S. M.; O'Reilly, J. C. & Nishikawa, K. C. (2001). The Evolution of the Motor Control of Feeding in Amphibians. *American Zoologist,* Vol. 41, pp. 1280-1298, ISSN 0003-1569

Douglas, W. H. (1996). Considerations for Modeling. *Dental Materials,* Vol. 12, pp. 203-207, ISSN 0109-5641

Druzinsky, R. E. (1993). The Time Allometry of Mammalian Chewing Movements: Chewing Frequency Scales with Body Mass in Mammals. *Journal of Theoretical Biology,* Vol. 160, No. 4, pp. 427-440, ISSN 0022-5193

Flavel, S.; Nordstrom, M. & Miles, T. (2002). A Simple and Inexpensive System for Monitoring Jaw Movements in Ambulatory Humans. *Journal of Biomechanics,* Vol. 35, pp. 573-577, ISSN 0021-9290

Gallo, L. M. (2005). Modeling of Temporomandibular Joint Function Using MRI and Jaw-Tracking Technologies--Mechanics. *Cells Tissues Organs,* Vol. 180, pp. 54-68, ISSN

Gerstner, G. & Fehrman, J. (1999). Comparison of Chin and Jaw Movement Parameters During Gum Chewing. *Journal of Prosthetic Dentistry,* Vol. 81, pp. 179-185, ISSN 1097-6841

Gerstner, G. & Goldberg, L. (1991). Genioglossus EMG Activity During Rhythmic Jaw Movements in the Anesthetized Guinea Pig. *Brain Research*, Vol. 562, pp. 79-84, ISSN 0006-8993

Gerstner, G. & Goldberg, L. (1994). Species-Specific Morphology of Masticatory Jaw Movements. *Behaviour*, Vol. 128, pp. 229-253, ISSN 0005-7959

Gerstner, G. & Kinra, D. (1999). Morphometric Analysis of Human Mastication. *Journal of Neuroscience Methods*, Vol. 88, pp. 171-179, ISSN 0165-0270

Gerstner, G.; Marchi, F. & Haerian, H. (1999). Relationship between Anteroposterior Maxillomandibular Morphology and Masticatory Jaw Movement Patterns. *American Journal of Orthodontics Dentofacial Orthopedics*, Vol. 115, pp. 258-266, ISSN 0889-5406

Gerstner, G. & Parekh, V. (1997). Evidence of Sex-Specific Differences in Masticatory Jaw Movement Patterns. *Journal of Dental Research*, Vol. 76, pp. 796-806, ISSN 0022-0345

Gerstner, G. E. & Gerstein, J. (2008). Chewing Rate Allometry among Mammalian Species. *Journal of Mammalogy*, Vol. 89, No. 4, pp. 1020-1030, ISSN 0022-2372

Gintof, G.; Konow, N.; Ross, C. F. & Sanford, C. P. (2010). Rhythmic Chewing with Oral Jaws in Teleost Fishes: A Comparison with Amniotes. *Journal of Experimental Biology*, Vol. 213, pp. 1868-1875, ISSN 1477-9145

Goldberg, L. & Chandler, S. (1990). Central Mechanisms of Rhythmic Trigeminal Activity, In: *Neurophysiology of the Jaws and Teeth*, (A. Taylor, ed.) pp. 268-293. MacMillan Press, ISBN-10: 0333423623, London

Hawthorne, A. J.; Booles, D.; Nugent, P. A.; Gettinby, G. & Wilkinson, J. (2004). Body-Weight Changes During Growth in Puppies of Different Breeds. *Journal of Nutrition*, Vol. 134, pp. 2027S - 2030S, ISSN 0022-3166

Herring, S. W.; Rafferty, K. L.; Liu, Z. J. & Marshall, C. D. (2001). Jaw Muscles and the Skull in Mammals: The Biomechanics of Mastication. *Comparative Biochemistry & Physiology Part A*, Vol. 131, pp. 207-219, ISSN 0300-9629

Hiiemae, K.; Heath, M. R.; Heath, G.; Kazazoglu, E.; Murray, J.; Sapper, D. & Hamblett, K. (1996). Natural Bites, Food Consistency and Feeding Behaviour in Man. *Archives of Oral Biology*, Vol. 41, No. 2, pp. 175-189, ISSN 0003-9969

Hiiemae, K. M. (1976). Masticatory Movements in Primitive Mammals, In: *Mastication*, (D.J. Anderson and B. Matthews, eds.), pp. 105-118. John Wright and Sons, ISBN 0-72360438X, Bristol

Hiiemae, K. M. (2000). Feeding in Mammals, In: *Feeding: Form, Function, and Evolution in Tetrapod Vertebrates*, (K. Schwenk, ed.) pp. 411-448. Academic Press, ISBN 0-12-632590-1, San Diego

Hylander, W. L.; Johnson, K. R. & Crompton, A. W. (1987). Loading Patterns and Jaw Movements During Mastication in Macaca Fascicularis: A Bone-Strain, Electromyographic, and Cineradiographic Analysis. *American Journal of Physical Anthropology*, Vol. 72, No. 3, pp. 287-314, ISSN 0002-9483

Iinuma, M.; Yoshida, S. & Funakoshi, M. (1994). A Role of Periodontal Sensation in Development of Rhythmical Chewing in Dogs. *Comparative Biochemistry & Physiology. Comparative Physiology*, Vol. 107, No. 2, pp. 389-395, ISSN 0300-9629

Iriki, A.; Nozaki, S. & Nakamura, Y. (1988). Feeding Behavior in Mammals: Corticobulbar Projection Is Reorganized During Conversion from Sucking to Chewing. *Brain Research. Developmental Brain Research*, Vol. 44, No. 2, pp. 189-196, ISSN 0165-3806

Kobayashi, M.; Masuda, Y.; Fujimoto, Y.; Matsuya, T.; Yamamura, K.; Yamada, Y.; Maeda, N. & Morimoto, T. (2002a). Electrophysiological Analysis of Rhythmic Jaw Movements in the Freely Moving Mouse. *Physiology & Behavior,* Vol. 75, No. 3, pp. 377-385, ISSN 0031-9384

Kobayashi, M.; Masuda, Y.; Kishino, M.; Ishida, T.; Maeda, N. & Morimoto, T. (2002b). Characteristics of Mastication in the Anodontic Mouse. *Journal of Dental Research,* Vol. 81, No. 9, pp. 594-597, ISSN 0022-0345

Korfage, J. A. M.; Koolstra, J. H.; Langenbach, G. E. J. & Van Eijden, T. M. G. J. (2005a). Fiber-Type Composition of the Human Jaw Muscles--(Part 1) Origin and Functional Significance of Fiber-Type Diversity. *Journal of Dental Research,* Vol. 84, pp. 774-783, ISSN 0022-0345

Korfage, J. A. M.; Koolstra, J. H.; Langenbach, G. E. J. & Van Eijden, T. M. G. J. (2005b). Fiber-Type Composition of the Human Jaw Muscles--(Part 2) Role of Hybrid Fibers and Factors Responsible for Inter-Individual Variation. *Journal of Dental Research,* Vol. 84, pp. 784-793, ISSN 0022-0345

Korioth, T. W. P. & Versluis, A. (1997). Modeling the Mechanical Behavior of the Jaws and their Related Structures by Finite Element (FE) Analysis. *Critical Reviews in Oral Biology & Medicine,* Vol. 8, pp. 90-104, ISSN 1045-4411

Langenbach, G. E. J. & Van Eijden, T. M. G. J. (2001). Mammalian Feeding Motor Patterns. *American Zoologist,* Vol. 41, pp. 1338-1351, ISSN 0003-1569

Larson, P. M. & Reilly, S. M. (2003). Functional Morphology of Feeding and Gill Irrigation in the Anuran Tadpole: Electromyography and Muscle Function in Larval Rana Catesbeiana. *Journal of Morphology,* Vol. 255, pp. 202-214, ISSN 0022-2887

Lund, J. P. (1991). Mastication and Its Control by the Brain Stem. *Critical Reviews in Oral Biology & Medicine,* Vol. 2, No. 1, pp. 33-64, ISSN 1045-4411

Lund, J. P. & Enomoto, S. (1988). The Generation of Mastication by the Mammalian Central Nervous System., In: *Neural Control of Rhythmic Movements in Vertebrates.,* (A.H. Cohen, S. Rossignol and S. Grillner, eds.), pp. 41-72. John Wiley and Sons, ISBN 0-471-81968-9, New York

Lund, J. P. & Kolta, A. (2006). Generation of the Central Masticatory Pattern and Its Modification by Sensory Feedback. *Dysphagia,* Vol. 21, pp. 167-174, ISSN 0179-051X

Marder, E.; Bucher, D.; Schulz, D. J. & Taylor, A. L. (2005). Invertebrate Central Pattern Generation Moves Along. *Current Biology,* Vol. 15, pp. R685-R699, ISSN 0960-9822

Masuda, Y.; Morimoto, T.; Hidaka, O.; Kato, T.; Matsuo, R.; Inoue, T.; Kobayashi, M. & Taylor, A. (1997). Modulation of Jaw Muscle Spindle Discharge During Mastication in the Rabbit. *Journal of Neurophysiology,* Vol. 77, No. 4, pp. 2227-2231, ISSN 0022-3077

McMahon, T. A. (1975). Using Body Size to Understand the Structural Design of Animals: Quadrupedal Locomotion. *Journal of Applied Physiology,* Vol. 39, pp. 619-827, ISSN 0021-8987

McMahon, T. A. (1984). *Muscles, Reflexes, and Locomotion*. Princeton University Press, ISBN 0-691-08322-3, Princeton

Morimoto, T.; Inoue, T.; Nakamura, T. & Kawamura, Y. (1984). Frequency-Dependent Modulation of Rhythmic Human Jaw Movements. *Journal of Dental Research,* Vol. 63, No. 11, pp. 1310-1314, ISSN 0022-0345

Morimoto, T.; Inoue, T.; Nakamura, T. & Kawamura, Y. (1985). Characteristics of Rhythmic Jaw Movements of the Rabbit. *Archives of Oral Biology,* Vol. 30, No. 9, pp. 673-677, ISSN 0003-9969

Nakamura, Y. (1985). Localization and Functional Organization of Masticatory Rhythm Generator in Lower Brain Stem Reticular Formation. *Neuroscience Letters,* Vol. 20, pp. S3-S4, ISSN 1872-7972

Nakamura, Y. & Katakura, N. (1995). Generation of Masticatory Rhythm in the Brainstem. *Neuroscience Research,* Vol. 23, pp. 1-19, ISSN 0168-0102

Narita, N.; Yamamura, K.; Yao, D.; Martin, R. E.; Masuda, Y. & Sessle, B. J. (2002). Effects on Mastication of Reversible Bilateral Inactivation of the Lateral Pericentral Cortex in the Monkey (Macaca Fascicularis). *Archives of Oral Biology,* Vol. 47, No. 9, pp. 673-688, ISSN 0003-9969

Ootaki, S.; Yamamura, K.; Inoue, M.; Amarasena, J. K.; Kurose, M. & Yamada, Y. (2004). Activity of Peri-Oral Facial Muscles and Its Coordination with Jaw Muscles During Ingestive Behavior in Awake Rabbits. *Brain Research,* Vol. 1001, pp. 22-36, ISSN 0006-8993

Peck, C. C. & Hannam, A. G. (2007). Human Jaw and Muscle Modelling. *Archives of Oral Biology,* Vol. 52, pp. 300-304, ISSN 0003-9969

Plesh, O.; Bishop, B. & McCall, W. (1987). Mandibular Movements and Jaw Muscles' Activity While Voluntarily Chewing at Different Rates. *Experimental Neurology,* Vol. 98, No. 2, pp. 285-300, ISSN 0014-4886

Plesh, O.; Bishop, B. & McCall, W. D., Jr. (1993). Kinematics of Jaw Movements During Chewing at Different Frequencies. *Journal of Biomechanics,* Vol. 26, No. 3, pp. 243-250, ISSN 0021-9290

Ross, C. F.; Baden, A. L.; Georgi, J.; Herrel, A.; Metzger, K. A.; Reed, D. A.; Schaerlaeken, V. & Wolff, M. S. (2010). Chewing Variation in Lepidosaurs and Primates. *Journal of Experimental Biology,* Vol. 213, pp. 572-584, ISSN 1477-9145

Ross, C. F.; Dharia, R.; Herring, S. W.; Hylander, W. L.; Liu, Z.-J.; Rafferty, K. L.; Ravosa, M. J. & Williams, S. H. (2007a). Modulation of Mandibular Loading and Bite Force in Mammals During Mastication. *Journal of Experimental Biology,* Vol. 210, pp. 1046-1063, ISSN 0022-0949

Ross, C. F.; Eckhardt, A.; Herrel, A.; Hylander, W. L.; Metzger, K. A.; Schaerlaeken, V.; Washington, R. L. & Williams, S. H. (2007b). Modulation of Intra-Oral Processing in Mammals and Lepidosaurs. *Integrative and Comparative Biology,* Vol. 47, pp. 118-136, ISSN 1557-7023

Ross, C. F.; Reed, D. A.; Washington, R. L.; Eckhardt, A.; Anapol, F. & Nazima Shahnoor, N. (2009). Scaling of Chew Cycle Duration in Primates. *American Journal of Physical Anthropology,* Vol. 138, pp. 30-44, ISSN 1096-8644

Schwartz, G.; Enomoto, S.; Valiquette, C. & Lund, J. P. (1989). Mastication in the Rabbit: A Description of Movement and Muscle Activity. *Journal of Neurophysiology,* Vol. 62, No. 1, pp. 273-287, ISSN 0022-3077

Sokal, R. R. & Braumann, C. A. (1980). Significance Tests for Coefficients of Variation and Variability Profiles. *Systematic Zoology,* Vol. 29, pp. 50-66, ISSN 0039-7989

Strait, D. S. ; Richmond, B. G.; Spencer, M. A.; Ross, C. F.; Dechow, P. C. & Wood, B. A. (2007). Masticatory Biomechanics and its Relevance to Early Hominid Phylogeny:

An Examination of Palatal Thickness Using Finite-Element Analysis. *Journal of Human Evolution,* Vol. 52, pp. 585-599, ISSN 1095-8606

Thexton, A. J.; Hiiemae, K. M. & Crompton, A. W. (1980). Food Consistency and Bite Size as Regulators of Jaw Movement During Feeding in the Cat. *Journal of Neurophysiology,* Vol. 44, No. 3, pp. 456-474, ISSN 0022-3077

Turvey, M. T.; Schmidt, R. C. & Rosenblum, L. D. (1988). On the Time Allometry of Co-ordinated Rhythmic Movements. *Journal of theoretical Biology,* Vol. 130, pp. 285-325, ISSN 0022-5193

Ungar, P. S. (2010). *Mammalian Teeth. Origin, Evolution, and Diversity.* The Johns Hopkins University Press, ISBN-13: 978-0-8018-9668-2, Baltimore

Van Eijden, T. M. G. J. (2000). Biomechanics of the Mandible. *Critical Reviews in Oral Biology & Medicine,* Vol. 11, pp. 123-136, ISSN 1045-4411

Wintergerst, A. M.; Buschang, P. H. & Throckmorton, G. S. (2004). Reducing within-Subject Variation in Chewing Cycle Kinematics-a Statistical approach. *Archives of Oral Biology,* Vol. 49, No. 12, pp. 991-1000, ISSN 0003-9969

Yamada, Y.; Haraguchi, N.; Oi, K. & Sasaki, M. (1988). Two-Dimensional Jaw Tracking and EMG Recording System Implanted in the Freely Moving Rabbit. *Journal of Neuroscience Methods,* Vol. 23, No. 3, pp. 257-261, ISSN 0165-0270

Yamada, Y. & Yamamura, K. (1996). Possible Factors Which May Affect Phase Durations in the Natural Chewing Rhythm. *Brain Research,* Vol. 706, No. 2, pp. 237-242, ISSN 0006-8993

Yamamura, K.; Narita, N.; Yao, D.; Martin, R. E.; Masuda, Y. & Sessle, B. J. (2002). Effects of Reversible Bilateral Inactivation of Face Primary Motor Cortex on Mastication and Swallowing. *Brain Research,* Vol. 944, No. 1-2, pp. 40-55, ISSN 0006-8993

13

Biomechanical, Respiratory and Cardiovascular Adaptations of Bats and the Case of the Small Community of Bats in Chile

Mauricio Canals L[1], Jose Iriarte-Diaz[2] and Bruno Grossi[1]
[1]*Department of Ecological Sciences, Faculty of Science. Universidad de Chile*
[2]*Department of organismal biology and anatomy, University of Chicago*
[1]*Chile*
[2]*USA*

1. Introduction

Bats are unique among mammals for their ability to fly. The acquisition of powered flight required a series of morphological and physiological changes in the basic mammal body plan. The structure of the limbs is the most obvious specialization, however, adaptations for powered flight encompass most organ systems, in particular the cardiovascular and respiratory apparatus. Flight performance is strongly determined by wing morphology, which in turn is associated with the biomechanics and energetics of flight, as well as ecological aspects such as foraging behavior and habitat selection.

In this chapter we focus on respiratory, cardiac and wing morphology characteristics of some bat species present in Chile, correlating the results with ecological and behavioral information. The small community of Chilean bat species shows a pattern similar to that found in other bat communities. With respect to wing morphology we found that *Tadarida brasiliensis*, *Desmodus rotundus* and *Mormopterus kalinowskii* have small wing areas, while molossids have high aspect ratios and that of *D. rotundus* is only moderate. *D. rotundus* has a smaller mass specific wing span, and the highest wing loading. *Myotis chiloensis* has a second moment of area of humerus (Ih), lower than expected from allometric predictions, suggesting poorer resistance. Based on these results four functional groups may be recognized: i) species with high wing loading and low wing span such as *D. rotundus*, capable of rapid flight with moderate power consumption, ii) species with high wing loading and high aspect ratio, such as the molossids *T. brasiliensis and M. kalinowski*, which are capable of fast flight and low power consumption, characteristic of foragers in open areas; iii) species with low wing loading and low wing span such as most vespertilionids, capable of slow and maneuverable flights in a bat that inhabits wooded areas; and iv) *L. cinereus*, forming an isolated group characterized by high speed and agility.

Also the respiratory and cardiovascular systems of bats are modifications or refinements that allow them to survive this extreme way of life. Bats have lung volumes about 72% greater than non-flying mammals of the same size. Pulmonary ventilation can rapidly increase 10 to 17 times as flight begins. These respiratory adaptations, along with structural changes of lungs, lead to higher oxygen consumption than other mammals of similar size, reaching up to 22 mlO_2/gh at low temperatures and during hovering. We found that the bronchial morphology of *T. brasiliensis* shows an optimization of the proximal airway with minimum entropy production during mechanical ventilation. In addition, bats have a very thin alveolar-capillary barrier, yielding an oxygen diffusion capacity similar to birds. Also, the heart of bats is larger than in all other mammals, representing about 1% of body weight, reaching in some cases 2%. Birds and bats reach very similar aerobic capacities. However, while birds have a large set of structural changes in their respiratory system, bats have a cardiorespiratory system optimized to their extreme life style.

The order Chiroptera ("winged hands") is practically defined by saying that it is constituted by flying mammals. These animals require deep structural changes associated with their lifestyle, but based on a mammalian model. Flight influences its main characteristic: wings formed by a membrane called a patagyum. The arms are the dominant limbs while legs are reduced, contributing to the reduction in body mass which is necessary for flight. These structural changes are also associated with the colonization of the crepuscular and nocturnal air space which required the specialization of the visual system in megachiropterans and the development of echolocation in michrochiropterans, where excepting macro chiropterans the vision contributes little, but where the emission and reception of ultrasound, or echolocation, allows the recognition of the surrounding environment; the ear is the main organ sense of the group.

2. Body size

Body size is associated with flight behavior, diet selection, reproductive behavior, physiology and practically all aspects of the biology of bats. (Swartz et al., 2003). Bat body sizes vary from 2 g and 16 cm wingspan in the mammal with the lowest body mass known *Craseonycteris thonglongyai*, to 1.5 Kg and 2 m wingspan in the Asian flying foxes (Megachiroptera; Pteropodidae) (Fenton, 1992).

The superior limit of body size is not imposed by flight, because among birds there are species which weigh up to 14 Kg, such as Koris`s bustard, and the extinct pterosaurs reached giant sizes. It is possible that in bats the superior limit to body mass is imposed by a combination of behavioral, ecological and physiological factors. Insectivorous bats would have aerodynamic and sensorial restrictions. Barclay & Brigham (1991) proposed that associated with an increase in the body mass there is a decrease in the maneuverability that prey detection at long distances requires. However, this would condition the use of low frequencies during echolocation, with a decrease in spatial resolution. Thus, the abundance of large prey could be a limiting factor of body size in these bats, which is corroborated in part by the positive correlation between prey size and body size of bats (Aldridge & Rautenbach 1987; O'Neil & Taylor, 1989). However, this does not apply to large fruit bats that do not use echolocation. In the latter restrictions derived from muscle physiology may operate; kinematics of flight or wing loading and mechanical stress imposed on the bones by flight (Marden, 1994). While the force per unit mass generated by a muscle is approximately constant, the mass-specific power to fly scales positively with mass, resulting in less lift generation per unit of muscle power (Marden, 1994). Similarly, the mechanical power required for flight grows faster (α Mb $^{1.185}$) than the oxygen consumption of bats (Maina et al., 1991; Maina 2000) helping to establish an upper limit of about 1.5 Kg for bats (Carpenter 1986, Maina 2000).

3. Limbs

Limbs of bats are completely conditioned by flight. While the forelimbs are large and strong, the legs are small, contributing to a reduced mass allowing flying. However, these latter have adaptations such as the joint mechanism of the claws, which pivot on the distal phalanges. While an elastic ligament extends the dorsal claw, the long plantar tendon inserts on the ventral side of the base of the claw, flexing it. Thus, when bats hang inverted during rest, the body weight flexes the claw and allows it to catch on a branch or a cliff (Neuweiler, 2000). In most mammals the diameter of the femur scales with body mass raised to the 1/3 power (geometric similarity), but in bats femur diameter is smaller than that of other mammals of similar size. An exception to this generalization is the vampire bat *Desmodus rotundus* in which the diameter of the femur follows the curve of non-flying mammals (Swartz, 1997). This species has a semi-quadrupedal locomotion while feeding, being able to travel on all four limbs and even start flight with a jump (Schutt et al., 1997).

The body and forelimbs are significantly modified for flight. The thin patagium is richly vascularized with muscles that allow tension and bending, thus contributing dynamically to flight. Occipitopollicalis muscles, Dorsoplagiopatagialis, Humeropatagialis, Coracocutaneus, Uropatagialis and Plagiopatagial Tensor contribute to this dynamic tension, while the adductor of the fifth digit causes the arched profile necessary for flight. While bird wing movement is controlled mainly by two muscles and the point of rotation of the wing is slightly medial or dorsal to the level of shoulder joint, in the bats this point is shifted ventrally to the sterno -clavicular articulation, allowing the scapula to participate in wing movements. In the movement of bat wings at least 17 muscles are involved (Neuweiler, 2000). The main lift muscles are the Trapezium, rhomboids, Acromiodeltoideus and Spinodeltoideus, while the lowering of the wings is controlled mainly by Pectoralis, Serratus, Clavodeltoid and Subscapularis. Extension and flexion of the wing are governed by a special muscle arrangement that automates these movements. Both the triceps (extensor, dorsal) and the biceps (flexor, ventral) are inserted from the scapula to the forearm, bypassing the humeral insertion. Also the extensor carpi radialis and flexor carpi ulnaris bypass the radius. Thus the contraction of the triceps causes the extension of the radio-carpal extensor and the whole wing in an almost automatic form (Neuweiler, 2000).

Wing morphology is highly variable, associated with the biomechanics and energetics of flight (Rayner 1979, 1982), and with ecological and behavioral factors such as flight pattern, foraging behavior and habitat selection (Norberg & Rayner 1987, Norberg 1994; Canals et al. 2001, Iriarte-Díaz et al. 2002, Canals et al., 2005).

There are four important parameters related to the aerodynamics of flight: 1) wing loading:

$$W_L = mg / S \quad (1)$$

which represents the weight per unit area (N/m^2) to be supported by the wings; 2) wingspan (B), corresponding to the length of the wings from tip to tip, 3) the aspect ratio:

$$AR = B^2 / S, \quad (2)$$

which is a dimensionless measure of the relative length to width of the wings, so high AR values correspond to long, thin wings and vice versa, and finally 4) wing acuity ratio (i.e., tip length ratio: TL = length of third finger / arm length) (Neuweiler, 2000) .

4. Flight

In its most simple terms, a bat must move the air with its wings in such a way as to produce aerodynamic force. The component of the aerodynamic force that propels the bat forward is thrust and the component that keeps the bat from falling is lift. These forces are opposed by drag (an aerodynamic force) and gravity, respectively. In contrast to planes that continuously produce thrust and lift (by their engines and the constant flow over the wings), bats generate aerodynamic force in a cyclic manner due to the flapping of the wings. Thus, flight in bats is dependent of an appropriate modulation of wing kinematics in order to generate enough aerodynamic force.

Unlike terrestrial locomotion, where limbs push against a solid substrate, aerial fliers use their wings to push against fluids, which distort and swirl to form a complex wake (Dickinson et al., 2000). Although it is the wing motion that is directly responsible for the generation of lift and thrust, we can estimate the aerodynamic forces by looking at the fluid motion left behind a flying animal. Newton's third law requires that the forces exerted by the air upon the wings must be equal and opposite to the forces exerted by the wings upon the air. The wake left behind the wing thus contains a complete 'footprint' of its force generation. An everyday example of this are the vapor trails left by airplane wings, the tip vortices, that arise directly from the aerodynamic forces produced as the plane moves through the atmosphere. Bats also leave an aerodynamic wake and this wake can be measured by looking at the movement of the air left behind.

An aerodynamic wake can be efficiently analyzed in terms of its *vortex structure*. Vorticity is the local angular or rotational velocity of the fluid, and a vortex is somewhat subjectively defined as a concentration of vorticity. Tornados and swirling motions of water draining are familiar examples of vortices. Visualization and quantification of these vortices can be used to estimate aerodynamic forces. Early studies of bat's wake structures, using helium-filled bubbles, suggested that the upstroke function and wingbeat gaits may vary to flight speed, with lift being produced during upstroke at high speeds but not during slow flights (Rayner et al., 1986). These differences in lift generation would be expressed as discrete vortex rings during slow flight in contrast to the ondulating but constant vortex lines observed at fast flight speeds (figure 1). Recent studies using digital particle image velocimetry (DPIV) have allow us to study the wake left behind flying bats with much higher temporal and spatial resolution than those original studies. The emerging picture of the aerodynamic footprint left by bats is that the wake structures are more complex than expected, potentially because of the more complex wing kinematics than that of birds and insects as well as the compliant characteristics of the wing membrane, and currently it is an area of very active research (e.g., Hedenström et al., 2007; Johansson et al., 2008; Muijres et al., 2008; Hedenström et al., 2009; Hubel et al., 2009; Hubel et al., 2010; Wolf et al., 2010).

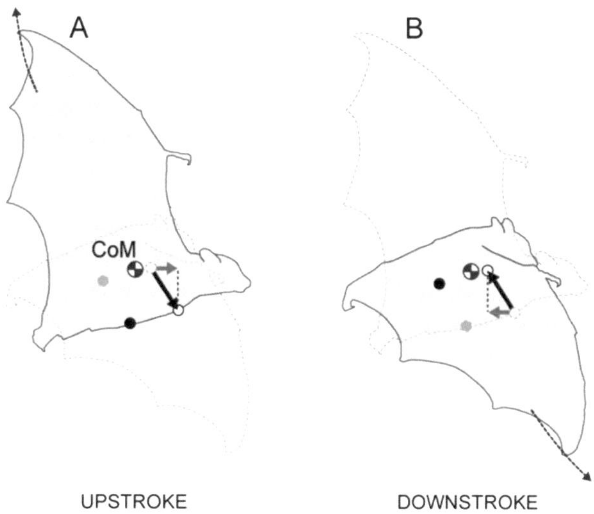

Fig. 1. Effect of the oscillation of the wings on the position of the center of mass (COM) and accelerations of the body. When external forces, such as aerodynamic and gravitational forces, are absent, the position of the COM will remain constant but the body moves in opposition to the flapping wings to conserve momentum. Closed and open symbols correspond to the pelvis and chest markers, respectively. During upstroke (A), the upward and backward acceleration of the wings will produce an inertial force (black arrow) that will move the body forward and downward with respect to the downstroke. This force will produce a forward-oriented component, or inertial thrust, during upstroke (grey arrow). During downstroke (B), the downward and forward acceleration of the wings will produce an inertial force (black arrow) that will move the body backward and upward while keeping the position of the COM constant. The horizontal component of this inertial force will produce negative inertial thrust during downstroke (grey arrow).

Aerodynamic theory predicts that the wing loading, the wing span and aspect ratio are significant parameters in determining performance in flight. For example, during flight the organism should generate sustained lift (L) to support body weight and thrust (T) to overcome drag (D). Thus, the power required to fly is:

$$P = D \cdot v = T \cdot v, \tag{3}$$

where v is the relative velocity of air over the wings. The cost of transport (C), which corresponds to the work done to move a unit of weight for a unit of distance is inversely proportional to the speed:

$$C = P / mgv = T / L, \tag{4}$$

with P = power, m the body mass and g gravity acceleration). Furthermore, the speed is proportional to $W_L{}^{1/2}$, so that both high wing loading and high flight speeds are associated with low transportation costs (Norberg 1987).

The energy per unit time (power) required to fly can be decomposed into that needed to move the wings (inertial power: P_{in}) and the power required to produce the aerodynamic force (R). The latter can be decomposed into the power required to overcome the resistance of the body (parasite power: P_{PAR}), the profile of the wings (Power Profile: P_{PRO}) and the power to generate lift and thrust (induced power: P_I). Thus the total aerodynamic power is the sum these:

$$P = (P_{PAR} + P_{PRO} + P_I) + P_{in} . \tag{5}$$

Plotting the power according to flight speed a typical "U" curve is obtained, whose minimum determines the speed at which it produces the minimum energy expenditure (V_{MP}). It is also possible to calculate the speed which determines the minimum cost of transport (V_{MR}), which is determined by the intersection between the curve and the tangent to it passing through the point (v = 0) (Norberg, 1987).

All these components of energy expenditure of flight are correlated with B and WL, for example $P_{par} \alpha\ v^3\ \alpha\ (W_L)^{3/2}$, $P_{pro}\ \alpha\ S(B/\tau)^3$ during hovering, where τ is the wing beat period, $P_I\ \alpha\ (Mg)^{3/2}/B$ during hovering and $P_I \alpha\ (Mg)^2/(B^2v)$ during forward flight, and $P_{in}\ \alpha\ B^2$ (Norberg, 1987). In addition, the minimum resistance (D_{min}) and the minimum power required to fly (P_{min}) are inversely correlated with the aspect ratio:

$$D_{\min} = 2mg(C_r / \pi AR)^{1/2} , \tag{6}$$

and

$$P_{\min} = [0.95(mg)^{3/2} C_r^{\ 1/4}] / B(AR)^{1/4} , \tag{7}$$

where C_r is the combined parasite and profile friction coefficient. Thus high values of AR are critical in reducing both parameters; AR is considered to be a measure of aerodynamic efficiency (Norberg, 1994). Another important aspect is the high wing acuity (i.e., TL) that allows adequate air movement dynamics around the wings without turbulence. By contrast, rounded wings can generate turbulent flow by increasing the resistance to movement and therefore P_{PRO}.

Norberg and Rayner (1987) attempted to establish a relationship between lifestyle and major aerodynamic parameters of wing morphology, being able to classify four groups of bats: i) bats of open space and faster flight have long and narrow wings, with high wing loadings up 20N/m² and aspect ratios as high as 14.3 in some Molossidae (Fenton 1992, Norberg & Rayner 1987), ii) slow-flying bats of forested areas with short and broad wings, with low wing loading, about 5 to 6 N/m², and low aspect ratios, about 5 (Canals et al. 2001, Iriarte-Díaz et al. 2002), iii) fast flying bats with stationary or short flights, which have high wing loading but low aspect ratios, and finally iv) slow-flying bats in open spaces, which have high aspect ratios but low wing loading (Figure 2).

Species that forage in and around foliage tend to have short, rounded wings with low values of AR and TL, which produces low wing loading. They have a relatively slow flight, between 2.5 and 6 m / s, and are very maneuverable (Neuweiler, 2000). Many of them can use hovering to locate and capture prey over the foliage or to feed on pollen or nectar. Species that forage on leaves are slender, with long, thin wings (high AR) and high wing loading. Their flight speed is high, between 9 and 15 m / s. These bats have less maneuverability. However, their agility, defined as the ability to accelerate and stop quickly, is increased, as is an ability related to wing loading (Norberg & Rayner, 1987). An example of such bats is the Molossidae, for example *Tadarida brasiliensis* in which the highest flight speed has been registered: 27 m / s (Neuweiler, 2000). Some species of bats feed by fishing or hunting on bodies of water, such as *Noctilio leporinus*, requiring a great generation of thrust (T) in flight, plus an important handling. Thus they have higher TL, AR moderate and relatively low wing loading.

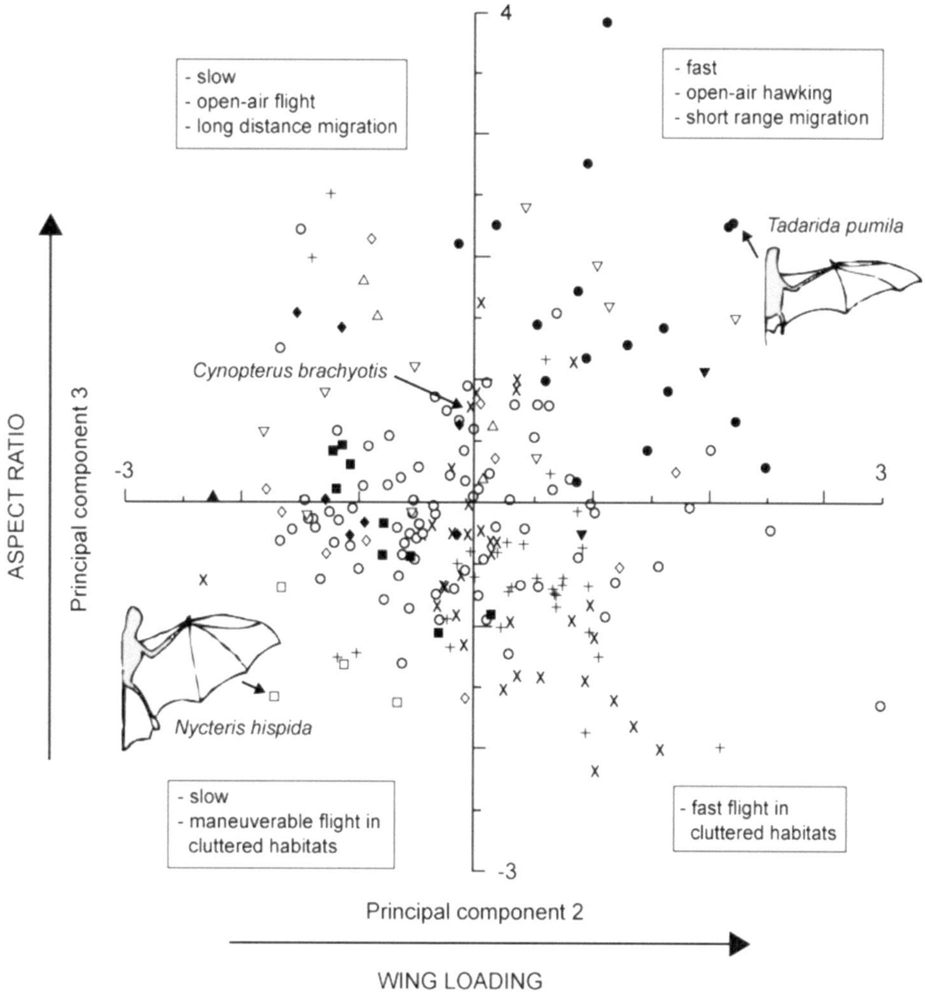

Fig. 2. Principal components for morphological characteristics in several bat species. The first component was explained for body mass, but second and third components are related with wing loading (WL) and the aspect ratio (AR) respectively. This analysis allow recognize different eco-morphological groups of bats. Modified from Wainwright & Reilly 1994.

Frugivorous bats usually fly long distances for foraging, occasionally flying over 27 km. This requires sustained flight and highly developed flight muscles that result in high wing loading, however, their wings are broad and rounded (Neuweiler 2000). The same is true in the vampire bat *Desmodus rotundus* (Canals et al., 2005). Bats which plane using convection currents such as some Pteropodidae usually have larger wingspan and wing loadings lower than those using flapping flight (Norberg et al., 2000).

4.1 Studies in Chile

In a series of studies, Canals et al (2001), Iriarte et al (2002) and Canals et al (2005) examined some aspects of the wing morphology of 8 species of bats present in Chile, correlating the results with available ecological information. They estimated aspect ratio, wingspan, wing surface, and wing loading of the molossids *Mormopterus kalinowskii* and *Tadarida brasiliensis*, the Phyllostomidae *Desmodus rotundus* and the vespertilionids *Myotis chiloensis, Histiotus montanus, Histiotus macrotus, Lasiurus borealis* and *Lasiurus cinereus* (Table 1).

Species	M_b (g)	B (cm)	S (cm^2)	W_L (N/m^2)	AR	I_h ($cm^4 x10^{-6}$)
Myotis chiloensis (49)	6.76 ± 0.18	23.69 ± 0.39	98.29 ± 3.47	6.8 ± 0.23	5.76 ± 0.16	3.89 ± 0.49
Histiotus montanus (1)	12.5	29.2	-	-	-	23.1
Histiotus macrotus (3)	9.37 ± 0.29	29.67 ± 0.58	129.67 ± 4.20	7.08 ± 0.19	6.78 ± 0.06	21.17 ± 3.52
Lasiurus borealis (3)	7.87 ± 1.12	25.37 ± 2.49	93.73 ± 8.87	8.20 ± 0.46	6.87 ± 0.70	12.68 ± 9.30
Lasiurus cinereus (2)	19.55 ± 6.58	30.20 ± 1.41	165.45 ± 52.07	15.42 ± 5.75	5.72 ± 1.29	26.78 ± 5.06
Tadarida brasiliensis (27)	11.95 ± 0.62	28.65 ± 0.63	100.14 ± 4.61	11.56 ± 0.66	8.12 ± 0.16	11.15 ± 2.61
Mormopterus kalinowskii (2)	3.10 ± 1.13	17.25 ± 0.35	32.4 ± 2.26	9.28 ± 2.77	9.20 ± 0.27	5.85 ± 5.98
Desmodus rotundus (1)	33.48	33.5	167.23	19.61	6.71	68.3
Histiotus montanus (1)	4.3	19.7	58.8	7.17	6.6	9.3
Lasiurus cinereus (4)	12.23 ± 2.71	27.33 ± 0.68	93.50 ± 8.18	12.74 ± 2.07	8.01 ± 0.44	21.24 ± 14.01

* From Iriarte-Díaz & Canals 2002 and Canals et al., 2005.

Mb = body mass, B = wing span, S = wing surface, W_L = wing loading, AR = aspect ratio and I_h = second moment of humeral area in median section. Asterisks indicate juvenile individuals. In one adult *H. montanus* it was not possible to estimate the wing surface. Numbers in parentheses indicate sample sizes.

Table 1. Summary of the aerodynamic characteristics of the wings of eight bats.

The free-tailed bat *T. brasiliensis* and *D. rotundus* have no tail membrane and a low wing area, but while the molossids have high aspect ratios, that of *D. rotundus* is only moderate. *D. rotundus* has a smaller wingspan for its body mass, and the highest wing loading. Furthermore, these authors estimated radiographically the second moment of area of humerus (I_h), which corresponds to a measure of bone strength to bending. *Myotis chiloensis* had a value lower than expected from allometric predictions, suggesting poor resistance. All other vespertilionids showed a high second moment of area, which may be explained by their costly form of locomotion, especially in species with high parasite load as a result of their long ears. The high I_h shown by *D. rotundus* may be explained by the low aspect ratio and high body mass, which increase the torque produced by the weight during quadrupedal locomotion.

The small community of Chilean bats showed a similar pattern to that found by Norberg and Rayner for many species, but at a small scale. Principal components analysis showed two axes, the first correlated positively with wing loading and negatively with wingspan and the second positively correlated with the aspect ratio. In these species 4 functional groups can be recognized, one for each quadrant in the graph:

i. *D. rotundus*, with high wing loading but low wingspan (relative to its body size), located in the high agility and rapid flight zone with moderate power consumption, which is likely related to long flights to their resting places and their particular form of locomotion;
ii. The molossids *T. brasiliensis* and *M. Kalinowski* in the area of high flight speed and low power consumption as is characteristic of high speed open area foragers;
iii. Most of vespertilionids in the zone of high maneuverability and low speed which correspond to bats which inhabit wooded areas;
iv. *L. cinereus* forming an isolated group in a zone of high speed and agility.

4.2 The mechanics of flight: Kinematics

The differences in flight performance observed in bats can be associated with higher energy expenditure efficiency as well as very high levels of maneuverability. For example, among animals of comparable body size, hovering flight of nectar-feeding bats is 40 and 60% less costly metabolically that that of hawkmoths and hummingbirds, respectively (Winter, 1998; Winter and von Helversen, 1998; Voigt and Winter, 1999), suggesting that bats have more efficient mechanisms of lift generation than member of other groups. Although the kinematics of hovering of bats differ from those of insects and hummingbirds, we lack experimental measurements that can explain such differences in efficiency. In a recent study using PIV methods, it was shown that bats can increase lift generation during slow flights by 40% by using attached leading-edge vortices around the wings (Muijres et al., 2008), similar to those used by insects (Fry et al., 2005) and hummingbirds (Warrick et al., 2005) during hovering flight. Why hovering flight in bats is energetically cheaper than that of insects and hummingbirds of similar size is still unclear.

4.3 Maneuvering during flight

The ability to quickly alter flight direction and speed is essential for bats to successfully navigate complex three-dimensional environments, to capture prey, and to avoid predators. Despite the importance of this task, maneuvering abilities and its mechanisms have been barely investigated. A flying organism has six degrees-of-freedom of movement: translation in three dimensions in space and rotation around three orthogonal axes centered on the center of mass, termed yaw, pitch, and roll.

In its most basic form, a turning maneuver requires the reorientation of the body in such a way that the net aerodynamic force is tilted laterally effectively producing a centripetal force that will drive the bat through the turn. The most common method in the literature is the bank turn. In this kind of turn, the body rolls into a bank, which orients the lift vector towards the direction of the turn, producing a centripetal force. When the turn is complete, the body rolls back into the unbanked position such that centripetal force is no longer produced. Airplanes use this mechanism, it has been observed in insects and birds, and it has been assumed that bats use it as well. If a flying organism performs a banked turn, then for any given lift coefficient and bank angle, the turning radius depends directly of the wing loading or body weight per unit wing

area; there is some evidence consistent with this relationship from bats in both field and obstacle course settings (Aldridge, 1986; Aldridge and Rautenbach, 1987; Stockwell, 2001).
However, growing evidence suggest that differences in turning techniques (e.g., gliding versus flapping turns, Aldridge, 1987b) and changes in wing posture throughout the turn (Lentink et al., 2007) can substantially alter the turning performance. The only study to investigate the mechanisms of turning in bats suggest a more complex mechanism. Detailed analysis of the wing motion and body orientation during 90-degree turns in the pteropodid *Cynopterus brachyotis* showed that during the upstroke the body rotates into the direction of the turn, a mix of roll and yaw rotations, without changes in flight direction. This body rotation allows the bat to use part of the thrust generated during the downstroke to enhance the centripetal force from the bank turn, thus allowing the bat to perform tighter turns than predicted by wing morphology alone (Iriarte-Díaz and Swartz, 2008). These results highlights the importance of studying the mechanics flight performance and that using morphological proxies to estimate performance (e.g., wing loading and aspect ratio) might severely underestimate flight abilities of bats.

4.4 The effect of wing inertia during flight

One aspect of flight performance that remains virtually unstudied is the importance of inertial forces generated by the flapping motion of relatively massive wings. The wings of bats comprise a significant portion of total body mass, ranging from 11 to 20% in a few measured species (Thollesson and Norberg, 1991; Watts et al., 2001) and consequently, inertial forces produced by accelerating these masses are expected to be high and the potential effect of these forces on flight performance is still not well understood. In a recent study, the effect of wing's inertial forces was studied on *C. brachyotis* during forward, steady flight (Iriarte-Díaz et al., 2011 in press). At any speed, the tip of the wings move upwards and backwards relatively to the body, but if the speed of the body is low enough, the tip can sometimes move backwards relatively to the still air during the upstroke. This backward movement of the wingtip has been called "tip-reversal upstroke" (Aldridge, 1987a) and for decades has been thought that it provides additional thrust to slow-flying bats, partially because the observation that the bat's trunk accelerate forward during upstroke. However, for *C. brachyotis*, the forward acceleration of the body is the result of forwardly directed inertial forces produced by the motion of the wings. When the wings swing backwards, approximately 20% of the bat's mass moves backward relative to the center of mass. In order to maintain the momentum, other portions of the body must move forward relative to the center of mass, which is reflected in the forward acceleration of the trunk. Using a model of the mass distribution of the trunk and wings, inertial accelerations were estimated and removed in order to estimate the acceleration of the center of mass. When inertial forces were removed, forward acceleration of the center of mass only occurred during the downstroke (Iriarte-Díaz et al., 2011). Thus, inertial forces may be potentially important during flight, although when and how they can be used is not known. Preliminary evidence suggest that inertial forces might be important during turning (Iriarte-Díaz and Swartz, 2008) and when performing landing maneuvers (Riskin et al., 2009).

5. Physiology and energy of bats

The first law of thermodynamics states that energy is neither created nor destroyed, only transformed. Living organisms as physical systems obey this principle, acquiring, converting, assigning, storing and dissipating energy. The transformation of energy plays a crucial role in the evolution, ecology and physiology of organisms. Thus the internal and external boundaries of the use and transformation of energy affect their fitness and may affect species richness, reproductive effort, activity patterns, habitat use and life history (McNab 2002, Cruz-Neto et al 2003; 2006).

Field metabolic rate (FMR) integrates all the energy costs of free-living organisms, including the costs of thermoregulation, locomotion etc. This has been quantified in the Australian bat *Syconycteris australis* with doubly labeled water, reaching 7 times the basal metabolic rate (Geiser & Coburn 1999), one of the highest values described in endotherms. This is attributable to the prolonged nocturnal flight (Geiser 2006). The mass specific metabolism of bats is 1.6 times that of non-flying mammals (Thomas, 1987). Also, during flight metabolism increases to 20 or 30 times the standard rate (Thomas, 1975). During flight, about 25% of metabolism is converted into work, so that 75% is dissipated as heat. This is done primarily in two ways: via airway and skin. The airway dissipates only about 15% because little or no frequency change is possible during flight, since there is a synchrony between wing beat and respiration. Thus the skin must remove the remaining heat (85%). Its large area and conductance allow this removal of heat by convection and radiation, which is favored by vasodilatation and opening of arteriovenous shunts in the wings and by the greater thermal difference between the body and the environment during nocturnal flying.

The thermal conductance of a microchiropteran of 10 g is about 6 times that of a mega-chiropteran of 500 g (Geiser 2006). Thus the maintenance of homeothermy is especially relevant in small bats with large membranous wings and large lungs. Bats have a respiratory area 6 times greater and a conductance between 1.5 and 4 times greater than non-flying mammals (Neuweiler, 2000), although the minimum conductance at rest appears to be similar (see Speakman & Thomas 2003). Despite this, bats can remain active and euthermic within wide temperature ranges.

To maintain their temperature bats may use different behavioral and physiological strategies. Behaviorally they can avoid overheating by wing movements that favor convection or licking the surface of their skin to increase evaporation, since they do not have sweat glands. Small bats find microenvironments with high thermal stability in caves or shelters, and can travel to other shelters to avoid overheating at times of high temperatures. Thus, the solitary bat *Syconycteris australis* resting under leaves selected thermal environments in the middle of wooded patches in spring and autumn, protected from the extreme temperatures, while in winter it moved to the extremes (Law 1993) . To avoid cold behaviorally, many species have a social grouping behavior (huddling) (Roveroud & Chappel 1991), or nest in caves forming large colonies of hundreds to millions of individuals, raising the temperature up to 8° C above that of the rest of the cave (Dwyer & Harris 1972).

The first physiological response to cold is to increase muscle tone generating heat, followed by shivering, which actually consists of rhythmic but asynchronous fibrillary muscle contractions. However, heat generation consumes so much energy that with limited resources it is not convenient for long periods.

When ambient temperatures fall below the lower limit of thermoneutrality, bats have the "option" to maintain their body temperature at a high energy cost, or to enter into torpor, maintaining a temperature similar to that of the environment with a significant decrease in energy expenditure. Entering into torpor seems to depend upon the interaction among resource availability, reproductive status and body size. McNab (1983) proposed a boundary line of endothermy, allometrically related to body size with an exponent -0.67, which intersects the Kleiber line for mass-specific metabolism at 37 g. Thus, individuals under this line and weighing less than 37 g may use torpor as a physiological response to save energy. During torpor, animals enter into a rhythmic pattern of breathing and apnea; the periods are longer as the temperature drops. . These periods allow the accumulation of CO_2 that triggers breathing and prevents evaporation in the lungs. The mechanism that triggers the awakening is still unknown. Many bats have facultative stupor, maintaining significant fluctuations of oxygen consumption and body temperature (heterothermy), saving a great amount of energy. Some examples of this behavior are found in *Eptesicus fuscus, Rhinolophus ferrunequinum, bechteinii Myotis, Myotis evotis, Lasiurus cinereus* (Willis 2006) and *Myotis chiloensis* (Bozinovic et al. 1985). These bats have different patterns, such as the presence of lethargy in the daily rhythm with no difference between sexes, preference in pregnant and breast-feeding and preference for males. These depend on the fine balance between the costs of endothermy, reproduction and locomotion costs imposed by the high wing loading in the pregnant females. For example, if the costs are very high, some bats prefer to rest in cold and go into torpor, avoiding the cost of endothermy and negative energy balance (Willis 2006).

Another long-term mechanism for energy saving is hibernation, in which metabolism falls to extremely low levels; heart rate can also decrease from more than 400 beats to a few beats per minute and the peripheral circulation and urine output may fall to almost nil. The respiratory quotient drops to 0.6-0.7, indicating that metabolism of lipids and blood glucose values may reach about 25 mg / dl. In contrast to torpor in which the values of Q10 (ratio of metabolic change with 10° C of temperature change) are around 2, during hibernation they are temperature-dependent, increasing from 2 to 4 with an increase of temperature, which suggests an active metabolic depression. For example at 20° C the metabolism of a bat in torpor is twice that of a hibernating bat.

This metabolic depression could be due to metabolic acidosis, low thyroid hormone or mediated by fatty acids (Neuweiler, 2000). The mechanisms that trigger hibernation have not been established, although it has been postulated that hibernation is regulated autonomously. Temperature, energy depletion and loss of water have been postulated as triggers that regulate arousal.

5.1 Energy balance: *Myotis chiloensis*, a case study

The perpetuation of animals over time requires an average positive energy balance, which is particularly difficult for small mammals such as the insectivorous bat *Myotis chiloensis*. Bozinovic et al (1985) studied the oxygen consumption of 25 individuals (5.78 ± 0.9g) at different temperatures. There were two responses: a) euthermic metabolic levels (36.6 ± 2.2° C) with an average oxygen consumption of 1.76 mlO_2/gh b) torpor metabolic levels, where the temperature was only 0.5° C above room temperature with metabolic reductions of 81 to 98% (Figure 3). In continuous records *M. chiloensis* showed a daily rhythm with only three hours in which animals were euthermic.

The torpor in *M. chiloensis* was as expected for a small mammal, under the endothermy limit proposed by McNab (1983); however it does not explain why this species does not maintain high metabolism all the time.

The answer seems to come from the energy balance

$$Intake - Egestion = M_{activity} + M_{euthermia} + M_{torpor} + E\,, \tag{8}$$

where M is metabolism and E the energy balance.

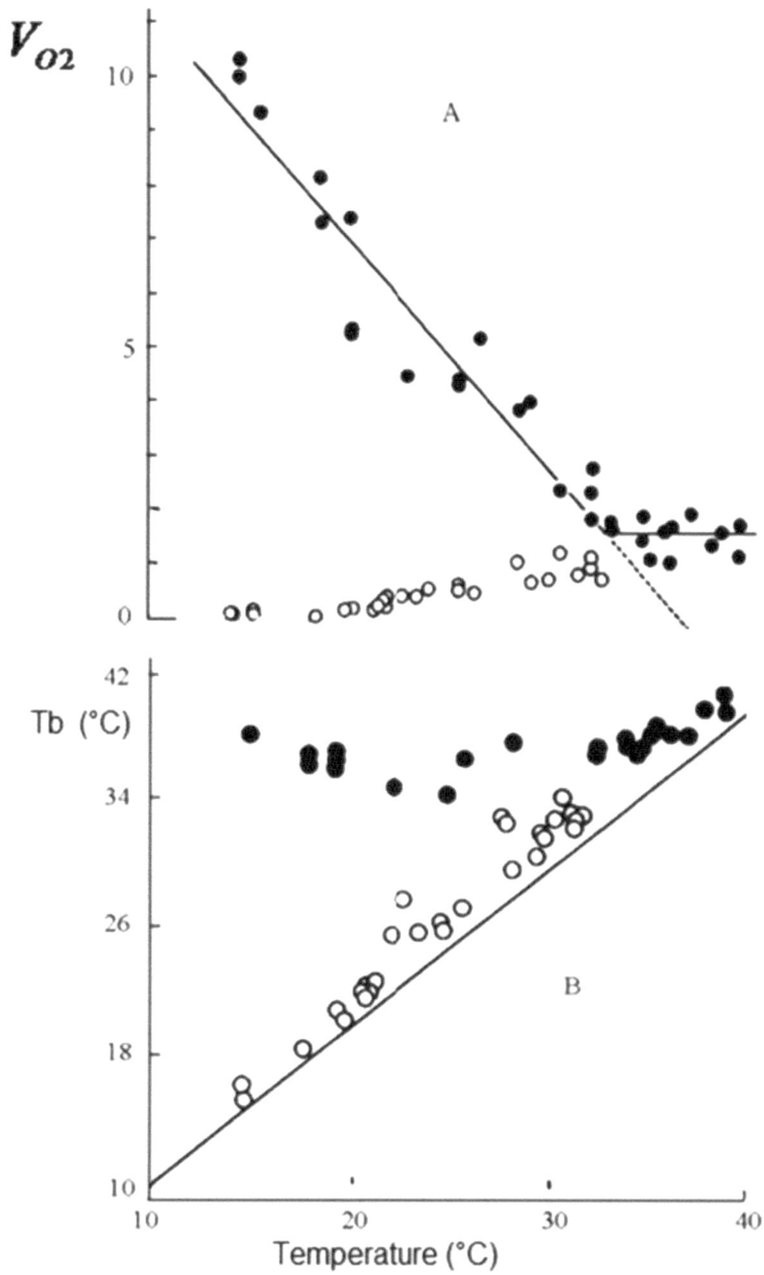

Fig. 3. A) Relation between ambient temperature and metabolism (MR, mlO_2/gh) and B) Relation between ambient temperature and body (Tb, °C) in *Myotis chiloensis* in euthermic state (black circles) and in torpor (white circles) (Modified from Bozinovic et al., 1985).

Data on the chemical composition of various flying insects indicates that their assimilated energy is approximately 5.3 Kcal / g; thus an individual of 5.8 g which ingested 11% of its weight in insects every day assimilates 5.8 x0, 11x5, 32 = 3.39 kcal / day. Therefore this individual may have two situations:

a. Euthermy: The temperature the shelters of *Myotis chiloensis* averages 19.5° C and metabolism at this temperature is 36 cal / gh, so that in the 21 hours of resting the minimal euthermic energy expenditure is 5.8 x36x21 = 4.38 kcal. The rest of the time (3 hours) *M. chiloensis* is flying and feeding. Assuming that the metabolic activity is at least three times BMR, the energetic cost would be 5.8 x36x3x3 = 1.88 kcal. Thus we have the following relationship: 3.39 = 4.38 + 1.88 + E, where the euthermic energy budget would be E = -2.87 kcal / day, i.e., the individual would have an energy imbalance equivalent to a mass loss of 5 to 10% per day.
b. Torpor: If instead it spends 20 hours in torpor with a metabolism of 1.2 cal / gh, 1 hour of euthermic rest (30 min before and after feeding) and the same three hours of activity, it would expend 5.8 x1, 2x20 = 0.14 Kcal in torpor, the same 1.88 Kcal during activity and 1x36x5, 8 = 0.21 Kcal at euthermic rest, giving a balance 3.39 = 0.21 + 1.88 + 0.14 + E. Now the energy budget is positive: E = +1.16 kcal / day.

6. The respiratory system

Endothermic animals depend on aerobic metabolism for most of their vital functions. The energy from food is allocated to different functions such as maintenance of homeostasis (i.e. temperature), reproduction, exchange mechanisms, maintenance of tone and locomotion. As most bats are small and therefore have a large surface area per unit volume, they have trouble maintaining their body temperature high and constant as consequence of the significant energy loss through the skin. Moreover, flight requires high energy expenditure, especially since many bats are exposed to cold nights and fly at high altitudes with low oxygen partial pressures (Harrison & Roberts 2000). In this sense bats may be considered as mammals adapted to extreme environments where oxygen management is crucial. Both the respiratory and cardiovascular systems undergo changes or refinements that allow them to optimize the acquisition and delivery of oxygen to tissues, and thus survive this extreme way of life.
Breathing in mammals consists basically of two connected events: ventilator convection and alveolar diffusion. The first is the displacement of a volume of air through the airway and the second in the effective exchange of oxygen and CO_2 at the alveolar level.

7. Ventilator convection

Alveolar ventilation ($\dot{V}$) may be expressed as the product of effective tidal volume (tidal volume (Vc) minus dead space (E)) and the respiratory rate (f_r):

$$\dot{V} = (Vc - E) \cdot f_r \,. \tag{9}$$

Thus increments in ventilation are possible only through effective tidal volume or respiratory rate increments. However, increasing alveolar ventilation may be costly in energetic terms as the movement of larger volumes of air results in greater breathing work. Moreover, the work of breathing (T_r) not only depends on the volume but also on the pressure necessary to mobilize this volume:

$$T_r = \int P dV \,. \tag{10}$$

This in turn is a direct function of the resistance to air movement which is influenced by a) a geometric factor:

$$R_g = \frac{8\eta l}{\pi r^4}, \tag{11}$$

(Poiseuille Law), where l is the length of the airway, η the air viscosity and r the radius of the bronchi, which basically indicates that the resistance to flow is inversely proportional to the fourth power of the radius, and b) a dynamic factor:

$$R_v = k_1 \cdot v + k_2 \cdot v^2 , \tag{12}$$

where v is the velocity of air flow, which indicates higher resistance at higher flow rates (or breathing rates). Thus the total resistance to airflow through the airway as a function of breath rate follows a U-shaped curve, determining for each species, according to the geometric characteristics of the airway, an optimal respiratory rate with minimal resistance. Murray (1926) and later Weibel and Gomez (1962) and Wilson (1967) established that respiratory geometry could be adapted to a minimum overall work of breathing and minimum entropy dissipation during mechanical ventilation, following approximately the Murray law "For minimum breathing work, ventilation (Q: minute volume) should be proportional to the third power of the radius (r):

$$Q = k \cdot r^3 \,. \tag{13}$$

However, mammals have considerable deviations from this pattern, especially due to the presence of asymmetries in diameter in the bronchial bifurcations and non-uniform length of segmental and subsegmental bronchi (Horstfield, 1990, Canals et al., 2002).

Bats have a much greater lung volume than non-flying mammals and they remove about 60% of the total lung capacity with each breath during flight (Neuweiler, 2000). Lung volume is about 72% greater than in non-flying mammals of similar weight (Canals et al, 2005a) (Table 2). At rest, pulmonary ventilation is similar to that of non-flying mammals. However, this can rapidly increase 10 to 17 times when flight begins (Thomas, 1987). This is due to increases of 3 to 5 times in breath rates and 2 to 4 times in tidal volume. The respiratory rate is synchronized to the wing beat frequency, reaching a value of 400 min^{-1}. These respiratory adaptations function together with structural changes of lung yield in oxygen consumption reaching to 2.5 to 3 times higher than mammals of equal size (Thomas, 1987) and high maximum oxygen consumption, which can reach 22 to mlO_2/gh at low temperatures (Canals et al., 2005b) and during hovering (Winter et al., 1998, Voigt & Winter, 1999; Voigt, 2004).

The morphology of the airways also appears to play a role in saving energy during flight. Canals et al. (2005) studied the airway of *Tadarida brasiliensis*, finding that this species showed fine adjustments in the geometry of the bronchial bifurcations leading to a better optimization of the proximal airway. As the airway is responsible for 80% of lung resistance and 80% of this is generated in the proximal airway, the optimization of the proximal airway can mean less energy loss during flight (Figure 4).

Species	Mb (g)	LV (cc)	RLV=LV/Mb (cc/g)
Tadarida brasiliensis	11.95 ± 1.36	0.654 ± 0.091	0.055 ± 0.011
Mormopterus kalinowski	3.1 ± 1.13	0.162 ± 0.024	0.054 ± 0.021
Myotis chiloensis	6.95 ± 0.54	0.406 ± 0.071	0.058 ± 0.009
Histiotus macrotus	9.80 ± 0.666	0.602 ± 0.094	0.061 ± 0.005
Histiotus montanus	12.5	0.696	0.056
Lasiurus borealis	6.8 ± 2.05	0.455	0.064 ± 0.004
Lasiurus cinereus	16.06 ± 7.62	1.025 ± 0.389	0.066 ± 0.010
Phyllostomus hastatus *	97.8 ± 2.56	4.95 ± 0.255	0.051 ± 0.007
Pteropus lyley *	456.0 ± 20.87	15.37 ± 1.93	0.034 ± 0.011
*Pteropus alecto**	667.0	22.20	0.033
Pteropus poliocephalus *	928.0	39.24	0.042

Table 2. Lung volume (LV) and relative lung volume (RLV) in several species of bats (from Canals et al 2005a and Maina et al., 1991*)

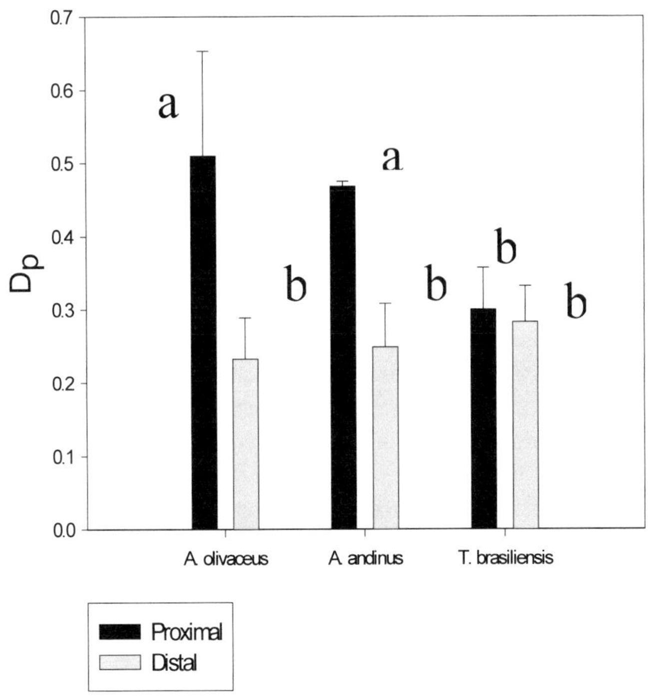

Fig. 4. Optimization of the proximal airway of *Tadarida brasiliensis. T. brasiliensis* is compared with the rodents *Abrothrix olivaceus* and *A. andinus.* The ordinate is the distance from the optimum value determined by the geometry of the bronchial bifurcations. While rodents have values farther from the optimum, *T. brasiliensis* shows a better optimization in the proximal zone, which is the key to a reduction in respiratory work, dissipating less energy. Different letters represent statistically significant differences

8. Alveolar diffusion

The diffusion of oxygen through the alveolar-capillary barrier depends directly on the gradient of partial pressure of oxygen between the alveoli and the capillary (ΔPO_2) and the respiratory surface (A), and inversely on the thickness of the alveolar-capillary membrane (τ_h) This can be expressed as:

$$\dot{V}_{O2} = \kappa \frac{dSa \cdot Vp}{\tau_h} \cdot \Delta PO_2, \tag{14}$$

where the alveolar surface is expressed as the product of lung volume (V_p) and the surface density per unit of lung volume (dSa), κ is Krogh's constant and VO_2 is the oxygen consumption (Weibel et al., 1981). Thus, high oxygen consumption may be achieved through increases in alveolar surface density or lung volume, or by reducing the thickness of the alveolar-capillary barrier. The factor:

$$DO_2 = \kappa \frac{dSa \cdot Vp}{\tau_h}, \tag{15}$$

is known as conductance or oxygen diffusing capacity (DO_2). As mentioned above, bats have a lung volume 1.72 to 1.75 times that of non-flying mammals, however, alveolar surface density is similar to that of non-flying mammals (Maina, 2000). As a result, the total respiratory area of bats is larger than in non-flying mammals. In addition, these animals have a very thin alveolar-capillary barrier (Maina et al., 1991; Maina, 2000a) that may reach a value of 0.1204 microns in *Phyllostomus hastatus*, the lowest measured in mammals. So bats have very high oxygen diffusion capacity, similar to those of birds (Table 3).

9. The cardiovascular system

Respiratory adaptations are insufficient to ensure adequate oxygen delivery to tissues, so these must be accompanied by changes in the cardiovascular system. Here the blood flow generated by the heartbeat, the resistance to flow, and transport of oxygen in the blood are all relevant.

9.1 The heart

Blood flow (Q) can be expressed as the product of volume ejected in each beat (V_E) and heart rate (f_c) or as the ratio between the gradient of pressure to generate the flow (ΔP) and peripheral resistance (R):

$$Q = V_E \cdot f_c = \Delta P / R. \tag{16}$$

Peripheral resistance follows a Poiseuille relationship and cardiac work, similar to respiratory work, depends on expulsive volume and pressure:

$$T_c = \int P dV. \tag{17}$$

Thus high flow is obtained by increasing the expulsive volume or heart rate and by decreasing peripheral resistance.

Rodents	Mb (g)	τh (μm)	Dsa (cm-1)	VLp (cm3)	DtO_2/Mb ($mlO_2\ s^{-1}\ Pa^{-1}\ g^{-1}$)
Abrothrix olivaceus	26.3 ± 2.00	0.303 ± 0.037	589.37 ± 45.26	0.846 ± 0.28	$2.565x10^{-6}$
Abrothrix andinus	25.48 ± 1.93	0.345 ± 0.057	791.8 ± 229.68	0.972 ± 0.12	$3.589x10^{-6}$
Phyllotis darwini	75.0 ± 4.96	0.223 ± 0.033	1140.5 ± 92.0	1.91 ± 0.17	$4.92\ x10^{-6}$
Bats					
Tadarida brasiliensis	11.25 ± 0.50	0.230 ± 0.086	690.28 ± 156.96	0.585 ± 0.09	$6.398x10^{-6}$
Myotis chiloensis	6 ± 0.10	0.219 ± 0.015	2020.3 ± 71.0	0.360 ± 0.01	$20.4x10^{-6}$
Birds					
Zenaida auriculata	142 ± 1.55	0.171 ± 0.026	3102.9 ± 175	3.77 ± 0.06	$9.28x10^{-6}$
Columbina picui	39.9± 1.4	0.302 ±0.118	2328.9 ±426.4	1.04± 0.04	$4.19x10^{-6}$
Metropelia melanoptera	78.4± 2.4	0.186± 0.008	2580.4± 190.3	2.11 ±0.07	$7.04\ x10^{-6}$
Notoprocta predicaría	398 ± 11.7	0.469 ± 0.019	1811.3 ± 27	11.32 ± 0.43	2.07x10-6

Table 3. Pulmonary parameters of some Chilean species rodents, bats and birds. Mb = body mass; τh6 = harmonic mean of alveolo-capillary barrier thickness; Dsa = density of respiratory surface; VLp = volume of lung parenchyma and DtO2/Mb = mass-specific oxygen diffusion capacity of the alveolo-capillary barrier (data from Canals et al., 2005b; Figueroa et al., 2006; Alfaro et al., 2010).

Bats have the largest hearts of mammals relative to body mass, usually representing about 1% of body weight (Neuweiler, 2000), but reaching 2% (Jurgens et al., 1981, Canals et al., 2005a) (Table 4). They have great development of the right ventricle associated with better lung perfusion and high density of capillaries per unit volume. They also have the highest level of energy reserves in the form of ATP that has been measured in the heart of any animal (Neuweiler, 2000). Despite increased cardiac output, the volume expelled is similar to other mammals, somewhat greater than 1.5 ml / kg, indicating that the increase in heart size is mainly at the expense of muscle hypertrophy. The heart rate is extremely variable and may range from a few beats per minute during hibernation to over 1000 beats per minute during flight (Wolf & Bogdanowics, 1987, Neuweiler, 2000).

Species	Mb (g)	Mh (g)	RHM=Mh/Mb (%)	Mh obs Mh exp
Tadarida brasiliensis	11.25 ± 1.13	0.145 ±0.033	1.29 ± 0.23	0.943 ± 0.176
Mormopterus kalinowski	3.1 ± 1.13	0.057 ± 0.018	1.88 ± 0.10	1.041 ± 0.022
Myotis chiloensis	6.88 ± 0.47	0.096 ± 0.0145	1.40 ± 0.20	0.921 ± 0.137
Histiotus macrotus	9.65 ± 0.61	0.166 ± 0.0350	1.71 ± 0.03	1.213 ± 0.237
Histiotus montanus	12.5	0.272	2.18	1.627 ± 0
Lasiurus borealis	7.87 ± 1.10	0.120 ± 0.02	1.55 ± 0.27	1.046 ± 0.169
Lasiurus cinereus	12.76 ± 2.74	0.173 ± 0.042	1.40 ± 0.04	1.042 ± 0.279
Pipistrellus pipistrellus *	4.85 ± 0.18	-	1.26 ± 0.24	-
Myotis myotis *	20.6 ± 0.9	-	0.98 ± 0.08	-
Molossus ater *	38.2 ± 1.4	-	0.97 ± 0.01	-
Phyllostomus discolor *	45.2 ± 1.34	-	0.94 ± 0.09	-
Rousettus aegyptiacus *	146.0 ± 7.5	-	0.84 ±0.08	-

Table 4. Heart size of several bat species. Mb = body mass; Mh = heart mass; RHM = relative heart mass; Mhobs/Mhexp = ratio of observed to that expected by allometry. (Data from Canals et al., 2005a; Jurgens et al., 1981*)

9.2 Vessels, the resistance to flow and oxygen transport in blood

The vessels of bats follow a mammalian pattern, with some arterial and venous modifications. Unlike other mammals, the venous return of the forelimbs occurs through two vena cava; inferior vena cava have a muscular zone that allow regulation of venous return, lower during rest and high during flight. The arteries of the wing branch into arterioles with a muscle base which can regulate the flow to the wings and maintain the arteriovenous differential pressure. There are also arteriovenous shunts and venous vessels with pulsating zones (venous hearts) that can regulate the return of blood from the wings. The volume of blood is similar to other mammals as well as the affinity of hemoglobin. However, bats have the highest levels of hematocrit measured in mammals and may reach values above 70% in *Tadarida brasiliensis* and *Miniopterus minor*. Red blood cells are smaller (Figueroa et al., 2007) and hemoglobin has been found in higher concentrations (18-24 g/100ml blood), similar to that found in hummingbirds (Johansen et al., 1987). Consequently, bats have a transport capacity of oxygen in the blood of 25 to 30%. In comparison, non-flying mammals have an oxygen-carrying capacity of about 18% (Thomas, 1987; Neuweiler, 2000).

10. The narrow-based, high keyed strategy

By comparing the structural and functional adaptations in birds and bats it can be established that they reach very similar aerobic capacities. However, strategies to achieve these high performances during flight are different. Birds have a large set of structural changes in their respiratory system, such as air bags, parabronchi systems, respiratory capillaries, cross-current flows, etc. In contrast, bats have a cardio-respiratory system fully modified to accomplish an extreme way of life. This mammalian structural base is highly refined, operating near maximum values (Maina, 1998) (Table 5). Thus, Maina (1998) comparing a set of 7 parameters including birds, bats and non-flying mammals, found that bats have higher "degrees" of optimization in 5 of them: resting respiratory rate, hematocrit, hemoglobin concentration, resting heart rate and blood count.

Optimization Strategy	
Respiratory Adaptations	**Cardiovascular Adaptations**
Increase of lung volumen	Increase of heart size
Thin alveolo-capillary membrane	Development of right half of the heart
Small alveoles	Regulation of venous return
High oxygen diffusing capacity	High hematocrit
High respiratory frequency	Small GR
Proximal airway adjusted to lower energy loss	Greater concentration of hemoglobin
	Greater oxygen transport capacity

Table 5. Strategy of respiratory and cardiovascular optimization in bats.

11. Acknowledgements

We thanks FONDECYT grants 100673, 1040649, 1080038 and 1110058.

12. References

Aldridge, H. D. J. N. 1986. Manoeuvrability and ecological segregation in the little brown (*Myotis lucifugus*) and Yuma (*M. yumanensis*) bats (Chiroptera: Vespertilionidae). *Canadian Journal of Zooogy* 64, 1878-1882.

Aldridge, H. D. J. N. 1987a. Body accelerations during the wingbeat in six bat species: the function of the upstroke in thrust generation. *Journal of Experimental Biology* 130, 275-293.

Aldridge, H. D. J. N. 1987b. Turning flight of bats. *Journal of Experimental Biology* 128, 419-425.

Aldridge, H. D. J. N. & rautenbach, I. L. 1987. Morphology, echolocation and resource partitioning in insectivorous bats. *Journal of Animal Ecology* 56, 763-778.

Alfaro, C., Figueroa, D., Sabat, P., Sallaberry, M. &Canals, M. 2010. Comparison of the oxygen difussion capacity of the picui ground dove (*Columbina picui*) with other doves of Chile. *International Journal of Morphology* 28(1), 127-133.

Barclay, R.M.R. & Brigham, R.M. 1991. Prey detection, dietary niche breath, and body size in bats: why are aerial insectivorous bats so small? *American Naturalist* 137, 693-703.

Bozinovic, F., Contreras, L.C., Rosenmann, M. & Torres-Mura, J.C. 1985. Bioenergética de Myotis chiloensis (Quiroptera: Vespertilionidae). *Revista Chilena de Historia Natural* 58, 39-45.

Canals, M., Atala, C., Olivares, R., Novoa, F.F. & Rosenmann, M. 2002. La asimetría y el grado de optimización del árbol bronquial en *Rattus norvegicus* y *Oryctolagus cuniculus. Revista Chilena de Historia Natural* 75, 271-282.

Canals, M., Atala, C., Grossi, B. 2005. Relative Size Of Hearts And Lungs Of Several Small Bats. *Acta Chiropterologica* 7, 65-72.

Canals, M., Atala, C., Olivares, R., Guajardo, F., Figueroa, D., Sabat, P., Rosenmann, M. 2005. Functional and structural optimization of the respiratory system of the bat Tadarida brasiliensis (Chiroptera; Molossidae): Does airway matter?. *Journal of Experimental Biology* 208, 3987-3995.

Canals, M., Iriarte-Díaz, J., Olivares, R. & Novoa, F.F. 2001. Comparación de la morfología alar de *Tadarida brasiliensis* (Chiroptera: Molossidae) y *Myotis chiloensis* (Chiroptera: Vespertilionidae), representantes de dos diferentes tipos de vuelo. *Revista Chilena de Historia Natural* 74, 699-704.

Canals, M., Grossi, M., Iriarte-Díaz, J. & Veloso, C. 2005. Biomechanical and ecological relationships of wing morphology of eight Chilean bats *Revista Chilena de Historia Natural* 78,215-227.

Carpenter, R.E. 1986. Flight physiology of intermediate sized fruit bats (Pteropodidae). *The Journal of Experimental Biology* 120, 79-103.

Cruz-Neto, A.P, Briani, D.C. & Bozinovic, F. 2003. La tasa metabólica basal: ¿una variable unificadora en energética animal? In *Fisiología ecólogica y evolutiva,* Bozinovic, F., Ediciones Universidad Católica de Chile, Santiago.

Cruz-Neto, A.P. & Jones, K.E. 2006. The evolution of basal metabolic rate in bats. In *Functional and evolutionary ecology of bats*, Zubaid, A., McCraken, G.F. & Kunz, T.H. 56-89, Oxford University Press.

Dickinson, M. H., Farley, C. T., Full, R. J., Koehl, M. A., Kram, R. & Lehman, S. 2000. How animals move: an integrative view. *Science* 288, 100-106.

Dwyer, P.D. & Harris, J.A. 1972. Behavioral acclimatization to temperature by pregnant *Miniopterus* (Chiroptera). *Physiological Zoology* 45, 14-21.

Fenton, M.B. 1992. *Bats*. Facts On File, Inc, New York.

Figueroa, D.P., Olivares, R., Sallaberry, M., Sabat, P., Canals, M. 2007. Interplay between the morphometry of the lungs and the mode of locomotion in birds and mammals. *Biological Research* 40, 193-201.

Findley. J.S., Studier, E.H. & Wilson, D.E. 1972. Morphologic properties of bat wings. *Journal of Mammalogy* 53, 429-444.

Fry, S. N., Sayaman, R.& Dickinson, M. H. 2005. The aerodynamics of hovering flight in *Drosophila. Journal of Experimental Biology* 208, 2303-2318.

Geiser, F. 2006. Energetics, thermal biology and torpor in Australian bats. In *Functional and evolutionary ecology of bats*, Zubaid, A., McCraken, G.F. & Kunz, T.H., 5-22. Oxford University Press.

Geiser, F. & Coburn, D.K. 1999. Field metabolic rates and water uptake in the blossom-bat *Syconycteris australis* (Mega chiroptera). *Journal of Comparative Physiology B* 169, 133-138.

Hedenström, A., Johansson, L. C., Wolf, M., Von Busse, R., Winter, Y. & Spedding, G. R. 2007. Bat flight generates complex aerodynamic tracks. *Science* 316, 894-897.

Hedenström, A., Muijres, F., Von Busse, R., Johansson, L., Winter, Y. & Spedding, G. 2009. High-speed stereo DPIV measurement of wakes of two bat species flying freely in a wind tunnel. *Experimental Fluids* 46, 923-932.

Hubel, T. Y., Hristov, N. I., Swartz, S. M. & Breuer, K. S. 2009. Time-resolved wake structure and kinematics of bat flight. *Experimental Fluids* 46, 933-943.

Hubel, T. Y., Riskin, D. K., Swartz, S. M. & Breuer, K. S. 2010. Wake structure and wing kinematics: the flight of the lesser dog-faced fruit bat, *Cynopterus brachyotis*. *Journal of Experimental Biology* 213, 3427-3440.

Iriarte-Díaz, J., Novoa, F.F. & Canals, M. 2002. Biomechanic consequences of differences in wing morphology between *Tadarida brasiliensis* and *Myotis chiloensis*. *Acta Theriologica* 47, 193-200.

Iriarte-Díaz, J., Riskin, D. K., Willis, D. J., Breuer, K. S. & Swartz, S. M. 2011. Whole-body kinematics of a fruit bat reveal the influence of wing inertia on body accelerations. *Journal of Experimental Biology* 214, 1546-1553.

Iriarte-Díaz, J. & Swartz, S. M. 2008. Kinematics of slow turn maneuvering in the fruit bat *Cynopterus brachyotis*. *Journal of Experimental Bioogy* 211, 3478-3489.

Johansson, L. C., Wolf, M., Von Busse, R., Winter, Y., Spedding, G. R. & Hedenstrom, A. 2008. The near and far wake of Pallas' long tongued bat (*Glossophaga soricina*). *Journal of Experimental Biology* 211, 2909-2918.

Maina, J.N. 2000. What it takes to fly: The structural and functional respiratory refinements in birds and bats *The Journal of Experimental Biology* 203, 3045-3064.

Maina, J.N., Thomas, S.P. & Dallas, D.M. 1991. A morphometric study of bats of different size: correlations between structure and function of the chiropteran lung. *Philosophical Transactions of The Royal Society of London B* 333, 31-50.

Harrison, J.F. & Roberts, S.P. 2000. Flight respiration and energetics. *Annual Review Physiology* 20, 179-205.

Johansen, K., Berger, M., Bicudo, J.E.P.W., Ruschi, A. & De Almeida, P.J. 1987. Respiratory properties of blood and myoglobin in hummingbirds. *Physiological Zoology* 60, 269-278.

Jürgens, J.D., Bartels, H. & Bartels, R. 1981. Blood oxygen transport and organ weight of small bats and small non-flying mammals. *Respiration Physiology* 45, 243-60.

Lentink, D., Muller, U. K., Stamhuis, E. J., De Kat, R., Van Gestel, W., Veldhuis, L. L. M., Henningsson, P., Hedenstrom, A., Videler, J. J. & Van Leeuwen, J. L. 2007. How swifts control their glide performance with morphing wings. *Nature* 446, 1082-1085.

Maina, J.N. 1998. The lungs of the flying vertebrates- birds and bats: is their structure optimized for this elite mode of locomotion? In *Principles of Animal design: The optimization and symmorphosis debate*, E.R. Weibel, C.R.Taylor, and L. Bolis, 177-185. Cambridge University Press, Cambridge.

Maina, J.N. 2000. What it takes to fly: The structural and functional respiratory refinements in birds and bats *The Journal of Experimental Biology* 203, 3045-3064.

Maina, J.N., Thomas, S.P. & Dallas, D.M. 1991. A morphometric study of bats of different size: correlations between structure and function of the chiropteran lung. Philosophical *Transactions of The Royal Society of London B* 333, 31-50.

Marden, J.H. 1994. From damselflies to pterosaurs: how burst and sustainable flight performance scale with size. *American Journal of Physiology* 266: R1077-R1984.

McNab, B.K. 1982. The physiological ecology of South America mammals. In *Mammalian Biology in South America*. Mares, M. & Genoways, H.H. : 187-207,

Pymatunig Laboratory of Ecology. University of Pittsburgh Special Publication.

McNab, B.K. 2002. *The Physiological ecology of vertebrales: a view from energetics*. Cornell University Press, Ithaca.

Muijres, F. T., Johansson, L. C., Barfield, R., Wolf, M., Spedding, G. R. & Hedenstrom, A. 2008. Leading-edge vortex improves lift in slow-flying bats. *Science* 319, 1250-1253.

Murray, C.D. 1926. The physiological principle of minimum work. *Proceedings of Natural Academy of Science USA* 12, 207-214.

Neuweiller, G. 2000. *The Biology of Bats*. Oxford University Press, Oxford.

Norberg, U.M. 1987. *Wing form and flight mode in bats*. In *Recent advances in the study of bats*: 43-57, M.B. Fenton, P. Racey & J.M.V. Rayner, Cambridge University Press, Cambridge.

Norberg, U.M. 1994. *Wing design, flight performance and habit use in bats*. In P.C. Wainwright & S.M. Reilly, *Ecological Morphology: integrative organismal biology*: 205-239. The University of Chicago Press, Chicago.

Norberg, U.M. & Rayner, J.M.V. 1987. Ecological, morphology and flight in bats (Mammalia: Chiroptera): Wing adaptations, flight performance, foraging strategy and echolocation. *Philosophical Transactions of the Royal Society of London B* 316: 335-427.

Norberg, U.M., Brooke, A.P. & Trewhella, W.J. .2000. Soaring and non-soaring bats of the family Pteropodidae (flying foxes, *Pteropus spp.*): wing morphology and flight performance. *Journal of Experimental Biology* 203, 651-664.

O`Neil, M.G. & Taylor, R.J. 1989. Feeding ecology of Tasmanian bat assemblages. *Australian Journal of Ecology* 14,19-31.

Rayner, L.M.V. 1979. A new approach to animal flight mechanics. *Journal of Experimental Biology* 80, 17-54.

Rayner, L.M.V. 1982. Avian flight energetics. *Annuals Review of Physiology* 44, 109-119.

Rayner, L.M.V. 1987. The mechanics of flapping flight in bats. In M.B. Fenton, P. Racey & J.M.V. Rayner, *Recent advances in the study of bats*: 23-42. Cambridge University Press, Cambridge.

Rayner, L.M.V., Jones, G. & Thomas, A. 1986. Vortex flow visualizations reveal change in upstroke function with flight speed in bats. *Nature* 321, 162-164.

Riskin, D. K., Bahlman, J. W., Hubel, T. Y., Ratcliffe, J. M., Kunz, T. H. & Swartz, S. M. 2009. Bats go head-under-heels: the biomechanics of landing on a ceiling. *Journal of Experimental Bioogy* 212, 945-953.

Roveroud, R.C. & Chappell, M.A. 1991. Energetic and thermoregulatory aspects of clustering behavior in the neotropical bat *Noctilio albiventer*. *Physiological Zoology* 64, 1527-1541.

Schutt, W.A.Jr., Altenbach, J.S., Chang, Y.H., Culliname, D.M., Hermanson, J.W., Murdali, F. & Bertram, J.E.A. 1997. The dynamics of flight-initiating jumps in the common vampire bat *Desmodus rotundus*. *The Journal of Experimental Biology* 200, 3003-3012.

Speakman, J.R. & Thomas, D.W. 2003. Physiological ecology and energetics of bats. In *Bat Ecology*, T.H. Kunz & M.B. Fenton: 430-492. University of Chicago Press, Chicago.

Stockwell, E. F. 2001. Morphology and flight manoeuvrability in New World leaf-nosed bats (Chiroptera: Phyllostomidae). *Journal of Zoology* 254, 505-514.

Swartz, S.M. 1997. Allometric pattering in the limb skeleton of bats: implications for the mechanics and the energetic of powered flight. *Journal of Morphology* 234, 277-294.

Swartz, S.M., Freeman, P.W. & Stockwell, E.F. 2003. Ecomorphology of bats: Comparative and experimental approaches relating structural design to ecology. In: Kunz, T.H. & M.B. Fenton, *Bat Ecology*, 257-301. The University of Chicago Press, Chicago and London.

Thollesson, M. & NORBERG, U. M. 1991. Moments of inertia of bat wings and body. *Journal of Experimental Biology* 158, 19-35.

Thomas, S.P. 1987. The physiology of bat flight. In *Recent advances in the study of bats*, M. B. Fenton, P. Racey, & J.M.V. Rayner, pp 75-99. Cambridge University press, Cambridge.

Thomas, S.P. 1975. Metabolism during flight in two species of bats, Phyllostomus hastatus and Pteropus gouldii. *Journal of Experimental Biology* 63, 273-293.

Vaugham, T.A. 1970. Adaptations for flight in bats. In: Slaughter, B.H. & D.W. Walton, *About bats*, 127-143. Southern Methodist University Press, Dallas, Texas.

Voigt, C.C. 2004. The power requirements (Glossophaginae: Phyllostomidae) innectar-feeding bats for clinging to flowers. *Journal of Comparative Physiology* 174, 541-548.

Voigt, C.C. & Winter, W. 1999. Energetic cost of hovering flight in nectar feeding bats (Phyllostomidae: Glossophaginae) and its scaling in moths, birds and bats. *Journal of Comparative Physiology B* 169, 38-48.

Warrick, D. R., Tobalske, B. W. & Powers, D. R. 2005. Aerodynamics of the hovering hummingbird. *Nature* 435, 1094-1097.

Watts, P., Mitchell, E. J. & Swartz, S. M. 2001. A computational model for estimating the mechanics of horizontal flapping flight in bats: model description and validation. *Journal of Experimental Biology* 204, 2873-2898.

Weibel, E.R. & Gomez , D.M. 1962. Architecture of the human lung. *Science* 137, 577-585.

Weibel, E.R., Gehr, P., Cruz-Ori, L., Muller, A.E., Mwangi, D.K. & Haussener, V. 1981. Design of the mammalian respiration system. IV. Morphometric estimation of pulmonary diffusing capacity: critical evaluation of a new sampling method. *Respiration Physiology* 44, 39-59.

Willis, C.K.R. 2006. Daily heterothermy by temperate bats using natural roosts. In *Functional and evolutionary ecology of bats*, Zubaid, A., McCraken, G.F. & Kunz, T.H. 38-55. Oxford University Press.

Wilson, T. 1967. Design of the bronchial tree. *Nature* 688-669.

Winter, Y., Voigt, C. & Von Helversen, O. 1998. Gas exchange during hovering flight in a nectar-feeding bat *Glossophaga soricina*. *Journal of Experimental Biology* 201, 237-244.

Winter, Y. 1998. Energetic cost of hovering flight in a nectar-feeding bat measured with fast-response respirometry. *Journal of Comparative Physiology B* 168, 434-444.

Winter, Y. & Von Helversen, O. 1998. The energy cost of flight: do small bats fly more cheaply than birds? *Journal of Comparative Physiology B* 168, 105-111

Wolf, M., Johansson, L. C., Von Busse, R., Winter, Y. & Hedenstrom, A. 2010. Kinematics of flight and the relationship to the vortex wake of a Pallas' long tongued bat (*Glossophaga soricina*). *Journal of Experimental Biology* 213, 2142-2153.

Wolk, E. & Bogdanowics, W. 1987. Hematology of the hibernating bat, *Myotis daubentoni*. *Comparative Biochemistry and Physiology* 88A, 637-39.

14

Factors Influencing Proprioception: What do They Reveal?

Fernando Ribeiro[1,2] and José Oliveira[2]
[1]*CESPU, Polytechnic Health Institute of the North, Physiotherapy Department*
[2]*University of Porto, Faculty of Sport, Research Centre in Physical Activity, Health and Leisure*
Portugal

1. Introduction

The term proprioception was coined in 1906 by the neurophysiologist Sir Charles Sherrington from the Latin "proprius," meaning "one's own," for sensory information derived from neural receptors embedded in joints, muscles, and tendons (Sherrington, 1906). Hence, proprioception was originally defined as "the perception of joint and body movement as well as position of the body, or body segments, in space"(Sherrington, 1906). Some years before, in 1880, Bastian introduced the term kinaesthesia, from the Greek "kinein" to move + "aisthēsis" sensation, to describe the role of the motor cortex in eliciting motor behaviors that coordinate specific and functionally appropriate somatosensory afferent patterns (Finger, 1994). Presently, "kinaesthesia" and "proprioception" are used practically synonymously to indicate the capability to appraise the configuration and movements of an organism's body parts.

At present, proprioception can be defined as the cumulative neural input to the Central Nervous System from specialized nerve endings called mechanoreceptors, which are located in the joint, capsules, ligaments, muscles, tendons, and skin (Carpenter, Blasier, & Pellizzon, 1998; Ribeiro & Oliveira, 2007; Voight, Hardin, Blackburn, Tippett, & Canner, 1996). Proprioception alludes to the perception of tension/force, body/joint movement, and limb relative position (Riemann & Lephart, 2002). Proprioception is generally divided in the sub modalities sense of tension (resistance), sense of movement, and joint position sense. Sense of resistance represents the ability to appreciate force generated within a joint. Sense of movement refers to the ability to appreciate joint movement, including the duration, direction, amplitude, speed, acceleration and timing of movements. Joint position sense determines the ability of the subject to perceive a presented joint angle and then, after the limb has been moved, to actively or passively reproduces the same joint angle. All three modalities can be appreciated consciously and unconsciously, contributing to automatic control of movement, balance, and joint stability, and thus being essential to carry out daily living tasks, walking, and sports activities (Riemann & Lephart, 2002).

Proprioceptive information is originated and perceived within an organism at the level of the mechanoreceptor, which are sensory neurons located in the muscle, tendon, fascia, joint capsule, ligament, and skin (Carpenter, et al., 1998; Voight, et al., 1996). The main receptors contributing to proprioceptive information are located in muscle, tendon, ligament, and capsule, while those located in the deep skin and fascial layers are traditionally considered as supplementary sources. Mechanoreceptors, as specialized sensory receptors, transduce the mechanical events, in general deformation of their host tissues, as frequency-modulated neural signals to the Central Nervous System throughout afferent sensory pathways (Grigg, 1994). The role of the different mechanoreceptors in the construction of proprioception has been actively debated in the literature, although current knowledge indicates that proprioception is primarily signaled by muscle receptors, namely muscle spindles (Proske, 2005, 2006). In fact, joint receptors seem to play a minor role through the midranges of motion, being only sufficiently stimulated in end ranges of motion in order to contribute substantially to proprioception (Burgess & Clark, 1969; Burke, Gandevia, & Macefield, 1988; Clark & Burgess, 1975; Grigg, 1975). Similar to joint receptors, cutaneous receptors have been hypothesized to respond only at the end ranges of motion (Burke, et al., 1988). In contrast, muscle spindles have been almost unanimously described as able to provide potent afferent information across the entire range of motion (Burgess, Wei, Clark, & Simon, 1982; Macefield, Gandevia, & Burke, 1990). In summary, muscle mechanoreceptors afferent information, specially arising from muscle spindles, is paramount to the mediation of proprioception, while other sources of proprioceptive information, including cutaneous and joint mechanoreceptors, seem to be also important for determining the position of distal body segments and/or signaling limits of range of motion (Goble, Coxon, Wenderoth, Van Impe, & Swinnen, 2009; Proske, 2005, 2006; Proske & Gandevia, 2009). The sense of tension is provided by muscle mechanoreceptors, namely Golgi tendon organs (Proske, 2005).

The sensory inputs received from mechanoreceptors are integrated and appreciated at three distinct levels of the Central Nervous System: at the spinal level, at the brain stem, and at the higher levels of the Central Nervous System such as the cerebral cortex and cerebellum (Myers & Lephart, 2000). At the spinal cord, the axons conveying proprioceptive information can be controlled via descending commands from the brain stem and cortex through interneurons and neurons connecting with higher Central Nervous System levels. Hence, the supraspinal regions of the Central Nervous System also play a role in the modulation of the proprioceptive information that enters the ascending tracts. Most proprioceptive information travels to the supraspinal regions of the Central Nervous System by both the dorsal lateral tracts that convey the signals to the somatosensory cortex and the spinocerebellar tracts that terminate in the cerebellum. The spinocerebellar tracts exhibit the fastest transmission velocities in the Central Nervous System and are associated with nonconscious proprioception, while the dorsal lateral tracts are responsible for the conscious perception of proprioception (Riemann & Lephart, 2002). The spinal level can contribute to functional joint stability by providing direct motor responses in the form of reflexes. At the brain stem, afferent information is integrated with visual and vestibular inputs in order to control automatic and stereotypical movement patterns, balance, and posture. The higher regions of the Central Nervous System, such as the cerebral cortex and cerebellum, elicit the conscious awareness of proprioception, thus contributing to the voluntary movements (Myers & Lephart, 2000). The integration of the proprioceptive input at these levels of the Central Nervous System aims to coordinate body stability ahead of movement execution (feedforward) as well as to correct for velocity and timing errors during its execution (feedback) (Batson, 2009).

Overall, undeniable evidence exists highlighting the importance of proprioception for the generation of smooth and coordinated movements, maintenance of normal body posture, regulation of balance and postural control, and influencing motor learning and relearning. These important roles were demonstrated in several studies evaluating deafferented patients (Ghez, Gordon, & Ghilardi, 1995; Ghez & Sainburg, 1995). Their data showed that without proprioception, the onset of movement is delayed and trajectory formation is impaired and highly inaccurate.

2. Techniques to measure proprioception

Several different testing techniques to assess joint proprioception have been reported in the literature. Despite proprioception being generally assessed by measuring both joint position sense and the sense of limb movement (Hiemstra, Lo, & Fowler, 2001), all three conscious sub modalities of proprioception can be assessed. Due to their nature, it is imperative to differentiate the modality been assessed.

Joint position sense measures the accuracy of position replication and can be conducted actively or passively in both open, and closed kinetic chain positions (D. M. Hopper, et al., 2003; Magalhaes, Ribeiro, Pinheiro, & Oliveira, 2010; Pickard, Sullivan, Allison, & Singer, 2003; Skinner, Wyatt, Hodgdon, Conard, & Barrack, 1986; Stillman & McMeeken, 2001; Torres, Vasques, Duarte, & Cabri, 2010). It can be also assessed using contralateral or ipsilateral matching responses (Bouet & Gahery, 2000). The accuracy of joint position sense has been measured directly, using goniometers, potentiometers and video analysis systems (Figure 1), and indirectly using visual analog scales (Barrett, 1991; Dover & Powers, 2004; D. Hopper, Whittington, & Davies, 1997; Miura, et al., 2004; Ribeiro, Mota, & Oliveira, 2007; Stillman, McMeeken, & Macdonell, 1998; Torres, et al., 2010; Tripp, Boswell, Gansneder, & Shultz, 2004; You, 2005).

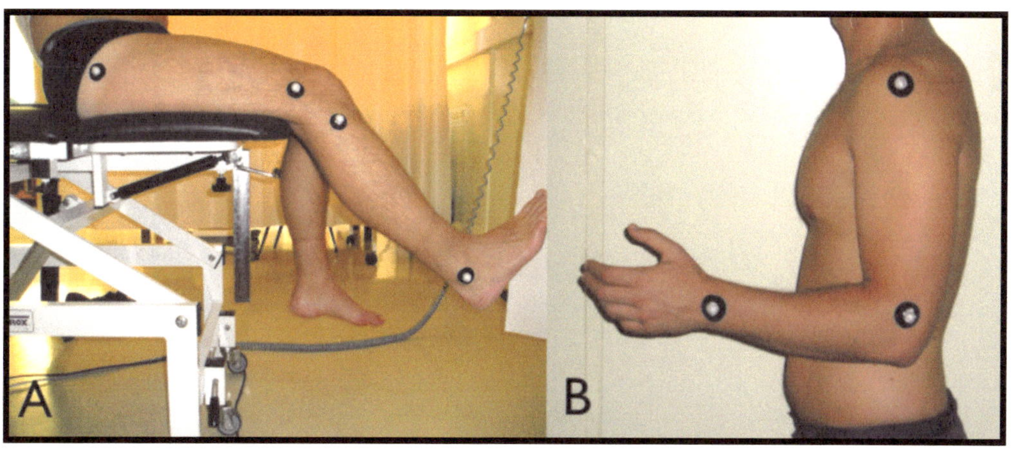

Fig. 1. Marker placement, according to four- (A) and three-point (B) model, for position sense assessment of individual joints using a video analysis system

The testing protocols usually comprise the definition of a target position that is identified and appreciated by the subjects, which are blindfolded. Then, the target position is reproduced passive or actively to the best of subjects' ability. Joint position sense is generally reported as the absolute angular error, defined as the absolute difference between the target position and the estimated position, the relative angular error, defined as the signed arithmetic difference between a test and response position, and the variable angular error, commonly represented by the standard deviation from the mean of a set of response errors. Importance should be paid to the quite different methods of joint position sense assessment employed in the literature, which make difficult to establish comparisons among the studies.

Sense of limb movement is evaluated by measuring the threshold to detection of passive motion (Allegrucci, Whitney, Lephart, Irrgang, & Fu, 1995; Carpenter, et al., 1998; Lephart, Giraldo, Borsa, & Fu, 1996; Li, Xu, & Hong, 2008; Skinner, et al., 1986; Torres, et al., 2010). Threshold to detection of passive motion quantifies a subject ability to consciously detect movement, as well as, its direction and is often performed on some type of proprioception testing device such as an isokinetic dynamometer (Figure 2).

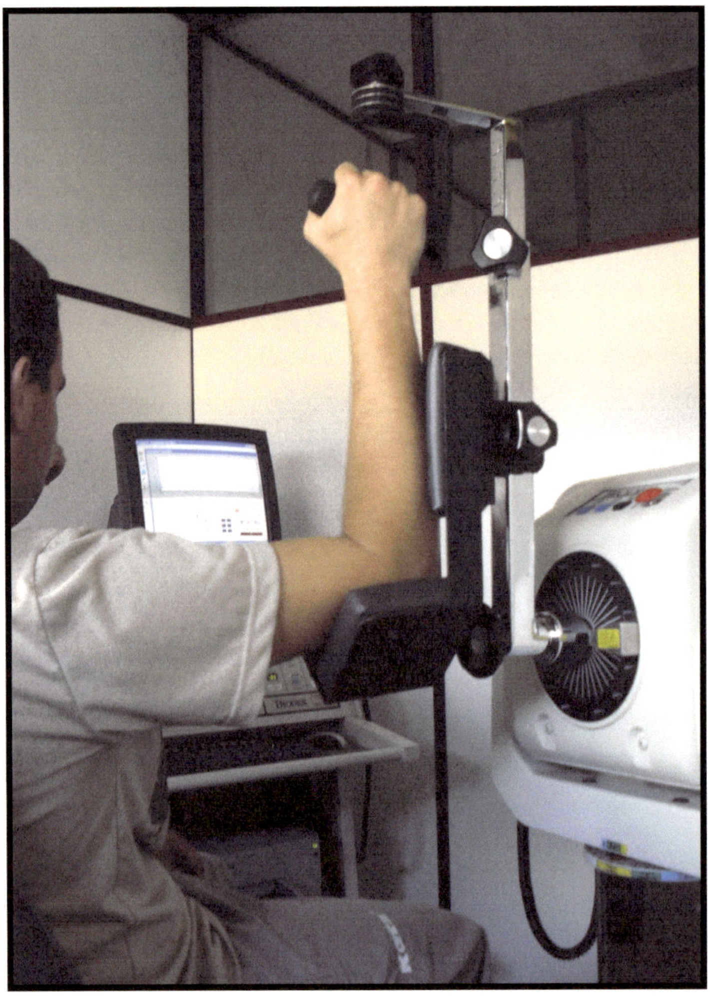

Fig. 2. The isokinetic dynamometer is used for assess joint position sense and sense of limb movement

In general, this procedure requires subjects to wear headphones, to be blindfolded to block visual input, and with a pneumatic sleeve to diminish tactile cues. The speeds used are slow, ranging from 0.5 to 2°/s, in order to target the slow-adapting mechanoreceptors (Riemann, Myers, & Lephart, 2002). The subject indicates (usually stops the device by pressing a "hold" button) when the passive movement is detected and the examiner records the amount of movement occurring before detection.

The sense of tension is assessed measuring the ability to reproduce torque magnitudes produced by a group of muscles (Riemann, et al., 2002; Torres, et al., 2010). The force-matching protocols are usually conducted without visual feedback and with low load, as the ability to reproduce force is associated with the recruitment of motor units and its firing frequency (Cafarelli, 1982). The difference between the target force and the torque produced is used to quantify the accuracy of sense of tension.

Despite different, all the above-mentioned proprioceptive testing methods rely on conscious appreciation of the mechanoreceptors input. Particular attention should be paid to several factors contributing to the wide variety of results reported in the literature, namely factors related with the testing device (eg, position of the patient with respect to gravity leading to different muscular actions during the reproduction movements), the assessment procedures (eg, angular positions, direction and speed of movement, ipsilateral or contralateral matching responses), and the study design (eg, experimental group compared with control group or bilateral comparison).

3. Factors influencing proprioception

A wealth of evidence exists pointing out several factors that induce transient or chronic changes in joint proprioception. In the following sections, we will focus the influence of aging, cryotherapy and acute bouts of exercise on proprioception.

3.1 Aging

A large body of evidence suggests that proprioceptive function declines during the aging process (Bullock-Saxton, Wong, & Hogan, 2001; Kaplan, Nixon, Reitz, Rindfleish, & Tucker, 1985; Pai, Rymer, Chang, & Sharma, 1997; Petrella, Lattanzio, & Nelson, 1997; Ribeiro & Oliveira, 2010; Skinner, Barrack, & Cook, 1984).

The deterioration of proprioception throughout the human lifespan has deleterious repercussions on motor coordination and balance (Shaffer & Harrison, 2007). Colledge et al. (1994) investigated the relative contribution of vision, proprioception, and vestibular system to the balance of different aged groups and reported that all aged groups rely more on proprioception than on vision for the maintenance of balance. This is exacerbated in subjects older than 80 years, in who the disruption of proprioceptive input seems to be a major determinant of quantitative balance performance (Camicioli, Panzer, & Kaye, 1997). In fact, impaired lower limb proprioception has been associated with balance deficits (Horak, Shupert, & Mirka, 1989; Lord & Ward, 1994; Manchester, Woollacott, Zederbauer-Hylton, & Marin, 1989; Woollacott, Shumway-Cook, & Nashner, 1986), which have, in turn, been associated with a higher incidence of falls (Lord, Rogers, Howland, & Fitzpatrick, 1999; Overstall, Exton-Smith, Imms, & Johnson, 1977; Sorock & Labiner, 1992; Tinetti, Speechley, & Ginter, 1988). Furthermore, decreased proprioception could lead to abnormal joint biomechanics during functional activities that over a period of time could result in degenerative joint disease (Skinner, 1993).

Proprioception acuity in the elderly has been extensively determined through cross-sectional studies comparing sense of position (Table 1) and/or limb movement in different age groups (Goble, et al., 2009; Ribeiro & Oliveira, 2007).

Among the first studies determining the effects of aging on proprioception are those performed by Kokmen and colleagues (1978) and Barrack and colleagues (Barrack, Skinner, & Cook, 1984; Skinner, et al., 1984). Skinner et al. (1984) compared knee proprioception under passive movement (threshold to detection of joint motion and the ability to reproduce passive knee positioning) between old and young subjects and found better proprioception in the young group. Similarly, Kaplan and colleagues, in 1985, determined the age-related changes in knee joint position sense using two techniques that required active movement, ipsilateral and contralateral matching repositioning, and observed reduced proprioception in older subjects. Interestingly, the source of acuity errors could be different for ipsilateral and contralateral matching. The contralateral matching limits the influence of eventual decreased memory abilities, as it relies greatly on interhemispheric communication, although the proprioceptive performance in this procedure could be influenced by decreased integrity of the corpus callosum or proprioceptive deficits in the contralateral leg (Goble, et al., 2009). A recent study, conducted by Ribeiro & Oliveira (2010), encompassing 129 subjects (69 older male adults aged 72.2 ± 5.0 years, and 60 young male adults aged 20.6 ± 3.0 years) and evaluating knee position sense with an open kinetic chain technique and active positioning also concluded that age has deleterious effects on position sense.

The different assessment methods employed in the above-mentioned studies and the different joints evaluated led to a wide range of acuity values, hence precluding the determination of normal values for elderly position sense acuity. Indeed, the methods used to assess position sense could have a direct influence in the acuity results. For instance, (i) active reproduction of joint position is more functional and accurate than passive reproduction (Bennell, Wee, Crossley, Stillman, & Hodges, 2005; Pickard, et al., 2003); (ii) weight bearing closed kinetic chain assessments enhance the position matching acuity (Bullock-Saxton, et al., 2001); and, (iii) target positions located farther from the starting joint position seem to increase the matching errors (Adamo, et al., 2007; Kaplan, et al., 1985). Despite using different methodological procedures, it is important to note that in general the direction of results allows to reach a similar conclusion: a significant deterioration of joint position sense is observed with advancing age.

Fewer studies have been conducted determining the effects of age on sense of movement in comparison with sense of position. Notwithstanding, they also clearly indicate that sense of movement is less accurate in old age subjects. In fact, studies conducted in the metacarpophalangeal and metatarsophalangeal (Kokmen, et al., 1978), knee (Barrack, et al., 1983; Skinner, et al., 1984), and ankle (Gilsing, et al., 1995; You, 2005) joints collectively highlight that the threshold to detection of passive motion increase with advancing age. In one of these studies (Skinner, et al., 1984), the decline in the acuity to detect passive motion was estimated to be, on average, 0.068° per year of adult life.

The mechanisms of proprioception deterioration with aging involve both central and peripheral nervous system changes. At the peripheral level, studies using animals and humans have shown anatomical and physiological age-related changes in several mechanoreceptors (Shaffer & Harrison, 2007). Aging changes the muscle spindles function by: (i) decreasing dynamic and static sensitivities (Miwa, Miwa, & Kanda, 1995); (ii) decreasing the total number of intrafusal muscle fibers and nuclear chain fibers per spindle (Kararizou, Manta, Kalfakis, & Vassilopoulos, 2005; Liu, Eriksson, Thornell, & Pedrosa-

Author	Joint	Assessment Procedures				Results (AAE)	
		Matching responses	Matching movement	Weight bearing	Target angle	Old	Young controls
Adamo, Martin, & Brown, 2007	Elbow	I	Active	No	10°	3.3°	1.6°
					30°	4.6°	3.3°
					60°	5.5°	4.0°
		C	Active	No	10°	3.8°	2.2°
					30°	5.1°	4.5°
					60°	6.6°	6.0°
Pickard, et al., 2003	Hip	I	Active (outer)	No	20°	~2.2°	~2.2°
			Active (inner)		20°	~1.8°	~1.8°
			Passive		20°	~2.4°	~2.4°
Ribeiro & Oliveira, 2010	Knee	I	Active	No	40°–60°	9.4 ± 4.3°	4.7 ± 2.7°*
Tsang & Hui-Chan, 2003	Knee	I	Passive	No	3°	4.0 ± 3.4°	-
Petrella, et al., 1997	Knee	I	Active	Yes	10°–60°	4.6 ± 1.9°	2.0 ± 0.5°*
Kaplan, et al., 1985	Knee	C	Active	No	15°	5°	3°
					30°	5°	3°
					70°	8°	4°
Barrack, Skinner, Cook, & Haddad, 1983	Knee	I	Active	No	5°–25°	4.6°	3.6°*
Verschueren, Brumagne, Swinnen, & Cordo, 2002	Ankle	I	Passive	No	10°	2.7°	2.2°*
You, 2005	Ankle	I	Active	Yes	2°–38°	2.6 ± 0.8°	1.4 ± 0.6°*
Lord, et al., 1999	Toe	C	Active	No	-	1.6°	-

Table 1. Summary of joint position sense results from studies in the elderly.
AAE – absolute angular error; C – contralateral; I – ipsilateral; * significantly better acuity in young vs. old subjects ($p<.05$)

Domellof, 2005; Miwa, et al., 1995; Swash & Fox, 1972); (iii) increasing spindle capsule thickness (Kararizou, et al., 2005; Liu, et al., 2005; Miwa, et al., 1995; Swash & Fox, 1972); (iv) deteriorating the spinal presynaptic inhibition pathways (Burke, Schutten, Koceja, & Kamen, 1996); and, (v) denervation due to spherical axonal swellings, expanded motor end plates, and group denervation atrophy (Swash & Fox, 1972). Cutaneous receptors, such as Meissner and Pacinian type corpuscles, also undergo structural modifications including a decrease in number and mean density of receptors per unit of skin area (Bolton, Winkelmann, & Dyck, 1966; Iwasaki, Goto, Goto, Ezure, & Moriyama, 2003). Changes in the number and morphology of joint mechanoreceptors, particularly in Ruffini, Pacinian and Golgi-tendon type receptors, are also reported in literature (Aydog, Korkusuz, Doral, Tetik, & Demirel, 2006; Morisawa, 1998). In addition to these peripheral modifications, the decline in proprioception as result of the aging process could be also consequence of changes in the Central Nervous System. Indeed, inadequate processing of proprioceptive input could be determined by numerous changes at central level, including decreased conductive function in the somatosensory pathways (Tanosaki, Ozaki, Shimamura, Baba, & Matsunaga, 1999), decreased grey matter in postcentral gyrus (Quiton, et al., 2007), progressive loss in the dendrite system of the motor cortex (Nakamura, Akiguchi, Kameyama, & Mizuno, 1985; Scheibel, Lindsay, Tomiyasu, & Scheibel, 1975), decline in the number of neurons and receptors, and neurochemical changes in the brain (Masliah, Mallory, Hansen, DeTeresa, & Terry, 1993; Pakkenberg & Gundersen, 1997; Strong, 1998). Central Nervous System alterations could also induce alterations in muscle spindle sensitivity, as supraspinally mediated changes in the gamma drive to the muscle spindle could have a direct effect on its sensitivity (Mynark, 2001).

3.2 Cryotherapy

Cool, in the form of cryotherapy, is one of the therapeutic modalities most extensively used in the treatment of acute and chronic injuries. Cryotherapy modalities comprise the application of ice (for instance crushed ice) (Oliveira, Ribeiro, & Oliveira, 2010), cold water immersion (Costello & Donnelly, 2011), commercially available cooling pads, and liquid cooling solutions (Leite & Ribeiro, 2010) aiming to reduce tissue temperature, metabolism, inflammation, pain, vasodilatation, and symptoms of delayed-onset muscle soreness. A number of studies have focused the effects of cryotherapy on proprioception (Costello & Donnelly, 2011; Dover & Powers, 2004; D. Hopper, et al., 1997; LaRiviere & Osternig, 1994; Oliveira, et al., 2010; Ozmun, Thieme, Ingersoll, & Knight, 1996; Uchio, et al., 2003; Wassinger, Myers, Gatti, Conley, & Lephart, 2007) and reported conflicting results (Table 2). Cryotherapy modalities varied from single joint ice-bag application to lower limb water immersion and durations ranging, in general, from 15 to 30 minutes. The ice bag modality was applied over the joint in all studies, with one study (Oliveira, et al., 2010) applying the ice bag also over the skeletal muscle. In general, the studies performed in this field assessed proprioception by measuring sense of position in different joints, including shoulder, knee, and ankle. All the studies (Dover & Powers, 2004; Thieme, et al., 1996; Wassinger, et al., 2007), but one (Oliveira, et al., 2010), using an ice bag application found no deleterious effect of cryotherapy on proprioception. Wassinger et al. (2007) applied an ice bag, filled with 1500 g of cubed ice, to the shoulder joint for 20 minutes and assessed active sense of position while standing in 2 target positions, 90° of shoulder flexion to 20° flexion and 20° of flexion to 90° of flexion. The authors found no differences in joint position sense after the ice application, but the results were reported in centimeters of vertical displacement, making those hard to interpret and compare with the literature.

Author	Joint	Cryotherapy application			Proprioception assessment	Results (AAE)	
		Modality	Local	Duration		Before	After
LaRiviere & Osternig, 1994	Ankle	Water immersion	Leg immersion to a distance of 4 cm distal from the knee joint line	20 min	Active JPS	3.8±2.0	3.7±2.3
Thieme, Ingersoll, Knight, & Ozmun, 1996	Knee	Ice bag	Knee joint	20 min	Active JPS	N/A	N/A
Hopper, et al., 1997	Ankle	Water immersion	Immersion to a depth of 5 cm above the medial malleolus	15 min	Active JPS	2.4^{o}	2.9^{o}*
Uchio, et al., 2003	Knee	Cooling pad	Knee joint	15 min	Active JPS	4.8±1.6^{o}	6.5±2.1*
Dover & Powers, 2004	Shoulder	Ice bag	Shoulder joint	30 min	Active JPS - IR Active JPS - ER	4.5±2.8^{o} 2.9±1.6	4.1±2.1^{o} 3.8±2.2^{o}
Oliveira, et al., 2010	Knee	Ice bag	Quadriceps muscle Knee joint	20 min 20 min	Active JPS Active JPS	4.7±3.0^{o} 4.6±2.9^{o}	6.9±4.8* 6.8±4.7*
Costello & Donnelly, 2011	Knee	Water immersion	Immersion to the level of the umbilicus	30 min	Active JPS: ~35° ~55° ~75°	 4.5±3.3^{o} 2.9±2.7^{o} 3.0±1.9^{o}	 5.4±2.5^{o} 5.6±3.1^{o} 3.2±2.9^{o}

Table 2. Summary of studies examining the effects of cryotherapy on proprioception. AAE - absolute angular error; ER - external rotation; IR - internal rotation; JPS - joint position sense; min - minutes; * significantly worse proprioception after cryotherapy application ($p<.05$)

The studies (Costello & Donnelly, 2011; D. Hopper, et al., 1997; LaRiviere & Osternig, 1994) using water-immersion cryotherapy protocols found similar results for lower limb proprioception. Indeed, despite using different immersion durations (15, 20 and 30 minutes), depths, and water temperatures (14°, 4°, 5°, respectively), and assessing different joints (ankle and knee), they reported no changes in position sense after water immersion (Costello & Donnelly, 2011; LaRiviere & Osternig, 1994) or have questioned the clinical significance of the changes (D. Hopper, et al., 1997).

In fact, Hopper et al. (1997) questioned if a 0.5° difference in ankle joint position sense following 15 minutes of ice bath immersion would be clinically relevant. Surenkok et al. (2008) investigated the effects of cold spray (ethyl chloride) application to the knee (until volunteers reported a feeling of cold) and a cooling pad (in two sessions 1-week apart) on passive knee joint position sense and concluded that both methods negatively affected position sense; despite these results, the efficacy of superficial applications of cryotherapy such as cold spray to decrease deep tissue sufficiently to elicit a reduction in proprioception is questionable (Costello & Donnelly, 2010). Moreover, the felling of cold could vary from individual to individual, and thus temperature decrease could not be uniform in all the subjects. Interestingly, Uchio et al. (2003) found a statistically significant decrease (1.7°) in knee joint position sense after 15 minutes of cooling, but reported position sense normalization at 15 minutes postcooling.

The authors reporting changes in proprioception after cryotherapy almost unanimously suggested the reduction of nerve conduction velocity, as the rationale for the observed decrease in proprioception. Indeed, a study reported an average reduction of 33 % and 17 % in nerve conduction velocity when the skin temperature was reduced to 10° C and 15 ° C, respectively, which relates to a 0.4 m/s decrease in nerve conduction velocity for each 1° C fall in skin temperature (Algafly & George, 2007).

In summary, the number of studies showing an increase in joint position sense error after cryotherapy is similar to the number of studies reporting no changes. Due to the limited number of investigations and the inconsistency of its results, which likely resulted from the methodological differences, the influence of cryotherapy on proprioception is still to be clearly ascertained. Since cryotherapy is a common therapeutic modality used in several settings, its impact on proprioception needs to be clearly determined in order to ensure its safety use before exercise without increasing the risk of injury due to inadequate proprioception and consequently impaired motor control.

3.3 Acute bouts of exercise

In this section we aim to discuss results of studies assessing the acute effects of pre-participation warm-up exercises and strenuous exercise inducing muscle fatigue on proprioception. The hypothesis underlying these studies is based on the proposition that if muscular mechanoreceptors were the most important afferent information contributors for proprioception, it would be expected that changes in the functional state of the muscle would have repercussions on proprioception acuity.

3.3.1 Pre-participation warm-up exercise

Warm-up exercise is acknowledged to have beneficial effects on athletic performance by reducing muscle stiffness, ameliorating the viscous elastic functioning of structures surrounding the joints, increasing neural conduction and velocity, and metabolic efficiency

(Bishop, 2003; Fradkin, Zazryn, & Smoliga, 2010). The general purposes of warm-up exercise are to increase muscle and tendon suppleness, muscle temperature, and blood flow to the periphery, and to enhance movement coordination (Fradkin, et al., 2010).

Since proprioception plays a vital role in the conscious and unconscious sensations, automatic control of movement, and motor coordination, improving proprioception in the course of warm-up might reduce the risk of injury and improve movement accuracy (Thacker, et al., 2003). Notwithstanding, few studies (Bartlett & Warren, 2002; Bouet & Gahery, 2000; Magalhaes, et al., 2010; Subasi, Gelecek, & Aksakoglu, 2008) investigated the impact of warm-up exercises on proprioception (Table 3). Indeed, the theoretical relation between warm-up, proprioception and reduced risk of sport injuries seems to be clearly established, however few studies determined the effect of pre-participation warm-up exercise on proprioception in athletes (Bartlett & Warren, 2002; Magalhaes, et al., 2010).

Regardless of using different warm-up protocols and assessment procedures to measure proprioception, the overall conclusions of all of the above-mentioned studies indicate an augment on joint proprioception after warm-up. Bouet and Gahéry, in 2000, tested the hypothesis that the accuracy of knee position sense would be better as the muscles worked under better conditions. The investigation involved 32 healthy subjects and comprised the assessment of knee position sense in two tasks (intramodal: using the contralateral leg, and crossmodal: using a scheme of a leg on a screen) with two ways of positioning (active and passive) before and after a moderate exercise consisting of pedaling during 10 minutes on a cycle ergometer. The results showed an improvement in position sense after warm-up only with the intramodal protocol combined with active positioning of the reference leg.

Bartlett and Warren (2002) evaluated the effects of a standardized four-minute duration warm up, consisting of jogging and stretching exercises, on passive knee position sense in 12 rugby players. The authors concluded that after a period of stretching and gentle exercise knee proprioception is improved, indicating an increase in sensitivity of proprioceptive mechanisms associated with the ligaments around the knee. More recently, Subasi et al. (2008) designed a study to determine the effects of different warming up periods on passive knee joint position sense of 30 healthy subjects. The 30 subjects were randomly distributed into a control (n = 10) and two exercise (each with n = 10) groups, which performed warm-up exercises of different lengths (5 and 10 minutes). Interestingly, the authors found that the 10-minute warm-up exercise period induced greater improvement in proprioception than the 5-minute warm-up period.

From the above-mentioned studies, only one (Magalhaes, et al., 2010) assessed proprioception, namely knee joint position sense, in closed kinetic chain, a procedure more close to the demands of sport and/or the exercises used in programs of proprioceptive training. The authors assessed knee joint position sense before and immediately after a warm-up program through active repositioning in open kinetic chain and closed kinetic chain in ten young amateur karatekas. Results showed that the warm-up program enhanced knee joint position sense only in closed kinetic chain.

The improvement of proprioception induced by pre-participation warm-up exercise involves exercise-related changes in both central and peripheral components of proprioception. At peripheral level, warm-up exercises may have positive impact on the function of muscular mechanoreceptors by improving the visco-elastic properties of muscular tissue, enhancing oxygenation, increasing nerve-conduction rate, and increasing body temperature due to vasodilatation (Bishop, 2003).

Author	Warm-up exercises	Warm-up duration
Bouet & Gahery, 2000	One-leg pedaling on a cycle ergometer without any imposed cadence and intensity	10 min
Bartlett & Warren, 2002	Jogging Stretching exercises (muscle group not specified)	4 min
Subasi, et al., 2008	Jogging (Protocol 1 - 2:30 min; Protocol 2 - 5 min) Stretching exercises Quadriceps muscle Hamstring muscle Gastrocnemius muscle	Protocol 1 - 5 min Protocol 2 - 10 min
Magalhaes, et al., 2010	Jogging and jumps Jogging end to end Backward running Forward running Jumping crossing the legs Skipping exercise Stretching exercises Quadriceps muscle Hamstring muscle Gastrocnemius muscle	10 min

Table 3. Summary of the warm-up procedures

At the level of Central Nervous System, warm-up exercises may also contribute to better proprioception by changing corollary discharges, likely involved in position sense (McCloskey & Torda, 1975), and/or fusimotor commands and, therefore, muscle spindle sensitivity (Bouet & Gahery, 2000).
Collectively, the available evidence supports that proprioceptive acuity is increased by pre-participation warm-up exercises.

3.3.2 Exercise-induced muscle fatigue

Per opposition to pre-participation warm-up exercises, high intensity exercise inducing muscle fatigue is associated with reduction of muscle force, joint range of motion and joint stability, and with clumsiness in movements demanding high levels of accuracy (Brockett, Warren, Gregory, Morgan, & Proske, 1997; Howell, Chleboun, & Conatser, 1993; Paschalis, et al., 2007; Proske, et al., 2003; Saxton, et al., 1995).
Fatigue is defined as an exercise-induced reduction in the ability of a muscle to generate force or power due to peripheral and/or central factors, related with an increase in perceived exertion, which can be defined as the intensity of subjective effort, strain, discomfort or fatigue sensation that one feels during exercise (Gandevia, 2001). The effects of exercise-induced muscle fatigue on joint proprioception have been extensively investigated in the last decades (Allen & Proske, 2006; Brockett, et al., 1997; Carpenter, et al., 1998; Forestier & Bonnetblanc, 2006; Forestier, Teasdale, & Nougier, 2002; Givoni, Pham, Allen, & Proske, 2007; Ju, Wang, & Cheng, 2010; Lattanzio, Petrella, Sproule, & Fowler, 1997;

Lee, Liau, Cheng, Tan, & Shih, 2003; Miura, et al., 2004; Myers, Guskiewicz, Schneider, & Prentice, 1999; Paschalis, et al., 2008; Paschalis, et al., 2007; Ribeiro, et al., 2007; Ribeiro, Santos, Gonçalves, & Oliveira, 2008; Ribeiro, Venâncio, Quintas, & Oliveira, 2011; Saxton, et al., 1995; Skinner, et al., 1986; Torres, et al., 2010; Tripp, et al., 2004; Vila-Cha, et al., 2011; Walsh, Hesse, Morgan, & Proske, 2004) (Table 4).

The majority of studies investigating the effects of exercise-induced fatigue on proprioception have been conducted in the knee joint. Sense of position, using active ipsilateral matching responses, has been the sub modality of proprioception mainly assessed.

The great majority of these studies induced muscle fatigue with laboratory protocols, often performed in an isokinetic dynamometer and involving isolated joint movements and muscle groups. The use of the information arising from laboratory studies is frequently difficult. Particularly in athletes, the use of exercise protocols that mimic the demands of sporting activity could have the advantage of reproducing more specifically the changes in neuromuscular control and proprioception observed in sport settings. Few studies have been conducted so far assessing changes in proprioception induced by sporting activity (Ribeiro, et al., 2008) or laboratory protocols replicating sporting activities (Tripp, et al., 2004). This issue is particularly relevant for athletes, as reduced proprioceptive acuity is an acknowledged risk factor for sport injuries (Barrack, Skinner, & Buckley, 1989). Additionally, it has been suggested that the higher number of injuries sustained during the last third of practice sessions or matches could be correlated with fatigue-induced alterations in lower limb neuromuscular control and joint dynamic stability due to changes in joint proprioception (Hiemstra, et al., 2001).

In general, the several studies performed in this field (Table 4), enrolling different populations (young and old-age subjects, male and female) and using distinct methodology in different joints, have demonstrated proprioceptive deficits, namely on joint position sense, as a consequence of exercise-induced muscle fatigue. The repercussions of muscle fatigue on elderly proprioception deserve singular interest, as altered proprioceptive input due to fatigue could result in deficits in neuromuscular and postural control, leading to increased risk of falls and consequently increasing the risk of osteoporotic fractures.

It has been theorized that muscle fatigue may impair the proprioceptive acuity by increasing the threshold of muscle spindle discharge and disrupting afferent feedback. Indeed, a plausible mechanism to explain the decrease in proprioception observed after fatiguing exercise could be the augmented intramuscular concentrations of several metabolites and inflammatory substances, which in turn have a direct impact on the discharge pattern of muscle spindles and alpha–gamma coactivation (Pedersen, Lonn, Hellstrom, Djupsjobacka, & Johansson, 1999; Pedersen, Sjolander, Wenngren, & Johansson, 1997). The direct impact of fatigue on the discharge patterns of muscle spindles was observed in an animal study (Pedersen, et al., 1997). In brief, in the fatigued muscle the nociceptors are activated by the end metabolic products (including bracykinin, arachidonic acid, prostaglandin E2, potassium, and lactic acid), which were produced during the previous muscular contractions. These metabolites and/or inflammatory substances within the muscle during fatiguing exercise modify the proprioceptive input by increasing the threshold for muscle spindle discharge (Djupsjobacka, Johansson, & Bergenheim, 1994; Djupsjobacka, Johansson, Bergenheim, & Wenngren, 1995; Pedersen, et al., 1997). On the other hand, changes in alpha/gamma co-activation or in alpha motoneuron activation induced by fatigue would alter muscle spindle excitability through stretch (Marks & Quinney, 1993). The decrease in proprioceptive acuity after fatiguing exercise may also be explained, at least partially, by changes in the central processing of proprioceptive signals, in result of Central Nervous System fatigue processes. It was reported that central fatigue may reduce the accuracy of motor control and interrupt voluntary muscle-stabilizing activity to resist imparted joint forces (Miura, et al., 2004).

Author	Joint	Sample	Exercise protocol	Proprioception assessment	Results
Saxton, et al., 1995	Elbow	12 subjects (6 female)	50 eccentric contractions of the forearm flexors	Sense of tension and active JPS (contralateral and ipsilateral matching)	Both parameters decreased when using contralateral matching
Brockett, et al., 1997	Elbow	13 subjects (7 female)	120 contractions at 20% of MVC	Sense of tension and active JPS (contralateral matching)	Decrease in sense of tension and JPS
Walsh, et al., 2004	Elbow	18 subjects (4 female)	2 protocols: 200-250 E or C contractions at 30% of MVC	Active JPS (contralateral matching)	Both protocols decreased JPS
Allen & Proske, 2006	Elbow	15 subjects (7 female)	Lifting a weight of 30% of MVC with elbow flexors until exhaustion	Active JPS (contralateral matching)	Decrease in JPS
Carpenter, et al., 1998	Shoulder	20 subjects (9 female)	C/C contractions of shoulder rotators until a PT drop of 50%	TTDPM of humeral rotation	Decrease of 73% in sense of movement
Lee, et al., 2003	Shoulder	11 male subjects	C/C contractions of external and internal rotators until a peak torque drop of 50%	Active and Passive JPS	Decrease in active but not in passive JPS
Skinner, et al., 1986	Knee	11 male subjects	3.75-mile run and exercise	Passive JPS and TTDPM	Decrease in JPS; no changes in TTDPM
Lattanzio, et al., 1997	Knee	16 subjects (8 female)	3 cycling protocols to maximal exhaustion	Active JPS	Decrease in JPS
Miura, et al., 2004	Knee	27 male subjects	2 protocols: local load and general load	Active JPS	Only general load decreased JPS
Ribeiro, et al., 2007	Knee	16 old-age male subjects	30 C/C contractions of the knee muscles	Active JPS	Decrease in JPS
Ribeiro, et al., 2008	Knee	17 young male athletes	Volleyball match (90 min duration)	Active JPS	Decrease in JPS

Author	Joint	Sample	Exercise protocol	Proprioception assessment	Results
Ribeiro, et al., 2011	Knee	40 male subjects	2 protocols: 30 C/E contractions of the knee extensors or flexors	Active JPS	Decrease in JPS on both protocols
Torres, et al., 2010	Knee	14 male subjects	E knee flexors contractions at 60% of PT until exhaustion	Active JPS, sense of tension, and TTDPM	Decreased acuity in all parameters
Forestier , et al., 2002	Ankle	8 male subjects	Isometric contractions of ankle flexor at 70% of MVC	Active JPS (contralateral matching)	Decrease in JPS
Forestier & Bonnetbl anc, 2006	Ankle	10 male subjects	Isometric contractions of ankle flexor at 70% of MVC	Active JPS (contralateral and ipsilateral matching)	Decreased JPS only when using contralateral matching

Table 4. Experimental evidence of the effects of exercise-induced muscle fatigue on joint proprioception. C - concentric; E - eccentric; JPS - joint position sense; MVC - maximum voluntary contraction; PT - peak torque; TTDPM - threshold to detection of passive motion.

Some authors, whose exercise protocols included eccentric contractions, have given as a reason for the proprioceptive deficits the exercise-induced muscle damage. In spite of this, it is pretty unlikely that the damage of muscle mechanoreceptors was the underlying cause of the changes observed, as studies using animal models revealed that, per opposition to extrafusal fibers, a series of eccentric contractions do not have any effect on intrafusal fibers of muscle spindles (Gregory, Morgan, & Proske, 2004) or on tendon organs (Gregory, Brockett, Morgan, Whitehead, & Proske, 2002).

4. Effects of regular physical activity and exercise on proprioception

It is widely acknowledged that regular physical activity and exercise generate an impressive collection of favorable effects in many physiologic systems. However, a pertinent question to be formulated is to whether physical activity performed on a regular basis is able to attenuate the age-related decline in proprioception?

The answer to this question is of crucial importance, since the only strategy that seems to retain/regain joint proprioception in old age subjects is regular physical exercise. The decline in proprioception in older adults, especially in lower limbs, is of great concern for several reasons: first, older adults rely more on proprioception than on vision (Colledge, et al., 1994); second, decreased proprioception has been related with disturbances in balance, which consequently increase the susceptibility to injurious falls (Lord, et al., 1999; Sorock & Labiner, 1992); and, third, decreased proprioception could lead to abnormal joint biomechanics during functional activities, which in turn could lead to, over a period of time, degenerative joint disease (Skinner, 1993).

Despite not consensual, the majority of studies pointed out the beneficial effect of regular physical activity and exercise on lower limb proprioception of older adults (Li, et al., 2008;

Petrella, et al., 1997; Pickard, et al., 2003; Ribeiro & Oliveira, 2010; Schmitt, Kuni, & Sabo, 2005; Tsang & Hui-Chan, 2003; Xu, Hong, Li, & Chan, 2004). Petrella et al. (1997) evaluated the influence of regular physical activity on proprioception by measuring knee joint proprioception among young volunteers and active and sedentary elderly volunteers. The authors reported significant differences between young (mean, 2.01 ± 0.46°) and active-old (mean, 3.12 ± 1.12°; $P < 0.001$), young and sedentary-old (mean, 4.58 ± 1.93°; $P < 0.001$), and active-old and sedentary-old ($P < 0.03$). Identical results were reported by Pickard et al. (2003), who found no differences when comparing hip joint position sense between sedentary-young and active-aged subjects (75 ± 6 years old). Some studies have also demonstrated a positive impact of Tai Chi, a Chinese mind-body exercise that puts a great emphasis on the exact joint position and direction, on proprioception, namely knee position sense (Tsang & Hui-Chan, 2003) and knee and ankle sense of movement (Li, et al., 2008; Xu, et al., 2004). More recently, Ribeiro and Oliveira (2010) tested the hypotheses that knee position sense declines with age and that regular exercise can attenuate that decline. The authors conducted a cross-sectional study encompassing 69 older and 60 young adults divided in four groups (exercised-old, N = 31; non-exercised-old, N = 38; exercised-young, N = 35; non-exercised-young, N = 25) according to chronological age and exercise practice in the past year and reported that compared to their non-exercised counterparts, exercised-old subjects exhibited better sense of position. Moreover, the proprioceptive acuity of exercised-old subjects was similar to non-exercised young subjects (Figure 3).

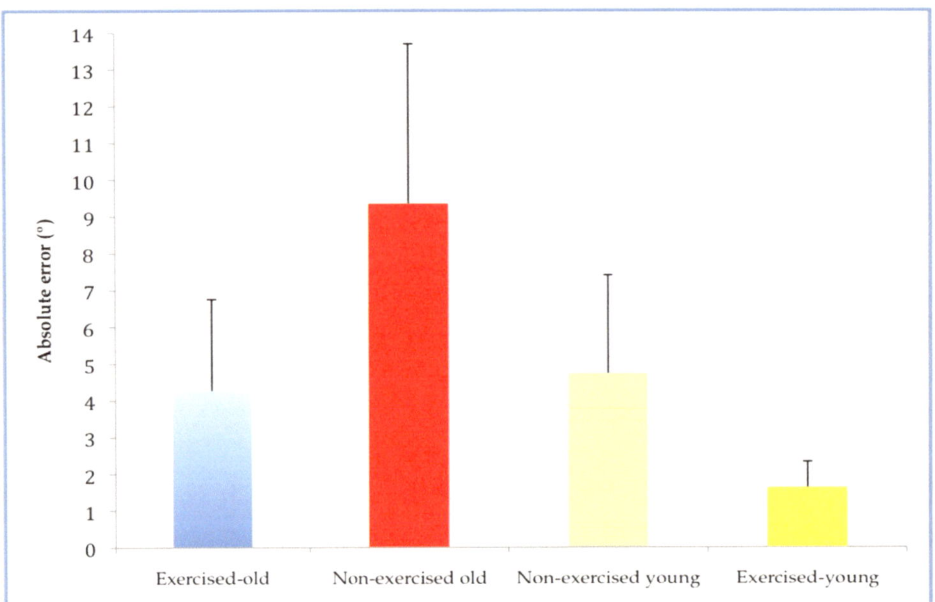

Fig. 3. Positive effects of regular physical exercise on knee joint position sense (adapted from Ribeiro & Oliveira, 2010)

Several mechanisms could be pointed towards to explain the positive impact of regular physical activity and exercise on joint proprioception. It is not surprising that being central and peripheral components of proprioception implicated in the age-related decline on proprioceptive function, they are also both potentially related to its improvement.

Physical exercise does not change the number of mechanoreceptors (Ashton-Miller, Wojtys, Huston, & Fry-Welch, 2001), but induces morphological adaptations in the muscle spindle (Hutton & Atwater, 1992). There are muscle spindle adaptations on a microlevel, the intrafusal muscle fibers could show some metabolic changes, and on a more macrolevel, the latency of the stretch reflex response decrease and the amplitude increase (Hutton & Atwater, 1992).

At central level, regular physical activity and exercise is able to change proprioception through the modulation of the muscle spindle gain and the induction of plastic modifications in the Central Nervous System. During physical activities an increase in the muscle spindle output through the γ route is observed, which facilitates the cortical projection of proprioception. Thus, by increasing the output of the muscle spindle over time, it is possible to induce plastic changes in the Central Nervous System, such as increased strength of synaptic connections and/or structural changes in the organization and numbers of connections among neurons (Ashton-Miller, et al., 2001). These plastic changes in the cortex would modify the cortical maps of the body over time, increasing the cortical representation of the joints and leading to enhanced joint proprioception (Ashton-Miller, et al., 2001).

5. Summary

In summary, this chapter highlighted the evidence that aging, cryotherapy, and exercise-induced fatigue have deleterious effects on joint proprioception, while moderate exercise or warm-up exercise enhances proprioceptive acuity. Additionally, it seems that regular physical activity and exercise play an undeniable role in the preservation of proprioceptive function.

6. References

Adamo DE, Martin BJ, Brown SH (2007). Age-related differences in upper limb proprioceptive acuity. *Percept Mot Skills* 104(3 Pt 2):1297-1309.

Algafly AA, George KP (2007). The effect of cryotherapy on nerve conduction velocity, pain threshold and pain tolerance. *Br J Sports Med* 41(6):365-369; discussion 369.

Allegrucci M, Whitney SL, Lephart SM, Irrgang JJ, Fu FH (1995). Shoulder kinesthesia in healthy unilateral athletes participating in upper extremity sports. *J Orthop Sports Phys Ther* 21(4):220-226.

Allen TJ, Proske U (2006). Effect of muscle fatigue on the sense of limb position and movement. *Exp Brain Res* 170(1):30-38.

Ashton-Miller JA, Wojtys EM, Huston LJ, Fry-Welch D (2001). Can proprioception really be improved by exercises? *Knee Surg Sports Traumatol Arthrosc* 9(3):128-136.

Aydog ST, Korkusuz P, Doral MN, Tetik O, Demirel HA (2006). Decrease in the numbers of mechanoreceptors in rabbit ACL: the effects of ageing. *Knee Surg Sports Traumatol Arthrosc* 14(4):325-329.

Barrack RL, Skinner HB, Buckley SL (1989). Proprioception in the anterior cruciate deficient knee. *Am J Sports Med* 17(1):1-6.

Barrack RL, Skinner HB, Cook SD (1984). Proprioception of the knee joint. Paradoxical effect of training. *Am J Phys Med* 63(4):175-181.

Barrack RL, Skinner HB, Cook SD, Haddad RJ, Jr. (1983). Effect of articular disease and total knee arthroplasty on knee joint-position sense. *J Neurophysiol* 50(3):684-687.

Barrett DS (1991). Proprioception and function after anterior cruciate reconstruction. *J Bone Joint Surg Br* 73(5):833-837.

Bartlett MJ, Warren PJ (2002). Effect of warming up on knee proprioception before sporting activity. *Br J Sports Med* 36(2):132-134.

Batson G (2009). Update on proprioception: considerations for dance education. *J Dance Med Sci* 13(2):35-41.

Bennell K, Wee E, Crossley K, Stillman B, Hodges P (2005). Effects of experimentally-induced anterior knee pain on knee joint position sense in healthy individuals. *J Orthop Res* 23(1):46-53.

Bishop D (2003). Warm up II: performance changes following active warm up and how to structure the warm up. *Sports Med* 33(7):483-498.

Bolton CF, Winkelmann RK, Dyck PJ (1966). A quantitative study of Meissner's corpuscles in man. *Neurology* 16(1):1-9.

Bouet V, Gahery Y (2000). Muscular exercise improves knee position sense in humans. *Neurosci Lett* 289(2):143-146.

Brockett C, Warren N, Gregory JE, Morgan DL, Proske U (1997). A comparison of the effects of concentric versus eccentric exercise on force and position sense at the human elbow joint. *Brain Res* 771(2):251-258.

Bullock-Saxton JE, Wong WJ, Hogan N (2001). The influence of age on weight-bearing joint reposition sense of the knee. *Exp Brain Res* 136(3):400-406.

Burgess PR, Clark FJ (1969). Characteristics of knee joint receptors in the cat. *J Physiol* 203(2):317-335.

Burgess PR, Wei JY, Clark FJ, Simon J (1982). Signaling of kinesthetic information by peripheral sensory receptors. *Annu Rev Neurosci* 5:171-187.

Burke D, Gandevia SC, Macefield G (1988). Responses to passive movement of receptors in joint, skin and muscle of the human hand. *J Physiol* 402:347-361.

Burke J, Schutten M, Koceja D, Kamen G (1996). Age-dependent effects of muscle vibration and the Jendrassik maneuver on the patellar tendon reflex response. *Arch Phys Med Rehabil* 77(6):600-604.

Cafarelli E (1982). Peripheral contributions to the perception of effort. *Med Sci Sports Exerc* 14(5):382-389.

Camicioli R, Panzer VP, Kaye J (1997). Balance in the healthy elderly: posturography and clinical assessment. *Arch Neurol* 54(8):976-981.

Carpenter JE, Blasier RB, Pellizzon GG (1998). The effects of muscle fatigue on shoulder joint position sense. *Am J Sports Med* 26(2):262-265.

Clark FJ, Burgess PR (1975). Slowly adapting receptors in cat knee joint: can they signal joint angle? *J Neurophysiol* 38(6):1448-1463.

Colledge NR, Cantley P, Peaston I, Brash H, Lewis S, Wilson JA (1994). Ageing and balance: the measurement of spontaneous sway by posturography. *Gerontology* 40(5):273-278.

Costello JT, Donnelly AE (2010). Cryotherapy and joint position sense in healthy participants: a systematic review. *J Athl Train* 45(3):306-316.

Costello JT, Donnelly AE (2011). Effects of cold water immersion on knee joint position sense in healthy volunteers. *J Sports Sci* 29(5):449-456.

Djupsjobacka M, Johansson H, Bergenheim M (1994). Influences on the gamma-muscle-spindle system from muscle afferents stimulated by increased intramuscular concentrations of arachidonic acid. *Brain Res* 663(2):293-302.

Djupsjobacka M, Johansson H, Bergenheim M, Wenngren BI (1995). Influences on the gamma-muscle spindle system from muscle afferents stimulated by increased intramuscular concentrations of bradykinin and 5-HT. *Neurosci Res* 22(3):325-333.

Dover G, Powers ME (2004). Cryotherapy does not impair shoulder joint position sense. *Arch Phys Med Rehabil* 85(8):1241-1246.

Finger S (1994). *Origins of Neuroscience*. New York: Oxford University Press.

Forestier N, Bonnetblanc F (2006). Compensation of lateralized fatigue due to referent static positional signals in an ankle-matching task. A feedforward mechanism. *Neurosci Lett* 397(1-2):115-119.

Forestier N, Teasdale N, Nougier V (2002). Alteration of the position sense at the ankle induced by muscular fatigue in humans. *Med Sci Sports Exerc* 34(1):117-122.

Fradkin AJ, Zazryn TR, Smoliga JM (2010). Effects of warming-up on physical performance: a systematic review with meta-analysis. *J Strength Cond Res* 24(1):140-148.

Gandevia SC (2001). Spinal and supraspinal factors in human muscle fatigue. *Physiol Rev* 81(4):1725-1789.

Ghez C, Gordon J, Ghilardi MF (1995). Impairments of reaching movements in patients without proprioception. II. Effects of visual information on accuracy. *J Neurophysiol* 73(1):361-372.

Ghez C, Sainburg R (1995). Proprioceptive control of interjoint coordination. *Can J Physiol Pharmacol* 73(2):273-284.

Gilsing MG, Van den Bosch CG, Lee SG, Ashton-Miller JA, Alexander NB, Schultz AB, Ericson WA (1995). Association of age with the threshold for detecting ankle inversion and eversion in upright stance. *Age Ageing* 24(1):58-66.

Givoni NJ, Pham T, Allen TJ, Proske U (2007). The effect of quadriceps muscle fatigue on position matching at the knee. *J Physiol* 584(Pt 1):111-119.

Goble DJ, Coxon JP, Wenderoth N, Van Impe A, Swinnen SP (2009). Proprioceptive sensibility in the elderly: degeneration, functional consequences and plastic-adaptive processes. *Neurosci Biobehav Rev* 33(3):271-278.

Gregory JE, Brockett CL, Morgan DL, Whitehead NP, Proske U (2002). Effect of eccentric muscle contractions on Golgi tendon organ responses to passive and active tension in the cat. *J Physiol* 538(Pt 1):209-218.

Gregory JE, Morgan DL, Proske U (2004). Responses of muscle spindles following a series of eccentric contractions. *Exp Brain Res* 157(2):234-240.

Grigg P (1975). Mechanical factors influencing response of joint afferent neurons from cat knee. *J Neurophysiol* 38(6):1473-1484.

Grigg P (1994). Peripheral neural mechanism in proprioception. *J Sport Rehabil* 3:2-17.

Hiemstra LA, Lo IK, Fowler PJ (2001). Effect of fatigue on knee proprioception: implications for dynamic stabilization. *J Orthop Sports Phys Ther* 31(10):598-605.

Hopper D, Whittington D, Davies J (1997). Does ice immersion influence ankle joint position sense? *Physiother Res Int* 2(4):223-236.

Hopper DM, Creagh MJ, Formby PA, Goh SC, Boyle JJ, Strauss GR (2003). Functional measurement of knee joint position sense after anterior cruciate ligament reconstruction. *Arch Phys Med Rehabil* 84(6):868-872.

Horak FB, Shupert CL, Mirka A (1989). Components of postural dyscontrol in the elderly: a review. *Neurobiol Aging* 10(6):727-738.

Howell JN, Chleboun G, Conatser R (1993). Muscle stiffness, strength loss, swelling and soreness following exercise-induced injury in humans. *J Physiol* 464:183-196.

Hutton RS, Atwater SW (1992). Acute and chronic adaptations of muscle proprioceptors in response to increased use. *Sports Med* 14(6):406-421.

Iwasaki T, Goto N, Goto J, Ezure H, Moriyama H (2003). The aging of human Meissner's corpuscles as evidenced by parallel sectioning. *Okajimas Folia Anat Jpn* 79(6):185-189.

Ju YY, Wang CW, Cheng HY (2010). Effects of active fatiguing movement versus passive repetitive movement on knee proprioception. *Clin Biomech (Bristol, Avon)* 25(7):708-712.

Kaplan FS, Nixon JE, Reitz M, Rindfleish L, Tucker J (1985). Age-related changes in proprioception and sensation of joint position. *Acta Orthop Scand* 56(1):72-74.

Kararizou E, Manta P, Kalfakis N, Vassilopoulos D (2005). Morphometric study of the human muscle spindle. *Anal Quant Cytol Histol* 27(1):1-4.

Kokmen E, Bossemeyer RW, Jr., Williams WJ (1978). Quantitative evaluation of joint motion sensation in an aging population. *J Gerontol* 33(1):62-67.

LaRiviere J, Osternig LR (1994). The effect of ice immersion on joint position sense. *J Sport Rehabil* 3(1):58-67.

Lattanzio PJ, Petrella RJ, Sproule JR, Fowler PJ (1997). Effects of fatigue on knee proprioception. *Clin J Sport Med* 7(1):22-27.

Lee HM, Liau JJ, Cheng CK, Tan CM, Shih JT (2003). Evaluation of shoulder proprioception following muscle fatigue. *Clin Biomech (Bristol, Avon)* 18(9):843-847.

Leite M, Ribeiro F (2010). Liquid Ice fails to cool the skin surface as effectively as crushed ice in a wet towel. *Physiother Theory Pract* 26(6):393-398.

Lephart SM, Giraldo JL, Borsa PA, Fu FH (1996). Knee joint proprioception: a comparison between female intercollegiate gymnasts and controls. *Knee Surg Sports Traumatol Arthrosc* 4(2):121-124.

Li JX, Xu DQ, Hong Y (2008). Tai Chi exercise and proprioception behavior in old people. *Med Sport Sci* 52:77-86.

Liu JX, Eriksson PO, Thornell LE, Pedrosa-Domellof F (2005). Fiber content and myosin heavy chain composition of muscle spindles in aged human biceps brachii. *J Histochem Cytochem* 53(4):445-454.

Lord SR, Rogers MW, Howland A, Fitzpatrick R (1999). Lateral stability, sensorimotor function and falls in older people. *J Am Geriatr Soc* 47(9):1077-1081.

Lord SR, Ward JA (1994). Age-associated differences in sensori-motor function and balance in community dwelling women. *Age Ageing* 23(6):452-460.

Macefield G, Gandevia SC, Burke D (1990). Perceptual responses to microstimulation of single afferents innervating joints, muscles and skin of the human hand. *J Physiol* 429:113-129.

Magalhaes T, Ribeiro F, Pinheiro A, Oliveira J (2010). Warming-up before sporting activity improves knee position sense. *Phys Ther Sport* 11(3):86-90.

Manchester D, Woollacott M, Zederbauer-Hylton N, Marin O (1989). Visual, vestibular and somatosensory contributions to balance control in the older adult. *J Gerontol* 44(4):M118-127.

Marks R, Quinney HA (1993). Effect of fatiguing maximal isokinetic quadriceps contractions on ability to estimate knee-position. *Percept Mot Skills* 77(3 Pt 2):1195-1202.
Masliah E, Mallory M, Hansen L, DeTeresa R, Terry RD (1993). Quantitative synaptic alterations in the human neocortex during normal aging. *Neurology* 43(1):192-197.
McCloskey DI, Torda TA (1975). Corollary motor discharges and kinaesthesia. *Brain Res* 100(2):467-470.
Miura K, Ishibashi Y, Tsuda E, Okamura Y, Otsuka H, Toh S (2004). The effect of local and general fatigue on knee proprioception. *Arthroscopy* 20(4):414-418.
Miwa T, Miwa Y, Kanda K (1995). Dynamic and static sensitivities of muscle spindle primary endings in aged rats to ramp stretch. *Neurosci Lett* 201(2):179-182.
Morisawa Y (1998). Morphological study of mechanoreceptors on the coracoacromial ligament. *J Orthop Sci* 3(2):102-110.
Myers JB, Guskiewicz KM, Schneider RA, Prentice WE (1999). Proprioception and neuromuscular control of the shoulder after muscle fatigue. *J Athl Train* 34(4):362-367.
Myers JB, Lephart SM (2000). The role of the sensorimotor system in the athletic shoulder. *J Athl Train* 35(3):351-363.
Mynark RG (2001). Effects of Age on the Spinal Stretch Reflex. *J Appl Biomech* 17(3):188-203.
Nakamura S, Akiguchi I, Kameyama M, Mizuno N (1985). Age-related changes of pyramidal cell basal dendrites in layers III and V of human motor cortex: a quantitative Golgi study. *Acta Neuropathol (Berl)* 65(3-4):281-284.
Oliveira R, Ribeiro F, Oliveira J (2010). Cryotherapy impairs knee joint position sense. *Int J Sports Med* 31(3):198-201.
Overstall PW, Exton-Smith AN, Imms FJ, Johnson AL (1977). Falls in the elderly related to postural imbalance. *Br Med J* 1(6056):261-264.
Ozmun JC, Thieme HA, Ingersoll CD, Knight KL (1996). Cooling Does Not Affect Knee Proprioception. *J Athl Train* 31(1):8-11.
Pai YC, Rymer WZ, Chang RW, Sharma L (1997). Effect of age and osteoarthritis on knee proprioception. *Arthritis Rheum* 40(12):2260-2265.
Pakkenberg B, Gundersen HJ (1997). Neocortical neuron number in humans: effect of sex and age. *J Comp Neurol* 384(2):312-320.
Paschalis V, Nikolaidis MG, Giakas G, Jamurtas AZ, Owolabi EO, Koutedakis Y (2008). Position sense and reaction angle after eccentric exercise: the repeated bout effect. *Eur J Appl Physiol* 103(1):9-18.
Paschalis V, Nikolaidis MG, Giakas G, Jamurtas AZ, Pappas A, Koutedakis Y (2007). The effect of eccentric exercise on position sense and joint reaction angle of the lower limbs. *Muscle Nerve* 35(4):496-503.
Pedersen J, Lonn J, Hellstrom F, Djupsjobacka M, Johansson H (1999). Localized muscle fatigue decreases the acuity of the movement sense in the human shoulder. *Med Sci Sports Exerc* 31(7):1047-1052.
Pedersen J, Sjolander P, Wenngren BI, Johansson H (1997). Increased intramuscular concentration of bradykinin increases the static fusimotor drive to muscle spindles in neck muscles of the cat. *Pain* 70(1):83-91.
Petrella RJ, Lattanzio PJ, Nelson MG (1997). Effect of age and activity on knee joint proprioception. *Am J Phys Med Rehabil* 76(3):235-241.

Pickard CM, Sullivan PE, Allison GT, Singer KP (2003). Is there a difference in hip joint position sense between young and older groups? *J Gerontol A Biol Sci Med Sci* 58(7):631-635.

Proske U (2005). What is the role of muscle receptors in proprioception? *Muscle Nerve* 31(6):780-787.

Proske U (2006). Kinesthesia: the role of muscle receptors. *Muscle Nerve* 34(5):545-558.

Proske U, Gandevia SC (2009). The kinaesthetic senses. *J Physiol* 587(Pt 17):4139-4146.

Proske U, Weerakkody NS, Percival P, Morgan DL, Gregory JE, Canny BJ (2003). Force-matching errors after eccentric exercise attributed to muscle soreness. *Clin Exp Pharmacol Physiol* 30(8):576-579.

Quiton RL, Roys SR, Zhuo J, Keaser ML, Gullapalli RP, Greenspan JD (2007). Age-related changes in nociceptive processing in the human brain. *Ann N Y Acad Sci* 1097:175-178.

Ribeiro F, Mota J, Oliveira J (2007). Effect of exercise-induced fatigue on position sense of the knee in the elderly. *Eur J Appl Physiol* 99(4):379-385.

Ribeiro F, Oliveira J (2007). Aging effects on joint proprioception: the role of physical activity in proprioception preservation. *Eur Rev Aging Phys Act* 4:71-76.

Ribeiro F, Oliveira J (2010). Effect of physical exercise and age on knee joint position sense. *Arch Gerontol Geriatr* 51(1):64-67.

Ribeiro F, Santos F, Gonçalves P, Oliveira J (2008). Effects of volleyball matchinduced fatigue on knee joint position sense. *Eur J Sport Sci* 8(6):397-402.

Ribeiro F, Venâncio J, Quintas P, Oliveira J (2011). The effect of fatigue on knee position sense is not dependent upon the muscle group fatigued. *Muscle and Nerve.* DOI 10.1002/mus.22018

Riemann BL, Lephart SM (2002). The Sensorimotor System, Part I: The Physiologic Basis of Functional Joint Stability. *J Athl Train* 37(1):71-79.

Riemann BL, Myers JB, Lephart SM (2002). Sensorimotor system measurement techniques. *J Athl Train* 37(1):85-98.

Saxton JM, Clarkson PM, James R, Miles M, Westerfer M, Clark S, Donnelly AE (1995). Neuromuscular dysfunction following eccentric exercise. *Med Sci Sports Exerc* 27(8):1185-1193.

Scheibel ME, Lindsay RD, Tomiyasu U, Scheibel AB (1975). Progressive dendritic changes in aging human cortex. *Exp Neurol* 47(3):392-403.

Schmitt H, Kuni B, Sabo D (2005). Influence of professional dance training on peak torque and proprioception at the ankle. *Clin J Sport Med* 15(5):331-339.

Shaffer SW, Harrison AL (2007). Aging of the somatosensory system: a translational perspective. *Phys Ther* 87(2):193-207.

Sherrington C (1906). *The Integrative Action of the Nervous System.* Cambridge, UK: Cambridge University Press.

Skinner HB (1993). Pathokinesiology and total joint arthroplasty. *Clin Orthop Relat Res*(288):78-86.

Skinner HB, Barrack RL, Cook SD (1984). Age-related decline in proprioception. *Clin Orthop Relat Res*(184):208-211.

Skinner HB, Wyatt MP, Hodgdon JA, Conard DW, Barrack RL (1986). Effect of fatigue on joint position sense of the knee. *J Orthop Res* 4(1):112-118.

Sorock GS, Labiner DM (1992). Peripheral neuromuscular dysfunction and falls in an elderly cohort. *Am J Epidemiol* 136(5):584-591.

Stillman BC, McMeeken JM (2001). The role of weightbearing in the clinical assessment of knee joint position sense. *Aust J Physiother* 47(4):247-253.

Stillman BC, McMeeken JM, Macdonell RA (1998). Aftereffects of resisted muscle contractions on the accuracy of joint position sense in elite male athletes. *Arch Phys Med Rehabil* 79(10):1250-1254.

Strong R (1998). Neurochemical changes in the aging human brain: implications for behavioral impairment and neurodegenerative disease. *Geriatrics* 53(1):S9-12.

Subasi SS, Gelecek N, Aksakoglu G (2008). Effects of different warm-up periods on knee proprioception and balance in healthy young individuals. *J Sport Rehabil* 17(2):186-205.

Surenkok O, Aytar A, Tuzun EH, Akman MN (2008). Cryotherapy impairs knee joint position sense and balance. *Isokinet Exerc Sci* 16(1):69-73.

Swash M, Fox KP (1972). The effect of age on human skeletal muscle. Studies of the morphology and innervation of muscle spindles. *J Neurol Sci* 16(4):417-432.

Tanosaki M, Ozaki I, Shimamura H, Baba M, Matsunaga M (1999). Effects of aging on central conduction in somatosensory evoked potentials: evaluation of onset versus peak methods. *Clin Neurophysiol* 110(12):2094-2103.

Thacker SB, Stroup DF, Branche CM, Gilchrist J, Goodman RA, Porter Kelling E (2003). Prevention of knee injuries in sports. A systematic review of the literature. *J Sports Med Phys Fitness* 43(2):165-179.

Thieme HA, Ingersoll CD, Knight KL, Ozmun JC (1996). Cooling Does Not Affect Knee Proprioception. *J Athl Train* 31(1).

Tinetti ME, Speechley M, Ginter SF (1988). Risk factors for falls among elderly persons living in the community. *N Engl J Med* 319(26):1701-1707.

Torres R, Vasques J, Duarte JA, Cabri JM (2010). Knee proprioception after exercise-induced muscle damage. *Int J Sports Med* 31(6):410-415.

Tripp BL, Boswell L, Gansneder BM, Shultz SJ (2004). Functional Fatigue Decreases 3-Dimensional Multijoint Position Reproduction Acuity in the Overhead-Throwing Athlete. *J Athl Train* 39(4):316-320.

Tsang WW, Hui-Chan CW (2003). Effects of tai chi on joint proprioception and stability limits in elderly subjects. *Med Sci Sports Exerc* 35(12):1962-1971.

Uchio Y, Ochi M, Fujihara A, Adachi N, Iwasa J, Sakai Y (2003). Cryotherapy influences joint laxity and position sense of the healthy knee joint. *Arch Phys Med Rehabil* 84(1):131-135.

Verschueren SM, Brumagne S, Swinnen SP, Cordo PJ (2002). The effect of aging on dynamic position sense at the ankle. *Behav Brain Res* 136(2):593-603.

Vila-Cha C, Riis S, Lund D, Moller A, Farina D, Falla D (2011). Effect of unaccustomed eccentric exercise on proprioception of the knee in weight and non-weight bearing tasks. *J Electromyogr Kinesiol* 21(1):141-147.

Voight ML, Hardin JA, Blackburn TA, Tippett S, Canner GC (1996). The effects of muscle fatigue on and the relationship of arm dominance to shoulder proprioception. *J Orthop Sports Phys Ther* 23(6):348-352.

Walsh LD, Hesse CW, Morgan DL, Proske U (2004). Human forearm position sense after fatigue of elbow flexor muscles. *J Physiol* 558(Pt 2):705-715.

Wassinger CA, Myers JB, Gatti JM, Conley KM, Lephart SM (2007). Proprioception and throwing accuracy in the dominant shoulder after cryotherapy. *J Athl Train* 42(1):84-89.

Woollacott MH, Shumway-Cook A, Nashner LM (1986). Aging and posture control: changes in sensory organization and muscular coordination. *Int J Aging Hum Dev* 23(2):97-114.

Xu D, Hong Y, Li J, Chan K (2004). Effect of tai chi exercise on proprioception of ankle and knee joints in old people. *Br J Sports Med* 38(1):50-54.

You SH (2005). Joint position sense in elderly fallers: a preliminary investigation of the validity and reliability of the SENSERite measure. *Arch Phys Med Rehabil* 86(2):346-352.

Part 5

Sport Biomechanics

15

Kinesiological Electromyography

Vladimir Medved[1] and Mario Cifrek[2]
[1]*University of Zagreb, Faculty of Kinesiology,*
[2]*University of Zagreb, Faculty of Electrical Engineering and Computing*
Croatia

1. Introduction

Sometimes even identified - albeit incorrectly - with biomechanics, kinesiology is a field relying heavily on biomechanical methodology. Borellian Rennaisance approach, enhanced in the past with seminal contributions by scientists such as Marey, Braune, and Fischer, followed further by the work of the Berkeley Group, and later by a number of modern authors, has put classical mechanics in the centre of a paradigm taken to understand, analyse and quantitatively assess human movement. As this framework sets both a geometrical and a dynamical definition of the spatial (three dimensional - 3D) movement of human body as a whole, an important further focus of the study may be directed to skeletal muscle itself, a basic actuator of movement and genuine biological system designed to produce mechanical force and cause movement. In this context, to monitor and evaluate human movement, we have a unique, second to none, method: electromyography (EMG); i.e. the recording of electrical activity of skeletal musculature. When studying kinesiological tasks, in particular, surface electromyography (sEMG) is the method's variant of choice. To quote Hess (Hess, 1954, as cited in Waterland, 1968): „The course of a movement is nothing else but a projection to the outside of a pattern of excitation taking place at a corresponding setting in the central nervous system". This thought reflects the importance of EMG signals as certain „windows" into the action of the central nervous system during the performance of a motor task.

Kinesiological electromyography is, therefore, an established subfield of modern locomotion biomechanics. We witness today a number of professional journals, conferences, organizations and university-level courses devoted to this subject around the world. At the University of Zagreb, in particular, courses of this kind are spread across several departments (Medved, 2007). At the intersection of physiology and biomechanics, and with strong quantitative aspect, this discipline significantly contributes to our understanding of human movement and is therefore used in a number of basic and applied fields. Consequently, due to its inter-disciplinary nature, it is used by different professionals; physical therapists, medical doctors of various specialties, electrical and biomedical engineers, kinesiologists, to name but a few.

To set the global framework, this chapter first shortly refers to the basics of methodology in biomechanical approach to human movement and of musculo-skeletal modelling. The method of surface electromyography is described next in some detail. Time domain signal processing methods are then presented, followed by the methods performed in the frequency domain; all with the vision towards applications in the field of kinesiology. Chapter concludes by pointing to modern engineering solutions for multichannel sEMG.

2. Multiple rigid body paradigm and neuro-muscular modelling

Biomechanical methodology for studying human movement is based on a multiple rigid body modelling paradigm in the representation of human body. Body segments are presumed to be rigid and interconnected by joints, so that a so-called kinematic chain is formed as a relevant description of movement of the body as a whole. At this level of abstraction (and simplification), the laws of classical mechanics may be applied to this system, whereby experimentally obtained (measured) kinematic data are combined with inertial properties of body segments, taking into account possible external acting forces and moments. The strict expression of quantitative relations in a system of this kind enables mathematical calculation of internal resultant (net) forces and moments acting in virtual joint centres, the procedure called inverse dynamic approach. Historically, the approach was first introduced by Braune and Fischer in Germany near to the end of 19th century, who have employed the method of photography to realize stereometry in movement recording and, consequently, implemented relevant Newtonian equations. The approach was later refined and perfected as technology for measurement and signal and data processing developed to our days. A detailed overview of the subject matter including exact mathematical formalisms describing the approach, as well as descriptions of a number of practical solutions, is available in representative journal papers (Cappozzo, 1984; a landmark paper) and in standard biomechanics literature (Medved, 2001; Rose & Gamble, 2006). This methodology forms the basis of modern biomechanics of human movement and locomotion, both in sportive and in medical applications.

Inverse dynamic approach is thus, to recapitulate, a vehicle to obtain quantitative estimates of internal resultant (net) forces and moments acting in the joints during movement of the body, idealized as a multi-segment mechanical system.

Skeletal muscle was researched the most during the 20th century, at the microstructural, biophysical, biochemical as well as at the control level. This was enabled by technological and methodological advancements such as the invention of electron microscopy, development of electrophysiological recording techniques, pursuing the concept of cybernetics, etc. Basic muscle contraction mechanism was elucidated and mathematically modelled: see, for instance, explanation of the Huxley's model of muscle contraction (McMahon, 1984). Up to the 1980es, therefore, theoretical basis was available for development of faithful quantitative models of the muscle-tendon complex (Zajac, 1989), based on which computer-supported quantitative and graphics-based solutions to model the neuro-musculo-skeletal system were realized (Delp et al., 1990). The approach has been broadly implemented until our days, not only in research, but entering the arena of clinical applications as well (Delp et al., 2000).

This methodological improvement has added to the classical inverse dynamic approach, enabling, in fact, further sub-division of calculated resultant (net) forces and moments in the joints into their components corresponding to particular muscles, resulting with a detailed and realistic biomechanical modelling and simulation possibilities of complex neuro-musculo-skeletal structures.

Skeletal muscle is a system characterized by mechanical, thermal and electrical energy outputs. Mechanical action of skeletal muscle as a whole is described well by the „tension-length" and „force-velocity" relations, its model including active, elastic and viscous components (Medved, 2001). EMG-supplied information is connected with fundamental muscle function. The active component, namely, is the one representing genuine feature of muscular tissue to mechanically contract, and this component is correlated with electrical events; being manifested ultimately as electromyographic signals (provided adequate detection and recording be secured). Contributions of elastic and viscous components of the model to the muscle force, on the contrary, are not „visible" in the EMG.

3. Surface electromyography

Electromyography means detection and recording the electrical activity of skeletal musculature. In kinesiology, predominantly surface recording technique is used due to the requirement of non-invasiveness. To correctly comprehend the method of electromyography, a certain level of understanding of signal genesis is necessary. Based on anatomico-physiological properties of neural and muscular tissues, the process may be mathematically modelled; a task accomplished successfully by Carlo De Luca, electrical and biomedical engineer, who in 1960es and 1970es gave a careful and systematic mathematical description of a so-called interference pattern - a resulting global electrical signal by the active muscle as a whole - and thus complemented the traditional anatomically-based approach. Interested reader is referred to original papers (De Luca, 1979, 1984, as well as to the book *„Muscles Alive: Their Functions Revealed by Electromyography"* (Basmajian & De Luca, 1985) - a classical reference in the field - where mathematical modelling of interference pattern is also reproduced.

3.1 On origin and properties of myoelectrical signal

Processes of depolarization and repolarization result with action potentials at the muscle fibre membrane. The depolarization–repolarization cycle forms a depolarization wave or electrical dipole travelling along the surface of a muscle fibre. Since a motor unit consists of a number muscle fibres, the electrode pair (detection electrodes issues will be discussed later) "sees" the potentials of all active fibres within this motor unit, depending on their spatial distance from the detection site. Typically, the action potentials sum up to a so-called Motor Unit Action Potential (MUAP), which differs in form and size depending on the geometrical fibre orientation with respect to the electrode(s) site. Within kinesiological studies, the MUAPs of all active motor units detectable under the electrode(s) site are electrically superimposed and observed as a bipolar signal with symmetric distribution of positive and negative amplitudes (mean value equals to zero). This is interference pattern (Konrad, 2005).

An unfiltered (exception: amplifier bandpass) and unprocessed signal comprising the superimposed MUAPs is called a raw EMG signal. In Fig. 1, a raw surface EMG (sEMG) recording is shown for three successive contractions of m. *rectus femoris*.

Raw EMG signal is, by its nature, of random shape (quasi-stochastic), meaning that one raw recording burst cannot be precisely reproduced in exact shape. This is due to the fact that the actual set of recruited motor units constantly changes within the matrix of available motor units: If occasionally two or more motor units fire at the same time, and they are located near the electrodes, they produce a strong superposition spike. By applying a smoothing algorithm (e.g. moving average) or yielding a proper amplitude parameter (e.g. area under the rectified curve), the non-reproducible contents of the signal is minimized.

Raw sEMG can range between ± 5 mV (maximum achieved in athletes) and typically the frequency contents ranges between 6 and 500 Hz, showing most power between ~ 20 and 250 Hz.

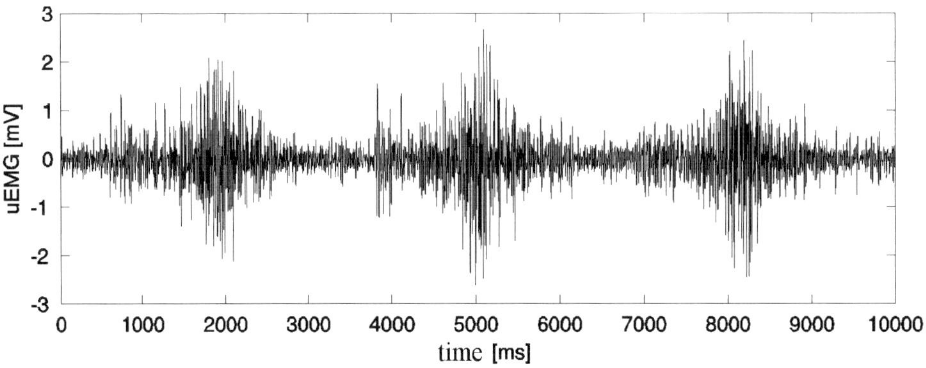

Fig. 1. Raw surface EMG recording for three successive contractions of m. *rectus femoris* (Cifrek, 1997).

3.2 Measurement of surface EMG signal

In majority of kinesiological studies surface electrodes are used due to their non-invasiveness. Offering the benefit of easy handling, their main limitation is that only surface muscles can be detected. For deeper muscles (covered by surface musculature or bones) fine-wire or needle electrodes are inevitable. (Fine-wire electrodes, being thin and flexible, are better suited to kinesiological applications than needle electrodes.)

Surface EMG electrodes can be classified considering the materials and the technologies adopted for their manufacturing (Merletti et al., 2009). One can distinguish between dry and non-dry or wet electrodes. Several types of dry electrodes exist: pin or bar electrodes made of noble metals (e.g. gold, platinum or silver), carbon electrodes, and sintered silver or silver chloride electrodes. Wet electrodes include a layer of conductive gel, hydrogel or sponge saturated with an electrolyte solution. These electrodes are often self-adhesive, so they can be easily applied and used for analysis of dynamic sEMG (Merletti et al., 2009).

Among surface electrodes, silver/silver chloride pre-gelled electrodes are the most often used ones and recommended for the general use (SENIAM, according to Hermens et al., 1999). The electrode diameter (conductive area) should be sized to 1 cm or smaller. Commercial disposable electrodes are manufactured as wet gel electrodes or adhesive gel electrodes. Generally wet gel electrodes have better conduction and impedance conditions (i.e. lower impedance) than adhesive gel electrodes. The latter one has the advantage that it can be repositioned in case of errors.

Electrodes are positioned in a so-called differential arrangement; meaning that to each specific skeletal muscle pair of electrodes is to be attached according to the standardized procedure regarding their location with respect to the muscle, and with standard spacing. It is common today to follow the SENIAM standards (Hermens et al., 1999). There is an on-going debate among the experts, however, regarding the actual positioning of the electrodes with regard to muscle for kinesiological measurements. The conservative opinion regarding two signal electrodes was that they have to be positioned at the midpoint, the most prominent part of muscle, at a distance of 15 to 30 mm (Nilsson et al., 1985). A more exact approach to electrode positioning, however, presupposes that the location of the motor point (plate) has been determined beforehand. This is accomplished by electrically stimulating the muscle and determining the location of stimulation where the muscle has the greatest mechanical response. For a long time the opinion held was that electrodes should be positioned as close as possible to the motor point (Viitasalo et al., 1980). Loeb and Gans explain this traditional attitude; they think that "electrodes have to be positioned reasonably close to the motor point with the goal of obtaining a signal of maximum and constant amplitude" (Loeb & Gans, 1986). But, from the point of view of signal stability, this location is the worst. In this region the action potentials travel caudally and rostrally along muscular tissue consisting of fibres, and so the positive and negative phases of the action potential are mutually neutralized. Basmajian and De Luca, therefore, are of the opinion that electrodes must be located approximately at the midpoint between the determined motor point location and the point where the muscle and tendon join because there signal properties are the most stable.

As far as interelectrode distance is concerned, De Luca and Knaflitz recommend a value of 10 mm centre to centre (De Luca & Knaflitz, 1992). Namely, the interelectrode distance influences signal spectrum (Lynn et al, 1978). It is therefore necessary to keep the distance fixed, so as to enable quantitative comparisons of measured values intra and inter-muscularly, as well as between subjects. A 10 mm distance is considered to be a good technical compromise because in this way a representative electrical muscle activity is detected during contraction (several cm^3 of muscular tissue), while the filtering effect of bipolar configuration is reduced at the same time (Lindström, 1973). But, in measuring dynamical muscle activity, it is often impossible to keep the interelectrode distance constant, introducing additional variability to the measurement procedure. It is customary to locate the third, neutral electrode as far away as possible from the muscle. As an addendum to experiment documentation, and in order to achieve repeatability of the measurement procedure, it is a common practice to take a photograph of the actual electrode setting. The dilemmas mentioned remain open. Besides the mentioned SENIAM protocol, valuable are also the Standards for Reporting EMG data (*Journal of Electromyography and Kinesiology*, February 1999; 9(1):III-IV).

After detection follow signal amplification and conditioning, bringing the signal into the volt range. Pre-amplifier is positioned as close as possible to detection site and is of a differential type. An important property of differential amplifier is high quality signal amplification with simultaneous suppression of noise (Medved, 2001). Interfaced to computer via analogue-to-digital (A/D) conversion, signals may be digitally processed, the task which can be accomplished either in the time domain or in the frequency domain.

Modern electromyograph devices secure high-quality signal recording with good noise suppression. Usually, they are designed as data-loggers or, alternatively, radiotelemetric systems (for example ZeroWire by Noraxon, FREEEMG 300 by BTS). Considering problems of muscle coordination and synchronisation when performing movement patterns, it is desirable to measure more EMG channels simultaneously. Modern electronics technology enables small and light detection-amplification devices as well as reliable signal transmission. Displaying a multichannel sEMG signal series provides a visually attractive means to monitor muscular activity, serving, as a first step, in qualitative analysis of multiple muscle action, be it isometric or dynamic.

4. SEMG signal processing in time domain: A muscle co-ordination issue

There are several typical time domain signal processing methods used in electromyography. All of them aim to simplify quantification and, subsequent, interpretation of signals recorded (Medved, 2001). (Raw EMG signals are, namely, of a quasi-stochastic and noise-like appearance: Fig. 1.) Among the proposed quantification methods pretending to offer indices correlating well with muscle force and energy, the most important one from the kinesiological point of view is signal smoothing (or averaging) which comprises full-wave rectification followed by low pass filtering. This kind of signal representation bears ressemblance to isometric muscular force signal - which, in principle, is not available - and can therefore in the first approximation be used as an indirect measure of muscular force (De Luca, 1997).
A number of kinesiological studies were realized in the past employing this rather non-invasive and elegant methodology to monitor muscular force(s). Spectrum of applications ranges from a number of medical rehabilitation examples, such as typically gait analysis (Fig. 2; see typical multichannel lower extremity EMG record of a walking child, Frigo & Crenna, 2009), over studies of sportive movement patterns, to various ergonomic problems. (Needless to say that a typical kinesiological experimental study incorporates, besides EMG, also other measurement quantities: kinematic and kinetic, depending upon availability.)

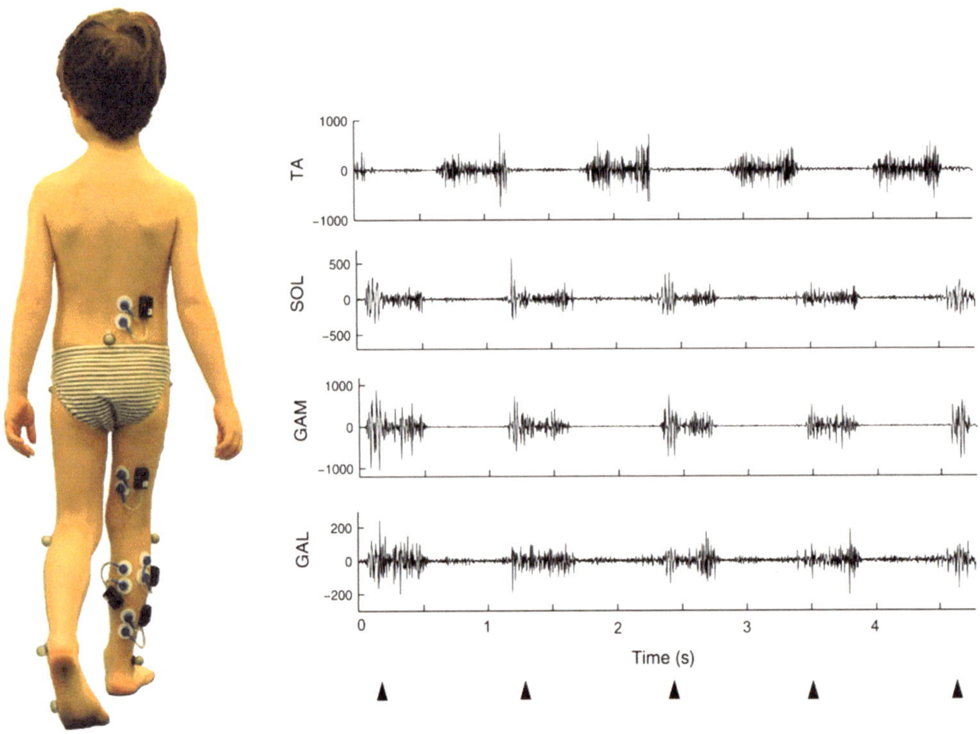

Fig. 2. Wireless sEMG recording in a 5 years old child. The picture on the left shows the electrodes and the self-powered cases, each one provided with preamplifier and antenna for independent transmission of myoelectric signals. Traces on the right-side are illustrative examples of EMG activities recorded during a tiptoe walking task from *tibialis anterior* (TA), *soleus* (SOL), *gastrocnemius medialis* (GAM), and *gastrocnemius lateralis* (GAL) (Frigo & Crenna, 2009).

Multichannel EMG may serve in studies of muscular coordination, enabling, in turn, certain evaluation of locomotor skill. An example of this kind of study whereby skilled artistic gymnastics movements were measured and analysed will be referred to (Medved & Tonković, 1991; Medved et al., 1995; reproduced in Medved, 2001). Gymnasts were instrumented with surface electrodes positioned at major lower extremity muscles (m. *gastrocnemius*, m. *tibialis anterior*, m. *rectus femoris*, m. *biceps femoris*). They were instructed to perform backward somersaults from the standing position with take-off from force platform (Fig. 3). Performances were graded by certified gymnastics judges. This gymnastics element of technique was chosen as it enabled insight into the level of acquired performance skill, because it concerns a complex movement structure. Gymnasts take a number of years of training to acquire a high-quality backward somersault and this element represents a significant component of the performance repertoire of their compositions.

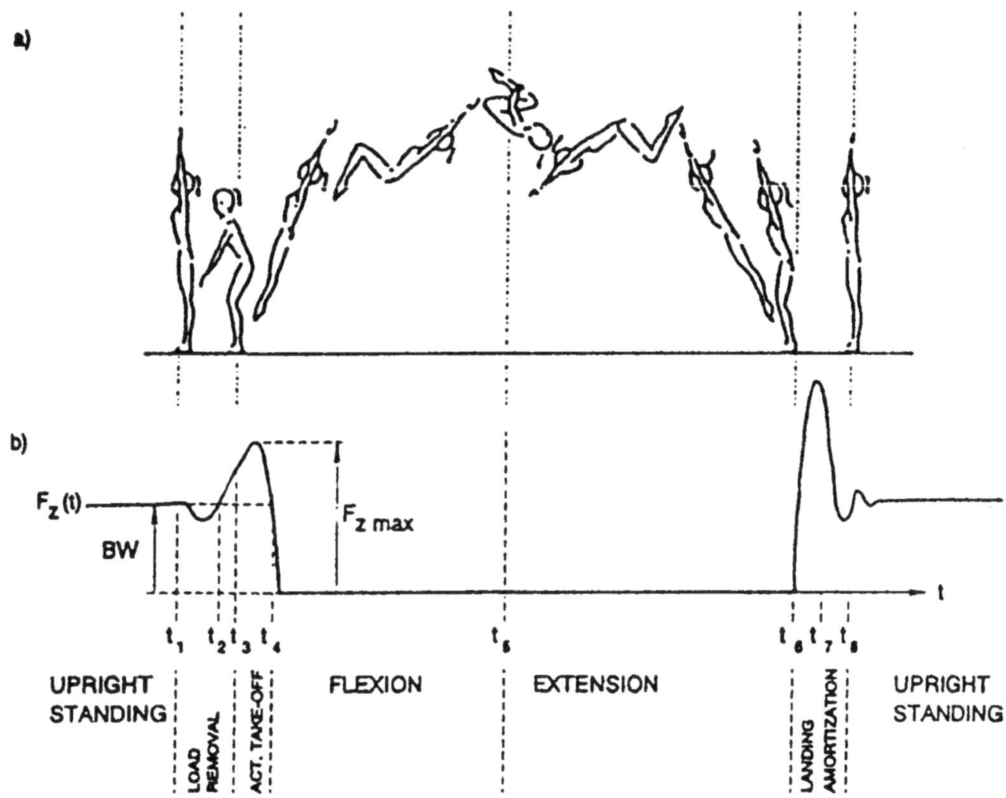

Fig. 3. a) Schematic sequential representation of the backward somersault kinematics b) Idealized waveform of the vertical component of ground reaction force vector F_Z (t), (BW= body weight, $F_{Z\,max}$ = maximum value of vertical force signal). Force signal waveform may be correlated to movement kinematics during the time period preceding airborne phase (Medved et al., 1995).

SEMG signals were detected, amplified and averaged on-line by analogue means, i.e. full-wave rectified and low pass filtered (analogue RC filter, 100 ms time constant), which was a part of the RM Beckman Dynograph device ("averaged" measurement mode). The upper frequency thus attained was 150 Hz. Signals were further digitized on-line and stored in computer memory. Quantification according to Gandy et al., (1980) was applied. The above procedure was thus: 1) measurement and signal acquisition, 2) signal pre-processing (i.e. signal smoothing), 3) statistical signal and data processing (i.e. calculation of correlation between smoothed signals, and of correlation between signal parameters and grades of performance) and 4) conclusion, i.e. determining quantitative skill criteria.

The experiments yielded the following quantitative criteria for the level of skill acquisition in the performance of the backward somersault from a standing position. The kinetic criterion of good quality performance is determined by values of the vertical force Fz impulse width < 300 ms and of ratio Fzmax/BW > 3 (Fig. 3), while the bioelectric criterion is determined by the value of the correlation coefficient of averaged EMG signals of the left and right m. *gastrocnemius* of ≥ 0.8, reflecting a high degree of symmetry in the activity of ankle extensor muscles (BW stands for body weight).

The bioelectrical criterion has been further elaborated into the so-called moving correlation function:

$$H(j)=\frac{\sum_{i=1}^{200}\left[A(i+j)-\bar{A}\right]\cdot\left[B(i+j)-\bar{B}\right]}{\sqrt{\sum_{i=1}^{200}\left[A(i+j)-\bar{A}\right]^2\cdot\sum_{i=1}^{200}\left[B(i+j)-\bar{B}\right]^2}} \tag{1}$$

The function $H(j)$, being a collection of scaled correlation coefficients, calculated one by one for each j shows the correlation between two selected averaged EMG signals. It is calculated by moving a 200 point window A over the original 300 point function B starting from the "-50 point" to the "+50 point" (Schwartz, 1975; Spiegel, 1992). The function $H(j)$ thus has 100 points in total (j = 100) with an expected maximum around or at the "50 point". Fig. 4 shows calculated moving correlation functions for the "top-level" and "poor" performer, that is, for performances by a top-level performer "at his best" and "deliberately poor", respectively. A good discriminability feature is observed in the procedure for the evaluation of skill level realized in this way; EMG signals have thus shown to be rather sensitive measures of neuro-muscular performance.

The method described serves as an example of possible use of multichannel sEMG signals as an indirect measure of multiple muscle force co-ordination pattern associated with particular skilled locomotion. It is potentially applicable in quantification of acquisition of other movement structures as well (presuming respective muscles are measured), and might also serve in monitoring the progress in motorics in course of particular diagnostics and/or treatment procedures in rehabilitation medicine.

Depending upon a kind of question attempted to be answered by EMG analysis, signal amplitude normalization might be necessary. This is for instance when inter-subject or inter-muscular (at the same subject) comparisons of EMG signals are to be made. Naturally, the value to which normalization is made (100%) must be determined precisely in a sense of defining actual kinesiological conditions of a corresponding movement or posture, and type of contraction performed (isometric, dynamic,...). There is no absolute consensus about this matter, however, and each investigator is responsible for correctness of his own measurement/experiment (Konrad, 2005; Medved, 2001).

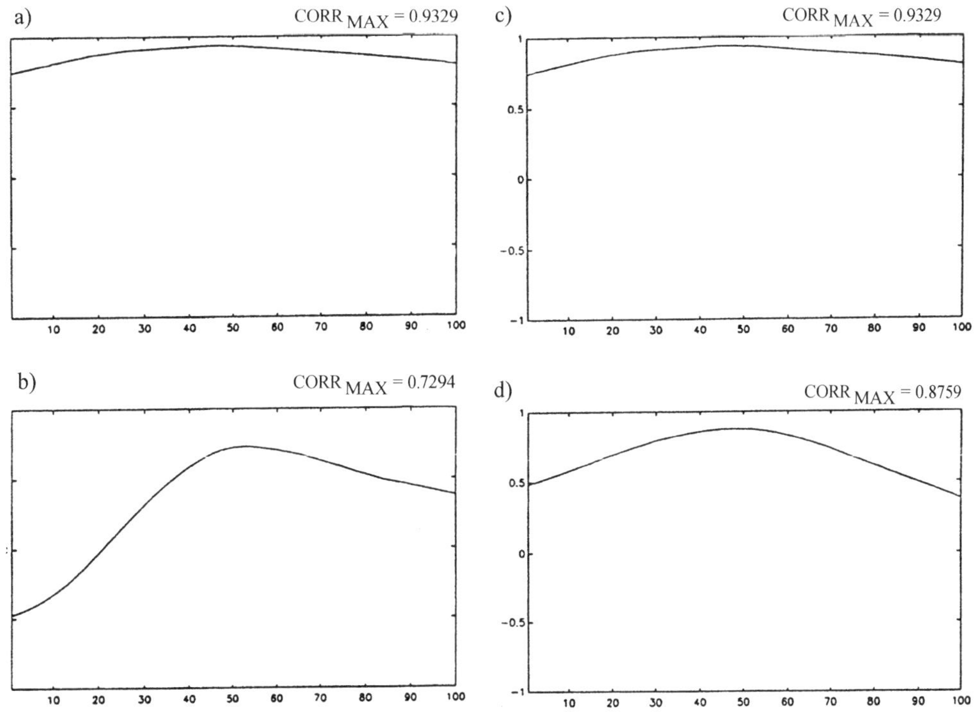

Fig. 4. Left column: correlation (L Ga vs. R Ga) functions *H(j)* of "top-level" performer (a) and "poor" performer (b). Right column: correlation (L Ga vs. R Ga) functions *H(j)* of top-level gymnast performing backward somersault "at his best" (c) and "deliberately poorly" (d) (Medved et al., 1995).

5. SEMG signal processing in frequency domain: A muscle fatigue issue

Given the recommended amplifier bandpass settings from 10 Hz high-pass up to at least 500 Hz low pass (SENIAM), most of the surface EMG frequency power is located between 20 and 250 Hz. Power distribution can be obtained by the Fourier Transformation (applying in practice Fast Fourier Transform (FFT) to a time represented signal) and graphically presented as EMG signal power density spectrum, which shows signal power distribution with regard to frequency (Fig. 5).

The dominant change in the EMG power density spectrum during sustained contractions is a compression of the signal spectrum toward lower frequencies, which is shown by curves on Fig. 5 a) and b). Measures of this compression are associated with metabolic fatigue in the underlying muscle.

Power spectrum density curve can be characterized by the following frequency parameters (Fig. 6): mean frequency, as the mathematical mean of the spectrum curve:

$$f_{mean} = \frac{\int_0^{f_s/2} fP(f)df}{\int_0^{f_s/2} P(f)df} \quad (2)$$

and median frequency as the parameter that divides the total power area into two equal parts:

$$\int_0^{f_{med}} P(f)df = \frac{1}{2}\int_0^{f_s/2} P(f)df \quad (3)$$

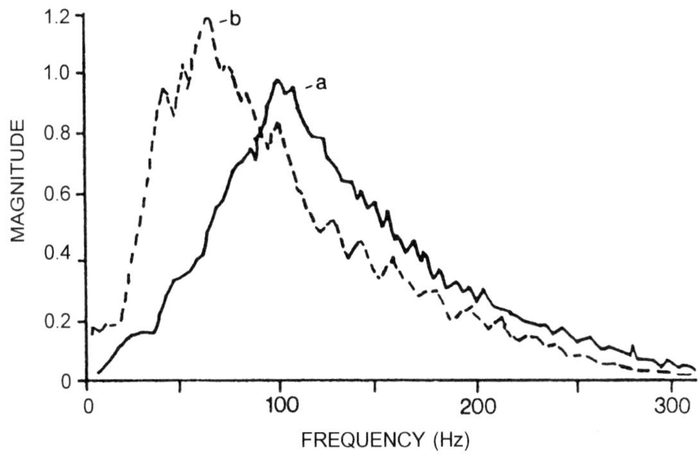

Fig. 5. SEMG power spectrum density - before (a) and after (b) fatiguing exercise (De Luca, 1984).

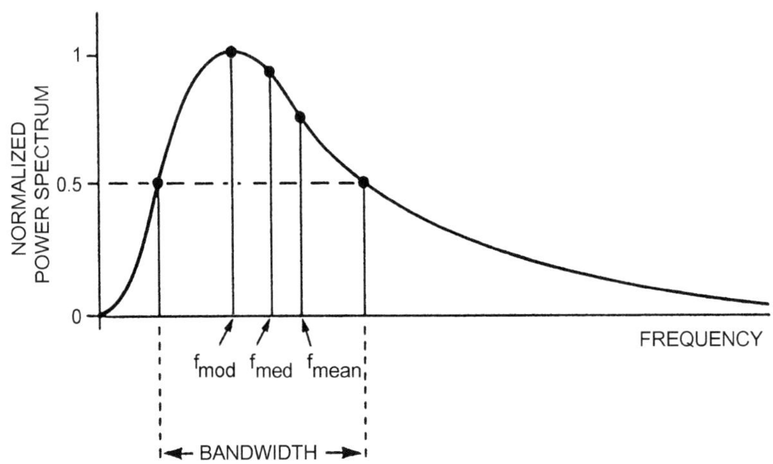

Fig. 6. Power spectrum density characteristic frequencies

Within applied EMG-frequency analysis the mean and median frequencies are the most important parameters, and their time domain changes in sustained contractions are monitored (fatigue studies).
(An alternative to the FFT based calculations was, historically, the simple counting of zero line crossings of the EMG signal, being highly correlated to the FFT based mean/median frequency values.)
Within static submaximal contractions both amplitude and frequency based analysis parameters show time domain changes due to muscular fatigue. The classical test requires a constant load level at a well defined angle position/muscular length. Due to recruitment of motor units, the amplitude shows an increase, whereas mean and median frequency of the power spectrum show a decrease over contraction time. The latter ones decline because - besides other reasons - the conduction velocity of the motor actions potentials at the muscle membrane decreases. This causes a shift to the left of the power density spectrum. The regression coefficient of the median or mean frequency slope towards lower values can be used as a non-invasive fatigue index for the investigated muscle.
The influence of muscle fatigue on the properties of the sEMG signal during isometric voluntary and electrically elicited contractions is clearly shown in Fig. 7 (Merletti & Lo Conte, 1997). In this example a subject maintained target torque level for 60 s before a mechanical manifestation of muscle fatigue occurred (healthy *tibialis anterior* muscle). Increase of the RMS value and decrease of CV and power spectrum mean frequency are evident from the beginning of the contraction. This is even more evident during electrically elicited contractions (*vastus medialis* stimulated for 30 s at 30 pulses/s), and it appears to be a combination of scaling (stretching in time and in amplitude) and a change of shape of the M-wave (myoelectric signal evoked by electrical stimulation).
Cifrek and colleagues (Cifrek, 1997; Cifrek et al., 1998, 2000) developed a method of surface myoelectric signal measurement and analysis aimed at evaluating muscle fatigue in healthy subjects during cyclic dynamic contractions of upper leg musculature in a simple cyclic flexion–extension movement of the lower leg, recorded during exercise on a training device (Fig. 8). The signal processing part of the method is schematically presented in Fig. 9. As an indicator of muscle fatigue a change in the power spectrum median frequency (MF), calculated from the spectrogram, was used. The authors also discussed the influence of analysis parameters on the results (Cifrek et al., 1999).
Merletti & Parker (2004) have edited a book providing a broad coverage of modern modelling and signal processing issues in the area of sEMG, among other also fatigue influences and means of quantification of this phenomenon. Cifrek et al. (2009), however, have recently presented a state of the art summary on the issue of sEMG based muscle fatigue evaluation. An overview is given of classical and modern signal processing methods and techniques from the standpoint of applicability to sEMG signals in fatigue-inducing situations relevant to the broad field of biomechanics. Time domain, frequency domain, time-frequency and time-scale representations, and other methods such as fractal analysis and recurrence quantification analysis are described succinctly and are illustrated with their biomechanical applications, research or clinical alike.
SEMG recordings during dynamic contractions are particularly characterised by non-stationary (and non-linear) features. Standard signal processing methods using Fourier and wavelet based procedures demonstrate well known restrictions on time–frequency resolution and the ability to process non-stationary and/or non-linear time series, thus aggravating the spectral parameters estimation. The Hilbert–Huang transform (HHT), comprising of the empirical mode decomposition (EMD) and Hilbert spectral analysis

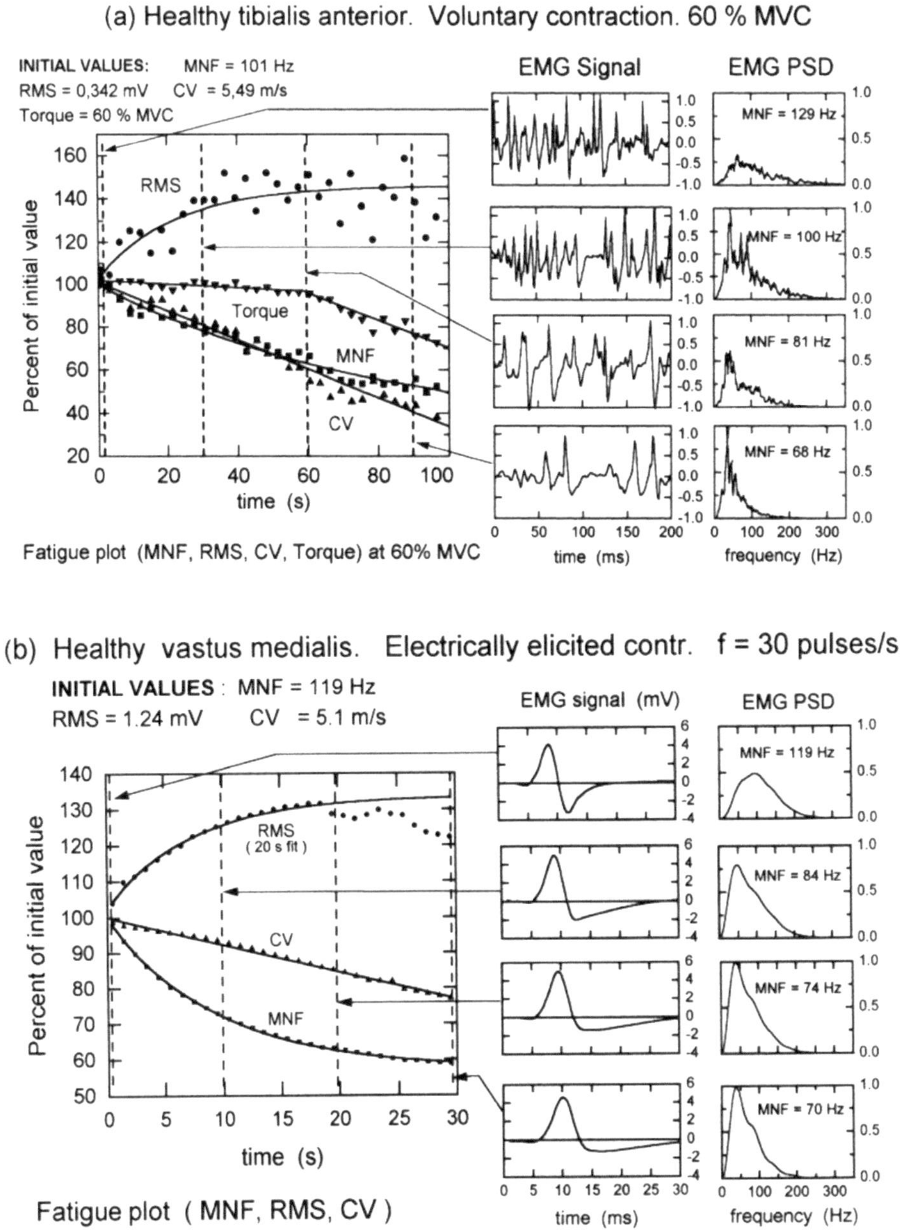

Fig. 7. Examples of fatigue plots showing the time course of the EMG signal variables during a sustained contraction, the EMG signal and its power spectral density (PSD) during specific time windows. (a) Voluntary contraction of a healthy *tibialis anterior* muscle sustained for 100 s with a target set at 60% MVC. For the sake of clarity a three-point moving average has been applied to the variables and one value every 3 s is displayed. Note the mechanical breakpoint at 60 s. (b) Electrically elicited contraction of a healthy *vastus medialis* stimulated for 30 s at 30 pulses/s. MNF = mean frequency of the PSD, RMS = root mean square value, CV = conduction velocity. From (Merletti & Lo Conte, 1997).

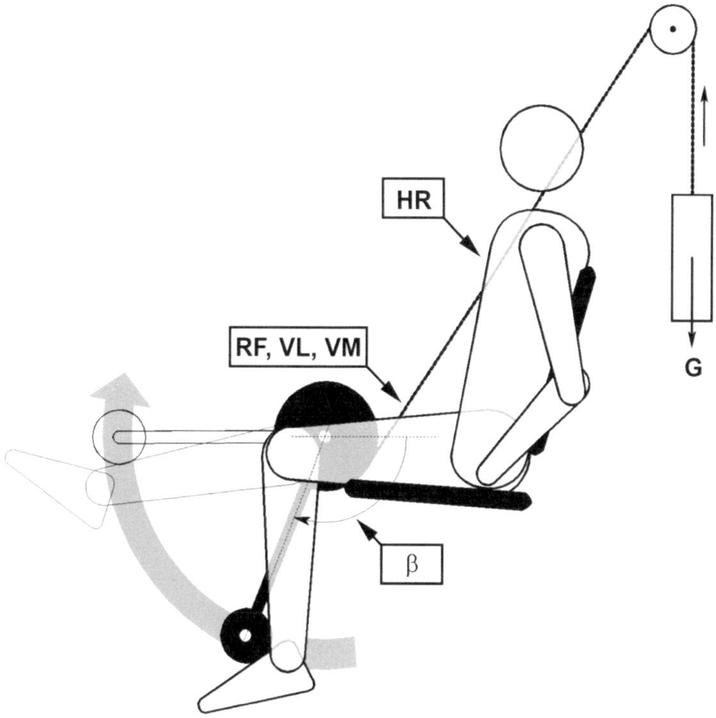

Fig. 8. Exercise on a "leg-extension" training device and measured quantities (HR=heart rate, RF = m. *rectus femoris*, VL = m. *vastus lateralis*, VM = m. *vastus medialis*, β = shaft angle) (Cifrek et al., 2000).

(HSA), provides a new approach to overcome these issues (Srhoj-Egerker at al., 2010). The time-dependent median frequency estimate is used as muscle fatigue indicator, and linear regression parameters are derived as fatigue quantifiers.
Moreover, emerging methods based on nonlinear signal analysis are being applied. These techniques, known as recurrence quantification analysis (RQA), are based on detecting deterministic structures in the signals that repeat throughout a contraction (Farina et al., 2002).

6. Conclusion

The presented methods of sEMG signal measurement and processing were based on a classical differential (bipolar) signal detection and amplification. Currently, improved measurement techniques, including multi-channel approaches targeted at a single muscle are being developed, shifting a focus from a one-dimensional signal-based considerations to two-dimensional surface-based approaches registering myoelectric phenomena (Fig. 10). Merging these new measurement possibilities with sophisticated mathematical methods and digital signal processing techniques provides a solid basis for validation, refinement and standardization of suitable new methods to be applied in biomechanical situations.
Methods for analyzing fatigue at the single motor unit level relying on non-invasive multichannel recordings and joint use of spatial filtering and spatial sampling are currently under study (Merletti et al., 2003; Farina et al., 2004).

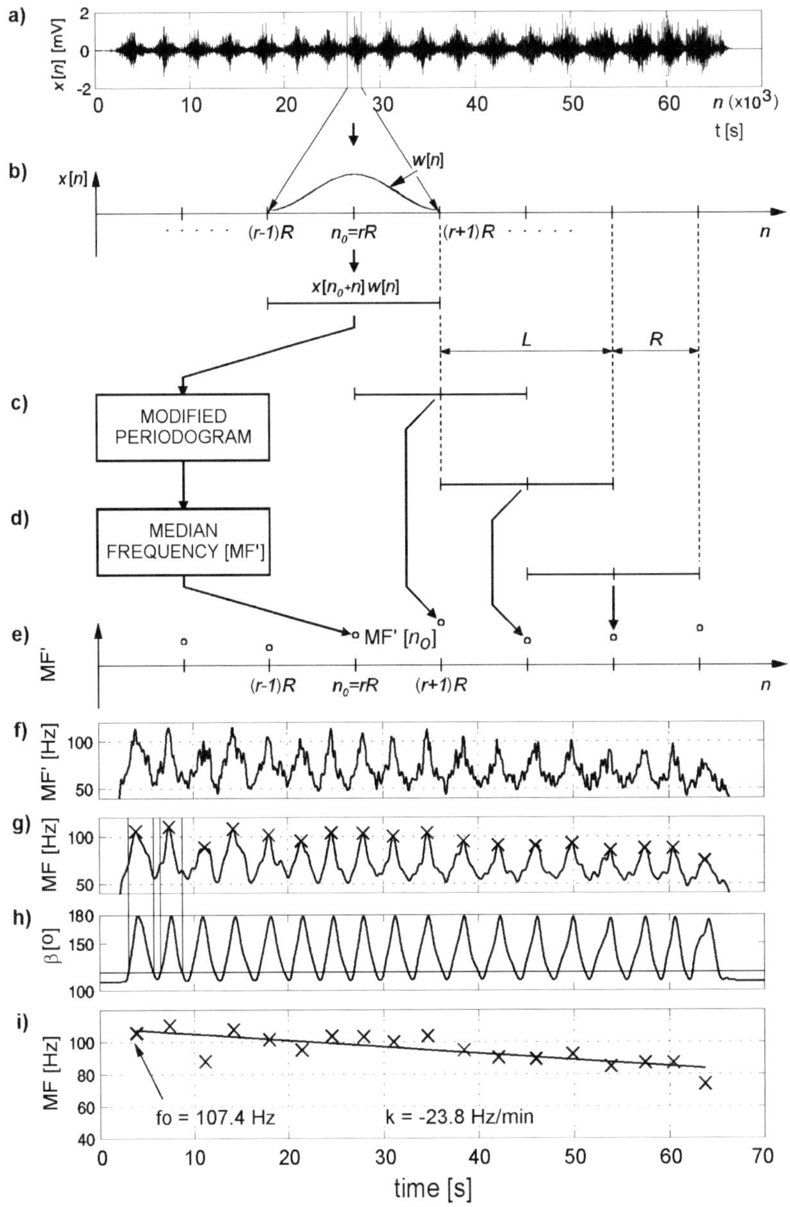

Fig. 9. Myoelectric signal spectral analysis for quantification of muscle fatigue during dynamic contractions: (a) sEMG signal x[n], raw data; (b) extracted data, using window sequence w[n] of length L, with shift of R samples (c), (d) and (e) estimation of median frequency (MF') using modified periodogram of windowed sequence, (f) course of median frequency (MF'), (g) after low-pass filtering, maximum values of MF during each contraction were calculated, (h) limits of contractions have been calculated using shaft angle data, (i) a slope of the regression line (k, expressed in Hz/min) that fits maximum values of MF in a least-square sense was used as a fatigue index. From regression line, the frequency at the beginning of exercise (f_0) was calculated (Cifrek et al., 2000).

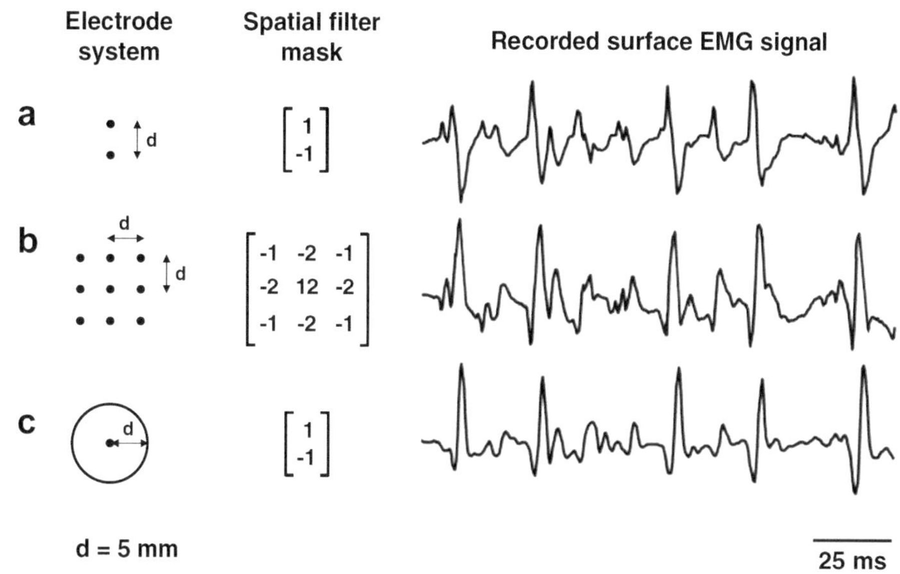

Fig. 10. Examples of sEMG signal recorded, during the same contraction, with different spatial filter configurations: (a) single differential system; (b) inverse binomial filter of the second order (IB2); (c) single ring concentric electrode system. In all cases, the interelectrode distance was 5 mm. The greater spatial selectivity of the concentric electrode system with respect to the other systems is evident (Merletti et al., 2009, redrawn and adapted from Farina & Cescon, 2001).

On the other hand, we feel confident that in realms of biomechanical research, the presented methods for muscle fatigue evaluation will be further developed, exercised, improved and standardized. In clinical diagnostic applications - both in sport and in medical rehabilitation contexts - standardization of modern methods embodied in a novel type of a "muscle fatigue monitor" device is yet to be realized. It may appear in a form of a compact device of portable design and makeup, offering a menu of several correlated fatigue indices, (including, possibly, some non-EMG based as well). This goes in line with the general feature of miniaturisation of biomedical electronics instrumentation, enabling its use in an increasing number of real-life situations.

7. Acknowledgment

The results presented are the product of a number of scientific projects including "Noninvasive measurements and procedures in biomedicine", "Automated motion capture and expert evaluation in the study of locomotion" and "Real-life data measurement and characterization", supported by The Ministry of Science, Education and Sports, Republic of Croatia.

8. References

Basmajian, J.V. & De Luca, C.J. (1985). *Muscles Alive: Their Functions Revealed by Electromyography.* Fifth Edition, Williams & Wilkins, ISBN 0-683-00414-X, Baltimore, Md., USA

Cappozzo, A. (1984). Gait Analysis Methodology. *Human Movement Science*, Vol.3, No.1-2, pp. 27-50, ISSN 0167-9457

Cifrek, M. (1997). *Myoelectric Signal Analysis during Dynamic Fatigue*. Ph.D. Dissertation. University of Zagreb, Faculty of Electrical Engineering and Computing (in Croatian).

Cifrek, M.; Tonković, S. & Medved, V. (1998). Surface Myoelectric Signal Spectral Analysis during Fatigued Dynamic Contractions of Quadriceps Muscle. In: R. Magjarević (Ed.), *Biomedical Measurement and Instrumentation: Proceedings of the 8th International IMEKO Conference on Measurement in Clinical Medicine*, Vol.3, KoREMA, Zagreb, pp. 98-101, ISBN 953-6037-26-2

Cifrek, M.; Tonkovic, S. & Medved, V. (1999). Surface EMG Spectrogram in Dynamic Muscle Fatigue Monitoring - Influence of Analysis Parameters. in: H. Hinrikus et al., (Eds.), *11th Nordic-Baltic Conference on Biomedical Engineering*, Tallin, Estonia, pp. 375-376, ISSN 01400118

Cifrek, M.; Tonkovic, S. & Medved, V. (2000). Measurement and Analysis of Surface Myoelectric Signals during Fatigued Cyclic Dynamic Contractions. *Measurement*, Vol.27, No.2, pp. 85-92, ISSN 0263-2241

Cifrek, M.; Medved, V.; Tonković, S. & Ostojić, S. (2009). Surface EMG Based Muscle Fatigue Evaluation in Biomechanics. *Clinical Biomechanics*, Vol.24, No.4, pp. 327-340, ISSN 0268-0033

De Luca, C. J. (1979). Physiology and Mathematics of Myoelectric Signals. *IEEE Transactions on Biomedical Engineering*, Vol.26, No.6, 313-326, ISSN 0018-9294

De Luca, C. J. (1984). Myoelectrical Manifestations of Localized Muscular Fatigue in Humans. *CRC Critical Reviews in Biomedical Engineering*, Vol.11, No.4, 251-279, ISSN 0278-940X

De Luca, C.J. (1997). The Use of Surface Electromyography in Biomechanics. *Journal of Applied Biomechanics*, Vol.13, 135-163, ISSN 1065-8483

De Luca, C.J. & Knaflitz, M. (1992). *Surface Electromyography: What's New?*, CLUT, Torino, Italy

Delp, S.L.; Loan, J.P.; Hoy, M.G.; Zajac, F.E.; Topp, E.L. & Rosen, J.M. (1990). An Interactive, Graphic-based Model of the Lower Extremity to Study Orthopaedic Surgical Procedures. *IEEE Transactions on Biomedical Engineering*, Vol.37, No.8, pp.757-767, ISSN 0018-9294

Delp, S.L.; Arnold, A.S. & Piazza, S.J. (2000). Clinical Applications of Musculoskeletal Models in Orthopedics and Rehabilitation, In: *Biomechanics and Neural Control of Posture and Movement*, J.M. Winters & P.E. Crago, (Eds.), 477-489, Springer-Verlag, ISBN 0387949747, New York-Berlin-Heidelberg

Gandy, M.; Johnson, S.W., Lynn, P.A.; Reed, G.A.L. & Miller, S. (1980). Acquisition and Analysis of Electromyographic Data Associated with Dynamic Movements of the Arm. *Medical & Biological Engineering & Computing*, Vol.18, No.1, pp. 57-64, ISSN 0140-0118

Farina, D.; Fattorini, L.; Felici, F. & Filligoi, G. (2002). Nonlinear Surface EMG Analysis to detect Changes of Motor Unit Conduction Velocity and Synchronization. *Journal of Applied Physiology*, Vol.93, No.5, pp. 1753-1763, ISSN 8750-7587

Farina, D.; Merletti, R., & Disselhorst-Klug, C. (2004). *Multi-Channel Techniques for Information Extraction from the Surface EMG, in: Electromyography - Physiology,*

Engineering, and Noninvasive Applications, 1 edn, R. Merletti & P. Parker, eds., John Wiley & Sons, Inc., ISBN 0-471-67580-6, Hogoken, New Jersey, pp. 169-203

Frigo, C. & Crenna, P. (2009). Multichannel SEMG in Clinical Gait Analysis: A Review and State-of-the-art. *Clinical Biomechanics*, Vol.24, No.3, pp. 236-245, ISSN 0268-0033

Hermens, J.; Freriks, B.; Merletti, R.; Stegman, D.; Blok, J.; Rau, G.; Disselhorst-Klug, C. & Hägg, G. (1999). *SENIAM 8: European Recommendations for Surface Electromyography*, Roessingh Research and Development b.v., ISBN 90-75452-15-2, The Netherlands.

Konrad, P. (2005). *The ABC of EMG. A Practical Introduction to Kinesiological Electromyography*, Version 1.0 April 2005, Noraxon INC. USA

Loeb, G. E. & Gans, C. (1986). *Electromyography for Experimentalists*, The University of Chicago Press, ISBN 0226490149, Chicago & London

Lindström, L. (1973). *A Model describing the Power Spectrum of Myoelectric Signals. Part I: Single Fiber Signal*. Chalmers University of Technology, Göteborg.

Lynn, P.A., Bettles, N. D., Hughes, A.D., Johnson, S.W. (1978) Influences of Electrode Geometry on Bipolar Recordings of the Surface Electromyogram. *Medical & Biological Engineering & Computing*, 16, 651-660, ISSN 0140-0118

McMahon, T.A. (1984). *Muscles, Reflexes, and Locomotion*, Princeton University Press, ISBN 0691083223, New Yersey, USA

Medved, V. (2001). *Measurement of Human Locomotion*, CRC Press, ISBN 0-8493-7675-0, Boca Raton, Fl., USA

Medved, V. (2007). From Research to Teaching Human Kinesiological Biomechanics: A Zagreb Experience. *Challenges in Remote Sensing. Proceedings of the 3rd WSEAS International Conference on Remote Sensing (REMOTE 07)*,pp. 43-46, ISBN 978-960-6766-17-6 ISSN: 1790-5117, Venice, Italy, November 21-23, 2007 (V Zanchi, R Revetria, A Cecchi, V Mladenov and A Zemliak (Eds.), WSEAS Press

Medved, V. & Tonković, S. (1991). Method to Evaluate The Skill Level in Fast Locomotion Through Myoelectric and Kinetic Signal Analysis, *Medical & Biological Engineering & Computing*, Vol.29, No.4, pp.406-412, ISSN 0140-0118

Medved, V.; Tonković, S. & Cifrek, M. (1995). Simple Neuro-mechanical Measure of the Locomotor Skill: An Example of Backward Somersault. *Medical Progress through Technology*, Vol.21, No.2, pp.77-84, ISSN 0047-6552

Merletti, R.; Botter, A.; Troiano, A.; Merlo, E. & Minetto, M.A. (2009). Technology and Instrumentation for Detection and Conditioning of the Surface Electromyographic Signal: State of the Art. *Clinical Biomechanics*, Vol.24, No.4, pp. 327-340, ISSN 0268-0033

Merletti, R.; Farina, D. & Gazzoni, M. (2003). The Linear Electrode Array: A useful Tool with many Applications, *Journal of Electromyography and Kinesiology*, Vol.13, No.1, pp. 37-47. ISSN 1050-6411

Merletti, R. & Lo Conte, L. R. (1997). Surface EMG Signal Processing during Isometric Contractions. *Journal of Electromyography and Kinesiology*, Vol.7, No.4, pp. 241-250, ISSN 1050-6411

Merletti, R. & Parker, P.A. (Eds.) (2004). *Electromyography - Physiology, Engineering, and Noninvasive Applications*, IEEE Press, John Wiley & Sons, ISBN 0-471-67580-6, Hoboken, New Jersey, USA

Nilsson, J.; Thorstensson, A. & Halbertsma, J. (1985). Changes in Leg Movements and Muscle Activity With Speed of Locomotion and Mode of Progression in Humans. *Acta Physiologica Scandinavica*, Vol.123, pp.457-475, ISSN 0001-6772

Rose, J. & Gamble, J.G. (Eds.) (2006). *Human Walking*. Third Edition, Lippincot Williams & Wilkins, ISBN 0781759544, Philadelphia, Pa., USA

Schwartz, M. (1975). *Signal Processing: Discrete Spectral Analysis, Detection, and Estimation*, Mc Graw Hill, Inc., ISBN 0-07-055662-8, New York, USA

Spiegel., M.R. (1992). *Theory and Problems in Statistics. Schaum's Outline Series*. Mc Graw Hill, Inc., ISBN 0070602344, New York, USA

Srhoj-Egerker, V.; Cifrek, M. & Medved, V. (2011). The Application of Hilbert-Huang Transform in the Analysis of Muscle Fatigue during Cyclic Dynamic Contractions. *Medical & Biological Engineering & Computing*, Vol.49, No.6, pp.659-669, ISSN 0140-0118

Viitasalo, J.T.; Saukkonen, S. & Komi, P.V. (1980). Reproducibility of Measurements of Selected Neuromuscular Performance Variables in Man. *Electromyography & Clinical Neurophysiology*, Vol.20, pp.487-501, ISSN 0301-150X

Waterland, J.C. (1968). Integration of Movement, In: *Biomechanics I: 1st International Seminar*, J. Wartenweiler, J.; E. Jokl & M. Hebbelnick (Eds.), 178-187, S. Karger, Basel, Switzerland

Zajac, F. E. (1989). Muscle and Tendon: Properties, Models, Scaling, and Application to Biomechanics and Motor Control, *CRC Critical Reviews in Biomedical Engineering*, Vol.17, No.4, pp.359-411, ISSN 0278-940X

16

Biomechanics of Competitive Swimming Strokes

Tiago M. Barbosa[1], Daniel A. Marinho[2], Mário J. Costa[3] and António J. Silva[4]
[1]*Polytechnic Institute of Bragança/CIDESD*
[2]*University of Beira Interior/CIDESD*
[3]*Polytechnic Institute of Bragança/CIDESD*
[4]*University of Trás-os-Montes and Alto Douro/CIDESD*
Portugal

1. Introduction

Competitive swimming is one of the most challenging sports to perform scientific research. Not only the research of human movement is quite complex, because human beings are not so determinists as other (bio)mechanical systems; but also, assessing human beings in aquatic environment becomes even more as this is not their natural environment and other physical principles have to be considered.

On regular basis, for human movement analysis, including the ones made on aquatic environments, experimental and numerical methods are used. Experimental methods are characterized by attaching bio-sensors to the subjects being analyzed, acquiring the bio-signal and thereafter processing it. Numerical methods are characterized by the introduction of selected input data, processing data according to given mechanical equations and thereafter collecting the output data. Both methods groups aim to perform kinematics analysis, kinetics analysis, neuromuscular analysis and anthropometrical/inertial analysis.

These method groups are also used for biomechanical analysis of competitive swimming. A swimming event can be decomposed in four moments or phases: (i) the starting phase; (ii) the swimming phase; (iii) the turning phase and; (iv) the finishing phase. During any swimming event, a swimmer spends most of his/her absolute or relative time in the swimming phase. Therefore, the swimming phase is the most (but not the only one) determinant moment of the swimming performance. In this sense, a large part of the biomechanical analysis of competitive swimming is dedicated to the four competitive swimming strokes: (i) the Front Crawl; (ii) the Backstroke; (iii) the Breaststroke and; (iv) the Butterfly stroke.

The aim of this chapter has two folds: (i): to perform a biomechanical characterization of the four competitive swimming strokes, based on the kinematics, kinetics and neuromuscular analysis; (ii) to report the relationships established between all the domains and how it might influence the swimming performance.

2. Competitive swimming strokes kinematics

Consistent swimming research started in the seventies. There is a significant increase on the scientific production about competitive swimming throughout the 1971-2006 period of time (Barbosa et al., 2010a) that continuous nowadays. A large part of the swimming research is dedicated to the swimming strokes kinematics. It can be considered that some topics are assessed on regular basis: (i) stroke cycle kinematics; (ii) limbs kinematics; (iii) hip and centre of mass kinematics.

2.1 Stroke cycle kinematics

Velocity (v) is the best variable to assess swimming performance. For a given distance, Front Crawl is considered the fastest swim stroke, followed by Butterfly, Backstroke and Breaststroke (Craig et al., 1985; Chengalur & Brown, 1992).

Swimming velocity can be described by its independent variables: stroke length (SL) and stroke frequency (SF). SL is defined as being the horizontal distance that the body travels during a full stroke cycle. SF is defined as being the number of full stroke cycles performed within a unit of time (strokes.min^{-1}) or Hertz (Hz). Increases or decreases in v are determined by combined increases or decreases in SF and SL, respectively (Tousaint et al., 2006; Craig et al., 1985; Kjendlie et al., 2006). Those are polynomial relationships for all swim strokes (Keskinen & Komi, 1988; Pendergast et al., 2006) (Fig. 1). For Craig and Pendergast (1979) the Front Crawl has the greatest SL and SF in comparison to remaining swimming techniques. Authors suggested similar behavior for the Backstroke except that at a given SF, the SL and v were less than for the Front Crawl. At Butterfly stroke, increases of the v were related almost entirely to increases in SF, except at the highest v. At Breaststroke increasing v was also associated with increasing in SF, but the SL decreased more than in the other swim strokes (Craig an Pendergast, 1979).

Throughout an event, the decrease of v is mainly related to the decrease of SL in all swim strokes (Hay & Guimarães, 1983). There is a "zig-zag" pattern for SF during inter-lap. The maximum SF on regular basis happens at the final lap (Letzelter & Freitag, 1983).

Comparing the swim strokes by distance, there is a trend for SF and v decrease and a slightly maintenance of SL with increasing distances (Jesus et al., 2011; Chollet et al., 1996). Swimmer must have a high SL and, therefore, v should be manipulated changing the SF (Craig & Pendergast, 1979).

One other variable often used to assess the stroke cycle kinematics is the stroke index (SI). SI is considered as an estimator for overall swimming efficiency (Costill et al., 1985). This index assumes that, at a given v, the swimmer with greater SL has the most efficient swimming technique. Regarding all the swimming strokes, Front Crawl is the one with the highest SI, followed by Backstroke, Butterfly and Breaststroke (Sánchez & Arellando, 2002). Analyzing it according to the distance, literature it not completely consensual. Sánchez and Arellano (2002) reported a trend for SI decrease from the 50 to the 400 m events, except at Breaststroke. On the other hand, Jesus et al. (2011) showed not so obvious decrease in SI from shorter to longer distances in the World Championships finalists. There was only a significant effect of distance in SI for the female swimmers.

2.2 Limbs kinematics

Stroke mechanics variables, including the SF and the SL are dependent from the limb's kinematics. That is the reason why some effort is done to understand the contribution of the limb's behavior. For instance, at Front Crawl, Deschodt et al. (1996) observed a significant relationship between the hip velocity and the horizontal and vertical motion of the upper limbs. As the upper limb's velocity increased, the horizontal velocity of the swimmers increased as well. Therefore, it can be argued that upper limbs velocity has a major influence in swimming performance. Indeed, Hollander et al. (1988) found a small contribution of the legs to propulsion (approximately 10%) at Front Crawl. However, Deschodt et al. (1999) reported a relative contribution of about 15%. To the best of our knowledge there is no study about the partial contribution of upper and lower limb's to total swim velocity in the remaining strokes.

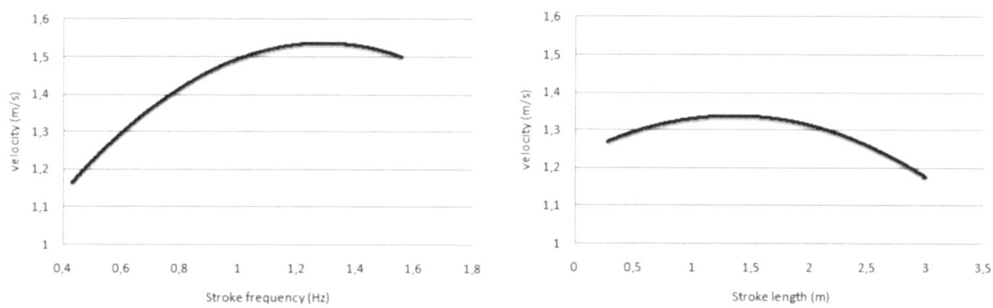

Fig. 1. The relationships between swimming velocity with stroke frequency and stroke length.

At Front Crawl another issue is the contribution of the body roll to the upper limb's kinematics and therefore to swim performance. Some researchers, such as Psycharakis and Sanders (2010), suggest a high contribution of the body roll and its relationship to breathing patterns to the limb's kinematics. A better body roll imposes a pronounced hand's "S" shape trajectory that increases the thrust.

At Backstroke the body roll is also a main issue. Good level swimmers should have a better streamlined position (Maglischo, 2003); plus a large body roll and a higher emphasis in the kicking actions (Cappaert et al., 1996). The "S" shape of the hand's path is also related to a higher thrust than other kind of trajectories (Ito, 2008).

At Breaststroke, the timing between the upper and lower limbs is a major concern. A significant relationship between upper and lower limbs coordination with swim velocity was verified (Chollet et al., 1999). Tourny et al. (1992) suggested that higher velocities might be achieved reducing the gliding phase. Nowadays, the total time gap between arms and legs propulsive actions is assessed on regular basis to understand this phenomenon (Seifert & Chollet, 2008).

At Butterfly stroke, main kinematic aspects are the trunk angle, the arm's full extension during the upsweep and the emphasis in the second kick. Higher trunk angle with horizontal plane will increase the projected surface area and the drag force. To decrease it some butterfliers breathe to the side (Barbosa et al., 1999) and others adopt a specific breathing pattern with no breathing in some cycles (Alves et al., 1999; Barbosa et al., 2003).

Butterfliers with increased velocities present a higher extension of the elbow at the upsweep, in order to increase the duration of this propulsive phase (Togashi & Nomura, 1992). Considering the lower limbs kinematics, the reduction of the kick amplitude plus the

increase of kick frequency, combined with the increase of the knee's angle during the downbeat, seems to be the best way to increase the swimmer's velocity (Arellano et al., 2003). Barbosa et al (2008a) found that a high segmental velocity of the legs during the downbeats, specially the second one, will decrease the speed fluctuation.
For all swim techniques, several manuscripts had demonstrated the importance of the last phases of the underwater stroke cycle for propulsion (Schleihauf, 1979; Schleihauf et al., 1988). So, higher swim velocities are achieved increasing the partial duration and the propulsive force during the final actions of the underwater curvilinear trajectories (Fig. 2).

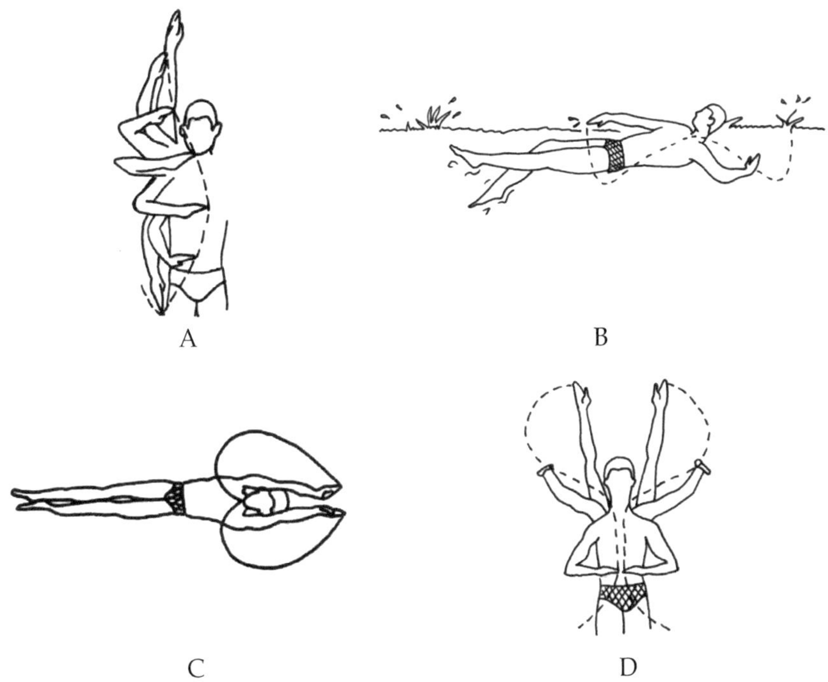

Fig. 2. The hand's underwater path at Front Crawl (panel A), Backstroke (panel B), Breaststroke (panel C) and Butterfly stroke (panel D).

2.3 Hip and centre of mass kinematics

Hip and/or centre of mass are considered as a way to analyze the body's kinematics. However, the hip is not validated as an appropriate estimator of the centre of mass kinematics (Mason et al., 1992; Barbosa et al., 2003; Psycharakis & Sanders 2009). The hip intra-cyclic velocity presents more variations than the centre of mass. Besides, the peaks and troughs do not temporally coincide throughout the stroke cycle. Inter-limbs actions during the stroke cycle constantly change the centre of mass position (Psycharakis & Sanders, 2009). The hip is not able to represent such variations since it is a fixed anatomical landmark. Although this bias, the assessment of the anatomical landmark is still an option for some research groups.
The most often assessed variable related to the hip and/or the centre of mass is the intra-cyclic variation of the horizontal velocity (dV). Throughout the stroke cycle, the body's velocity is not uniform. There are increases and decreases of the body's velocity due to the limb's actions. Indeed, the dV has been considered as one of the most important biomechanical variables to be assessed in competitive swimming (Komolgorov & Duplisheva, 1992).

From a mathematical point of view, the dV is described with non-linear functions. Nevertheless, determination coefficients from those models are moderate, since swimmers present different individual dV curves. Individual curve present some changes in comparison to mean curves from several subjects, expressing his/her interpretation of the swim technique (Barbosa et al., 2010b).

At Front Crawl, dV has a multi-model profile (Barbosa et al., 2010c) (Fig. 3, panel A). Higher peaks are related to arm's actions and lower peaks to leg's actions. For some individual curve it can be noticed two higher peaks with different velocities. Those peaks are related to the most propulsive phases of each arm. Moreover, it seems that there is for some subjects an asymmetrical application of propulsive force from both arms. A similar trend can be verified for the Backstroke dV's (Fig. 3, panel B).

At Breaststroke, dV is characterized by a bi-modal profile (Barbosa et al., 2010c) (Fig. 3, panel C). One peak is related to arm's actions and the other to the leg's action. Both peaks should be more or less even, but with a higher value for the leg's peak followed. After that peak, the gliding phase happens with a v decrease. Indeed, the gliding phase is another issue to consider regarding the Breaststroke dV. Subjects should know the exact moment to start a new stroke cycle, avoiding a major decrease of the instantaneous v (Capitão et al., 2006).

At Butterfly stroke, dV presents a tri-modal profile (Barbosa et al., 2003) (Fig. 3, panel D). The first peak is due to the leg's first downbeat, a second peak related to the arm's insweep, a last and highest peak during the arm's upsweep. The arm's recovery is a phase when the instantaneous velocity rapidly decreases.

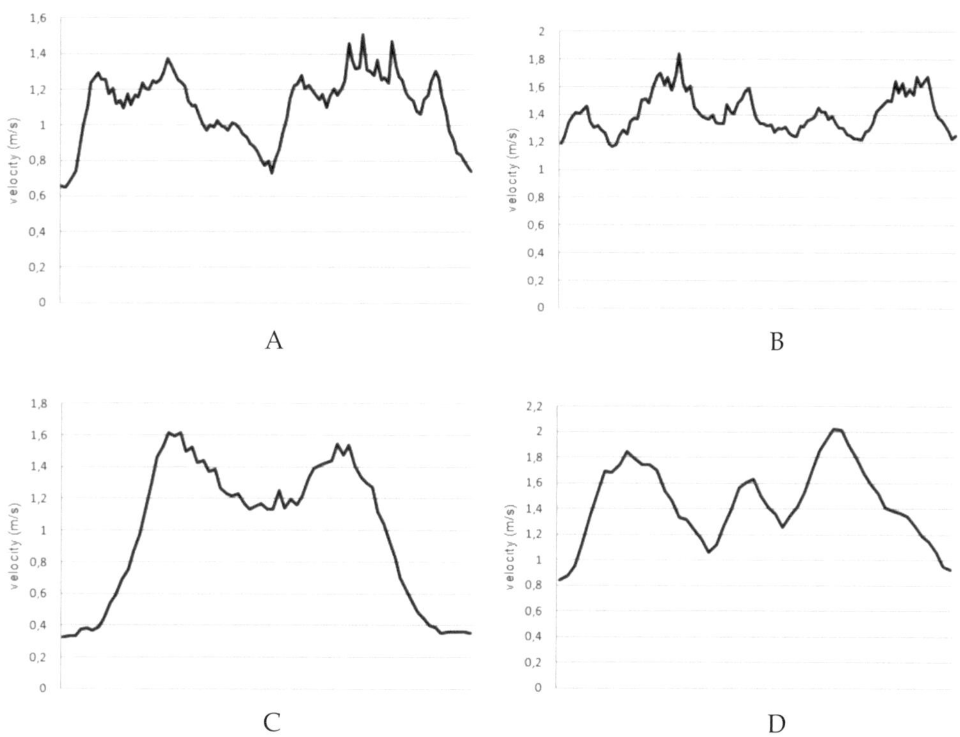

Fig. 3. The intra-cyclic variation of the horizontal velocity at Front Crawl (panel A), Backstroke (panel B), Breaststroke (panel C) and Butterfly stroke (panel D).

There is a relationship between dV and v, as well as, between dV and the swimming energy cost. There is a polynomial relationship between dV and v in the four competitive swim strokes (Barbosa et al., 2006). The dV increases to a given point with increasing v and then starts to decrease. So, high velocities seem to impose a lower dV. Added to that, increasing dV will lead to an increase in the energy cost of swimming, even controlling the effect of the v (Barbosa et al., 2005; 2006). In this sense, in all the four competitive strokes, a low dV leads to higher swim efficiency. For instance, at Breaststroke more pronounced body waving imposed a decreased dV (Persyn et al., 1992; Sanders et al., 1998; Silva et al., 2002). At Butterfly stroke, a low velocity during hand's entry, a high hand's velocity during the upsweep and a high velocity of the second downbeat will decrease the dV (Barbosa et al., 2008). So, some specific limb's actions in each swim stroke are able to decrease the dV and, therefore, to increase the swim efficiency and by this way enhancing performance.

3. Competitive swimming strokes kinetics

For a long time kinetic assessment was made adopting experimental research designs. Since the beginning of the XXth century some research was done to estimate the drag submitted and the propulsion produced by a swimmer. Houssay in 1912, Cureton in 1930 and Karpovich and Pestrecov in 1939 are considered the pioneers in this kind of research (Lewillie, 1983). One hundred years later, in the beginning of the XXIth century, new research trends, based on computational simulation techniques (Bixler & Riewald, 2002; Bixler et al., 2007; Marinho et al., 2008) and particle image velocimetry (Kamata et al., 2006) have started.
Kinetics analysis in swimming has addressed to understand two main topics of interest: (i) the propulsive force generated by the propelling segments and; (ii) the drag forces resisting forward motion, since the interaction between both forces will influence the swimmer's speed.

3.1 Propulsive force

The swimmers' performance is limited by their ability to produce effective propulsive force (the component of the total propulsive force acting in the direction of moving). The measurement of the propulsive forces generated by a swimmer has been of interest to sports biomechanics for many years. Despite the task of directly measuring the propulsive forces acting on a freely swimming subject is practically impossible, Hollander et al. (1986) developed a system for measuring active drag (MAD system) by determining the propulsive force applied to underwater push-off pads by a swimmer performing the Front Crawl arm action only. However, the intrusive nature of the device disables its use during competition and reduces its ecological validity (Payton & Bartlett, 1995). A non-intrusive method of estimating propulsive hand forces during free swimming was developed by Schleihauf (1979) and was the basis of several studies (Berger et al., 1995; Sanders, 1999). In this method the instantaneous propulsive forces are estimated according to vectorial analysis of forces combination's acting on model hands in an open-water channel and the recordings of underwater pulling action of a swimmer. Using a plastic resin model of an adult human hand, Schleihauf (1979) measured forces for known orientations to a constant water flow, determining drag and lift coefficients for specific orientations. These data were then used together with digitized kinematic data of the hand to estimate the lift, drag and resultant force vectors produced during the stroke cycle of the swimmers.

The relative contribution of drag and lift forces to overall propulsion is one of the most discussed issues in swimming hydrodynamics research. Regarding the water channel analysis, Schleihauf (1979) reported that lift coefficient values increased up to an attack angle around 40° and then decreased, although some differences with respect to the sweepback angle were observed. Drag coefficient values increased with increasing the attack angle and were less sensitive to sweepback angle changes. In a more detail analysis, Bixler and Riewald (2002) evaluated the steady flow around a swimmer's hand and forearm at various angles of attack and sweep back angles. Force coefficients measured as a function of angle of attack showed that forearm drag was essentially constant and forearm lift was almost zero (Figs. 4 and 5). Moreover, hand drag presented the minimum value near angles of attack of 0° and 180° and the maximum value was obtained near 90°, when the model is nearly perpendicular to the flow. Hand lift was almost null at 95° and peaked near 60° and 150°.

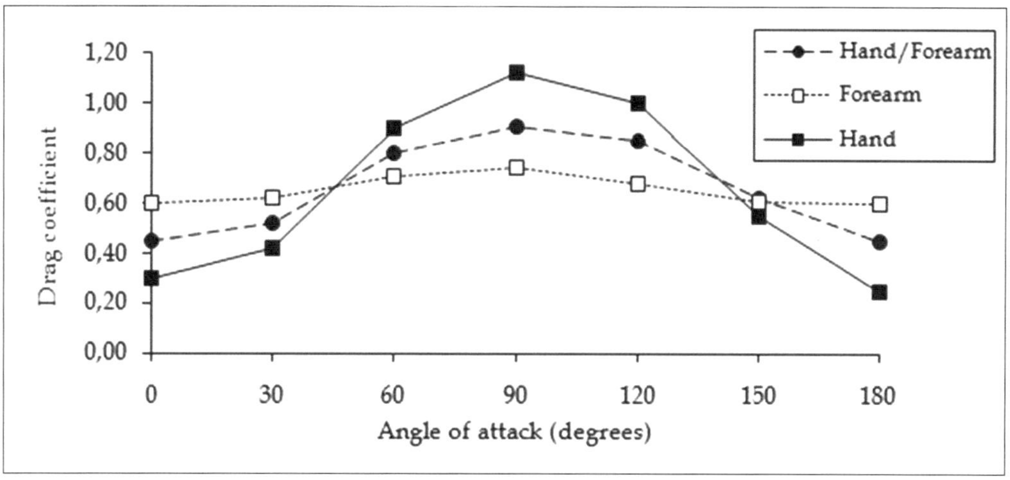

Fig. 4. Drag coefficient *vs.* angle of attack for the digital model of the hand, forearm and hand/forearm (Sweep back angle = 0°). Adapted from Bixler and Riewald (2002).

When the sweep back angle is considered, it is interesting to notice that more lift force is generated when the little finger leads the motion than when the thumb leads (Bixler & Riewald, 2002; Silva et al., 2008).

Another important issue is related to the contribution of arms and legs to propulsion. It is almost consensual that most of propulsion is generated by the arms' actions. In Front Crawl swimming, it was found (Hollander et al., 1988; Deschodt, 1999) that about 85 to 90% of propulsion is produced by the arms' movements. Accordingly, the majority of the research under this scope is performed on arm's movements. Nevertheless, leg's propulsion should not be disregarded and future studies under this field should be addressed, helping swimmers to enhance performance. Regarding arms' actions, a large inter-subject range of fingers relative position can be observed during training and competition, regarding thumb position and finger spreading. Although some differences in the results of different studies (Schleihauf, 1979; Takagi et al., 2001; Marinho et al., 2009), main results seemed to indicate that when the thumb leads the motion (sweep back angle of 0°) a hand position with the thumb abducted would be preferable to an adducted thumb position. Additionally, Marinho et al. (2009) found, for a sweep back angle of 0°, that the position with the thumb abducted presented higher values than the positions with the thumb partially abducted and adducted at angles of attack of 0° and 45°. At an angle of attack of 90°, the position with the thumb adducted presented the highest value of resultant force.

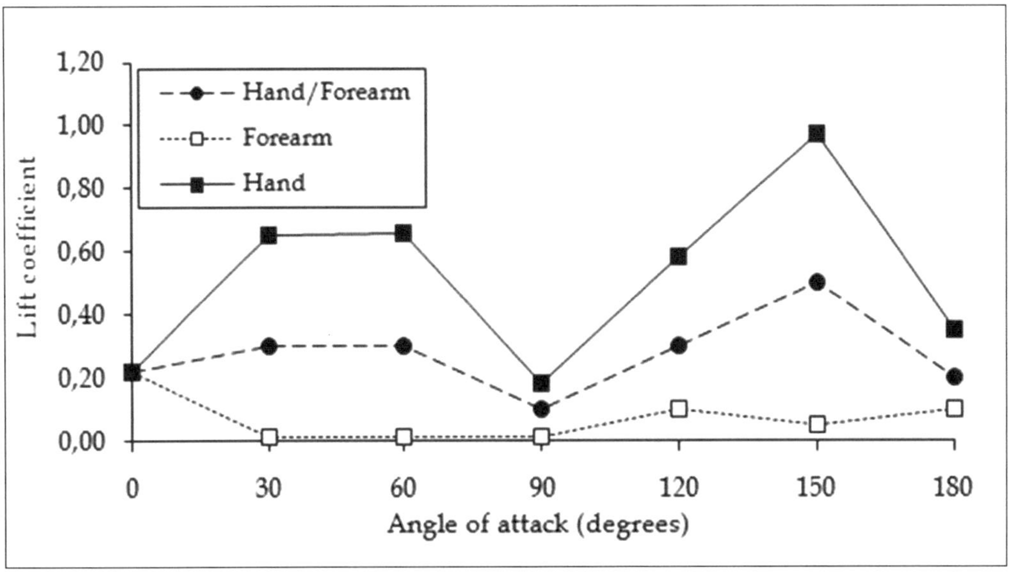

Fig. 5. Lift coefficient *vs.* angle of attack for the digital model of the hand, forearm and hand/forearm (Sweep back angle = 0°). Adapted from Bixler and Riewald (2002).

When considering different finger spreading, Marinho et al. (2010a), using a numerical analysis, studied the hand with: (i) fingers close together, (ii) fingers with little distance spread (a mean intra finger distance of 0.32 cm, tip to tip), and (iii) fingers with large distance spread (0.64 cm, tip to tip), following the same procedure of Schleihauf (1979) research. Marinho et al. (2010a) found that for attack angles higher than 30°, the model with little distance between fingers presented higher values of drag coefficient when compared with the models with fingers closed and with large finger spread. For attack angles of 0°, 15° and 30°, the values of drag coefficient were very similar in the three models of the swimmer's hand. Moreover, the lift coefficient seemed to be independent of the finger spreading, presenting little differences between the three models. Nevertheless, Marinho et al. (2010a) were able to note slightly lower values of lift coefficient for the position with larger distance between fingers. These results suggested that swimmers to create more propulsive force could use fingers slightly spread.

However, these studies were conducted only under steady state flow conditions and as mentioned above one knows (Schleihauf et al., 1988) that swimmers do not move their arms/hands under constant velocity and direction motions. Therefore, some authors (e.g., Sanders, 1999; Bixler & Riewald, 2002; Sato & Hino, 2003; Rouboa et al., 2006) referred that it is important to consider unsteady effects when swimming propulsion is analysed. For instance, Sato and Hino (2003) using also numerical and experimental data showed that the hydrodynamic forces acting on the accelerating hand was much higher than with a steady flow situation and these forces amplifies as acceleration increases.

3.2 Drag force

Regarding the hydrodynamic drag, this force can be defined as an external force that acts in the swimmer's body parallel but in the opposite direction of his movement direction. This resistive force is depending on the anthropometric characteristics of the swimmer, on the characteristics of the equipment used by the swimmers, on the physical characteristics of the water field, and on the swimming technique.

The hydrodynamic drag resisting forward motion (*D*) can be expressed by Newton's equation:

$$D = \tfrac{1}{2}\, C_D\, \rho\, S\, v^2 \qquad (1)$$

Where ρ represents the fluid density, C_D represents the drag coefficient, S represents the projection surface of the swimmer and v represents the swimming velocity.

The evaluation of the intensity of the hydrodynamic drag during swimming represents an important aim in swimming biomechanics. Drag determined by towing a non-swimming subject through the water (passive drag) has been studied for a long time (Karpovich, 1933). However, passive drag analysis does not consider the drag that the swimmer creates when he produces thrust to overcome the drag, i.e., during actual swimming (active drag). Thus, one of the most important parameters in the swimming hydrodynamics scope is to determine the drag of a body that is actively swimming. This assumption resulted in attempts to determine the drag of a person who is actively swimming. Indeed, passive drag is lower than active drag for the same subject (Kjendlie & Stallman, 2008).

Aiming to achieve this goal, techniques to assess active drag were developed by several research groups in the 70s, based on interpolation techniques (e.g., Clarys & Jiskoot, 1975; di Prampero et al., 1974). These methods involved indirect calculations based upon changes in oxygen consumption, as additional loads were placed on the swimmer (Marinho et al., 2010b). Later on, Hollander et al. (1986) developed the MAD-system (measurement of active drag), relying on the direct measurement of the push-off forces while swimming the Front Crawl stroke only with arms. In the 90s, Kolmogorov and Duplishcheva (1992) designed another method to determine the active drag: the velocity perturbation method, also known as the method of small perturbations. In this approach, subjects swim a lap twice at maximal effort: (i) free swimming; and (ii) swimming while towing a hydrodynamic body that creates a known additional drag. For both trials, the average velocity is calculated. Under the assumption that in both swims the power output to overcome drag is maximal and constant, drag force can be determined considering the difference in swimming velocity. In contrast to the interpolation techniques and the MAD-system, that required heavy and costly experimental procedures, the velocity perturbation method just required the use of the hydrodynamic body device and a chronometer to assess active drag. Additionally, this approach can be applied to measure active drag in the four competitive strokes. Other methods can only be applied to the Front Crawl (e.g., the MAD-system, Hollander et al., 1986) and the swimmer presents some segmental constrains, since legs are not taken into account, as they are hold by a pull buoy. Using this approach several studies has been conducted to evaluate active drag in swimming (e.g., Kjendlie & Stallman, 2008; Marinho et al., 2010b). Kjendlie and Stallman (2008) found that active drag in adults was significantly higher than in children. This difference between adults and children was mostly due to the different size and velocity during swimming. Marinho et al. (2010b) also studied active drag comparing boys and girls, reporting that there were no differences between boys and girls.

A possible explanation may be related to the similar values of body mass and height in boys and girls found in this study. However, girls tended to have lower drag values than boys, which can be also related to the lower velocities achieved by the first ones.
The total drag consists of the frictional, form and wave drag components. Frictional drag is depending on water viscosity and generates shear stress in the boundary layer. The intensity of this component is mainly due to the wetted surface area of the body, the characteristics of this surface and the flow conditions inside the boundary layer. Form drag is the result of a pressure differential between the front and the rear of the swimmer, depending on the velocity, the density of water and the cross sectional area of the swimmer. Near the water surface, due to the interface between two fluids of different densities, the swimmer is constrained by the formation of surface waves leading to wave drag (Toussaint & Truijens, 2005).
The contribution of form, friction and wave drag components to total drag during swimming is an interesting topic in sports biomechanics. Data available from several experimental studies show some difficulties involved in the evaluation of the contribution of each drag component (Bixler et al., 2007). It is mostly accepted that frictional drag is the smallest component of total drag, especially at higher swimming velocities, although this drag component should not be disregarded in elite level swimmers. Bixler et al. (2007) using numerical simulation techniques found that friction drag represented about 25% of total drag when the swimmer is gliding underwater. Zaidi et al. (2008) also found an important contribution of friction drag to the total drag when the swimmer is passively gliding underwater. These authors found that friction drag represented about 20% of the total drag. In this sense, issues such as sports equipments, shaving and the decrease of immersed body surface should be considered with detail, since this drag component seems to influence performance especially during the underwater gliding after starts and turns. In addition, form and wave drag represent the major part of total hydrodynamic drag, thus swimmers must emphasize the most hydrodynamic postures during swimming (Toussaint, 2006; Marinho et al., 2009). Although wave drag represents a huge part of total drag during swimming (Kjendlie & Stallman, 2008); when gliding underwater there is a tremendous reduction of this drag component. For instance, Lyttle et al. (1999) concluded that there is no significant wave drag when a typical adult swimmer is at least 0.6 m under the water's surface. Moreover, Vennell et al. (2006) found that a swimmer to avoid wave effects must be deeper than 1.8 and 2.8 chest depths below the surface for velocities of 0.9 m s^{-1} and 2.0 m s^{-1}, respectively.

4. Competitive swimming strokes neuromuscular response

Since the early sixties some research was done regarding the swimming neuromuscular activity (Ikai et al., 1964). However, for a long time such research was merely qualitative, with a reduce focus quantifying this phenomena. For instance, Ikai et al (1964) qualitatively showed that the bicep braquialis, the triceps braquialis, the deltoid and grand dorsal were highly activate during the strokes. On the other hand, for a quantitative perspective, the authors verified that the elbow extensors presented a higher activation than the elbow flexors at Front Crawl, Breaststroke and Butterfly stroke. Indeed this electromyographic (EMG) assessment from Ikai et al. (1964) was thereafter the basis for the swimming stroke descriptions popularized in some swimming textbooks including the ones from Counsilman (1968) or Catteau and Garrof (1968). In the late sixties a research trend more focus in quantifying the EMG signal was started by Lewillie (1967; 1973) and followed by Clarys (1983; 1988). Comparing to kinematics and kinetics researches, neuromuscular assessments are the less used approach for competitive swimming.

4.1 Qualitative assessment

Qualitative EMG relies on judgment of wave form patterns from neuromuscular activity in graphical demonstration. Based on the visual interpretation of the gross EMG signal it is possible to describe the neuromuscular activation according to the temporal domain. In most circumstances, the bio-signal amplitude and the duration are used as variables for a temporal interpretation. The amplitude is roughly proportionally to the force exerted by the underlying muscle. This relationship can be easily appreciated by viewing the EMG signal in real-time while the intensity of the muscular contraction increases. However, the EMG signal is not an estimation of the muscle force produced. On the other hand, analyzing the duration of muscular activation it is possible to observe whether a muscle is active or inactive. Moreover, it is possible to establish timing patterns for dynamic movements and the co-activation of several opossite muscle groups.

For swimming researchers the main focus relies in understanding the dynamics of neuromuscular activity between strokes during the limbs and trunk actions.

Lewillie (1973) conducted a case study in the four strokes at three conditions (slow, normal, fast). The highest neuromuscular activation was observed for the Butterfly stroke at fast condition. Increasing intensity imposed an increase in the anterior rectum and triceps surae activation for all strokes. Nuber et al. (1986) observed high activation of the supraspinatus, infraspinatus, middle deltoid, and serratus anterior during the recovery phases of the Front Crawl, Breaststroke and Butterfly. On the other hand, the latissimus dorsi and pectoralis major were predominately pull-through phase muscles (Nuber et al., 1986). Latter, similar activation during Front Crawl was reported by Pink et al. (1991) for the pectoralis major and latissimus dorsi to propel the body and for the infraspinatus to externally rotate the arm at middle of the arm's recovery. Authors also observed high activation for the three heads of the deltoid and the supraspinatus during the arm's entry and exit.

A study in breaststrokes demonstrated consistently activation for the serratus anterior and teres minor muscles throughout the stroke cycle (Ruwe et al., 1994). Barthels and Adrian (1971) found a great activity for the rectus abdominus and for the spine erector, suggesting that the trunk movement in Butterfly stroke is associated to the lower limbs action. Concerning the upper lims propulsion, Pink et al (1993) reported that the serratus anterior and the subscapularis maintained a high level of activation, being highly susceptible to fatigue and vulnerable to injury.

4.2 Quantitative assessment

The quantitative EMG analyzes the subtle changes on wave form patterns that normally are missed or not appreciated by qualitative EMG. This approach combines graphical interpretation with numerical processing data to describe the neuromuscular activation. The amplitude and duration analysis are improved using several data analysis procedures. On a regular basis, researchers use some quantified variables, including the root mean square (RMS) and threshold models for that purpose in the time domain. The RMS is considered to be the most meaningful technique, since it gives a measure of the power of the signal. Threshold intervals are also helpful because they more clearly demarcate the beginning and

end of each muscle contraction. Both techniques require the use of automated algorithms that extract and analyze motor unit action potentials. The algorithms can simultaneously identify several different motor units' wave forms from the EMG signal to facilitate the acquisition of more data in less time (Stálber et al., 1996).
One other approach used in the quantitative EMG assessment is the spectral analysis. This approach allows to change the signal from temporal domain to frequency domain. Essentially it gives an evaluation of what contribution each frequency has to the original sign. To evaluate the different frequencies contents of maximal voluntary contraction the usual procedure is to use the Fourier transformation. However, new spectral indices (e.g. FInsmk) have been proposed and considered to be valid, reliable and more sensitive than those traditionally used for competitive swimming Dimitrov, 2006; Figueiredo et al., 2010).
Generally, the mean and median frequencies of the EMG signal decrease with time during a task that induces fatigue. The pratical aplication for spectral analysis in swimming is to study muscle fatigue and its relationship to limb's kinematics. Monteil et al. (1996) analyzing the fatigue at the beginning and at the end of a 400m Front Crawl bout in a flume found a data decrease during the insweep phase followed by an increase during the outsweep. Authors indicated a shift of the force production from the insweep to the outsweep and a decrease of hand velocity during the insweep phase. A similar phenomenon was observed by Aujouannet et al. (2006). EMG spectral parameters of the biceps brachii and triceps brachii demonstrated a shift toward lower frequency before and after a maximal 4*50m swimming test (Aujouannet et al., 2006). In a fatigue state, the spatial hand path remained unchanged, with a greater duration of the catch, the insweep and the outsweep phases (Aujouannet et al., 2006). A 4*100 Front Crawl test until exhaustion demonstrated larger muscular recruitments obtained during the insweep phase and the antagonist activities increases (Rouard et al., 1997). Caty et al. (2007) found an important stabilization of the wrist and high antagonist flexor and extensor carpi activity during the insweep phase (Caty et al., 2007). On the other hand, in outsweep phase, less stabilization and lower antagonist activities were noted (Caty et al., 2007). Fatigue analysis showed an increase in latissimos dorsi and triceps braquialis during 100m all out Front Crawl (Stirn et al., 2010). When increasing distance to 200m, the inability to maintain swimming velocity in the last laps was coincident with the increase of the fatigue indices for the flexor carpi radialis, biceps brachii, triceps brachii, pectoralis major, upper trapezius, rectus femoris and biceps femoris (Figueiredo et al., 2010).

5. Competitive swimming strokes biomechanics and performance

The main focus of swimming researchers is to enhance performance. From a historic perspective, a large part of the research dedicated to competitive swimming aims to identify variables that determine the performance. This can be considered as an exploratory research trend. Very recently, confirmatory data analysis became another topic of interest. In such research designs, researchers try to understand the relationships between the variables identified in previous researches and model the links among them and performance (Barbosa et al., 2010b).

5.1 Exploratory research

With exploratory research the aim is to identify from several biomechanical variables those that are associated or related to the swimming performance. This kind of research has been developed based on (Barbosa et al., 2010b): (i) comparing cohort groups; (ii) applying exploratory regression models and; (iii) implementing neural network procedures.

The comparison of cohort groups is done comparing mean values or analyzing the variation of some selected biomechanical variables between different competitive level sub-sample groups. For instance, compare expert versus non-expert swimmers, national level versus international/elite level swimmers or, world championships and Olympic Games finalists versus non-finalists. It is obvious that better competitive level is related to a higher swim velocity. On the other hand, higher swim velocity, from better swimmers, is achieved by an increasing stroke length than remain swimmers (Craig et al., 1985; Vilas-Boas, 1996; Leblanc et al., 2007; Seifert et al., 2007). Higher level swimmers also present a higher efficiency, which is expressed by a higher stroke index (Sánchez et al., 2002; Jesus et al., 2011). During high-standard competitions, world-ranked swimmers already maintain a high stroke length. Therefore their biomechanical strategy to increase the swim velocity is to increase as well the stroke rate (Jesus et al., 2011). At least one study attempted to compare the stroke cycle kinematics between World championships medalists versus remaining finalists. There were no significant differences in the stroke kinematics between medallists and non-medallists. As both cohort groups have a very small gap performance, differences between them might be explained by other variables (Jesus et al., 2011). There are also some limb's kinematics differences according to competitive level. The elite swimmers posses a great strength and power to accelerate through the water. They present a limb's kinematics making them able to apply it effectively. Plus, the same limb's kinematics also aims to maintain a better body streamlining position to reduce drag force (Cappaert et al., 1996). For instance, comparing elite versus non-elite swimmers, participating in world championships and Olympic Games (Cappaert et al., 1996;): (i) the trunk angle is lower and there is a higher elbow extension during the finish phase of the pulling pattern for elite than for non-elite swimmers swimming Butterfly stroke; (ii) there is a higher body roll and a higher emphasis in the kicking for elite backstrokes than non-elite ones; (iii) in Breaststroke, timing between arm's and leg's actions is a key factor as non-elite swimmers sometimes achieve a null body velocity within a stroke cycle; (iv) a higher elbow position is required to achieve higher propulsion and a higher body roll in Front Crawl, as done by elite swimmers in comparison to non-elite. Few studies suggest that better competitive level swimmers also present a lower intra-cyclic variation of the body's swimming velocity (Manley and Atha, 1996; Takagi et al., 2004). This seems consistent in Breaststroke but less obvious in remaining swim strokes and should be clear out in near future.

Another possibility is to develop statistical models to identify the best biomechanical predictors of swimming performance. Stroke length was related to swimming economy (Costill et al., 1985) and this one to swimming performance. One attempted was made to determine the stroke cycle variables that are related to Olympic swimmers performance. However, stroke rate, stroke length and stroke index did not correlated significantly with the performance (Arellano et al., 2001). As reported in the previous paragraph, the arguably best swimmers in the world make it difficult to see trends in these variables on the basis of stroke variations. Some papers report the prediction of children swimming performance. The stroke index for the boys (Saavedra et al., 2003; 2010; Vitor & Bohem, 2010) and the mean velocity of a 50-m maximal bout for girls were included in the final models (Saavedra et al., 2003). In both genders, from 9 to 22 years-old, for the 50-m freestyle event, increases in the swim velocity happen due to increases in the stroke length and stroke index (Morales et al., 2010).

Neural network is a somewhat recent approach to solve complex problems to model a given phenomena (Fig. 6). Few attempts were made to apply this data analysis procedure to model swimming performance (Pffier & Hohmann, in press). Modeling the 400-m freestyle performance in young male swimmers, based on several variables including kinetic and kinematical ones, the estimation error was 7±7.8% and for the 200-m medley performance 1.7±13.3% (Silva et al., 2007). Same trend was reported in another couple of papers that included Front crawl and Backstroke techniques, gliding in supine and back positions to predict the 50-m Backstroke (Lobenius, 2003) and the stroke rate, swim velocity to predict the 50-m freestyle event (Hohman & Seidel, 2010).

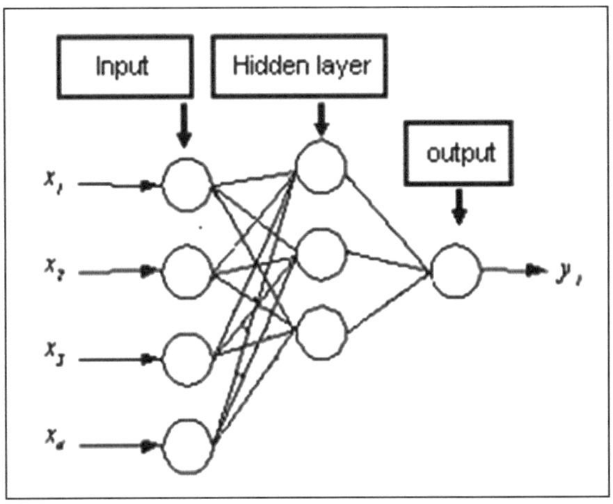

Fig. 6. Example of a performance modeling accomplished by a feed forward neural network with three neurons in a single hidden layer.

5.2 Confirmatory research

This procedure consists of a mathematical approach for testing and estimating causal relationships using a combination of statistical data and qualitative causal assumptions previously defined by the researcher to be (or not to be) confirmed. This approach rather than to identify variables, suggests the kind of interplay existing among them (Barbosa et al., 2010d). Hence, structural equating modeling allows analyzing the hypothetical relationships between several biomechanical variables with swim performance and the model's good-of-fit. Indeed this approach is often used on other scientific domains although it is not so popular in the sport's performance, including competitive swimming. To the best of our knowledge this procedure only was applied for young swimmers.

One paper reported the development of a path-flow analysis model for young male swimmers' performance based on biomechanical and energetics variables (Fig. 7). The model included variables such as the stroke length, stroke rate, stroke index, and swim velocity. The confirmatory model explained 79% of the 200-m freestyle performance and being suitable of the theory presented (Barbosa et al., 2010d). One other study developed a structural equation modeling for active drag force based on anthropometric, hydrodynamic (i.e., frontal surface area, drag coefficient) and biomechanical variables (i.e., stroke length, stroke rate and swim velocity) in young boys (Barbosa et al., 2010e). The confirmatory model explained 95% of the active drag after the elimination of the frontal surface area.

Main limitation of the model is related to the frontal surface area estimation equation that does not fit in the model. The confirmatory model included all selected anthropometrical variables, prone gliding test, stroke length, stroke frequency and velocity. Final model excluded the vertical buoyancy test. The confirmatory path-flow model good-of-fit was considered as being very close to the cut-off value, but even so not suitable of the theory. Vertical buoyancy and prone gliding tests are easy and cheap procedures to assess swimmer's kinetics. However, both procedures are not the best techniques to assess the swimmer's hydrostatic and hydrodynamic profile, respectively. Hohmann and Seidel (2010) predicted 41% of girl's 50-m freestyle performance based on psychological, technique (i.e., stroke rate, swim velocity, limb's coordination), physical conditioning and anthropometrical variables.

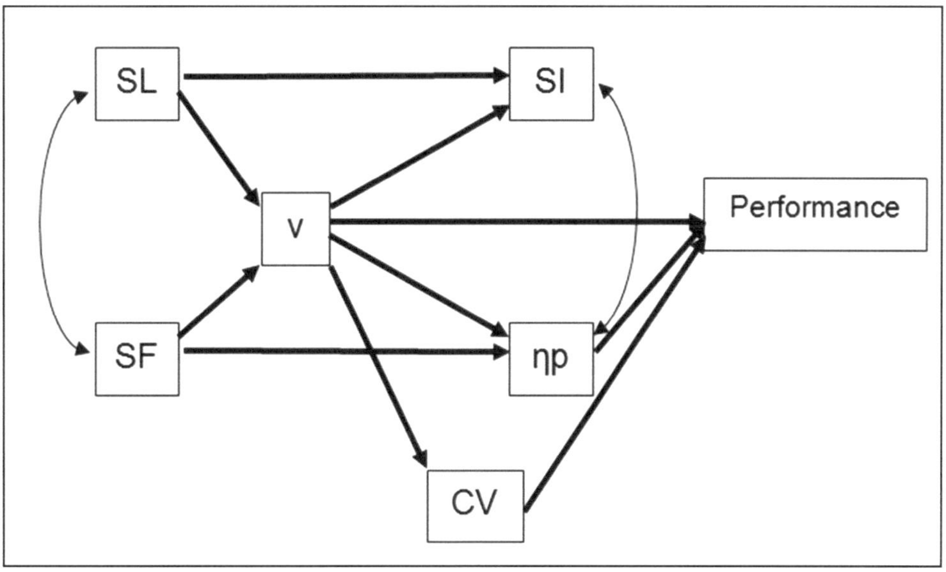

Fig. 7. The final confirmatory model about the relationship between biomechanics, energetics and swimming performance. The model includes the stroke length (SL), stroke frequency (SF), swimming velocity (v), stroke index (SI), propulsive efficiency (ηp), critical velocity (CV) and performance.

6. Conclusion

There are several biomechanical variables determining the competitive swimmer's performance. For instance, some of those are kinematics variables (e.g., stroke length, stroke frequency, speed fluctuation, limbs' kinematics), kinetics variables (e.g., propulsive drag, lift force, drag force) and neuromuscular variables.

Attempts are being made nowadays to understand the links between all these variables and how it is possible to enhance performance manipulating it. Some models about these relationships are already at the disposal of practitioners. Moreover, a great effort is done by researchers and coaches to assess, to compare and to manipulate these variables from times to times to define goals, establish milestones in the periodization program or even predict the swimmers performance.

7. References

Alves, F.; Cunha, P. & Gomes-Pereira, J. (1999). Kinematic changes with inspiratory actions in butterfly swimming, In: *Biomechanics and Medicine in Swimming VIII,* K.L. Keskinen, P.V. Komi & P.A. Hollander, (Eds.), 9-14, Gummerus Printing, Jyvaskyla

Aujouannet, Y.A.; Bonifazi, M.; Hintzy, F.; Vuillerme, N. & Rouard, A.H. (2006). Effects of a high-intensity swim test on kinematic parameters in high-level athletes. *Applied Physiology Nutrition and Metabolism*, 3, 150-158

Barbosa, T.M.; Sousa, F. & Vilas-Boas, J.P. (1999). Kinematical modifications induced by the introduction of the lateral inspiration in butterfly stroke, In: *Biomechanics and Medicine in Swimming VIII,* K.L. Keskinen, P.V. Komi & P.A. Hollander, (Eds.), 15-19, Gummerus Printing, Jyvaskyla

Barbosa, T.M.; Santos Silva, J.; Sousa, F. & Vilas-Boas, J.P. (2003). Comparative study of the response of kinematical variables from the hip and the center of mass in butterfliers, In: *Biomechanics and Medicine in Swimming IX*, J.C. Chatard, (Ed.), 93-98, University of Saint-Etienne, Saint-Etienne

Barbosa, T.; Keskinen, K.L.; Fernandes, R.J.; Colaço, P.; Lima, A.B. & Vilas-Boas, J.P. (2005). Energy cost and intracyclic variation of the velocity of the centre of mass in butterfly stroke. *European Journal of Applied Physiology*, 93, pp. 519-523

Barbosa, T.M.; Lima, F.; Portela, A.; Novais, D.; Machado, L.; Colaço, P.; Gonçalves, P.; Fernandes, R.J. & Vilas-Boas, J.P. (2006). Relationships between energy cost, swimming velocity and speed fluctuation in competitive swimming strokes, In: *Biomechanics and Medicine in Swimming X*, J.P. Vilas-Boas, F. Alves & A. Marques (Eds.), 192-194, Portuguese Journal of Sport Science, Porto

Barbosa, T.M.; Fernandes, R.J.; Morouço, P. & Vilas-Boas, J.P. (2008). Predicting the intra-cyclic variation of the velocity of the centre of mass from segmental velocities in butterfly stroke: a pilot study. *Journal of Sports Science & Medicine*, 7, pp. 201-209

Barbosa, T.M.; Pinto, E.; Cruz, A.M.; Marinho, D.A.; Silva, A.J.; Reis, V.M.; Costa, M.J. & Queirós, T.M. (2010a). The Evolution of Swimming Science Research: Content analysis of the "Biomechanics and Medicine in Swimming" Proceedings Books from 1971 to 2006, In: *Biomechanics and Medicine in Swimming XI,* P.L., Kjendlie, R.K. Stallman & J. Cabri (Eds.), 312-314, Norwegian School of Sport Sciences, Oslo

Barbosa, T.M.; Bragada, J.A.; Reis, V.M.; Marinho, D.A.; Carvalho, C. & Silva, J.A. (2010b). Energetics and biomechanics as determining factors of swimming performance: updating the state of the art. *Journal of Science and Medicine in Sports*, 13, pp. 262-269

Barbosa, T.M.; Silva, A.J.; Reis, A.M.; Costa, M.J.; Garrido, N.; Policarpo, F. & Reis, V.M. (2010c). Kinematical changes in swimming front crawl and breaststroke with the AquaTrainer (R) snorkel. *European Journal of Applied Physiology*, 109, pp. 1155-1162

Barbosa, T.M.; Costa, M.J.; Coelho, J.; Moreira, M. & Silva, A.J. (2010d). Modeling the links between young swimmer's performance: energetic and biomechanics profile. *Pediatric Exercise Science*, 22, pp. 379-391

Barbosa, T.M.; Costa, M.J.; Marques, M.C.; Silva, A.J. & Marinho, D.A. (2010e). A model for active drag force exogenous variables in young swimmers. *Journal of Human Sports & Exercise*, 5, pp. 379-388

Barthels, K.M. & Adrina, M.J. (1971). Variability in the dolphin kick under four conditions. In: *First International Symposium on "Biomechanics in Swimming, Waterpolo and Diving,*

L. Lewillie & J.P. Clarys, (Eds.), 105-118. Université Libre de Bruxelles, Laboratoire de L'effort. Bruxelles.

Berger, M.A.M.; de Groot, G. & Hollander, P. (1995). Hydrodynamic drag and lift forces on human hand/arm models. *Journal of Biomechanics,* 28, pp. 125-133

Bixler, B.S. & Riewald, S. (2002). Analysis of swimmer's hand and arm in steady flow conditions using computational fluid dynamics. *Journal of Biomechanics,* 35, pp. 713–717.

Bixler, B.; Pease, D. & Fairhurst, F. (2007). The accuracy of computational fluid dynamics analysis of the passive drag of a male swimmer. *Sports Biomechanics,* 6, pp. 81–98

Capitão F, Lima AB, Gonçalves P, Morouço P, Silva M, Fernandes R, Vilas-Boas JP. 2006. Videogrametrically and acelorimetrically assessment intra-cyclic variations of the velocity in breaststroke, In: *Biomechanics and Medicine in Swimming X,* J.P. Vilas-Boas JP, F. Alves F & A. Marques (Eds.), 212-214, Portuguese Journal of Sport Science, Porto

Catteau, R. & Garoff, G. (1968). *L'enseignement de la natation,* Edition vigot, Paris

Cappaert, J.; Pease, D. & Troup, J. (1996). Biomechanical highlights of world champion and Olympic swimmers. In: *Biomechanics and Medicine in Swimming VII,* J. Troup, A. Hollander, D. Strasse, S. Trappe, J. Cappaert & T. Trappe (Eds.), 76-80, E & FN SPON, London

Caty, V.; Aujouannet, Y.A.; Hintzy, F.; Bonifazi, M.; Clarys, J.P. & Rouard, A.H. (2007). Wrist stabilisation and forearm muscle coactivation during freestyle swimming. *Journal of Electromyography and Kinesiology,* 17, 285-291

Chengalur, S. & Brown, P. (1992). An analysis of male and female Olympic swimmers in the 200m events. *Canadian Journal of Sport Science,* 17, pp. 104-109

Chollet, D.; Pelayo, P.; Tourney, C. & Sidney, M. (1996). Comparative analysis of 100 m and 200 m events in the four strokes in top level swimmers. *Journal of Hum Movement Studies,* 31, pp. 25-37

Chollet, D.; Tourny-Chollet, C. & Gleizes, F. (1999). Evolution of co-ordination in fl at breaststroke in relation to velocity, In: *Biomechanics and Medicine in Swimming VIII,* K.L. Keskinen, P.V. Komi & P.A. Hollander, (Eds.), 29-32, Gummerus Printing, Jyvaskyla

Clarys, J.P. & Jiskoot, J. (1975). Total resistance of selected body positions in the front crawl, In: *Swimming II.* J.P. Clarys & L. Lewillie, (Eds.), 110-117, University Park Press, Baltimore

Clarys, J.P. (1983). A review of EMG in Swimming: explanation of facts and/or feedback information. In: *Biomechanics and Medicine in Swimming,* A.P. Hollander, P.A. Huijing & G. de Groot (Eds.), 123-135. Human Kinetics Publishers, Illinois

Clarys, J.P. (1988). The Brussels Swimming EMG project. In: *Swimming Science V,* B. Ungerechts, K. Wilke & K. Reischle (Eds.), 157-172, Human Kinetics Books, Illinois

Costill, D.; Kovaleski, J.; Porter, D.; Fielding, R. & King, D. (1985). Energy expenditure during front crawl swimming: predicting success in middle-distance events. *International Journal of Sports Medicine,* 6, pp. 266-270

Counsilman, J. (1968). *The Science of Swimming.* Prentice Hall. Englewood Cliffs, New york.

Craig, A. & Pendergast, D. (1979). Relationships of stroke rate, distance per stroke and velocity in competitive swimming. *Medicine and Science Sports Exercise,* 11, pp. 278-283

Craig, A.; Skehan, P.; Pawelczyk, J. & Boomer W. (1985). Velocity, stroke rate and distance per stroke during elite swimming competition. *Medicine and Science Sports Exercise,* 17, pp. 625-634

Deschodt V, Rouard A, Monteil K (1996). Relationship between the three coordinates of the upper limb joints with swimming velocity. In: Troup JP, Hollander AP, Strasse D, Trappe SW, Cappaert JM, Trappe TA (Eds). *Biomechanics and Medicine in Swimming VII.* London: E & FN Spon, 52-58.

Deschodt, V. (1999). Relative contribution of arms and legs in human to propulsion in 25 m sprint front crawl swimming. *European Journal of Applied Physiology,* 80, pp. 192-199

Dimitrov, G.V.; Arabadzhiev, T.I.; Mileva, K.N.; Bowtell, J.L.; Crichton, N. & Dimitrova, N.A. (2006). Muscle fatigue during dynamic contractions assessed by new spectral indices. *Medicine Science and Sports Exercise,* 38, 1971-1979

Di Prampero, P.E.; Pendergast, D.R.; Wilson, D.W. & Rennie, D.W. (1974). Energetics of swimming in man. *Journal of Applied Physiology* 37, pp. 1-5

Figueiredo, P.; Sousa, A.; Goncalves, P.; Pereira, S.M.; Soares, S.; Vilas-Boas, J.P. & Fernandes, R.J. (2010). Biophysical Analysis of the 200m Front Crawl Swimming: a Case Study. In: *Biomechanics and Medicine in Swimming XI,* P.L., Kjendlie, R.K. Stallman & J. Cabri (Eds.), 79-81, Norwegian School of Sport Sciences, Oslo

Hay, J. & Guimarães, A. (1983). A quantitative look at swimming biomechanics. *Swimming Technique,* 20, pp. 11-17

Hohmann, A. & Seidel, I. (2010). Talent Prognosis in Young Swimmers, In: *Biomechanics and Medicine in Swimming XI,* P.L., Kjendlie, R.K. Stallman RK & J. Cabri (Eds.), 262-264, Norwegian School of Sport Sciences, Oslo

Hollander, A.P. ; de Groot, G. ; Van Ingen Schenau, G.L. ; Toussaint, H.M. ; de Best, H. & Peeters, W. (1986). Measurement of active drag during crawl arm stroke swimming. *Journal of Sports Sciences,* 4, pp. 21-30

Hollander, A.P., de Groot, G., van Ingen Schenau, G., Kahman, R. & Toussaint, H. (1988) Contribution of thr legs to propulsion in Front Crawl swimming. In: *Swimming Science V,* B. Ungerechts, K. Wilke & K. Reischle, (Eds.), 39-43, Human Kinetics Books, Illinois

Ikai, M.; Ishii, K. & Miyashita, M. (1964). An electromyographic study of Swimming. *Journal of Physical Education,* 7, pp. 47-54

Ito, S. (2008). Analysis of the optimal arm stroke in the backstroke. In: *The Book of Proceedings of the 1st International Scientific Conference of Aquatic Space Activities,* T. Nomura & B.E. Ungerechts, (Eds.), 362-367, University of Tskuba, Tskuba

Jesus, S.; Costa, M.J.; Marinho, D.A.; Garrido, N.D.; Silva, A.J. & Barbosa, T.M. (20010). 13th FINA World Championship finals: stroke kinematics and race times according to performance, gender and event, In: *Proceedings of the International Symposium in Biomechanics of Sports,* J.P. Vilas-Boas, & A. Veloso, (Eds.), Portuguese Journal of Sport Science, Porto

Lyttle, A.D.; Blanksby, B.A.; Elliott, B.C. & Lloyd, D.G. (1999). Optimal depth for streamlined gliding, In: *Biomechanics and Medicine in Swimming VIII,* K.L. Keskinen, P.V. Komi & P.A. Hollander, (Eds.), 165-170, Gummerus Printing, Jyvaskyla

Kamata E, Miwa T, Matsuuchi K, Shintami H, Nomura T. Analysis of sculling propulsion mechanism using two-components particle image velocimetry. In: Vilas-Boas JP,

Alves F, Marques A, editors. *Biomechanics and Medicine in Swimming X*. Porto: Portuguese Journal of Sports Sciences; 2006. Supl 2: 50-52

Karpovich, P. (1933). Water resistance in swimming. *Research Quarterly*, 4, pp. 21-28

Keskinen, K.L. & Komi, P.V. (1988). The stroking characteristics in four different exercises in freestyle swimming. In: *Biomechanics XI-B,* G. de Groot, P.A. Hollander , P. Huijing & G. van Ingen Schenau, (Eds.), 839-843, Free University Press, Amsterdam

Kjendlie, P.L.; Haljand, R.; Fjortoft, O. & Stallman RK. (2006). Stroke frequency strategies of international and national swimmers in 100-m races In: *Biomechanics and Medicine in Swimming X,* J.P. Vilas-Boas JP, F. Alves F & A. Marques (Eds.), 52-54, Portuguese Journal of Sport Science, Porto

Kjendlie, P.L. & Stallman, R. (2008). Drag characteristics of competitive swimming children and Adults. *Journal of Applied Biomechanics* 24, pp. 35-42

Kolmogorov, S. & Duplischeva, O. (1992). Active drag, useful mechanical power output and hydrodynamic force coeffi cient in different swimming strokes at maximal velocity. *Journal of Biomechanics,* 25, pp. 311–318

Leblanc H, Seifert L, Tourny-Chollet C, Chollet D. Intra-cyclic distance per stroke phase, velocity fluctuation and acceleration time ratio of a breaststroker's hip: a comparison between elite and non elite swimmers at different race paces. *Int J Sports Med* 2007; 28:140-147

Letzelter, H. & Freitag, W. Stroke length and stroke frequency variations in men's and women's 100m freestyle swimming. In: Hollander AP, Huijing PA, de Groot G, editors. *Biomechanics and Medicine in Swimming*. Illinois: Human Kinetics Publishers; 1983. p.315-322

Lewillie, L. (1967). Analyse télemétrique de l'electromyogramme du nageur. *Societé Médicine Belge Education Physique Sport*, 20, pp. 174-177

Lewillie, L. (1973). Muscular activity in swimming. In: *Biomechanics III*, 440-445, Karger, Basel.

Lewillie, L. (1983). Research in swimming: historical and scientific aspects, In: *Biomechanics and Medicine in Swimming,* A. Hollander, P. Huijing & G. de Groot, (Eds.), 7-16, Human Kinetics Publishers, Illinois

Lobenius, K. (2003). The employment of regression analysis and neural networks in the prognosis of competitive swimming performance, In: *Biomechanics and Medicine in Swimming IX*, J.C. Chatard, (Ed.), 545-550, University of Saint-Etienne, Saint-Etienne

Maglischo, E. (2003). *Swimming fastest.* Human Kinetics Champaign, Illinois

Manley, P. & Atha J. (1992). Intra-stroke velocity fluctuations in paces breaststroke swimming, In: *Biomechanics and Medicine in Swimming VI, D.* MacLaren, T. Reilly & A. Lees, (Eds.), 151-160, E & FN Spon, London

Marinho, D.A.; Reis, V.M.; Alves, F.B.; Vila-Boas, J.P.; Machado, L.; Rouboa, A.I. & Silva, A.J. (2008). The analysis of swimming propulsion under unsteady flow conditions. *Journal of Sports Science,* 26(S1), pp. 10

Marinho, D.A.; Rouboa, A.I.; Alves, F.B.; Vilas-Boas, J.P.; Machado, L.; Reis, V.M., & Silva, A.J. (2009). Hydrodynamic analysis of different thumb positions in swimming. *Journal of Sports Science and Medicine,* 8, pp. 58-66

Marinho, D.A.; Barbosa, T.M.; Reis, V.M.; Kjendlie, P.L.; Alves, F.B.; Vilas-Boas, J.P.; Machado, L.; Rouboa, A.I. & Silva, A.J. (2010a). Swimming propulsion forces are enhanced by a small finger spread. *Journal of Applied Biomechanics,* 26, pp. 87-92

Marinho, D.A.; Barbosa, T.M.; Costa, M.J.; Figueiredo, C.; Reis, V.M.; Silva, A.J. & Marques, M.C. (2010b). Can 8-weeks of training affect active drag in age-group swimmers? *Journal of Sport Science and Medicine*, 9, pp. 71-78

Monteil, K.M.; Rouard, A.H.; Dufour, A.B.; Cappaert, J.M. & Troup, J.P. (1996). Swimmers'shoulder: EMG of the rotators during a flume test. In: *Biomechanics and Medicine in Swimming VII*, J. Troup, A. Hollander, D. Strasse, S. Trappe, J. Cappaert & T. Trappe (Eds.), 83-89, E & FN SPON, London

Morales, E.; Arellano, R.; Famia, P. & Mercades J. (2010). Regression Analysis Model Applied to Age-Group Swimmers: Study of Stroke Rate, Stroke Length and Stroke Index, In: *Biomechanics and Medicine in Swimming XI,* P.L., Kjendlie, R.K. Stallman RK & J. Cabri (Eds.), 129-132, Norwegian School of Sport Sciences, Oslo

Nuber, G.W.; Jobe, F.W.; Perry, J.; Moynes, D.R. & Antonelli D. (1986). Fine wire electromyography analysis of muscles of the shoulder during swimming. *American journal of Sports Medicine*,14, 7-11

Rouboa, A.I.; Silva, A.J.; Leal, L.; Rocha, J. & Alves, F. (2006). The effect of swimmer's hand/forearm acceleration on propulsive forces generation using computational fluid dynamics. *Journal of Biomechanics, 39*, pp. 1239-1248

Payton, C., & Bartlett, R. (1995). Estimating propulsive forces in swimming from three-dimensional kinematic data. *Journal of Sports Sciences, 13*, pp. 447-454

Pendergast, D.R.; Capelli, C.; Craig, A.B.; di Prampero, P.E.; Minetti, A.E.; Mollendorf, J.; Termin, .I.I. & Zamparo, P. (2006). Biophysics in swimming, In: *Biomechanics and Medicine in Swimming X*, J.P. Vilas-Boas, F. Alves & A. Marques (Eds.), 185-189, Portuguese Journal of Sport Science, Porto

Persyn, U.; Colman, V. & van Tilborg, L. (1992). Movement analysis of flat and undulating breaststroke patterns, In: *Biomechanics and Medicine in Swimming VI, D.* MacLaren, T. Reilly & A. Lees, (Eds.), 75-80, E & FN Spon, London

Pfeiffer, M. & Hohmann A. (2011). Applications of neural networks in training science. *Human Movement Science*, Epub ahead of print

Pink, M.; Perry, J.; Browne, A.; Scovazzo, M.L. & Kerrigan, J. (1991). The normal shoulder during freestyle swimming. An electromyographic and cinematographic analysis of twelve muscles. *American journal of Sports Medicine,* 19, 569-576

Psycharakis, S.G. & Sanders, R.H. (2009) Validity of the use of a fixed point for intracycle velocity calculations in swimming. *Journal of Science and Medicine in Sport*, 12, pp. 262–526

Psycharakis, S.G. & Sanders, R.H. (2010). Body roll in swimming: a review. *Journal of Sports Science*, 28, pp. 229-236

Rouard, A.H.; Billat, R.P.; Deschodt, V. & Clarys, J.P. (1997). Muscular activations during repetitions of sculling movements up to exhaustion in swimming. *Archives of Physiology and Biochemistry*, 105, 655-662

Ruwe, P.A.; Pink, M.; Jobe, F.W.; Perry, J. & Scovazzo, M.L. (1994). The normal and the painful shoulders during the breaststroke. Electromyographic and cinematographic analysis of twelve muscles. *American journal of Sports Medicine,* 22, 789-796

Sánchez, J. & Arellano, R. (2002). Stroke index values according to level, gender, swimming style and event race distance, In: *Proceedings of the XXth International Symposium on Biomechanics in Sports,* K. Gianikellis, (Ed.), 56-59, Universidad de Extremadura, Cáceres

Sanders, R.; Cappaert, J. & Pease, D. (1998). Wave characteristics of Olympic breaststroke swimmers. *Journal of Applied Biomechanics*, 14, pp. 40-51

Saavedra, J.; Escalante, Y. & Rodriguez, F. (2003). Multidimensional evaluation of peripubertal swimmers: multiple regression analysis applied to talent selection, In: *Biomechanics and Medicine in Swimming IX*, J.C. Chatard, (Ed.), 551-556, University of Saint-Etienne, Saint-Etienne

Saavedra, J.M.; Escalante, Y. & Rodríguez, F.A. (2010). A multivariate analysis of performance in young swimmers. *Pediatric Exercise Science*, 22, pp. 135-151

Sanders, R.H. (1999). Hydrodynamic characteristics of a swimmer's hand. *Journal of Applied Biomechanics, 15*, pp. 3-26

Sato, Y. & Hino, T. (2003). Estimation of thrust of swimmer's hand using CFD, In: *Proceedings of second international symposium on aqua bio-mechanisms*, 81-86, Honolulu

Schleihauf, R.E. (1979). A hydrodynamic analysis of swimming propulsion, In: *Swimming III*, J. Terauds & E.W. Bedingfield, (Eds.), 70-109, University Park Press, Baltimore

Seifert, L. ; Chollet, D. & Chatard, J.C. (2007). Kinematic change during a 100-m Front Crawl: effects of performance level and gender. *Medicine Science Sports Exercise*, 39, pp. 1784-1793

Seifert, L. & Chollet, D. (2008). Inter-limb coordination and constraints in swimming: a review. In: *Physical Activity and Children*, N.P. Beaulieu, (Ed.), 65-93, Nova Science Publishers, New York

Silva, A.J.; Colman, V.; Soons, B.; Alves, F. & Persyn, U. (2002). Movement variables important for effectiveness and performance in breaststroke, In: *Proceedings of the XXth International Symposium on Biomechanics in Sports*, K. Gianikellis, (Ed.), 39-42, Universidad de Extremadura, Cáceres

Silva, A.J.; Costa, A.M.; Oliveira, P.M.; Reis, V.M.; Saavedra, J.; Perl, J.; Rouboa, A.I. & Marinho, D.A. (2007). The use of neural network technology to model swimming performance. *Journal of Sports Science & Medicine*, 6, pp. 117-125

Silva, A.J.; Marinho, D.A.; Reis, V.M.; Alves, F.B.; Vilas-Boas, J.P.; Machado, L. & Rouboa, A.I. (2008). Study of the propulsive potential of the hand and forearm in swimming. *Medicine Science and Sport Exercise*, 40, pp. S212

Stalber, E.; Nandedkar, S.; Sanders, D. & Falck, B. (1996). Quantitative motor unit potencial analysis. *Journal of Clinical Neurophysiology*, 13, 401-422

Stirn I, Jarm T, Kapus V, Strojnik V. 2010. Fatigue Analysis of 100 Meters All-Out Front Crawl Using Surface EMG. In: *Biomechanics and Medicine in Swimming XI*, P.L., Kjendlie, R.K. Stallman & J. Cabri (Eds.), 168-170, Norwegian School of Sport Sciences, Oslo

Takagi, H.; Shimizu, Y.; Kurashima, A. & Sanders, R. (2001). Effect of thumb abduction and adduction on hydrodynamic characteristics of a model of the human hand, In: *Proceedings of swim sessions of the XIX international symposium on biomechanics in sports*, J. Blackwell & R. Sanders, (Eds.), 122-126, University of San Francisco, San Francisco

Takagi, H.; Sugimoto, S.; Nishijma, N. & Wilson, B. (2004). Differences in stroke phases, arm-leg coordination and velocity fluctuation due to event, gender and performance level in breaststroke. *Sports Biomechanics*, 3, pp. 15-27

Togashi, T. & Nomura, T. (1992). A biomechanical analysis of the swimmer using the butterfl y stroke. analysis of the swimmer using the butterfly stroke, In:

Biomechanics and Medicine in Swimming VI, D. MacLaren, T. Reilly & A. Lees, (Eds.), 87-91, E & FN Spon, London

Tourny, C.; Chollet, D.; Micallef, J. & Macabies, J. (1992). Comparative analysis of studies of speed variations within a breaststroke cycle, In: *Biomechanics and Medicine in Swimming VI, D.* MacLaren, T. Reilly & A. Lees, (Eds.), 161-166, E & FN Spon, London

Toussaint, H. & Truijens, M. (2005). Biomechanical aspects of peak performance in human swimming. *Animal Biology*, 55, 1, 17-40

Toussaint, H.; Carol, A.; Kranenborg, H. & Truijens, M. (2006). Effect of fatigue on stroking characteristics in an arms-only 100-m front-crawl race. *Medicine Science Sports Exercise,* 38, pp. 1635-1642

Vennell, R.; Pease, D.L. & Wilson, B.D. (2006). Wave drag on human swimmers. *Journal of Biomechanics*, 31, pp. 664-671

Vilas-Boas, J.P. (1996). Speed fluctuations and energy cost of different breaststroke techniques. In: *Biomechanics and Medicine in Swimming VII*, J.P. Troup, A.P. Hollander, D. Strasse, S.W. Trappe, J.M. Cappaert & T.A. Trappe, (Eds.), 167-171, E & FN Spon, London

Vitor, Fde.M. & Böhme, M.T. (2010). Performance of young male swimmers in the 100-meters front crawl. *Pediatric Exercise Science*, 22, pp. 278-87

Zaidi, H.; Taiar, R.; Fohanno, S. & Polidori, G. (2008). Analysis of the effect of swimmer's head position on swimming performance using computational fluid dynamics. *Journal of Biomechanics*, 41, pp. 1350-1358

17

Investigation of the Unsteady Mechanism in the Generation of Propulsive Force While Swimming Using a Synchronized Flow Visualization and Motion Analysis System

Kazuo Matsuuchi and Yuki Muramatsu
University of Tsukuba
Japan

1. Introduction

The highly efficient locomotion of birds, insects and fish is based on unsteady dynamics. The central mechanism in their locomotion is related to the unsteady behaviour of vortices such as the formation and shedding of boundary layers developed on their bodies. The relation between an object and vortex movement was first noticed in the field of aeronautics. The problem of a thin aerofoil performing small lateral oscillations in a uniform stream of an incompressible fluid, which is at the heart of all flutter prediction, has received interest for many years. A great deal of research within the scope of the linear perturbation theory has been published in past times. Well-documented summaries can be seen in Bisplinghoff et al. (1955).

Recently, significant attention has been given to the lift-sustaining flight of insects and birds despite their weight, and many fruitful discoveries have been made. Flow unsteadiness was found to play an important role in the flights. However, the unsteady mechanism in swimming propulsion has received relatively little interest. The first important contribution related to the mechanism of propulsion in a swimming stroke was made by Counsilman (1971), who divided the force of a swimming stroke into two components: a lift component normal to the hand motion and a drag component parallel to it. He pointed out the greater importance of lift force rather than drag force. The next critical contribution was made by Schleihauf (1979), who measured the lift and drag forces on hand models for various geometrical configurations of flow. Berger et al. (1995) carried out similar measurements using hand and arm models in fixed geometrical configurations within a flow and obtained the results consistent with those of Schleihauf. Subsequently, Bixler and Riewald (2002) used a numerical approach under a scenario similar to the experiments described above. Each of the approaches mentioned above can be termed a *quasi-steady analysis*, which depends on the assumption that the flow at each instance is nearly steady.

Studies using flow visualisation have revealed the importance of a rotating water mass (Ungerechts (1981)), which focused attention on the contribution of vortices in propulsion.

Ungerechts (1986) also pointed out the importance of the turning phase of the leg kick during a breast stroke and found that the acceleration peak of the body is in approximate agreement with the turning phase of the feet. This observation suggests that vortices generated during this phase are related to the body force or its acceleration. Arellano (1999) investigated the vortices generated while swimming underwater, and showed that the size and the movement of the vortex seem to be related to the propulsion obtained through the hand and foot movements. Arellano et al. (2002) also described the difference between efficient and less efficient swimmers from the perspective of generated vortex patterns of vortices. Colwin (2002) provided several detailed sketches of vortices generated during various stroke patterns. Recently, a method approaching the unsteadiness has been actively developed by numerically solving the Navier-Stokes equations; however, its reliability is somewhat poor and there are many cases in which the experimental validation is needed.

The only method for analyzing quantitatively an unsteady flow is particle image velocimetry (PIV). This method is used to determine the displacement of particles dispersed in water within a short time interval. This method was successfully used in the fields of insect and fish locomotion. Even with the use of this sophisticated method, however, it is difficult to measure an entire flow field directly around a human hand and foot. Using PIV Matsuuchi et al. (2004) first demonstrated the flow field occurring around a moving hand while swimming, which may be the main source of propulsion for the crawl stroke. Momentum generation was estimated from this flow field obtained through PIV (Matsuuchi et al. (2009). According to Newton's second law of motion, the increment of momentum leads directly to the force generation. A remarkable amount of momentum was found to be produced in the transition phase from an in-sweep to out-sweep motion during a crawl stroke.

However, since the hand motion and flow field were measured separately, or independently, our knowledge on the instance when the vortices of coherent structure are generated was limited. To determine the mechanism on force generation in more detail, we have developed a new PIV system combined with the motion analysis, called SMAP (**S**ynchronized System of **M**otion **A**nalysis and **P**IV). This system is synchronized with the direct linear transformation (DLT) method for motion analysis. In the motion analysis we used two high-speed cameras which are available to a 3D analysis. The system can measure the flow fields, i.e., velocity and vorticity fields and the geometrical configuration of hand simultaneously.

2. Importance of unsteady behavior

It is well known that the unsteady mechanism plays a crucial role in the the generation of propulsive force in birds, insects and fish (for example, see Dickinson(1996)). In most cases vortex behaviors such as formation and shedding are important.

Before introducing our system and its results, we illustrate the importance of unsteadiness using an example of a flow field around a human hand. First we show an example of velocity field in a horizontal plane around a hand during a crowl stroke (see Fig. 1). The subject is a female Olympic swimmer in a flume set at a velocity 1.5 m/s. She swims from right to left. The generation of momentum can be seen in the direction opposite to her swimming direction, i.e., from the left to right. It is easy to see that the momentum is generated between a pair of vortices. This generation of momentum leads directly to the propulsive force in swimming. In the figure, the mean velocity averaged over the entire plane has already been subtracted from the real velocity. This subtraction was made to emphasize the deviation from the mean velocity. The asterisk in the figure marks the location of the tip of the middle finger. Next in Fig. 2 we pick up an image file from which the Fig. 1 is drawn. This figure also shows the locations of the swimmer's hand 1/15 s before and after the instant the image was taken, which are depicted by cross marks. In addition to these locations, a predicted trace of the finger is depicted by a dotted line.

From the figure it is easy to see that two problems arise. One problem is the uncertainty of the finger positions and also the hand orientation. This problem is fatal, as a detailed hand orientation is important to determine the unsteady mechanism of force production. The other problem is that the 1/15 s interval of two subsequent events is too long to know the precise variation of a hand motion. The latter problem is very difficult to overcome, as shorter intervals are difficult to choose in a usual PIV system. However, the former problem is easily resolved by appying motion analysis with a high-speed camera, as will be mentioned in the next section.

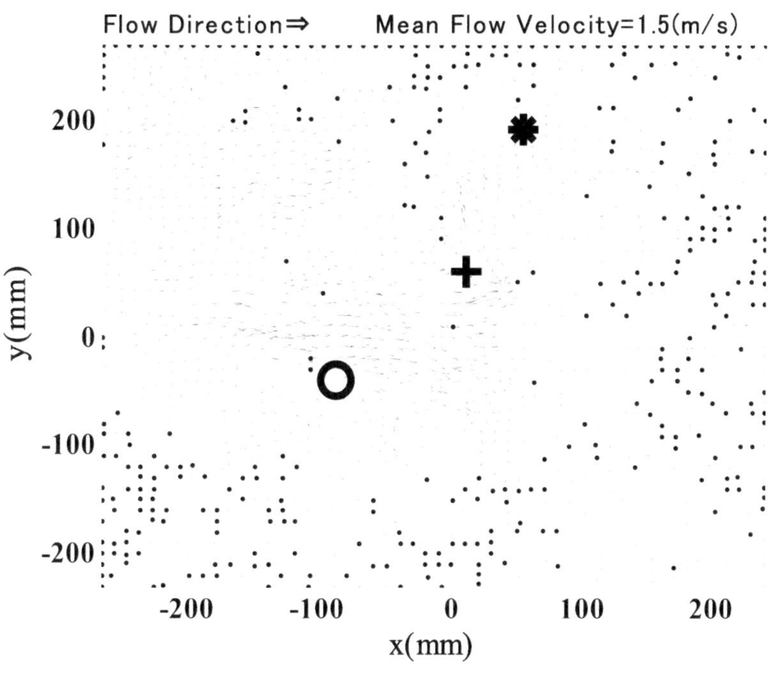

Fig. 1. Velocity field near a hand position, the third finger of which is located at the position shown by the asterisk. The cross mark and open circle denote the locations of vortices rotating anticlockwise and clockwise, respectively.

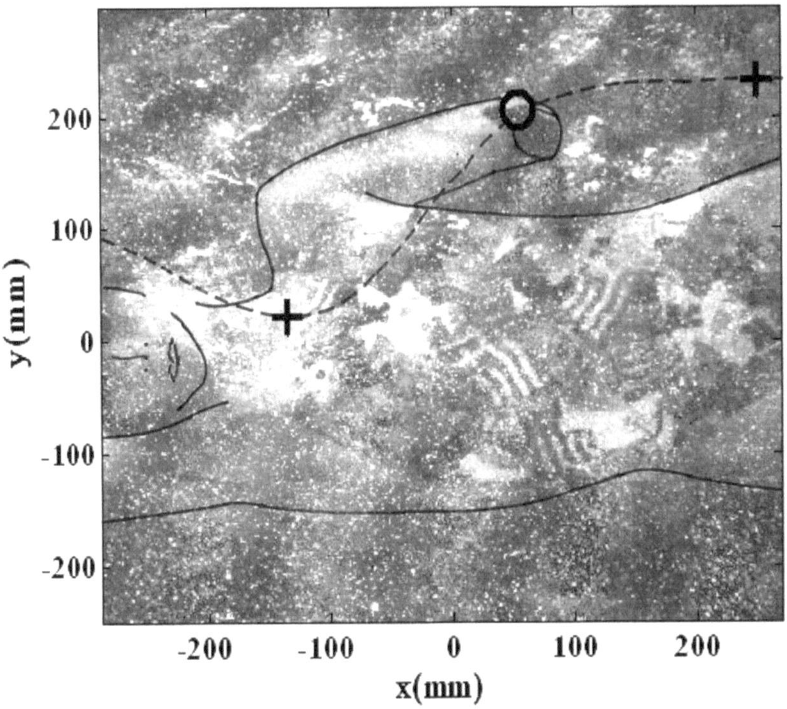

Fig. 2. Image of the swimmer as viewed from below. The outline of the swimmer is also depicted to clarify the posture. The open circle denotes the position of the tip of middle finger at this instant and the two cross marks the positions 1/15 s before and after this instant.

3. Particle image velocimetry

PIV is the most sophisticated method for measuring unsteady flow fields. In this method, a laser sheet illuminates tracer particles diffused in water. Two subsequent images of the particles are captured by a CCD camera and the path of the particle movement within a short interval is calculated. PIV has been frequently used to analyze the unsteady behavior of fish, insects and other creatures. For application of a flow field around a hand, it should be noted that the laser light must be intense as the flow field is not small.

3.1 Characteristic features

PIV is a global measurement technique used to trace a group of particles and determine their velocity through image processing. This technique has been developed owing to the rapid shortening in computer processing times, and is now widely used in the area of turbulence and heat transfer as a replacement for point measurements such as a hot-wire anemometry.

As will be mentioned in the next subsection, the principle is very simple: the velocity is taken as the moving distance devided by a short time interval. Since various global measurement techniques have been developed thus far, many researches using PIV have been published and systems installed using PIV have become a commercial reality. The merits and demerits of the PIV are as follows:

Merits:

- It is non-disturbing owing to its contact-free setup.
- It has a fast response and can hence capture rapid changes of velocity and temperature.
- The instantaneous velocity, vorticity, and heat flux rates may be measured, as the velocity and temparature gradients can be measured instantaneously.
- Lagrangean measurements are possible including Lagrangean correlation and Lagrangean vector measurements.
- Without the movement of probes such as hot wires, the mean velocity and temperature are also easily obtainable.
- Multi-dimensional measurements are possible.

Demerits:

- Calibration is necessary.
- Tracer particles have to be diffused in water.
- The time resolution is poor.
- The dynamic range of the velocity is low.

3.2 Principle

Tracer particles diffused in water are illuminated by a laser sheet and an image is taken by a CCD camera. From two subsequential images within a certain small area at t_0 and $t_0 + \Delta t$ the correlation function is calculated by traversing the area in the searching region. The area that gives the maximum correlation is simply the one that includes particles corresponding to those at $t = t_0$ (see Fig.3). The moving distance of each particle $(\Delta x, \Delta y)$ is then determined. The velocity vector (u, v) in the two-dimensional plane is thus calculated by dividing the distance by the time interval Δt, i.e.,

$$u = \lim_{\Delta t \to 0} \frac{\Delta x}{\Delta t} \tag{1}$$

$$v = \lim_{\Delta t \to 0} \frac{\Delta y}{\Delta t} \tag{2}$$

Vorticity is a vector quantity that has three components and is a measure of the magnitude of fluid rotation. The concept of vorticity is important in the mechanism of an unsteady flow force. The simplest example for demonstrating vorticity is the lift force acting on an aerofoil. This force is generated by a starting vortex and a bound vortex around an aerofoil (see, for example, Lamb (1932) and Izumi and Kuwahara (1983)).

In this study we consider a two dimensional flow on a laser sheet. For this reason, only the *z*-component of the vorticity ζ is considered, which is simply defined as

$$\varsigma = \frac{\partial v}{\partial x} - \frac{\partial u}{\partial y} \tag{3}$$

The clockwise and anti-clockwise rotations of a fluid correspond to negative and positive values, respectively. The absolute value of ζ provides a measure of the rotation intensity.

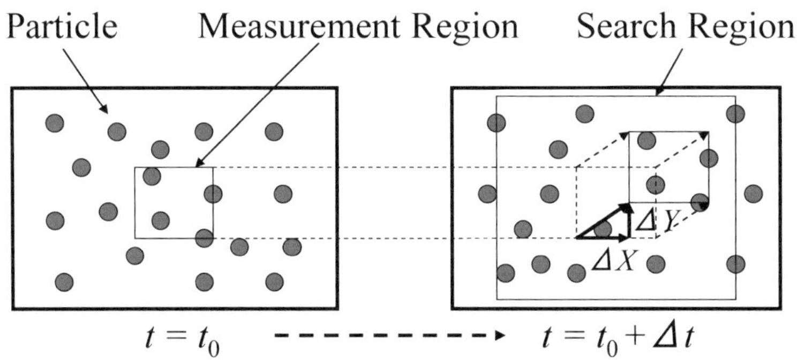

Fig. 3. Principle of determining velocity through PIV.

4. Motion analysis

Human movement constitutes of the superpositions of many rotating motions around a joint. In general, the motion of the center of gravity in human movement is not in a two-dimensional plane but in a three-dimensional space. Accordingly, the human body, in this case swimmer's hand, should be captured correctly as a function of time in a three-dimensional space.

To determine the coordinates in a three-dimensional space from video-recorded images, multiple images taken from video recordings in different directions relative to the subject are necessary. For this goal, we used a direct linear transformation (DLT) (Shapiro (1978), Abel-Aziz and Karana (1971)), which is used in the field of sports biomechanics. This DLT method has an advantage in the real positioning of cameras. Camera constants such as the direction of the optical axis and the focal length are not necessary to know. Instead the relationship between known coordinates in a real space and coordinates in a two-dimensional image is calibrated in advance. The relationships of several images, usually two images, determine the coordinates in a real three-dimensional space. The limitation of the optical axes are somewhat moderate. When two cameras are used, the angle between the two optical axes is about 30 to 150 deg. This method has been widely used in this respect.

5. Simultaneous measurement of hand motion and flow field

5.1 Synchronization between PIV and DLT

As shown in the previous section, PIV is a powerful method for visualizing the flow field around a swimmer, particularly around the hand. Considering the mechanism of propulsive force through hand movement, however, information on the precise formation and orientation of the hand is critical. PIV does not provide correct information on the hand motion. The DLT method, however, combined with high-speed cameras is useful for the determination of hand motion. However, correspondence of flow field by the hand motion and hence the force generation is still unclear. To determine the mechanism for the generation of propulsive force it is necessary to synchronize the DLT method with PIV. To know the instant when a force becomes strong and why the force is generated by the flow field, we have built a new system combining the two methods, which we call SMAP.

5.2 Separation of PIV and DLT in frequency range

PIV measurements are usually carried out in a dark room, with the use of only a laser light. On the other hand, the DLT method is usually applied under bright circumstances to digitize the position of the marker attached to the hand surface. To synchronize the two methods, the frequency range has to be separated into two ranges, one each for the PIV and DLT methods.

The remaining problem is how to synchronize the timing of the two measurements. We performed this operation using a pulse generator.

6. Experimental setup

We performed experiments using a flume installed at the University of Tsukuba (Igarashi Industrial Works Co., Ltd.). The test section is 4.6 m long, 2 m wide, and 1.5 m high with a 1.2 m water depth. It can provide a maximum flow of 2.5 m/s. The flow speed was set at 1.0 m/s.

6.1 Subject

The subject is a male triathlete of the Univesity of Tsukuba volunteered for the present purpose. We explained the aim, procedure and the risk, and got his approval to the cooperation.

6.2 Method

We used an Nd-YAG laser with a sufficiently high intensity (Solo PIV 120; New Wave Research Inc.). Under the flume a CCD camera (ES1.0, Eastman Kodak Co.) for PIV was set. This camera captures the images reflected by a mirror (see Fig. 4). Two high-speed cameras (FASTCAM-512PCI, Photron) for DLT were set as shown in Fig. 4. We paid attention only to the swimmer's right hand for the present experiment. The subject wore glasses for protection against the strong laser light and also a black globe made from silicon rubber to avoid halation. The tracer particles and data aquisition procedure were quite simiar to those in previous experiments (Matsuuchi et al. (2009)).

During the motion analysis, we captured 1088 frames at one time. We digitized images from the video using 2D and 3D video analysis software (Frame DIAS version 3, DKH Co., Ltd), and determined the traces of the hand, the velocity and the geometry of the palm. The points digitized are the metacarpopharangeal joints of the second and fifth fingers and the tip of the third finger. Fig. 5 shows the points and a local coordinate system (X, Y, Z) fixed to the palm. The coordinates are related to the global coordinates (x, y, z) fixed to the flume. As will be explained later, x is the flow direction; y the horizontal backward direction; and z vertically upward. The global coordinates (x, y, z) were measured directly by the CCD cameras, and the local coordinates (X, Y, Z) of the specified three points of the palm were calculated. The identification of these palm points gives the geometrical configuration of the palm. On the other hand, in the PIV measurements 128 images, or 64 pairs, were taken. Each pair taken at 1 ms interval represents a set of two kinds of fields - velocity and vorticity fields. In the PIV measurements the relationship between the real coordinates and two-dimensional image data needs to be determined in advance. Calibrations were carried out for this purpose.

To determine the global coordinates (*x*, *y*, *z*) from the two-dimensional data captured by CCD cameras, it is necessary to obtain in advance the relationship between the coordinates (*x*, *y*, *z*) and the two-dimensional image data through a calibration procedure.

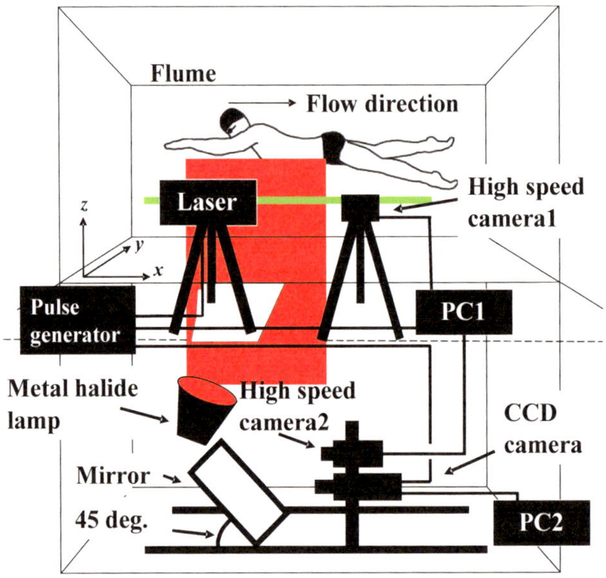

Fig. 4. Experimental configuration and setup.

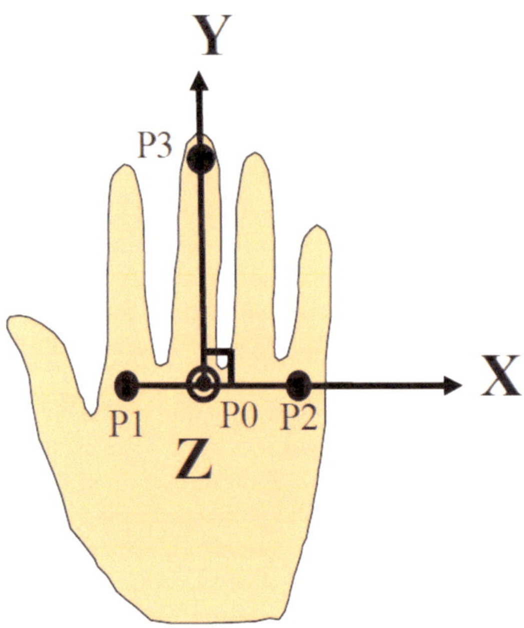

Fig. 5. Local coordinates fixed on the palm.

To combine the two methods we used two kinds of light with different spectrum characteristics. One is an Nd-YAG laser, and the other the light of a metal halide lamp. The metal halide lamp was covered with a red film for the DLT. For this method, band-pass filters that pass through a light at a wavelength of 640 to 700 nm are attached to the front of the lens of the CCD cameras for DLT method. On the other hand, for PIV a band-pass filter ranging between 532+2 and 532-2 nm was used. The wavelength of 532 nm corresponds to that of the Nd-YAG laser. The ranges of the wavelength utilized for the two methods are illustrated in Fig. 6. The first wavelength was used for PIV and was created using a line band-pass filter, whereas the second wavelength was created using a red band-pass filter and was used for the DLT method.

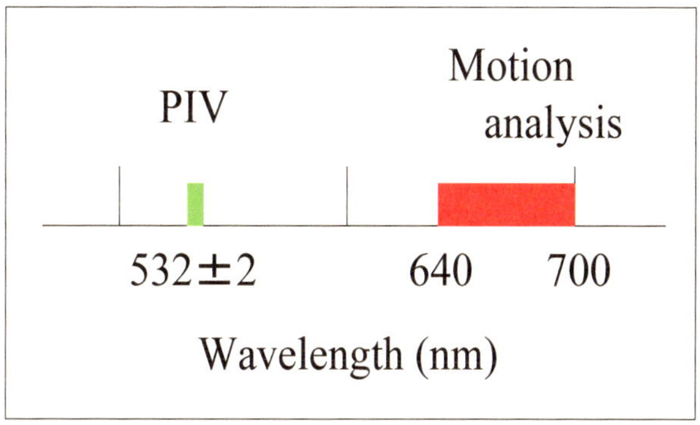

Fig. 6. Separation of ranges of wavelength - for PIV and for motion analysis.

The timing was synchronized with pulses generated by a pulse generator. Our PIV system is capable of capturing images at a minimum of every 1/15 of a second, whereas the high-speed cameras are able to take photos within shorter periods. To synchronize two signals, we chose $\Delta t = 0.068$ s for PIV, while setting the period at 0.004 s for the DLT. A timing chart is shown in Fig. 7.

As mentioned before, two subsequent images taken within a short interval determine the velocity field. The timing is also controlled by two pulses, Pulse 1 and Pulse 2, generated by the pulse generator. The interval of the two pulses was set at 1 ms in the experiments.

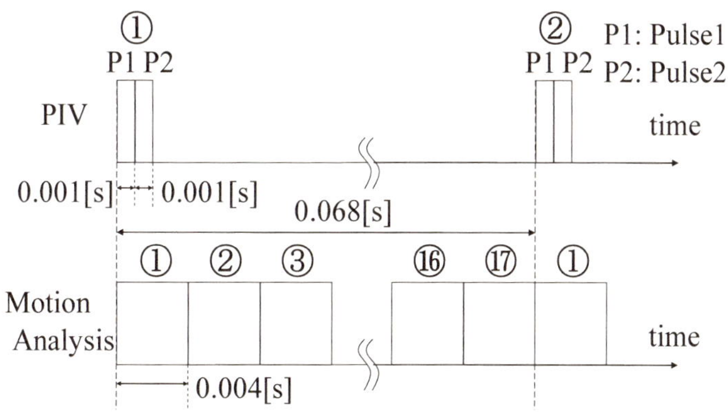

Fig. 7. Timing chart of the dual analysis system. The time interval used for obtaining the flow field using PIV was set at 68 ms, while the motion analysis using high-speed cameras set at 4 ms.

7. Results

Our SMAP system can be used to determine the flow field and hand movement of a swimmer simultaneously using geometrical configurations. It is a start of thinking of the mechanism of propulsive force generation in swimming. This mechanism will be discussed in terms of the unsteady properties of the flow field and hand motions. The results teach us many things about the mechanism of how vortices are created and how the momentum leading to thrust force is generated. While this mechanism is very complex, it is quite interesting although a high-level of knowledge on fluid mechanics is needed for proper understanding.

7.1 Motion analysis

First, we show the the changes of hand orientation in a three-dimensional space. Our system determines the variations of hand orientation accurately, as shown in Fig. 8. The thick lines corresponds to the instants at which the PIV determines the velocity and vorticity fields, i.e., t = 0.036, 0.104, and 0.172 s. The initial time t = 0 chosen arbitrarily is different for each event. A complex change in the hand path can be easily seen, which makes it difficult to interpret its role in force generation.

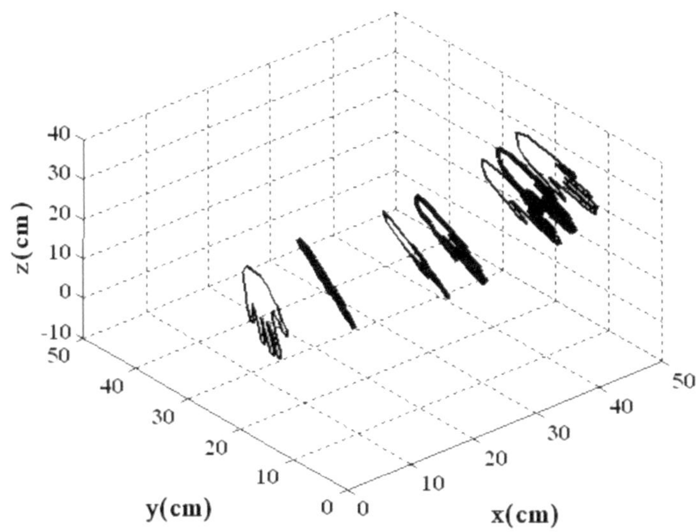

Fig. 8. Three-dimensional path of hand and the variations in the palm orientation. Rapid changes of the hand path and orientation can be seen.

While our motion analysis system can be used to determine the coordinates of the palm in a three dimensional space, the interpretation of the unsteady mechanism of force generation in a three-dimensional space is very complex and difficult to understand. Therefore, in this report, only a two dimensional field in a laser sheet is discussed for simplicity. A hand path in the transition phase from in-sweep to out-sweep and the definition of the angle are shown in Fig. 9. During this phase, it is plausible that a significant generation of momentum can be produced. The pitch angle, which is the flow direction measured from the normal to the palm, was chosen as an important parameter to determine the circulation of the palm. It was noted that if we view the palm as an aerofoil, the leading edge changes from the thumb side to the fifth finger side. This indicates that a change in the sign of the circulaltion around the palm occurs (see Prandtl and Tiejens (1934) for further details). This change is important to determine the generation of forces that occur from vortex motions (see Matsuuchi et al., 2009). The change of the leading edge durintg the phase is a critical difference in the generation of unsteady forces created from flight or locomotion in insects and birds.

Real variations of the palm projected on the horizontal x-y plane are shown in Fig. 10. Variations of the flow direction relative to the hand are crucial for understanding of the generation of vortices and thus the production of force. Time variations of the hand velocity and pitch angle measured in the frame relative to water are illustrated in Fig. 11. The thick vertical lines correspond to the instants at which PIV measurements were made, i.e., at t = 0.036, 0.104, and 0.172 s. During the period from t = 0.104 to 0.172 s, the velocity is decreased by about 1 m/s and the pitch angles vary largely. The magnitude of the angle variation is as large as 120 deg. This is simply the transition phase in the hand stroke from an in-sweep to an out-sweep. These variations of hand velocity and pitch angle are essential during the transition phase in the crawl stroke. We now calculate rotational velocity compared to the uniform velocity, which is usually called the reduced frequency. If this rate is small, the flow is considered to be steady. If we set the chord length as 10 cm, the reduced frequency is calculated as 3.1. This value is too high to neglect the unsteadiness.

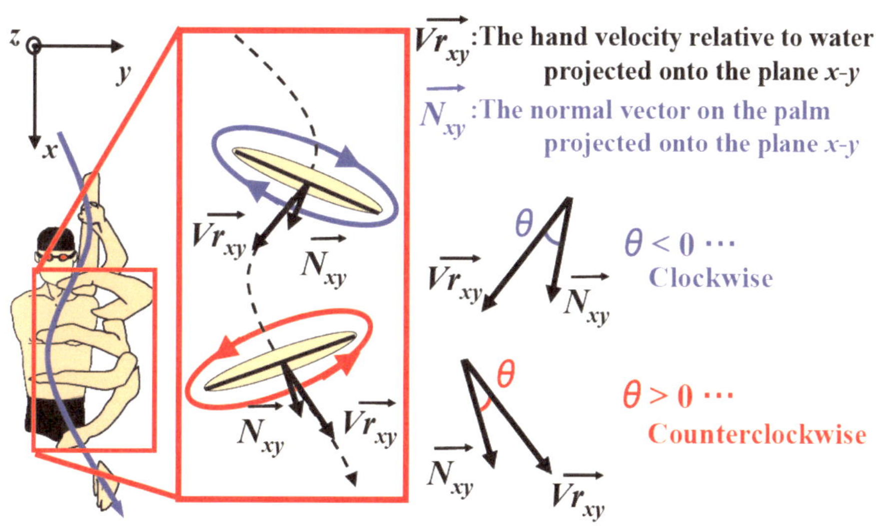

Fig. 9. Definition of and change in the angle of pitch along the hand path.

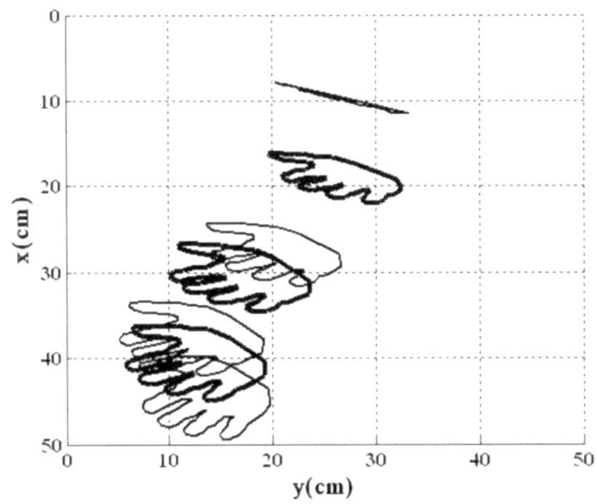

Fig. 10. Temporal variations of hand configuration in the *x-y* plane. The thick lines correspond to the instants at 0.036, 0.104, and 0.172 s. The corresponding configurations at other instants are also superposed using thin lines to facilitate an understanding of the variations in the characteristics of a hand motion.

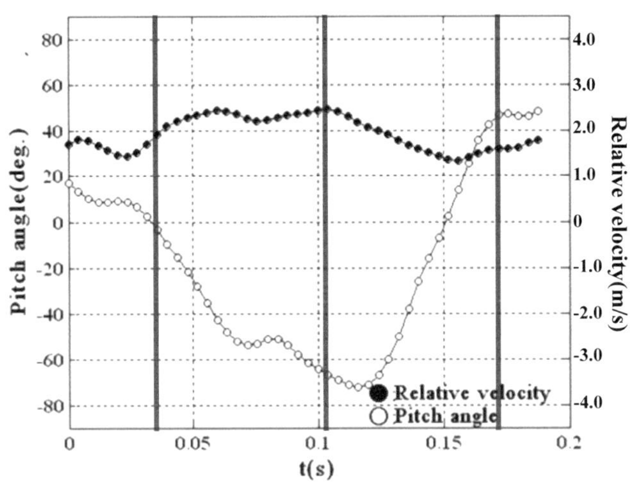

Fig. 11. Variations of pitch angle and hand velocity. The three vertical lines drawn in bold indicate instants of 0.036, 0.104, and 0.172 s

Thus far, the hand paths have been drawn in a three-dimensional space fixed to the flume. However, the real swimming is performed in still water. In this meaning, it seems to be better to depict the path relative to the running water. The palm paths in the *x-y* and *x-z* planes of the transformed coordinates of still water are picked up and shown in Figs. 12 (a) and (b), respectively. In the figure, the green colored palms correspond to those at the instant PIV works. The vectors in red denote the movement direction, while the vectors in blue are unit normals to the palm. A red vector of 3 m/s is also drawn in the corner as a reference. Remarkable and rapid changes of the palm orientation can clearly be seen from these figures.

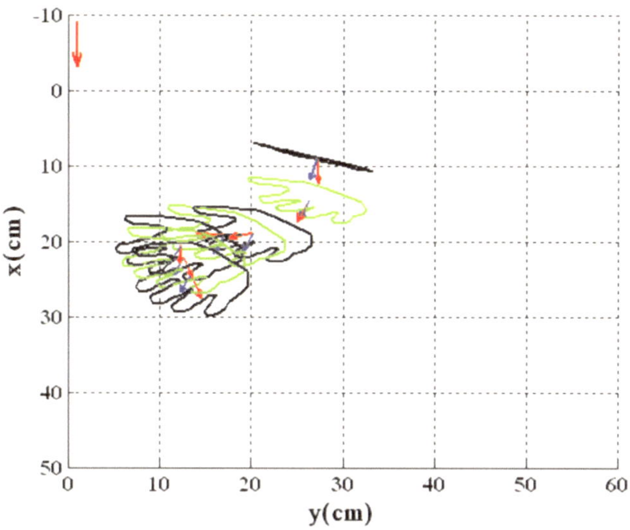

(a)

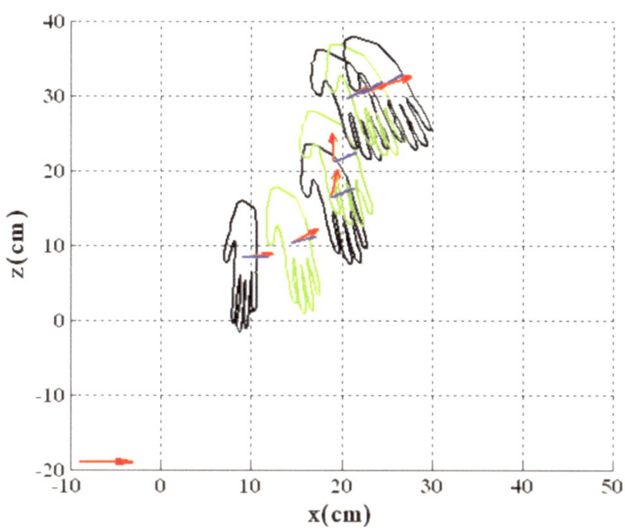

(b)

Fig. 12. Palm outlines relative to water are depicted. The red arrows denote the velocity of the palm relative to the water. The subject moves his hand in a complex manner, and rapidly changes the orientation in both planes.

7.2 Visualization of flow field

In Fig. 13, first we show a hand position and body viewed from the bottom at 0.036 s. Note here that although it appears to be the left arm owing to mirror imaging, the arm shown in the figure is actually the right one. The hand position relative to the aswimmer's trunk can easily be seen. The velocity and vorticity fields corrresponding to those at the instant depicted in Fig. 13 are shown in Figs. 14(a) and (b), respectively. To clarify the generation of velocity fluctuations from the hand movement the mean velocity was subtracted from the real velocity vectors. At this stage, no remarkable increments in velocity or no strong generation of momentum occured. Only a weak positive rotation, shown in white, can be seen near the little finger.

Velocity and vorticity fields at an instant 0.068 s later are depicted in Fig. 15. The positive rotation that appeared in the previous instant shown in Fig. 14 remains in the place where it existed at the previous instant. More intense rotations of positive and negative signs are found to be produced adjacent to the hand. It can be seen that the generation of momentum in the positive x-direction can be detected between two vortices; the positive vortex produced at the previous instant and a newly produced negative rotation. Such momentum generation simply corresponds to the production of force, which is a reduction from Newton's second law of motion. A similar but simple circumstance occurs when an aerofoil is suddenly started (Lamb (1932)). In Fig. 16 the velocity field obtained at t = 0.172 s through PIV is shown as a solid line and hand positions at two other instants, t = 0.036 and 0.104 s are shown as broken lines. The generation of momentum in the positive x-direction can be clearly seen in the figure. Note that this direction is opposite to the negative x-direction, which is the swimming direction. The generation of momentum is the result of a pair of vortices rotating in opposite directions. Such momentum generation leads to a thrust force by the hand, which is indeed a consequence of Newton's second law of motion, as already explained.

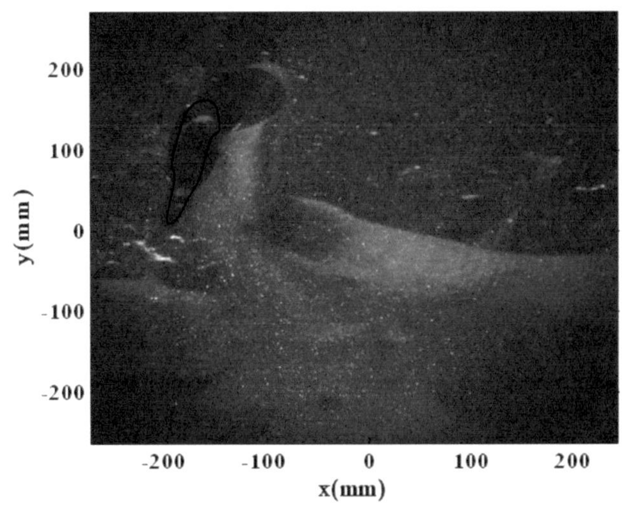

Fig. 13. Swimmer viewed from below at 0.036 s. The closed curve in the solid line indicates the near side of the palm on the laser sheet.

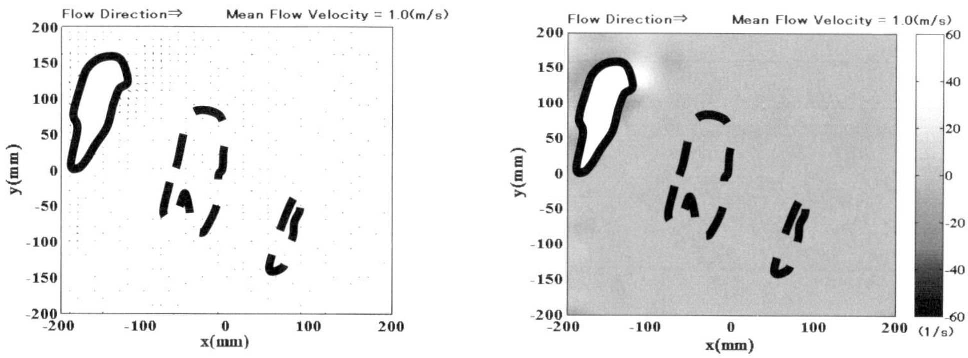

(a) (b)

Fig. 14. Velocity (a) and vorticity (b) fields at 0.036 s are shown. The solid line corresponds to the outline of the hand at this instant and the other two broken lines show the outlines at instants 0.068 s and 0.136 s later.

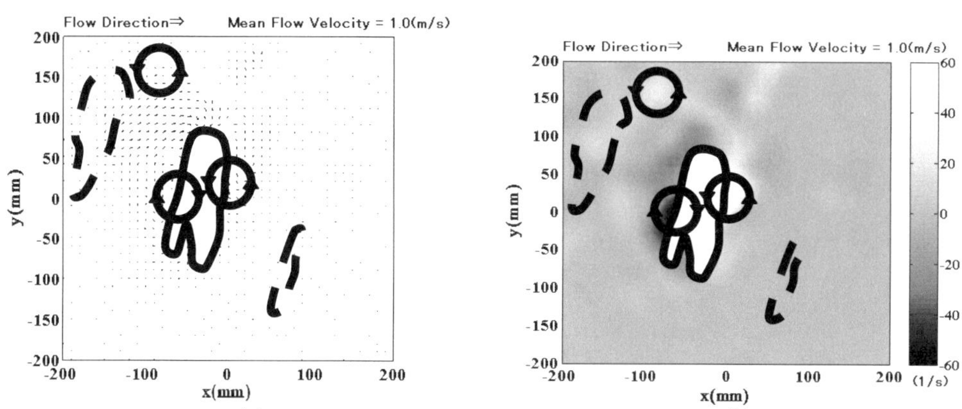

(a) (b)

Fig. 15. Velocity (a) and vorticity (b) fields in the x-y plane at 0.104 s. The solid line corresponds to the outline of the hand cross section at this instant and the two broken lines show the outlines at 0.036 s and 0.172 s. The three circles with arrows indicate the vortices.

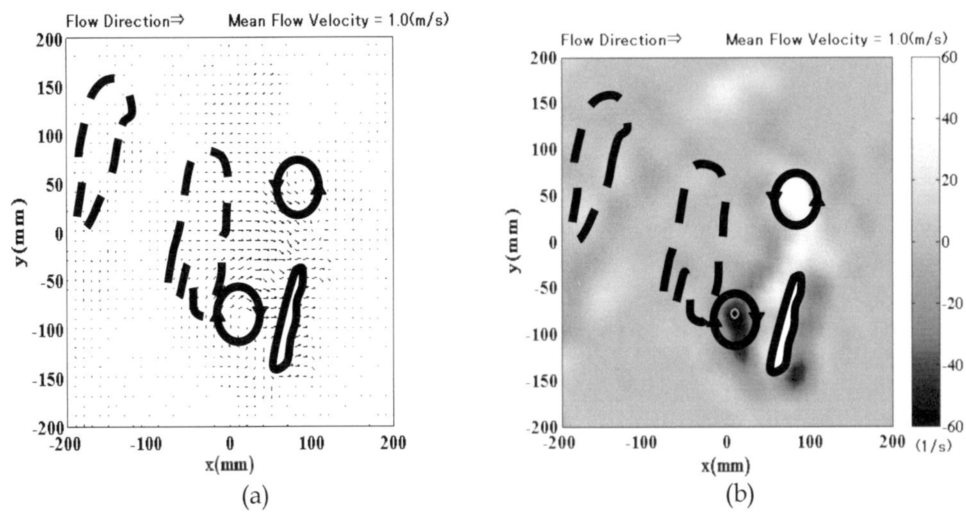

Fig. 16. Velocity (a) and vorticity (b) fields in the x-y plane at the instant 0.172 s. The solid line is an outline of the cross section at this instant, and the two broken lines are those at 0.036 and 0.104 s. The two circles with arrows indicate vortices generating momentum in the positive x-direction.

8. Discussions

Our main concern is to find the source of propulsive force arising from hand movements. To obtain a better understanding of the source, a synchronized system for the visualization of flow fields and hand motions was established.

The orientation of the palm was found to vary in a complex manner. When hand orientation changes rapidly, vortex generation and shedding, and consequently momentum generation are found to occur in the flow field. Such a vortex behavior makes the flow fields unsteady. The introduction of unsteadiness in the generation of propulsive force while swimming is a newly developed idea. Thus far, an approach for understanding the mechanism of propulsive force has been developed in many researches on the basis of the concept that the motions of the hand and foot seem to be steady. This approach is called the quasi-steady theory. Several authors have pointed out that quasi-steady results lead to an underestimation of force magnitude (Sanders (1999), Toussaint, Van den Berg and Beek (2002)). The results of the present research will provide important information on the momentum generation and force production due to the flow unsteadiness.

However, some problems remain. The most serious one is the limitation of the sampling time when using PIV. The movement of a human swimmer is not too slow, but our sampling interval is only 66 ms at minimum. Therefore, it is difficult to trace the details of a flow field. While there is a way to overcome this difficulty, it is not easy to implement owing to the high costs involved. The other problem is the limitation of the obserbvation area, i.e., observations using a laser are essentially limited to only the area within the laser sheet, i.e., they are two dimensional observations. Observational data accumulated in many horizontal planes could provide sufficeint information. However, if we could make experiments simultaneously in many horizontal planes, the task were not tolerable to make.

Before concluding this section, we will now introduce a new approach called stereoscopic PIV (see Prasad and Adrian (1993), Prasad and Jensen (1995), in addition, for the case of turning fish, see Sakakibara et al.(2004)). This technique can be used to reconstruct a quasi three-dimensional flow field.

Fig. 17 shows the results obtained through stereoscopic PIV are shown. The subject is an elite short-distance swimmer from Japan, who swam in the flume at a velocity of 1.0 m/s. The laser sheet is placed in a vertical plane normal to the swimming direction. The figure shows the velocity field in the y-z plane, or in a vertical plane. The first picture in Fig. 17(a) shows a photo taken obliquely behind the subject, while the right image is the flow field at the initial instant t = 0. The color bar represents the magnitude of the velocity component in the x-direction, i.e., the direction opposite to the swimming one. The vectors are the velocity vectors in the y-z plane. The instant t = 0 is the moment when the hand passes through the laser sheet. In this stage the velocity component in the flow direction induced from the hand motion appears to be slight.

At the next instant, t = 0.067 s (b), when the hand passes away from the laser, the area of strong axial velocity (in the x-direction) increases. This means that the momentum increases together with a strong clockwise rotation leading to the propulsive force. At the instant t = 0.134 s (c) an area with a strong rotation flows downstream and a weak area remains there.

In the above three stages were picked up. If we could obtain sequential velocility fields at a shorter time intervals, it would be possible to reconstruct three-dimensional velocity or vorticity fields by applying Taylor's frozen-flow hypothesis. We will be able to obtain important information from the three-dimensional structure of vortices and velocities induced by hand movement. This three-dimensional data is expected to give a definitive answer to the problems for the generation mechanism and time variations of a propulsive force.

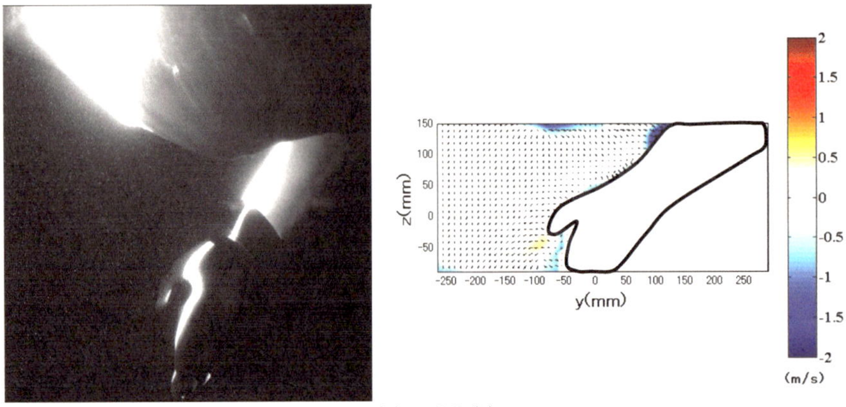

(a) t=0.0 (s)

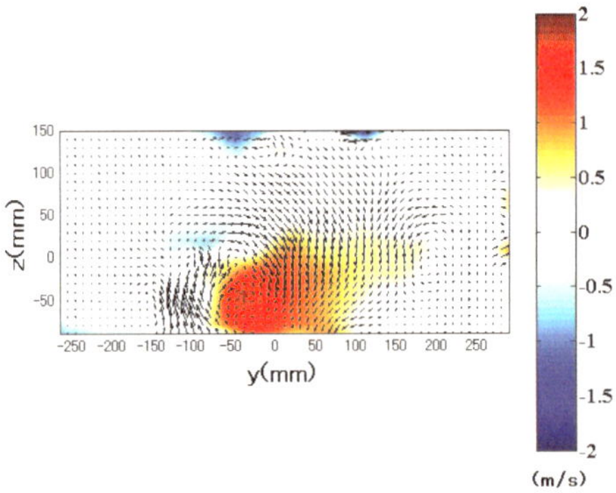

(b) t=0.067 (s)

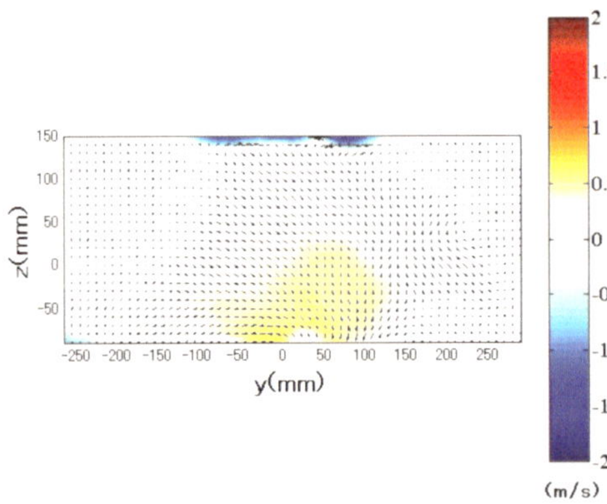

(c) t=0.134 (s)

Fig. 17. Flow field in the y-z plane obtained through the stereoscopic PIV method. The vectors denote the velocities in the plane, while the colors represent the magnitude induced by the hand motion opposite to the swimming direction, i.e., the x-direction.

9. Concluding remarks

Our system SMAP method can provide us with significant information for understanding the mechanism of force. This system can be used to quantitatively evaluate an unsteadiness such as a reduced frequency and from the flow field we can determine the instants of large momentum and hence the produced propulsive force of significant magnitude.

In most cases, however, our data is still limited to that obtained from two-dimensional information. To adopt the present approach for real swimming and traiming routines, many more experiments need to be carried out and much more information is required.

Our system, which combines two different methods, has room for modification. Three dimensionality and a shorter acquisition are included in the new system. Such a modified system is expected to provide us knowledge useful for improving swimming techniques and to become a powerful tool for refining or reforming efficient swimming form.

10. Acknowledgements

This study was supported by a Grant-in-Aid for Scientific Research ((B)21300228) from the Japan Society for the Promotion of Science.

11. References

Abdel-Aziz, Y.I., Karana, H. M. (1971). Direct Linear Transformation from Comparator Coordinates into Object Space in Close-range Photogrammetry. ASP Symposium on Close-Range Photogrammetry, American Society of Photogrammetry, Falls Church

Arelllano, R. (1999). Vortices and Propulsion. In: Applied Proceedings of the XVII International Symposium on Biomechanics in Sports, 53-66

Arelllano, R., Pardillo, S., Gavilan, S. (2002). Underwater Undulatory Swimming: Kinematic Characteristics, Vortex Generation and Application during the Start, Turn and Swimming Strokes. In: Proceedings of the XXth International Symposium on Biomechanics in Sports, Universidad de Granada

Berger, M.A.M., de Groot, G., Hollander, A. P. (1995). Hydrodynamic Drag/Lift Forces on Human Hand/Arm Models, *Journal of Biomechanics*, 28, 125-133

Bisplinghoff, R. L., Ashley, H., Halfman, R.L. (1955). *Aeroelasticity*, Chap. 5, Addison-Wesley Pub.

Bixler, B., Riewald, S. (2002). Analysis of a Swimmer's Hand and Arm in Steady Flow Conditions Using Computational Fluid Dynamics, *Journal of Biomechanics* 28, 125-133

Colwin, C.M. (2002). *Breakthrough Swimming*, Chap.5, Human Kinetics

Counsilman, J.E. (1971). The Application of Bernoulli's Principle to Human Propulsion in Water, *Swimming* 1, Eds. Lewillie, L. and Clarys , J.P., University Park Press, 59-71

Dickinson, M. (1996). Unsteady Mechanisms of Force Generation in Aquatic and Aerial Locomotion, American Zoologist, 36, 537-554

Izumi, K., Kuwahara, K. (1983). Unsteady Flow Field, Lift and Drag Measurements of Impulsively Started Elliptic Cylinder and Circular-Arc Airfoil, *AIAA*-83-1711

Lamb, H. (1932). *Hydrodynamics*, 6th Ed., Art. 157, Cambridge Univ. Press

Matsuuchi, K., Miwa, T., Nomura, T., Sakakibara, J., Shintani, H., Ungerechts, B.E. (2004). Unsteady Flow Measurement around a Human Hand in Swimming Using PIV, *9th Annual Congress of the ECSS*, CDROM.

Matsuuchi, K., Miwa, T., Nomura, T., Sakakibara, J., Shintani, H., Ungerechts, B.E. (2009). Unsteady Flow Field around a Human Hand and Propulsive Force in Swimming, *Journal of Biomechanics*, 42, 42-47

Prandtl, L., Tiejens, O. G. (1934). *Applied Hydro- and Aeromechanics*, Chap. 6, Dover Pub.

Prasad, A. K., and Adrian, R. J. (1993). Stereoscopic Particle Image Velocimetry Applied to Liquid Flows, *Experiments in Fluids*, 15, 49-60

Prasad, A.K., Jensen, K. (1995). Scheimpflug Stereocamera for Particle Image Velocimetry in Liquid Flows, *Applied Optics*, 34, 7092-7099

Sakakibara, J., Nakagawa, M., Yoshida, M. (2004). Stereo-PIV Study of Flow around a Maneuvering Fish, *Experiments in Fluids*, 36, 282-293

Sanders, R. H. (1999). Hydrodynamic Characteristics of a Swimmer's Hand, *Journal of Applied Biomechanics*, 15, 3-26

Schleihauf, R. E. (1979). A Hydrodynamic Analysis of Swimming Propulsion, *Swimming III*, 70-109

Shapiro, R. (1978). The Direct Linear Transformation Method for Three-Dimensional Cinematography, *Research Quarterly*, 49, 197-205

Toussaint, H. M., Van den Berg, C., Beek, W.J. (2002). ``Pumped-Up Propulsion" during Front Crawl Swimming. *Medicine and Science in Sports and Exercise*, 34, 314-319

Ungerechts, B. E. (1981). Propulsive Principle of Fast Swimming Vertebrates Analysed by Flow Visualizing Techniques, In: Abstracts of the VIIIth International Congress of Biomechanics, Nagoya, Japan, 165

Ungerechts, B.E. (1992). The Interrelationship of Hydrodynamical Forces and Swimming Speed in Breaststroke. In: D. MacLaren, T. Reilly & A. Lees (eds.), *Biomechanics and Medicine in Swimming -Swimming Science* VI. E. & FN Spon, London, 69-73